Casarett & Doull's
Essentials of Toxicology

Casarett & Doull's
Essentials of Toxicology

Second Edition

Editors

Curtis D. Klaassen, PhD

University Distinguished Professor and Chair
Department of Pharmacology, Toxicology, and Therapeutics
University of Kansas Medical Center
Kansas City, Kansas

John B. Watkins III, PhD

Assistant Dean and Director
Professor of Pharmacology and Toxicology
Medical Sciences Program
Indiana University School of Medicine
Bloomington, Indiana

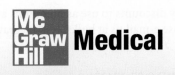

New York   Chicago   San Francisco   Lisbon   London   Madrid   Mexico City
Milan   New Delhi   San Juan   Seoul   Singapore   Sydney   Toronto

Casarett & Doull's Essentials of Toxicology, Second Edition

Copyright © 2010, by The McGraw-Hill Companies, Inc. All rights reserved. Printed in China. Except as permitted under the United States Copyright Act of 1976, no part of this publication may be reproduced or distributed in any form or by any means, or stored in a data base or retrieval system, without the prior written permission of the publisher.

7 8 9 10 CTP/CTP 17 16 15 14

ISBN 978-0-07-162240-0
MHID 0-07-162240-3

This book was set in Minion Pro by Thomson Digital.
The editors were James Shanahan and Christie Naglieri.
The production supervisor was Sherri Souffrance.
Project management was provided by Aakriti Kathuria, Thomson Digital.
The text designer was Elise Lansdon.
The cover designer was Margaret Webster-Shapiro.
The index was prepared by Thomson Digital.
China Translation & Printing, Ltd. was the printer and binder.

This book is printed on acid-free paper.

Library of Congress Cataloging-in-Publication Data

Casarett & Doull's essentials of toxicology/editors, Curtis D. Klaassen, John B. Watkins III.—2nd ed.
     p. ; cm.
  Includes bibliographical references and index.
  Summary: "We are delighted to present an updated full color, edition of Essentials of Toxicology, which distills the major principles and concepts of toxicology that were described in detail in the seventh edition of Casarett & Doull's Toxicology: The Basic Science of Poisons. We are grateful to the colleagues who contributed to the seventh edition of Casarett & Doull's Toxicology: The Basic Science of Poisons; their contributions to the parent text served as the foundation for the chapters in this edition of Essentials of Toxicology. Essentials of Toxicology concisely presents the broad science of toxicology. Important concepts from anatomy, physiology and biochemistry have been included to facilitate the understanding of the principles and mechanisms of toxicant action on specific organ systems. It is hoped that the book will be useful to students in undergraduate and graduate courses in toxicology, as well as students from other disciplines, who want to have a strong foundation in toxicologic concepts and principles"—Provided by publisher.
  ISBN-13: 978-0-07-162240-0 (pbk. : alk. paper)
  ISBN-10: 0-07-162240-3 (pbk. : alk. paper)
  ISBN-10: (invalid) 0-07-174274-0 (international ed.)
  1. Toxicology—Textbooks. I. Klaassen, Curtis D. II. Watkins, John B. (John Barr)
III. Casarett, Louis J. IV. Title: Casarett & Doull's essentials of toxicology.
V. Title: Essentials of toxicology.
  [DNLM: 1. Poisons—toxicity. 2. Toxicology—methods. QV 600 C3349 2010]
  RA1211.C298 2010
  615.9—dc22
                                    2009047866

McGraw-Hill books are available at special quantity discounts to use as premiums and sales promotions, or for use in corporate training programs. To contact a representative please e-mail us at bulksales@mcgraw-hill.com.

International Edition ISBN 978-0-07-174274-0; MHID 0-07-174274-3
Copyright © 2010. Exclusive rights by The McGraw-Hill Companies, Inc. for manufacture and export. This book cannot be re-exported from the country to which it is consigned by McGraw-Hill. The International Edition is not available in North America.

Contents

Contributors

Michael Aschner, PhD
Gray E.B. Stahlman Chair in Neuroscience,
Professor of Pediatrics and Pharmacology and
Senior Investigator of the Kennedy Center,
Vanderbilt University, Nashville, Tennessee

S. Satheesh Anand, PhD
Research Toxicologist, DuPont Haskell Laboratory for
Health and Environmental Sciences, Newark, Delaware

John C. Bloom, VMD, PhD
Executive Director, Distinguished Medical Fellow,
Diagnostic and Experimental Medicine,
Eli Lilly and Company, Indianapolis, Indiana

William K. Boyes, PhD
Neurotoxicology Division
National Health and Environmental Effects Research
Laboratory, Office of Research and Development,
U.S. Environmental Protection Agency, Durham,
North Carolina

John T. Brandt, MD
Medical Fellow II, Diagnostic and Experimental
Medicine, Eli Lilly and Company, Indianapolis, Indiana

James V. Bruckner, PhD
Department of Pharmaceutical and Biomedical
Sciences, College of Pharmacy, University of Georgia,
Athens, Georgia

George A. Burdock, PhD, DABT, FACN
President, Burdock Group, Vero Beach, Florida

Louis R. Cantilena, Jr. MD, PhD
Professor of Medicine and Pharmacology,
Director, Division of Clinical Pharmacology
and Medical Toxicology, Uniformed Services University,
Bethesda, Maryland

Charles C. Capen, DVM, MSc, PhD
Distinguished University Professor, The Ohio State
University, Department of Veterinary Biosciences,
Columbus, Ohio

Lucio G. Costa, PhD
Professor, Department of Environmental and
Occupational Health Sciences, University of Washington,
Seattle, Washington

Daniel L. Costa, ScD
National Program Director for Air Research,
Office of Research and Development,
U.S. Environmental Protection Agency,
Research Triangle Park, North Carolina

Robert T. Di Giulio, PhD
Professor, Nicholas School of the Environment and Earth
Sciences, Duke University, Durham, North Carolina

David L. Eaton, PhD
Professor of Environmental and Occupational Health
Sciences and Public Health Genetics, School of Public
Health and Community Medicine; and Associate Vice
Provost for Research, University of Washington,
Seattle, Washington

Elaine M. Faustman, PhD, DABT
Professor and Director, Institute for Risk Analysis and
Risk Communication, Department of Environmental
and Occupational Health Sciences, University of
Washington, Seattle, Washington

Paul M.D. Foster, PhD
National Toxicology Program, National Institute of
Environmental Health Sciences, Research Triangle Park,
North Carolina

Donald A. Fox, PhD
Professor of Vision Sciences, Biology and Biochemistry,
and Pharmacology, University of Houston, Houston, Texas

Michael A. Gallo, PhD
UMDNJ-Robert Wood Johnson Medical School,
Piscataway, New Jersey

Steven G. Gilbert, PhD, DABT
Director, Institute of Neurotoxicology and Neurological
Disorders (INND), Affiliate Associate Professor,
Department of Environmental and Occupational Health
Sciences, University of Washington, Seattle, Washington

Robert A. Goyer, MD
Professor Emeritus Department of Pathology, University of Western Ontario, London, Ontario, Canada

L. Earl Gray, Jr. PhD
NHEERL Reprotoxicology Division Endocrinology Branch, U.S. Environmental Protection Agency, Research Triangle Park, North Carolina

Zoltán Gregus, MD, PhD, DSc, DABT
Department of Pharmacology and Therapeutics, Toxicology Section, University of Pécs, Medical School, Pécs, Hungary

Naomi H. Harley, PhD
New York University School of Medicine, Department of Environmental Medicine, New York, New York

George R. Hoffman, PhD
Professor, Department of Biology, College of Holy Cross, Worcester, Massachusetts

Michael P. Holsapple, PhD, FATS
Executive Director, ILSI Health and Environmental Sciences Institute (HESI), Washington, District of Columbia

Hartmut Jaeschke, PhD
Professor, Department of Pharmacology, Toxicology and Therapeutics, University of Kansas Medical Center, Kansas City, Kansas

Lisa M. Kamendulis, PhD
Assistant Professor, Department of Pharmacology and Toxicology, Indiana University School of Medicine, Indianapolis, Indiana

Norbert E. Kaminski, PhD
Professor, Pharmacology & Toxicology, Director, Center for Integrative Toxicology, Michigan State University, East Lansing, Michigan

Y. James Kang, DVM, PhD, FATS
Professor, Departments of Medicine, and Pharmacology and Toxicology University of Louisville School of Medicine, Louisville, Kentucky

Barbara L. Faubert Kaplan, PhD
Assistant Professor, Center for Integrative Toxicology, Michigan State University, East Lansing, Michigan

Robert J. Kavlock, PhD
National Health and Environmental Effects Research Laboratory, U.S. Environmental Protection Agency, Research Triangle Park, North Carolina

James E. Klaunig, PhD
Robert B. Forney Professor of Toxicology, Director, Center for Environmental Health, Associate Director, IU Cancer Center, School of Medicine, Indiana University, Indianapolis, Indiana

Frank N. Kostonis, PhD
Department of Food Microbiology and Toxicology, Food Research Institute, University of Wisconsin, Madison, Wisconsin

Jerold A. Last, PhD
Professor, Department of Pulmonary and Critical Care Medicine, University of California, Davis, California

Lois D. Lehman-McKeeman, PhD
Distinguished Research Fellow, Discovery Toxicology, Bristol-Myers Squibb Company, Princeton, New Jersey

Jie Liu, PhD
Staff Scientist, Inorganic Carcinogenesis, Laboratory of Comparative Carcinogenesis, National Cancer Institute at NIEHS, Research Triangle Park, North Carolina

Theodora M. Mauro, MD
Associate Professor in Residence and Vice Chairman, Department of Dermatology, University of California, San Francisco; and Service Chief, Department of Dermatology, VA Medical Center San Francisco, San Francisco, California

Virginia C. Moser, PhD, DABT
Toxicologist, Neurotoxicology Division, National Health and Environmental Effects Research Laboratory, U.S. Environmental Protection Agency, Research Triangle Park, North Carolina

Michael C. Newman, PhD
Professor of Marine Science, School of Marine Science, College of William and Mary, Gloucester Point, Virginia

Stata Norton, PhD
Emeritus Professor, Department of Pharmacology, Toxicology and Therapeutics, University of Kansas Medical Center, Kansas City, Kansas

Brian W. Ogilvie, BA
Director of Drug Interactions, XenoTech, LLC, Lenexa, Kansas

Gilbert S. Omenn, MD, PhD
Professor of Internal Medicine, Human Genetics, Public Health and Computational Biology, University of Michigan, Ann Arbor, Michigan

Andrew Parkinson, PhD
Chief Executive Officer, XenoTech, LLC, Lenexa, Kansas

Martin A. Philbert, PhD
Professor and Senior Associate Dean for Research, University of Michigan School of Public Health, Ann Arbor, Michigan

Kent E. Pinkerton, PhD
Professor, Center for Health and the Environment, University of California, Davis, California

Alphonse Poklis, PhD
Professor of Pathology, Director of Toxicology, Department of Pathology, Virginia Commonwealth University, Richmond, Virginia

R. Julian Preston, PhD
Associate Director for Health, National Health and Environmental Effects Laboratory, U.S. Environmental Protection Agency, Research Triangle Park, North Carolina

Rudy J. Richardson, SD, DABT
Professor of Toxicology, Department of Environmental Health Sciences, School of Public Health, University of Michigan, Ann Arbor, Michigan

Robert H. Rice, PhD
Professor, Department of Environmental Toxicology, University of California, Davis, Davis, California

John M. Rogers, PhD
Chief, Developmental Biology Branch, Reproductive Toxicology Division, National Health and Environmental Effects Research Laboratory, Office of Research and Development, U.S. Environmental Protection Agency, Research Triangle Park, North Carolina

Rick G. Schnellmann, PhD
Professor and Chair, Department of Pharmaceutical Sciences, Medical University of South Carolina, Charleston, South Carolina

Danny D. Shen, PhD
Professor, Department of Pharmacy and Pharmaceutics, School of Pharmacy, University of Washington, Seattle, Washington

Peter S. Thorne, PhD
Professor and Director, Environmental Health Sciences Research Center, The University of Iowa, Iowa City, Iowa

Laura S. Van Winkle, PhD
Associate Adjunct Professor, Department of Anatomy, Physiology and Cell Biology, School of Veterinary Medicine; and Center for Health and the Environment, University of California at Davis, Davis, California

Michael P. Waalkes, PhD
Chief Inorganic Carcinogenesis Section, Laboratory of Comparative Carcinogenesis, National Cancer Institute at the National Institute of Environmental Health Sciences, Research Triangle Park, North Carolina

D. Alan Warren, MPH, PhD
Program Director, Environmental Health Science, University of South Carolina Beaufort, Beaufort, South Carolina

John B. Watkins III, PhD, DABT
Assistant Dean and Director, Professor of Pharmacology and Toxicology, Medical Sciences Program, Indiana University School of Medicine, Bloomington, Indiana

Hanspeter R. Witschi, MD, DABT, FATS
Professor of Toxicology, Institute of Toxicology and Environmental Health and Department of Molecular Biosciences, School of Veterinary Medicine, University of California, Davis, California

Preface

We are delighted to present an updated full-color edition of *Essentials of Toxicology*, which distills the major principles and concepts of toxicology that were described in detail in the seventh edition of *Casarett & Doull's Toxicology: The Basic Science of Poisons*. We are grateful to the colleagues who contributed to the seventh edition of *Casarett & Doull's Toxicology: The Basic Science of Poisons*; their contributions to the parent text served as the foundation for the chapters in this edition of *Essentials of Toxicology*.

Essentials of Toxicology concisely presents the broad science of toxicology. Important concepts from anatomy, physiology, and biochemistry have been included to facilitate the understanding of the principles and mechanisms of toxicant action on specific organ systems. It is hoped that the book will be useful to students in undergraduate and graduate courses in toxicology, as well as students from other disciplines, who want to have a strong foundation in toxicologic concepts and principles.

The book is organized into seven units: (1) General Principles of Toxicology; (2) Disposition of Toxicants; (3) Nonorgan-directed Toxicity; (4) Target Organ Toxicity; (5) Toxic Agents; (6) Environmental Toxicology; and (7) Applications of Toxicology. A summary of important points is included at the beginning of each chapter, and a set of review questions is provided at the end of each chapter. We invite our readers to send us their suggestions of ways to improve this text and we appreciate the thoughtful suggestions that we received on the last edition.

We would like to acknowledge all individuals who were involved in this project. We particularly give a heartfelt and sincere thanks to our families for their love, patience, and support during the preparation of this book. We especially appreciate Ronnie Hamrick, Greg Dowling, Todd Dejulio, and Ruth Sanders who provided invaluable assistance on this project. The capable advice, guidance, and assistance of the McGraw-Hill staff is gratefully acknowledged. Finally, we thank our students for their enthusiasm for learning and what they have taught us during their time with us.

Curtis D. Klaassen
John B. Watkins III

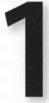

C H A P T E R

History and Scope of Toxicology

Michael A. Gallo

HISTORY OF TOXICOLOGY

    Antiquity

    Middle Ages

    Renaissance

        Paracelsus

    Age of Enlightenment

MODERN TOXICOLOGY

AFTER WORLD WAR II

KEY POINTS

- Toxicology is the study of the adverse effects of xenobiotics on living systems.
- Toxicology assimilates knowledge and techniques from biochemistry, biology, chemistry, genetics, mathematics, medicine, pharmacology, physiology, and physics.

- Toxicology applies safety evaluation and risk assessment to the discipline.

HISTORY OF TOXICOLOGY

Modern toxicology goes beyond the study of the adverse effects of exogenous agents by assimilating knowledge and techniques from most branches of biochemistry, biology, chemistry, genetics, mathematics, medicine, pharmacology, physiology, and physics and applies safety evaluation and risk assessment to the discipline. In all branches of toxicology, scientists explore the mechanisms by which chemicals produce adverse effects in biological systems. Activities in these broad subjects complement toxicologic research, thereby contributing to the application of this knowledge to the science and art of toxicology.

Antiquity

Knowledge of animal venoms and plant extracts for hunting, warfare, and assassination presumably predate recorded history. One of the oldest known writings, the Ebers Papyrus (circa 1500 B.C.), contains information pertaining to many recognized poisons, including hemlock, aconite, opium, and metals such as lead, copper, and antimony. Whereas the *Book of Job* (circa 1400 B.C.) speaks of poison arrows (Job 6:4), Hippocrates (circa 400 B.C.) added a number of poisons and clinical toxicology principles pertaining to bioavailability in therapy and overdosage. Theophrastus (370–286 B.C.), a student of Aristotle, included numerous references to poisonous plants in *De Historia Plantarum*. Dioscorides, a Greek physician in the court of the Roman emperor Nero, made the first attempt at classifying poisons into plant, animal, and mineral poisons in his book *De Materia Medica*, which contains reference to some 600 plants.

One legend tells of Roman King Mithridates VI of Pontus, who was so fearful of poisons that he regularly ingested a mixture of 36 ingredients as protection against assassination. On the occasion of his imminent capture by enemies, his attempts to kill himself with poison failed because of his successful antidote concoction. This tale leads to use of the word mithridatic as an antidote or protective mixture. Because poisonings in politics became so extensive, Sulla issued the *Lex Cornelia* (circa 82 B.C.), which appears to be the first law against poisoning and later became a regulatory statute directed at careless dispensers of drugs.

Middle Ages

The writings of Maimonides (Moses ben Maimon, A.D. 1135–1204) included a treatise on the treatment of poisonings from insects, snakes, and mad dogs (*Poisons and their Antidotes,* 1198). Maimonides described the subject of bioavailability, noting that milk, butter, and cream could delay intestinal absorption. In the early Renaissance and under the guise of delivering provender to the sick and the poor, Catherine de Medici tested toxic concoctions, carefully noting the rapidity of the toxic response (onset of action), the effectiveness of the compound (potency), the degree of response of the parts of the body (specificity and site of action), and the complaints of the victim (clinical signs and symptoms).

Renaissance

All substances are poisons; there is none that is not a poison. The right dose differentiates a poison from a remedy.

Paracelsus

Philippus Aureolus Theophrastus Bombastus von Hohenheim-Paracelsus (1493–1541) was pivotal, standing between the philosophy and magic of classic antiquity and the philosophy and science willed to us by figures of the seventeenth and eighteenth centuries. Paracelsus, a physician-alchemist, formulated many revolutionary views that remain integral to the structure of toxicology, pharmacology, and therapeutics today. He focused on the primary toxic agent as a chemical entity, and held that (1) experimentation is essential in the examination of responses to

chemicals, (2) one should make a distinction between the therapeutic and toxic properties of chemicals, (3) these properties are sometimes but not always indistinguishable except by dose, and (4) one can ascertain a degree of specificity of chemicals and their therapeutic or toxic effects. These principles led Paracelsus to articulate the dose–response relation as a bulwark of toxicology.

> Come bitter pilot, now at once run on
> The dashing rocks thy seasick weary bark!
> Here's to my love! O true apothecary!
> Thy drugs are quick. Thus with a kiss I die.
> *Romeo and Juliet,* act 5, scene 3

Although Ellenbog (circa 1480) warned of the toxicity of mercury and lead from goldsmithing and Agricola published a short treatise on mining diseases in 1556, the major work on the subject, *On the Miners' Sickness and Other Diseases of Miners* (1567), was published by Paracelsus. This treatise addressed the etiology of miners' disease, along with treatment and prevention strategies. Occupational toxicology was further advanced by the work of Bernardino Ramazzini when he published in 1700 his *Discourse on the Diseases of Workers,* which discussed occupations ranging from miners to midwives and including printers, weavers, and potters. Percival Pott's (1775) recognition of the role of soot in scrotal cancer among chimney sweeps was the first report of polyaromatic hydrocarbon carcinogenicity. These findings led to improved medical practices, particularly in prevention.

Age of Enlightenment

Experimental toxicology accompanied the growth of organic chemistry and developed rapidly during the nineteenth century. Magendie (1783–1885), Orfila (1787–1853), and Bernard (1813–1878) laid the groundwork for pharmacology, experimental therapeutics, and occupational toxicology.

Orfila, a Spanish physician in the French court, used autopsy material and chemical analysis systematically as legal proof of poisoning. His introduction of this detailed type of analysis survives as the underpinning of forensic toxicology. Orfila published a major work devoted expressly to the toxicity of natural agents in 1815. Magendie, a physician and experimental physiologist, studied the mechanisms of action of emetine and strychnine. His research determined the absorption and distribution of these compounds in the body. One of Magendie's more famous students, Claude Bernard, contributed the classic treatise, *An Introduction to the Study of Experimental Medicine.*

German scientists Oswald Schmiedeberg (1838–1921) and Louis Lewin (1850–1929) made many contributions to the science of toxicology. Schmeideberg trained approximately 120 students who later populated the most important laboratories of pharmacology and toxicology throughout the world. Lewin published much of the early work on the toxicity of narcotics, methanol, glycerol, acrolein, and chloroform.

MODERN TOXICOLOGY

Toxicology has drawn its strength and diversity from its proclivity to borrowing from almost all the basic sciences to test its hypotheses. This fact, coupled with the health and occupational regulations that have driven toxicology research since 1900, has made this discipline exceptional in the history of science.

With the advent of anesthetics and disinfectants in the late 1850s, toxicology as it is currently understood began. The prevalent use of "patent" medicines led to several incidents of poisonings from these medicaments, which, when coupled with the response to Upton Sinclair's exposé of the meat-packing industry in *The Jungle,* culminated in the passage of the Wiley Bill in 1906, the first of many U.S. pure food and drug laws.

During the 1890s and early 1900s, the discovery of radioactivity and the vitamins, or "vital amines," led to the use of the first large-scale bioassays (multiple animal studies) to determine whether these "new" chemicals were beneficial or harmful to laboratory animals.

One of the first journals expressly dedicated to experimental toxicology, *Archiv für Toxikologie,* began publication in Europe in 1930. That same year the National Institutes of Health (NIH) was established in the United States. As a response to the tragic consequences of acute kidney failure after taking sulfanilamide in glycol solutions, the Copeland bill was passed in 1938. This was the second major bill involving the formation of the U.S. Food and Drug Administration (FDA). The first major U.S. pesticide act was signed into law in 1947. The significance of the initial Federal Insecticide, Fungicide, and Rodenticide Act was that for the first time in U.S. history a substance that was neither a drug nor a food had to be shown to be safe and efficacious.

AFTER WORLD WAR II

You too can be a toxicologist in two easy lessons, each of ten years.
Arnold Lehman (circa 1955)

The mid-1950s witnessed the strengthening of the U.S. FDA's commitment to toxicology. The U.S. Congress passed and the president of the United States signed the additives amendments to the Food, Drug, and Cosmetic Act. The Delaney clause (1958) of these amendments stated broadly that any chemical found to be carcinogenic in laboratory animals or humans could not be added to the U.S. food supply. Delaney became a battle cry for many groups and resulted in the inclusion at a new level of biostatisticians and mathematical modelers in the field of toxicology. Shortly after the Delaney amendment, the first

American journal dedicated to toxicology, *Toxicology and Applied Pharmacology,* was launched. The founding of the Society of Toxicology followed shortly afterward.

The 1960s started with the tragic thalidomide incident, in which several thousand children were born with serious birth defects, and the publication of Rachel Carson's *Silent Spring* (1962). Attempts to understand the effects of chemicals on the embryo and fetus and on the environment as a whole gained momentum. New legislation was passed, and new journals were founded. Cellular and molecular toxicology developed as a subdiscipline, and risk assessment became a major product of toxicologic investigations.

Currently, many dozens of professional, governmental, and other scientific organizations with thousands of members and over 120 journals are dedicated to toxicology and related disciplines. In addition, the International Congress of Toxicology is made up of toxicology societies from Europe, South America, Asia, Africa, and Australia, which brings together the broadest representation of toxicologists.

Toxicology has an interesting and varied history. Perhaps as a science that has grown and prospered by borrowing from many disciplines, it has suffered from the absence of a single goal, but its diversification has allowed for the interspersion of ideas and concepts from higher education, industry, and government. This has resulted in an exciting, innovative, and diversified field that is serving science and the community at large. Few disciplines can point to both basic sciences and direct applications at the same time. Toxicology—the study of the adverse effects of xenobiotics—may be unique in this regard.

BIBLIOGRAPHY

Bryan CP: *The Papyrus Ebers.* London: Geoffrey Bales, 1930.
Carson R: *Silent Spring.* Boston: Houghton Mifflin, 1962.
Gunther RT: *The Greek Herbal of Dioscorides.* New York: Oxford University Press, 1934.
Guthrie DA: *A History of Medicine.* Philadelphia: Lippincott, 1946.
Hays HW: *Society of Toxicology History, 1961–1986.* Washington, DC: Society of Toxicology, 1986.
Munter S (ed): *Treatise on Poisons and their Antidotes. Vol. II of the Medical Writings of Moses Maimonides.* Philadelphia: Lippincott, 1966.
Pagel W: *Paracelsus: An Introduction to Philosophical Medicine in the Era of the Renaissance.* New York: Karger, 1958.
Thompson CJS: *Poisons and Poisoners: With Historical Accounts of Some Famous Mysteries in Ancient and Modern Times.* London: Shaylor, 1931.

QUESTIONS

1. Which one of the following statements regarding toxicology is true?
   a. Modern toxicology is concerned with the study of the adverse effects of chemicals on ancient forms of life.
   b. Modern toxicology studies embrace principles from such disciplines as biochemistry, botany, chemistry, physiology, and physics.
   c. Modern toxicology has its roots in the knowledge of plant and animal poisons, which predates recorded history and has been used to promote peace.
   d. Modern toxicology studies the mechanisms by which inorganic chemicals produce advantageous as well as deleterious effects.
   e. Modern toxicology is concerned with the study of chemicals in mammalian species.

2. Knowledge of the toxicology of poisonous agents was published earliest in the:
   a. Ebers papyrus.
   b. *De Historia Plantarum.*
   c. *De Maateria Medica.*
   d. *Lex Cornelia.*
   e. *Poisons and their Antidotes.*

3. Paracelsus, a physician-alchemist, formulated many revolutionary views that remain integral to the structure of toxicology, pharmacology, and therapeutics today. He focused on the primary toxic agent as a chemical entity and articulated the dose–response relation. Which one of the following statements is not attributable to Paracelsus?
   a. Natural poisons are quick in their onset of actions.
   b. Experimentation is essential in the examination of responses to chemicals.
   c. One should make a distinction between the therapeutic and toxic properties of chemicals.
   d. These properties are sometimes but not always indistinguishable except by dose.
   e. One can ascertain a degree of specificity of chemicals and their therapeutic or toxic effects.

4. The art of toxicology requires years of experience to acquire, even though the knowledge base of facts may be learned more quickly. Which modern toxicologist is credited with saying that "you can be a toxicologist in two easy lesions, each of 10 years?"
   a. Claude Bernard.
   b. Rachel Carson.
   c. Upton Sinclair.
   d. Arnold Lehman.
   e. Oswald Schmiedeberg.

5. Which of the following statements is correct?
   a. Claude Bernard was a prolific scientist who trained over 120 students and published numerous contributions to the scientific literature.
   b. Louis Lewin trained under Oswald Schmiedeberg and published much of the early work on the toxicity of narcotics, methanol, and chloroform.
   c. *An Introduction to the Study of Experimental Medicine* was written by the Spanish physician Orfila.
   d. Magendie used autopsy material and chemical analysis systematically as legal proof of poisoning.
   e. Percival Potts was instrumental in demonstrating the chemical complexity of snake venoms.

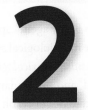

Principles of Toxicology

David L. Eaton and Steven G. Gilbert

- A *poison* is any agent capable of producing a deleterious response in a biological system.
- A *mechanistic toxicologist* identifies the cellular, biochemical, and molecular mechanisms by which chemicals exert toxic effects on living organisms.
- *Toxicogenomics* permits mechanistic toxicologists to identify and protect genetically susceptible individuals from harmful environmental exposures, and to customize drug therapies based on their individual genetic makeup.
- A *descriptive toxicologist* is concerned directly with toxicity testing, which provides information for safety evaluation and regulatory requirements.
- A *regulatory toxicologist* both determines from available data whether a chemical poses a sufficiently low risk to be marketed for a stated purpose and establishes standards for the amount of chemicals permitted in ambient air, industrial atmospheres, and drinking water.

- *Selective toxicity* means that a chemical produces injury to one kind of living matter without harming another form of life even though the two may exist in intimate contact.
- The individual or "graded" dose–response relationship describes the response of an *individual* organism to varying doses of a chemical.
- A quantal dose–response relationship characterizes the distribution of responses to different doses in a *population* of individual organisms.
- Hormesis, a "U-shaped" dose–response curve, results with some xenobiotics that impart beneficial or stimulatory effects at low doses but adverse effects at higher doses.
- Descriptive animal toxicity testing assumes that the effects produced by a compound in laboratory animals, when properly qualified, are applicable to humans, and that exposure of experimental animals to toxic agents in high doses is a necessary and valid method of discovering possible hazards in humans.

INTRODUCTION TO TOXICOLOGY

Toxicology is the study of the adverse effects of chemicals on living organisms. A *toxicologist* is trained to examine the nature of those effects (including their cellular, biochemical, and molecular mechanisms of action) and assess the probability of their occurrence.

Different Areas of Toxicology

A *mechanistic toxicologist* identifies the cellular, biochemical, and molecular mechanisms by which chemicals exert toxic effects on living organisms (see Chapter 3 for a detailed discussion of mechanisms of toxicity). Mechanistic data may be useful in the design and production of safer chemicals and in rational therapy for chemical poisoning and treatment of disease. In risk assessment, mechanistic data may be very useful in demonstrating that an adverse outcome observed in laboratory animals is directly relevant to humans. *Toxicogenomics* permits mechanistic toxicologists to identify and protect genetically susceptible individuals from harmful environmental exposures, and to customize drug therapies based on their individual genetic makeup. Numerous genetic tests can identify susceptible individuals in advance of pharmacological treatment.

A *descriptive toxicologist* is concerned directly with toxicity testing, which provides information for safety evaluation and regulatory requirements. Toxicity tests (described later in this chapter) in experimental animals are designed to yield information that can be used to evaluate risks posed to humans and the environment by exposure to specific chemicals.

A *regulatory toxicologist* has the responsibility for deciding, on the basis of data provided by descriptive and mechanistic toxicologists, whether a drug or another chemical poses a sufficiently low risk to be marketed for a stated purpose. Regulatory toxicologists are involved in the establishment of standards for the amount of chemicals permitted in foods, drugs, ambient air, industrial atmospheres, and drinking water (see Chapter 4).

Forensic toxicology is a hybrid of analytic chemistry and fundamental toxicologic principles that focuses primarily on the medicolegal aspects of the harmful effects of chemicals on humans and animals (see Chapter 31).

Clinical toxicology is concerned with disease caused by or uniquely associated with toxic substances (see Chapter 32).

Environmental toxicology focuses on the impacts of chemical pollutants in the environment on biological organisms, specifically studying the impacts of chemicals on nonhuman organisms such as fish, birds, terrestrial animals, and plants. *Ecotoxicology*, a specialized area within environmental toxicology, focuses specifically on the impacts of toxic substances on population dynamics in an ecosystem (see Chapter 29).

Developmental toxicology is the study of adverse effects on the developing organism that may result from exposure to chemical or physical agents before conception (either parent), during prenatal development, or postnatally until the time of puberty. *Teratology* is the study of defects induced during development between conception and birth (see Chapter 10).

Reproductive toxicology is the study of the occurrence of adverse effects on the male or female reproductive system that may result from exposure to chemical or physical agents (see Chapter 20).

Toxicology and Society

Knowledge about the toxicologic effect of a compound affects consumer products, drugs, manufacturing processes, waste cleanup, regulatory action, civil disputes, and broad policy decisions. The expanding influence of toxicology on societal issues is accompanied by the responsibility to be increasingly sensitive to the ethical, legal, and social implications of toxicologic research and testing.

The convergence of multiple elements has highlighted the following ethical dynamics of toxicology. First, experience and new discoveries in the biological sciences have emphasized the need for well-articulated visions of human, animal, and environmental health. Second, experience with the health consequences of exposure to such things as lead, asbestos, and tobacco has precipitated many regulatory and legal actions and public policy decisions. Third, we have an increasingly well-defined framework for discussing our social and ethical responsibilities. Fourth, all research involving humans or animals must be conducted in a responsible and ethical manner. Fifth, the uncertainty and biological variability inherent in the biological sciences requires decision making with limited or uncertain information. And finally, individuals involved in toxicologic research must adhere to the highest ethical standards of the profession.

General Characteristics of the Toxic Response

One could define a *poison* as any agent capable of producing a deleterious response in a biological system. Virtually every known chemical has the potential to produce injury or death if it is present in a sufficient amount. Table 2–1 shows the dosage of chemicals needed to produce death in 50 percent of treated animals (LD_{50}). It should be noted that measures of acute lethality such as LD_{50} may not accurately reflect the full spectrum of toxicity, or hazard, associated with exposure to a chemical. For example, some chemicals with low acute toxicity may have carcinogenic or teratogenic effects at doses that produce no evidence of acute toxicity.

CLASSIFICATION OF TOXIC AGENTS

Toxic agents are classified depending on the interests and needs of the classifier. These agents may be discussed in terms of their target organs, use, source, and effects. The term *toxin* generally refers to toxic substances that are produced by biological systems such as plants, animals, fungi, or bacteria. The term *toxicant* is used in speaking of toxic substances that are produced by or are a by-product of human activities. Toxic agents also may be classified in terms of their physical state,

TABLE 2–1 Approximate acute LD_{50} of some representative chemical agents.

Agent	LD_{50}, mg/kg[1]
Ethyl alcohol	10,000
Sodium chloride	4,000
Ferrous sulfate	1,500
Morphine sulfate	900
Phenobarbital sodium	150
Picrotoxin	5
Strychnine sulfate	2
Nicotine	1
Tubocurarine	0.5
Hemicholinium-3	0.2
Tetrodotoxin	0.10
Dioxin (TCDD)	0.001
Botulinum toxin	0.00001

[1]LD_{50} is the dosage (mg/kg body weight) causing death in 50 percent of exposed animals.

chemical stability or reactivity, general chemical structure, or poisoning potential.

SPECTRUM OF UNDESIRED EFFECTS

The spectrum of undesired effects of chemicals is broad. In therapeutics, for example, each drug produces a number of effects, but usually only one effect is associated with the primary objective of the therapy; all the other effects are referred to as *undesirable* or *side effects*. However, some of these side effects may be desired for another therapeutic indication. Some side effects of drugs are always deleterious to the well-being of humans. These are referred to as the *adverse, deleterious,* or *toxic* effects of the drug.

Allergic Reactions

Chemical allergy is an immunologically mediated adverse reaction to a chemical resulting from previous sensitization to that chemical or to a structurally similar one. The terms *hypersensitivity, allergic reaction,* and *sensitization reaction* are used to describe this situation (see Chapter 12). Once sensitization has occurred, allergic reactions may result from exposure to relatively very low doses of chemicals. However, for a given allergic individual, allergic reactions are dose-related. Sensitization reactions are sometimes very severe and may be fatal.

Most chemicals and their metabolic products are not sufficiently large to be recognized by the immune system as a foreign substance and thus must first combine with an endogenous protein to form an antigen (or immunogen). Such a molecule is called a *hapten*. The hapten–protein complex (antigen) is then capable of eliciting the formation of antibodies. Subsequent exposure to the chemical results in an antigen–antibody interaction, which provokes the typical manifestations of allergy that range in severity from minor skin disturbance to fatal anaphylactic shock.

Idiosyncratic Reactions

Chemical idiosyncrasy refers to a genetically determined abnormal reactivity to a chemical. The response observed is usually qualitatively similar to that observed in all individuals but may take the form of extreme sensitivity to low doses or extreme insensitivity to high doses of the chemical. For example, individuals abnormally sensitive to nitrites readily oxidize the iron in hemoglobin to produce *methemoglobin*, which is incapable of transporting oxygen to tissues. Consequently, they may suffer from tissue hypoxia after exposure to doses of methemoglobin-producing chemicals that would be harmless to normal individuals.

Immediate versus Delayed Toxicity

Immediate toxic effects occur or develop rapidly after a single administration of a substance, whereas delayed toxic effects occur after the lapse of some time. Most substances produce immediate toxic effects. However, carcinogenic effects of chemicals usually have long latency periods, often 20 to 30 years after the initial exposure, before tumors are observed in humans.

Reversible versus Irreversible Toxic Effects

Some toxic effects of chemicals are reversible, and others are irreversible. If a chemical produces pathological injury to a tissue, the ability of that tissue to regenerate largely determines whether the effect is reversible or irreversible. For liver tissue, with its high regeneration ability, most injuries are reversible, whereas injury to the CNS is largely irreversible because its differentiated cells cannot be replaced. Carcinogenic and teratogenic effects of chemicals, once they occur, are usually considered irreversible toxic effects.

Local versus Systemic Toxicity

Another distinction between types of effects is made on the basis of the general site of action. Local effects occur at the site of first contact between the biological system and the toxicant. In contrast, systemic effects require absorption and distribution of a toxicant from its entry point to a distant site, at which deleterious effects are produced. Most substances, except for highly reactive materials, produce systemic effects. For some materials, both effects can be demonstrated.

Most chemicals that produce systemic toxicity usually elicit their major toxicity in only one or two organs, which are referred to as the *target organs* of toxicity of a particular chemical. The target organ of toxicity is often not the site of the highest concentration of the chemical.

Target organs in order of frequency of involvement in systemic toxicity are the CNS; the circulatory system; the blood and hematopoietic system; visceral organs such as the liver, kidney, and lung; and the skin. Muscle and bone are seldom target tissues for systemic effects.

Interaction of Chemicals

Chemical interactions can occur via various mechanisms, such as alterations in absorption, protein binding, and the biotransformation and excretion of one or both of the interacting toxicants. In addition to these modes of interaction, the response of the organism to combinations of toxicants may be increased or decreased because of toxicologic responses at the site of action.

An *additive* effect, most commonly observed when two chemicals are given together, occurs when the combined effect of two chemicals is equal to the sum of the effects of each agent given alone. A *synergistic* effect occurs when the combined effects of two chemicals are much greater than the sum of the effects of each agent given alone (example: 2 + 2 = 20). *Potentiation* occurs when one substance does not have a toxic effect on a certain organ or system but when added to another chemical makes that chemical much more toxic (example: 0 + 2 = 10). Isopropanol, for example, is not hepatotoxic, but when it is administered in addition to carbon tetrachloride, the hepatotoxicity of carbon tetrachloride is much greater than that when it is given alone. *Antagonism* occurs when two chemicals administered together interfere with each other's actions or one interferes with the action of the other. There are four major types of antagonism: functional, chemical, dispositional, and receptor. *Functional antagonism* occurs when two chemicals counterbalance each other by producing opposite effects on the same physiologic function. For example, the marked fall in blood pressure during severe barbiturate intoxication can be effectively antagonized by the intravenous administration of a vasopressor agent such as norepinephrine or metaraminol. *Chemical antagonism* or *inactivation* is simply a chemical reaction between two compounds that produces a less toxic product. For example, chelators of metal ions decrease metal toxicity and antitoxins antagonize the action of various animal toxins. *Dispositional antagonism* occurs when the absorption, biotransformation, distribution, or excretion of a chemical is altered so that the concentration and/or duration of the chemical at the target organ are diminished. *Receptor antagonism* occurs when two chemicals that bind to the same receptor produce less of an effect when given together than the addition of their separate effects (example: 4 + 6 = 8) or when one chemical antagonizes the effect of the second chemical. Receptor antagonists are often termed *blockers*.

Tolerance

Tolerance is a state of decreased responsiveness to a toxic effect of a chemical resulting from prior exposure to that chemical or to a structurally related chemical. Two major mechanisms are responsible for tolerance: one is due to a decreased amount of toxicant reaching the site where the toxic effect is produced (*dispositional tolerance*) and the other is due to a reduced responsiveness of a tissue to the chemical.

CHARACTERISTICS OF EXPOSURE

Toxic effects in a biological system are not produced by a chemical agent unless that agent or its metabolic breakdown (biotransformation) products reach appropriate sites in the body at a concentration and for a length of time sufficient to produce a toxic manifestation. Whether a toxic response occurs is dependent on the chemical and physical properties of the agent, the exposure situation, how the agent is metabolized by the system, and the overall susceptibility of the biological system or subject.

Route and Site of Exposure

The major routes (pathways) by which toxic agents gain access to the body are the gastrointestinal tract (ingestion), lungs (inhalation), skin (topical, percutaneous, or dermal), and other parenteral (other than intestinal canal) routes. Toxic agents generally produce the greatest effect and the most rapid response when given directly into the bloodstream (the intravenous route). An approximate descending order of effectiveness for the other routes would be inhalation, intraperitoneal, subcutaneous, intramuscular, intradermal, oral, and dermal. The "vehicle" (the material in which the chemical is dissolved) and other formulation factors can markedly alter absorption. In addition, the route of administration can influence the toxicity of agents. For example, an agent that acts on the CNS, but is efficiently detoxified in the liver, would be expected to be less toxic when given orally than when inhaled, because the oral route requires that nearly all of the dose pass through the liver before reaching the systemic circulation and then the CNS.

Duration and Frequency of Exposure

Toxicologists usually divide the exposure of experimental animals to chemicals into four categories: acute, subacute, subchronic, and chronic. *Acute* exposure is defined as exposure to a chemical for less than 24 h. While acute exposure usually refers to a single administration, repeated exposures may be given within a 24-h period for some slightly toxic or practically nontoxic chemicals. Acute exposure by inhalation refers to continuous exposure for less than 24 h, most frequently for 4 h. Repeated exposure is divided into three categories: subacute, subchronic, and chronic. *Subacute exposure* refers to repeated exposure to a chemical for 1 month or less, *subchronic* for 1 to 3 months, and *chronic* for more than 3 months.

In human exposure situations, the frequency and duration of exposure are usually not as clearly defined as in controlled animal studies, but many of the same terms are used to describe general exposure situations. Thus, workplace or environmental exposures may be described as *acute* (occurring from a single incident or episode), *subchronic* (occurring repeatedly over several weeks or months), or *chronic* (occurring repeatedly for many months or years).

For many agents, the toxic effects that follow a single exposure are quite different from those produced by repeated exposure. Acute exposure to agents that are rapidly absorbed is likely to produce immediate toxic effects but also can produce delayed toxicity that may or may not be similar to the toxic effects of chronic exposure. Conversely, chronic exposure to a toxic agent may produce some immediate (acute) effects after each administration in addition to the long-term, low-level, or chronic effects of the toxic substance. The other time-related factor that is important in the temporal characterization of repeated exposures is the frequency of exposure. The relationship between elimination rate and frequency of exposure is shown in Figure 2–1. A chemical that produces severe effects with a single dose may have no effect if the same total dose is given in several intervals. For the chemical depicted by line B in Figure 2–1, in which the half-life for elimination (time necessary for 50 percent of the chemical to be removed from the bloodstream) is approximately equal to the dosing frequency, a theoretical toxic concentration of 2 U is not reached until the fourth dose, whereas that concentration is reached with only two doses for chemical A, which has an elimination rate much slower than the dosing interval (time between each repeated dose). Conversely, for chemical C, where the elimination rate is much shorter than the dosing interval, a toxic concentration at the site of toxic effect will never be reached regardless of how many doses are administered. Of course, it is possible that residual cell or tissue damage occurs with each dose even though the chemical itself is not accumulating. The important consideration, then, is whether the interval between doses is sufficient to allow for complete repair of tissue damage. Chronic toxic effects may occur, therefore, if the chemical accumulates in the biological system (rate of absorption exceeds the rate of biotransformation and/or excretion), if it produces irreversible toxic effects, or if there is insufficient time for the system to recover from the toxic damage within the exposure frequency interval. For additional discussion of these relationships, consult Chapters 5 and 7.

DOSE–RESPONSE

The characteristics of exposure and the spectrum of effects come together in a correlative relationship customarily referred to as the *dose–response relationship*. Whatever response is selected for measurement, the relationship between the degree of response of the biological system and the amount of toxicant administered assumes a form that occurs so consistently as to be considered the most fundamental and pervasive concept in toxicology.

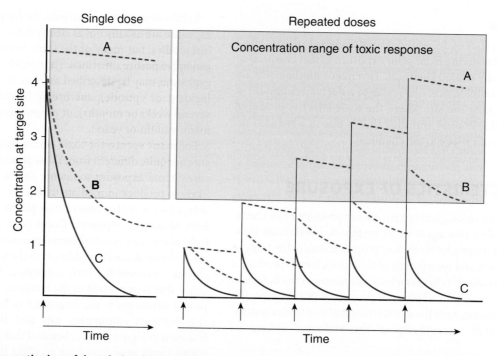

FIGURE 2–1 **Diagrammatic view of the relationship between dose and concentration at the target site under different conditions of dose frequency and elimination rate.** *Line A.* A chemical with very slow elimination (e.g., half-life of 1 year). *Line B.* A chemical with a rate of elimination equal to frequency of dosing (e.g., 1 day). *Line C.* Rate of elimination faster than the dosing frequency (e.g., 5 h). Purple-shaded area is representative of the concentration of chemical at the target site necessary to elicit a toxic response.

From a practical perspective, there are two types of dose–response relationships: (1) the individual dose–response relationship, which describes the response of an *individual* organism to varying doses of a chemical, often referred to as a "graded" response because the measured effect is continuous over a range of doses, and (2) a quantal dose–response relationship, which characterizes the distribution of responses to different doses in a *population* of individual organisms.

Individual, or Graded, Dose–Response Relationships

Individual dose–response relationships are characterized by a dose-related increase in the severity of the response. For example, Figure 2–2 shows the dose–response relationship between different dietary doses of the organophosphate insecticide chlorpyrifos and the extent of inhibition of two different enzymes in the brain and liver: acetylcholinesterase and carboxylesterase. In the brain, the degree of inhibition of both enzymes is clearly dose-related and spans a wide range, although the amount of inhibition per unit dose is different for the two enzymes. From the shapes of these two dose–response curves, it is evident that, in the brain, cholinesterase is more easily inhibited than carboxylesterase. The toxicologic response that results is directly related to the degree of cholinesterase enzyme inhibition in the brain. It should be noted that most toxic substances have multiple sites or mechanisms of toxicity, each with its own "dose–response" relationship and subsequent adverse effect.

Quantal Dose–Response Relationships

In contrast to the "graded" or continuous-scale dose–response relationship that occurs in individuals, the dose–response relationships in a *population* are by definition quantal—or "all or none"—in nature; that is, at any given dose, an individual in the population is classified as either a "responder" or a "nonresponder." Although these distinctions of "quantal population" and "graded individual" dose–response relationships are useful, the two types of responses are conceptually identical. The ordinate in both cases is simply labeled *the response*, which may be the degree of response in an individual or system or the fraction of a population responding, and the abscissa is the range in administered doses.

The LD_{50} is the statistically derived single dose of a substance that can be expected to cause death in 50 percent of the animals tested. The top panel of Figure 2–3 shows that quantal dose–responses such as lethality exhibit a normal or Gaussian distribution. The frequency histogram in this panel also shows the relationship between dose and effect. The bars represent the percentage of animals that died at each dose minus the percentage that died at the immediately lower dose. One can clearly see that only a few animals responded to the lowest dose and the highest dose. Larger numbers of animals responded to doses intermediate between these two extremes, and the maximum frequency of response occurred in the middle portion of the dose range. Thus, we have a bell-shaped curve known as a *normal frequency distribution*. The reason for this normal distribution is that there are differences in

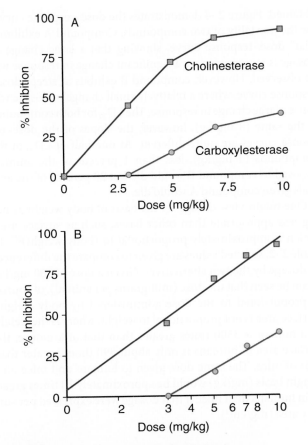

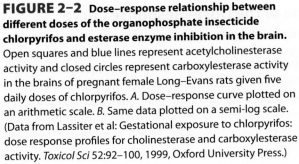

FIGURE 2–2 **Dose–response relationship between different doses of the organophosphate insecticide chlorpyrifos and esterase enzyme inhibition in the brain.** Open squares and blue lines represent acetylcholinesterase activity and closed circles represent carboxylesterase activity in the brains of pregnant female Long–Evans rats given five daily doses of chlorpyrifos. *A.* Dose–response curve plotted on an arithmetic scale. *B.* Same data plotted on a semi-log scale. (Data from Lassiter et al: Gestational exposure to chlorpyrifos: dose response profiles for cholinesterase and carboxylesterase activity. *Toxicol Sci* 52:92–100, 1999, Oxford University Press.)

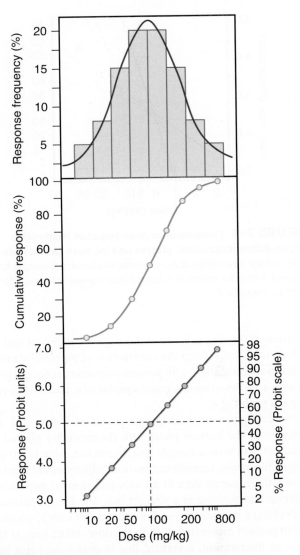

FIGURE 2–3 **Diagram of a quantal dose–response relationship.** The abscissa is a log dosage of the chemical. In the top panel the ordinate is mortality frequency, in the middle panel the ordinate is percent mortality, and in the bottom panel the mortality is in probit units (see text).

susceptibility to chemicals among individuals. Animals responding at the left end of the curve are referred to as *hypersusceptible,* and those at the right end of the curve are called *resistant.* If the numbers of individuals responding at each consecutive dose are added together, a cumulative, quantal dose–response relationship is obtained. When sufficient doses are used with a large number of animals per dose, a sigmoid dose–response curve is observed, as depicted in the middle panel of Figure 2–3. With the lowest dose (6 mg/kg), 1 percent of the animals die. A normally distributed sigmoid curve such as this one approaches a response of 0 percent as the dose is decreased and approaches 100 percent as the dose is increased, but—theoretically—it never passes through 0 and 100 percent. However, the minimally effective dose (ED) of any chemical that evokes a stated all-or-none response is called

the *threshold dose* even though it cannot be determined experimentally.

The sigmoid curve has a relatively linear portion between 16 and 84 percent. These values represent the limits of 1 standard deviation (SD) of the mean (and the median) in a population with truly normal distribution. In a normally distributed population, the mean ±1 SD represents 68.3 percent of the population, the mean ±2 SD represents 95.5 percent of the population, and the mean ±3 SD equals 99.7 percent of the population. Because quantal dose–response phenomena are usually normally distributed, one can convert the percent response to units of deviation from the mean or normal equivalent deviations (NEDs). Thus, the NED for a 50 percent response is 0; an NED of +1 is equated with an 84.1 percent response. Units of NED can be converted by the

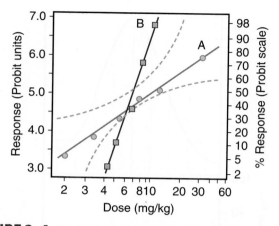

FIGURE 2–4 **Comparison of dose–response relationship for two different chemicals, plotted on a log dose–probit scale.** Note that the slope of the dose–response relationship is steeper for chemical B than for chemical A. Dotted lines represent the confidence limits for chemical A.

addition of 5 to the value to avoid negative numbers and be called *probit units* (from the contraction of *prob*ability un*it*). In this transformation, a 50 percent response becomes a probit of 5, a +1 deviation becomes a probit of 6, and a –1 deviation is a probit of 4.

The data given in the top two panels of Figure 2–3 are replotted in the bottom panel with the mortality plotted in probit units to form a straight line. In essence, what is accomplished in a probit transformation is an adjustment of mortality or other quantal data to an assumed normal population distribution, resulting in a straight line. The LD_{50} is obtained by drawing a horizontal line from the probit unit 5, which is the 50 percent mortality point, to the dose–effect line. At the point of intersection, a vertical line is drawn, and this line intersects the abscissa at the LD_{50} point. In addition to the LD_{50}, the slope of the dose–response curve can also be

obtained. Figure 2–4 demonstrates the dose–response curves for the mortality of two compounds. Compound A exhibits a "flat" dose–response curve, showing that a large change in dosage is required before a significant change in response will be observed. However, compound B exhibits a "steep" dose–response curve, where a relatively small change in dosage will cause a large change in response. The LD_{50} for both compounds is the same (8 mg/kg); however, the slopes of the dose–response curves are quite different. At one-half of LD_{50} of the compounds (4 mg/kg), less than 1 percent of the animals exposed to compound B would die but 20 percent of the animals given compound A would die.

One might view dosage on the basis of body weight as being less appropriate than other bases, such as surface area, which is approximately proportional to (body weight)$^{2/3}$. In Table 2–2, selected values are given to compare the differences in dosage by the two alternatives. Given a dose of 100 mg/kg, it can be seen that the dose (milligrams per animal), of course, is proportional to the dose administered by body weight. Surface area is not proportional to weight: whereas the weight of a human is 3500 times greater than that of a mouse, the surface area of humans is only about 390 times greater than that of mice. The same dose given to humans and mice on a weight basis (mg/kg) would be approximately 10 times greater in humans than mice if that dosage were expressed per surface area (mg/cm²).

Shape of the Dose–Response Curve

Essential Nutrients—The shape of the dose–response relationship has many important implications in toxicity assessment. For example, for substances that are required for normal physiologic function and survival (e.g., vitamins and essential trace elements such as chromium, cobalt, and selenium), the shape of the "graded" dose–response relationship in an individual over the entire dose range is actually U-shaped

TABLE 2–2 **Allometric scaling of dose across different species.**

Species	Weight (kg)	Surface Area (cm²)*	Fold Difference, Relative to Humans, Normalized by Body Weight		
			mg/kg	(BW)$^{2/3}$	(BW)$^{3/4}$
Mouse	0.02	103	1	13.0	7.0
Rat	0.2	365	1	6.9	4.3
Guinea pig	0.4	582	1	5.5	3.6
Rabbit	1.5	1,410	1	3.5	2.6
Cat	2	1,710	1	3.2	2.4
Monkey	4	2,720	1	2.6	2.0
Dog	12	5,680	1	1.8	1.5
Human	70	18,500	1	1.0	1.0

*Surface area of animals is closely approximated by the formula: SA = 10.5 × (body weight [in grams])$^{2/3}$.

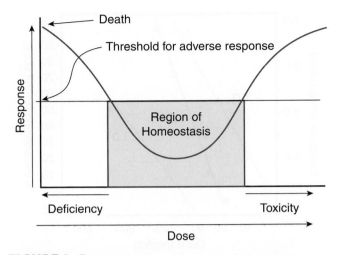

FIGURE 2–5 **Individual dose–response relationship for an essential substance such as a vitamin or trace element.** It is generally recognized that, for most types of toxic responses, a threshold exists such that at doses below the threshold, no toxicity is evident. For essential substances, doses below the minimum daily requirement, as well as those above the threshold for safety, may be associated with toxic effects. The purple-shaded region represents the "region of homeostasis"—the dose range that results in neither deficiency nor toxicity.

(Figure 2–5). That is, at very low doses (or deficiency), there is a high level of adverse effect, which decreases with an increasing dose. As the dose is increased to a point where the deficiency no longer exists, no adverse response is detected and the organism is in a state of homeostasis. However, as the dose is increased to abnormally high levels, an adverse response (usually qualitatively different from that observed at deficient doses) appears and increases in magnitude with increasing dose.

Hormesis—Some nonnutritional toxic substances may also impart beneficial or stimulatory effects at low doses but, at higher doses, they produce adverse effects. This concept of "hormesis" may also result in a U-shaped dose–response curve. For example, chronic alcohol consumption is well recognized to increase the risk of esophageal cancer, liver cancer, and cirrhosis of the liver at relatively high doses, and this response is dose-related (curve A, Figure 2–6). However, there is substantial clinical and epidemiologic evidence that low to moderate consumption of alcohol reduces the incidence of coronary heart disease and stroke (curve B, Figure 2–6). Thus, when all responses are plotted on the ordinate, a U-shaped dose–response curve is obtained (curve C, Figure 2–6).

Threshold—Another important aspect of the dose–response relationship at low doses is the concept of the threshold, some dose below which the probability of an individual responding is zero. For the individual dose–response relationship, thresholds for most toxic effects certainly exist, although inter-individual variability in response and qualitative changes in response

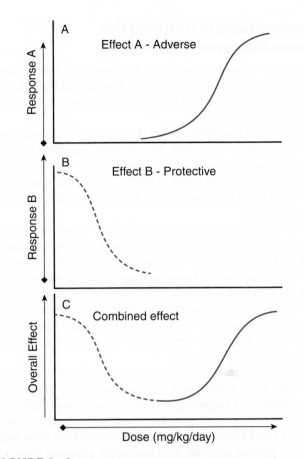

FIGURE 2–6 **Hypothetical dose–response relationship depicting characteristics of hormesis.** Hormetic effects of a substance are hypothesized to occur when relatively low doses result in the stimulation of a beneficial or protective response (*B*), such as induction of enzymatic pathways that protect against oxidative stress. Although low doses provide a potential beneficial effect, a threshold is exceeded as the dose increases and the net effects will be detrimental (*A*), resulting in a typical dose-related increase in toxicity. The complete dose–response curve (*C*) is conceptually similar to the individual dose–response relationship for essential nutrients shown in Figure 2–5.

pattern with dose makes it difficult to establish a true "no effects" threshold for any chemical. In the identification of "safe" levels of exposure to a substance, it is important to determine the absence or presence of a threshold.

In evaluating the shape of the dose–response relationship in populations, it is realistic to consider inflections in the shape of the dose–response curve rather than absolute thresholds. That is, the slope of the dose–response relationship at high doses may be substantially different from the slope at low doses, usually because of dispositional differences in the chemical. Saturation of biotransformation pathways, protein-binding sites or receptors, and depletion of intracellular cofactors represent some reasons why sharp inflections in the dose–response relationship may occur.

Assumptions in Deriving the Dose–Response Relationship

A number of assumptions must be considered before dose–response relationships can be used appropriately. The first is that the response is due to the chemical administered, a cause-and-effect relationship.

The second assumption is that the magnitude of the response is in fact related to the dose. This assumes that: there is a molecular target site (or sites) with which the chemical interacts to initiate the response, which is related to the concentration of the agent at the target site, which, in turn, is related to the dose administered.

The third assumption in using the dose–response relationship is that there exists both a quantifiable method of measuring and a precise means of expressing the toxicity. A given chemical may have a family of dose–response relationships, one for each toxic endpoint. For example, a chemical that produces cancer through genotoxic effects, liver damage through inhibition of a specific enzyme, and CNS effects via a different mechanism may have three distinct dose–response relationships, one for each endpoint.

With a new substance, the customary starting point is a single dose acute toxicity test designed to provide preliminary identification of target organ toxicity. Studies specifically designed with lethality as an endpoint are no longer recommended by United States or international agencies. Data from acute studies provide essential information for choosing doses for repeated dosing studies, as well as choosing specific toxicologic endpoints for further study. From these studies, clues as to the direction of further studies come about in two important ways. An acute toxicity study ordinarily is supported by histologic examination of major tissues and organs for abnormalities. From these observations, one can usually obtain more specific information about the events leading to the lethal effect, the target organs involved, and often a suggestion about the possible mechanism of toxicity.

Evaluating the Dose–Response Relationship

Comparison of Dose–Responses—Figure 2–7 illustrates a hypothetical quantal dose–response curve for a desirable effect of a chemical ED such as anesthesia, a toxic dose (TD) effect such as liver injury, and the lethal dose (LD). Even though the curves for ED and LD are parallel, the mechanism by which the drug works is not necessarily that by which the lethal effects are caused. The same admonition applies to any pair of parallel "effect" curves or any other pair of toxicity or lethality curves.

Therapeutic Index—The hypothetical curves in Figure 2–7 illustrate two other interrelated points: the importance of the selection of the toxic criterion and the interpretation of comparative effect. The *therapeutic index* (TI) is defined as the ratio of the dose required to produce a toxic effect and the dose needed to elicit the desired therapeutic response. Similarly, an index

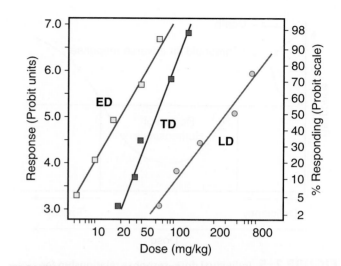

FIGURE 2–7   **Comparison of effective dose (ED), toxic dose (TD), and lethal dose (LD).** The plot is of log dosage versus percentage of population responding in probit units.

of comparative toxicity is obtained by the ratio of doses of two different materials to produce an identical response or the ratio of doses of the same material necessary to yield different toxic effects.

The most commonly used index of effect, whether beneficial or toxic, is the median dose—that is, the dose required to result in a response in 50 percent of a population (or to produce 50 percent of a maximal response). The TI of a drug is an approximate statement about the relative safety of a drug expressed as the ratio of the TD (historically the LD) to the therapeutic dose:

$$TI = \frac{TD_{50}}{ED_{50}}$$

From Figure 2–7, one can approximate a TI by using these median doses. The larger the ratio is, the greater the relative safety. The ED_{50} is approximately 20, and the TD_{50} is about 60; thus, the TI is 3, a number indicating that reasonable care in exposure to the drug is necessary to avoid toxicity. However, median doses tell nothing about the slopes of the dose–response curves for therapeutic and toxic effects.

Margins of Safety and Exposure—One way to overcome this deficiency is to use the ED_{99} for the desired effect and the LD_1 for the undesired effect. These parameters are used to calculate the margin of safety:

$$\text{Margin of safety} = \frac{LD_1}{ED_{99}}$$

For nondrug chemicals, the term *margin of safety* is an indicator of the magnitude of the difference between an estimated "exposed dose" to a human population and the no observable

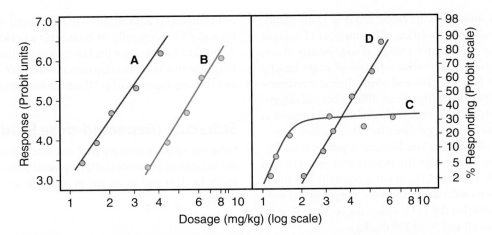

FIGURE 2–8 Schematic representation of the difference in the dose–response curves for four chemicals (A–D), illustrating the difference between potency and efficacy (see text).

adverse effect level (NOAEL) determined in experimental animals.

Potency versus Efficacy—To compare the toxic effects of two or more chemicals, the dose–response to the toxic effects of each chemical must be established. The potency and maximal efficacy of the two chemicals to produce a toxic effect can be explained by reference to Figure 2–8. Chemical A is said to be more potent than chemical B, and C is more potent than D, because of their relative positions along the dosage axis. Potency thus refers to the range of doses over which a chemical produces increasing responses. Maximal efficacy reflects the limit of the dose–response relationship on the response axis to a certain chemical. Chemicals A and B have equal maximal efficacy, whereas the maximal efficacy of C is less than that of D.

VARIATION IN TOXIC RESPONSES

Selective Toxicity

Selective toxicity means that a chemical produces injury to one kind of living matter without harming another form of life even though the two may exist in intimate contact. By taking advantage of biological diversity, it is possible to develop agents that are lethal for an undesired species and harmless for other species. Such selective toxicity can be due to differences in distribution (absorption, biotransformation, or excretion) or to differing biochemical processing of the toxicant by different organisms.

Species Differences

Although a basic tenet of toxicology is that "experimental results in animals, when properly qualified, are applicable to humans," it is important to recognize that both quantitative and qualitative differences in response to toxic substances may occur among different species. Identifying the mechanistic basis for species differences in response to chemicals establishes the relevance of animal data to human response.

Individual Differences in Response

Even within a species, large interindividual differences in response to a chemical can occur because of subtle genetic differences referred to as *genetic polymorphisms*. These may be responsible for idiosyncratic reactions to chemicals and for interindividual differences in toxic responses.

DESCRIPTIVE ANIMAL TOXICITY TESTS

Two main principles underlie all descriptive animal toxicity testing. The first is that the effects produced by a compound in laboratory animals, when properly qualified, are applicable to humans. The second principle is that exposure of experimental animals to toxic agents in high doses is a necessary and valid method of discovering possible hazards in humans because the incidence of an effect in a population is greater as the dose or exposure increases. Obtaining statistically valid results from the small groups of animals used in toxicity testing requires the use of relatively large doses so that the effect will occur frequently enough to be detected. However, the use of high doses can create problems in interpretation if the response(s) obtained at high doses does not occur at low doses.

Toxicity tests are not designed to demonstrate that a chemical is safe but to characterize the toxic effects a chemical can produce. There are no set toxicology tests that have to be performed on every chemical intended for commerce. Depending on the eventual use of the chemical, the toxic effects produced by structural analogs of the chemical, as well as the toxic effects produced by the chemical itself, contribute to the determination of the toxicology tests that should be performed.

Acute Lethality

The first toxicity test performed on a new chemical is acute toxicity. The LD_{50} and other acute toxic effects are determined after one or more routes of administration (one route being oral or the intended route of exposure) in one or more species, usually the mouse and rat, but sometimes the rabbit and dog. Daily examination of the animals and tabulation of the number of animals that die in a 14-day period after a single dosage occurs. Acute toxicity tests (1) give a quantitative estimate of acute toxicity (LD_{50}), (2) identify target organs and other clinical manifestations of acute toxicity, (3) identify species differences and susceptible species, (4) establish the reversibility of the toxic response, and (5) provide dose-ranging guidance for other studies.

Determination of the LD_{50} has become a public issue because of increasing concern for the welfare and protection of laboratory animals. Because LD_{50} is not a constant and many variables influence its estimation, for most purposes it is only necessary to characterize the LD_{50} within an order of magnitude range (e.g., 5 to 50 and 50 to 500 mg/kg).

If there is a reasonable likelihood of substantial exposure to the material by dermal or inhalation exposure, acute dermal and acute inhalation studies are performed. When animals are exposed acutely to chemicals in the air they breathe or the water they (fish) live in, the lethal concentration 50 (LC_{50}) is usually determined for a known time of exposure, that is, the concentration of chemical in the air or water that causes death to 50 percent of the animals. The acute dermal toxicity test is usually performed in rabbits. The site of application is shaved, and the substance is applied and covered for 24 h, and then removed. The skin is cleaned and the animals observed for 14 days to calculate LD_{50}. Acute inhalation studies are performed that are similar to other acute toxicity studies except that the route of exposure is inhalation for 4 h.

Acute lethality studies are essential for characterizing the toxic effects of chemicals and their hazard to humans. The most meaningful scientific information derived from acute lethality tests comes from clinical observations and postmortem examination of animals rather than from the specific LD_{50} value.

Skin and Eye Irritations

For the dermal irritation test (Draize test), the skin of rabbits is shaved, the chemical applied to one intact and two abraded sites and covered for 4 h. The degree of skin irritation is scored for erythema (redness), eschar (scab), edema (swelling) formation, and corrosive action. These dermal irritation observations are repeated at various intervals after the covered patch has been removed. To determine the degree of ocular irritation, the chemical is instilled into one eye of each test rabbit. The contralateral eye is used as the control. The eyes of the rabbits are then examined at various times after application.

Alternative in vitro models, including epidermal keratinocyte and corneal epithelial cell culture models, have been developed for evaluating cutaneous and ocular toxicity of substances.

Sensitization

Information about the potential of a chemical to sensitize skin is needed in addition to irritation testing for all materials that may repeatedly come into contact with the skin. In general, the test chemical is administered to the shaved skin of guinea pigs topically, intradermally, or both, over a period of 2 to 4 weeks. About 2 to 3 weeks after the last treatment, the animals are challenged with a nonirritating concentration of the test substance and the development of erythema is evaluated.

Subacute (Repeated-dose Study)

Subacute toxicity tests are performed to obtain information on the toxicity of a chemical after repeated administration for typically 14 days and as an aid to establish doses for subchronic studies.

Subchronic

Subchronic exposure usually lasts for 90 days. The principal goals of the subchronic study are to establish a "lowest observed adverse effect level" (LOAEL) and a NOAEL, and to further identify and characterize the specific organ or organs affected by the test compound after repeated administration.

A subchronic study is usually conducted in two species (rat and dog for FDA; mouse and rat for EPA) by the route of intended exposure. At least three doses are employed (a high dose that produces toxicity but less than 10 percent fatalities, a low dose that produces no apparent toxic effects, and an intermediate dose). Animals should be observed once or twice daily for signs of toxicity. All premature deaths should be recorded and necropsied. Severely moribund animals should be terminated immediately to preserve tissues and reduce unnecessary suffering. At the end of the 90-day study, all the remaining animals should be terminated and blood and tissues should be collected for further analysis. The gross and microscopic conditions of the organs and tissues are recorded and evaluated. Hematology, blood chemistry, and urinalysis measurements are usually done before, in the middle of, and at the termination of exposure. Hematology measurements usually include hemoglobin concentration, hematocrit, erythrocyte counts, total and differential leukocyte counts, platelet count, clotting time, and prothrombin time. Clinical chemistry determinations commonly include glucose, calcium, potassium, urea nitrogen, alanine aminotransferase (ALT), serum aspartate aminotransferase (AST), gamma-glutamyltranspeptidase (GGT), sorbitol dehydrogenase, lactic dehydrogenase, alkaline phosphatase, creatinine, bilirubin, triglycerides, cholesterol, albumin, globulin, and total protein. Urinalysis includes determination of specific gravity or osmolarity, pH, proteins, glucose, ketones, bilirubin, and urobilinogen as well as microscopic examination of formed elements. If humans are likely to have significant exposure to the chemical by dermal contact or inhalation, subchronic dermal and/or inhalation experiments may also be required.

Chronic

Long-term or chronic exposure studies are performed similarly to subchronic studies except that the period of exposure is usually for 6 months to 2 years. Chronic toxicity tests are often designed to assess both the cumulative toxicity and the carcinogenic potential of chemicals. Both gross and microscopic pathological examinations are made not only on animals that survive the chronic exposure, but also on those that die prematurely.

Dose selection is critical to ensure that premature mortality from chronic toxicity does not limit the number of animals that survive to a normal life expectancy. Most regulatory guidelines require that the highest administered dose be the estimated maximum tolerable dose (MTD), that is, the dose that suppresses body weight gain slightly in a 90-day subchronic study. Generally, one or two additional doses, usually one-half and one-quarter MTD, and a control group are tested.

Chronic toxicity assays commonly evaluate the potential oncogenicity of test substances. Both benign and malignant tumors must be reported. Properly designed chronic oncogenicity studies require a concurrent control group matched for variables such as age, diet, and housing conditions.

Other Tests

The effects of chemicals on reproduction and development are discussed in Chapters 10 and 20. Oncogenicity bioassays are introduced in Chapter 8. Mutagenicity is discussed in detail in Chapter 9. Information on methods, concepts, and problems associated with inhalation toxicology is provided in Chapters 15 and 28. A discussion of neurotoxicity and behavioral toxicology can be found in Chapter 16. Immunotoxicity assessment is mentioned in Chapter 12.

TOXICOGENOMICS

Toxicogenomics defines the interaction between genes and toxicants in toxicity etiology. Transcript, protein, and metabolite profiling is combined with conventional toxicology. The human genome consists of approximately 3 billion base pairs of deoxyribonucleotides. The differential expression of genes in a given cell is largely responsible for the diverse function of the thousands of different cells, tissues, and organs that constitute an individual organism. Experimental data on how a toxicant affects gene expression (transcriptomics), protein production (proteomics), and small molecule metabolism and function (metabolomics) from a test species (rat/mouse, etc.) can be combined with those of humans and analyzed with the computational tools of bioinformatics to ascertain unique or predictive patterns of toxicity.

BIBLIOGRAPHY

Boverhoff DR, Zacharewski TR: Toxicogenomics in risk assessment: applications and needs. *Toxicol Sci* 89:352–360, 2006.

Calabrese EJ, Blain R: The occurrence of hormetic dose responses in the toxicological literature, the hormesis database: an overview. *Toxicol Appl Pharmacol* 202:289–301, 2005.

Davila JC, Rodriguez RJ, Melchert RB, et al: Predictive value of in vitro model systems in toxicology. *Annu Rev Pharmacol Toxicol* 38: 63–96, 1998.

Hayes AW (ed): *Principles and Methods of Toxicology,* 4th ed. New York: Taylor and Francis, 2001.

Kitchin KT (ed): *Carcinogenicity Testing: Predicting & Interpreting Chemical Effects.* New York: Marcel Dekker, 1999.

Tennant RW, Stasiewicz S, Mennear J, et al: Genetically altered mouse models for identifying carcinogens. *IARC Sci Publ* 146:123–150, 1999.

Walsh CT, Schwartz-Bloom RD, Levine RR: *Levine's Pharmacology: Drug Actions and Reactions,* 7th ed. London: Taylor and Francis, 2005.

Waters MD, Fostel JM: Toxicogenomics and systems toxicology: aims and prospects. *Nat Rev Genet* 5:936–948, 2004.

Williams PD, Hottendorf GH (eds): *Toxicological Testing and Evaluation.* Volume 2 in Sipes GI, McQueen CA, Gandolfi AJ (eds): *Comprehensive Toxicology,* New York: Pergamon Press, 1997.

QUESTIONS

1. Five identical experimental animals are treated with 1 mg of one of the following toxins. The animal treated with which toxin is most likely to die?
   a. ethyl alcohol (LD_{50} = 10,000 mg/kg).
   b. botulinum toxin (LD_{50} = 0.00001 mg/kg).
   c. nicotine (LD_{50} = 1 mg/kg).
   d. ferrous sulfate (LD_{50} = 1500 mg/kg).
   e. picrotoxin (LD_{50} = 5 mg/kg).

2. Place the following mechanisms of toxin delivery in order from most effective to least effective—1: intravenous; 2: subcutaneous; 3: oral; 4: inhalation; 5: dermal.
   a. 1, 5, 2, 4, 3.
   b. 4, 1, 2, 3, 5.
   c. 1, 4, 2, 3, 5.
   d. 4, 2, 1, 5, 3.
   e. 1, 4, 3, 2, 5.

3. A toxin with a half-life of 12 h is administered every 12 h. Which of the following is true?
   a. The chemical is eliminated from the body before the next dose is administered.
   b. The concentration of the chemical in the body will slowly increase until the toxic concentration is attained.
   c. A toxic level will not be reached, regardless of how many doses are administered.
   d. Acute exposure to the chemical will produce immediate toxic effects.
   e. The elimination rate of the toxin is much shorter than the dosing interval.

4. Urushiol is the toxin found in poison ivy. It must first react and combine with proteins in the skin in order for the immune system to recognize and mount a response against it. Urushiol is an example of which of the following?
   a. antigen.
   b. auto-antibody.
   c. superantigen.
   d. hapten.
   e. cytokine.

5. Toxic chemicals are most likely to be biotransformed in which of the following organs?
   a. central nervous system.
   b. heart.
   c. lung.
   d. pancreas.
   e. liver.

6. When chemicals A and B are administered simultaneously, their combined effects are far greater than the sum of their effects when given alone. The chemical interaction between chemicals A and B can be described as which of the following?
   a. potentiative.
   b. additive.
   c. antagonistic.
   d. functionally antagonistic.
   e. synergistic.

7. With respect to dose–response relationships, which of the following is true?
   a. Graded dose–response relationships are often referred to as "all or nothing" responses.
   b. Quantal dose–response relationships allow for the analysis of a population's response to varying dosage.
   c. Quantal relationships characterize the response of an individual to varying dosages.
   d. A quantal dose–response describes the response of an individual organism to varying doses of a chemical.
   e. The dose–response always increases as the dosage is increased.

8. When considering the dose–response relationship for an essential substance:
   a. there are rarely negative effects of ingesting too much.
   b. the curve is the same for all people.
   c. adverse responses increase in severity with increasing or decreasing dosages outside of the homeostatic range.
   d. the relationship is linear.
   e. deficiency will never cause more harm than over-ingestion.

9. The therapeutic index of a drug:
   a. is the amount of a drug needed to cure an illness.
   b. is lower in drugs that are relatively safer.
   c. describes the potency of a chemical in eliciting a desired response.
   d. describes the ratio of the toxic dose to the therapeutic dose of a drug.
   e. explains the change in response to a drug as the dose is increased.

10. Penicillin interferes with the formation of peptidoglycan cross-links in bacterial cell walls, thus weakening the cell wall and eventually causing osmotic death of the bacterium. Which of the following is true?
   a. Treatment with penicillin is a good example of selective toxicity.
   b. Penicillin interferes with human plasma membrane structure.
   c. Penicillin is a good example of a drug with a low therapeutic index.
   d. Penicillin is also effective in treating viral infections.
   e. Penicillin is completely harmless to humans.

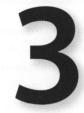

Mechanisms of Toxicity

Zoltán Gregus

KEY POINTS

- Toxicity involves toxicant delivery to its target or targets and interactions with endogenous target molecules that may trigger perturbations in cell function and/or structure or that may initiate repair mechanisms at the molecular, cellular, and/or tissue levels.
- Biotransformation to harmful products is called *toxication* or *metabolic activation*.
- Biotransformations that eliminate the ultimate toxicant or prevent its formation are called *detoxications*.
- Apoptosis, or programmed cell death, is a tightly controlled, organized process whereby individual cells break into small fragments that are phagocytosed by adjacent cells or macrophages without producing an inflammatory response.

- Sustained elevation of intracellular Ca^{2+} is harmful because it can result in (1) depletion of energy reserves by inhibiting the ATPase used in oxidative phosphorylation, (2) dysfunction of microfilaments, (3) activation of hydrolytic enzymes, and (4) generation of reactive oxygen and nitrogen species (ROS and RNS).
- Cell injury progresses toward cell necrosis (death) if molecular repair mechanisms are inefficient or the molecular damage is not readily reversible.
- Chemical carcinogenesis involves insufficient function of various repair mechanisms, including (1) failure of DNA repair, (2) failure of apoptosis (programmed cell death), and (3) failure to terminate cell proliferation.

An understanding of the mechanisms of toxicity provides a rational basis for interpreting descriptive toxicity data. The cellular mechanisms that contribute to the manifestation of toxicities are overviewed by relating a series of events that begins with exposure, involves a multitude of interactions between the invading toxicant and the organism, and culminates in a toxic effect.

As a result of the huge number of potential toxicants and the multitude of biological structures and processes that can be impaired, there are a tremendous number of possible pathways that may lead to toxicity (Figure 3–1). Commonly, a toxicant is delivered to its target, reacts with it, and the resultant cellular dysfunction manifests itself in toxicity. Sometimes a xenobiotic does not react with a specific target molecule but rather adversely influences the biological environment, causing molecular, organellar, cellular, or organ dysfunction leading to deleterious effects.

The most complex path to toxicity involves more steps (Figure 3–1). First, the toxicant is delivered to its target or targets (step 1), interacting with endogenous target molecules (step 2a) or altering the environment (step 2b), triggering perturbations in cell function and/or structure (step 3), which initiate repair mechanisms at the molecular, cellular, and/or tissue levels (step 4). When the perturbations induced by the toxicant exceed repair capacity or when repair becomes malfunctional, toxicity occurs. Tissue necrosis, cancer, and fibrosis are examples of chemically induced toxicities that follow this four-step course.

STEP 1—DELIVERY: FROM THE SITE OF EXPOSURE TO THE TARGET

Theoretically, the intensity of a toxic effect depends on the concentration and persistence of the ultimate toxicant at its site of action. The ultimate toxicant is the chemical species that reacts with the endogenous target molecule or critically alters the biological environment, initiating structural and/or functional alterations that result in toxicity. The ultimate toxicant can be the original chemical to which the organism is exposed (parent compound), a metabolite or a reactive oxygen or nitrogen species (ROS or RNS) generated during the biotransformation of the toxicant, or an endogenous molecule.

The concentration of the ultimate toxicant at the target molecule depends on the relative effectiveness of the processes that increase or decrease its concentration at the target site (Figure 3–2). Increased concentration is facilitated by absorption, distribution to the site of action, reabsorption, and toxication, while presystemic elimination, distribution away from the site of action, excretion, and detoxication will decrease the toxicant concentration at its target.

Absorption versus Presystemic Elimination

Absorption—The transfer of a chemical from the site of exposure, usually an external or internal body surface, into the systemic circulation is called *absorption*. Factors that influence absorption include concentration, surface area of exposure, characteristics of the epithelial layer through which the toxicant is being absorbed, and, usually most important, lipid solubility because lipid-soluble molecules are absorbed most easily into cells.

Presystemic Elimination—During transfer from the site of exposure to the systemic circulation, toxicants may be eliminated. This is common for chemicals absorbed from the gastrointestinal (GI) tract because they must first pass through the GI mucosal cells, liver, and lung before being distributed to the rest of the body by the systemic circulation. The GI mucosa and the liver may eliminate a significant fraction of a toxicant during its

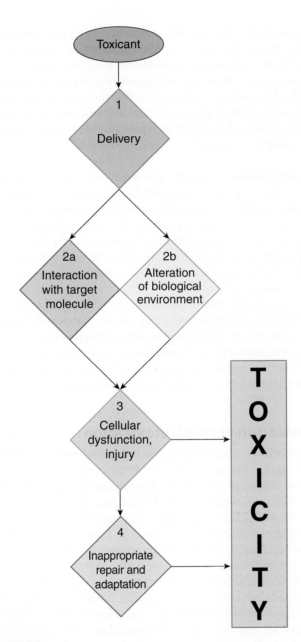

FIGURE 3–1 Potential stages in the development of toxicity after chemical exposure.

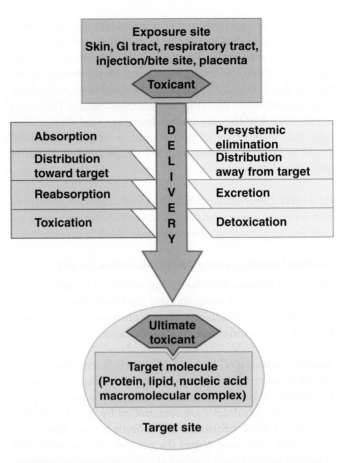

FIGURE 3–2 The process of toxicant delivery is the first step in the development of toxicity. Delivery—that is, movement of the toxicant from the site of exposure to the site of its action in an active form—is promoted by the processes listed on the left and opposed by the events indicated on the right.

or sites of toxication, usually an intracellular enzyme, where the ultimate toxicant is formed through biotransformation.

Mechanisms Facilitating Distribution to a Target

Porosity of the Capillary Endothelium—Endothelial cells in the hepatic sinusoids and in the renal peritubular capillaries have large fenestrae (50 to 150 nm in diameter) that permit passage of even protein-bound xenobiotics. This favors the accumulation of chemicals in the liver and kidneys.

Specialized Transport across the Plasma Membrane—Specialized ion channels and membrane transporters can contribute to the delivery of toxicants to intracellular targets. Na$^+$,K$^+$-ATPase, voltage-gated Ca^{2+} channels, carrier-mediated uptake, endocytosis, and membrane recycling facilitate the entry of toxicants into specific cells, rendering those cells targets. Endocytosis of some toxicant–protein complexes occurs in some cells as well.

Accumulation in Cell Organelles—Amphipathic xenobiotics with a protonatable amine group and lipophilic character

passage through these tissues. Presystemic or first-pass elimination generally reduces the toxic effects of chemicals that reach their target sites by way of the systemic circulation, but may contribute to injury of the digestive mucosa, the liver, and the lungs because these processes promote toxicant delivery to those sites.

Distribution to and away from the Target

Toxicants exit the blood during the distribution phase, enter the extracellular space, and reach their site or sites of action, usually a macromolecule on either the surface or the interior of a particular type of cell. Chemicals also may be distributed to the site accumulate in lysosomes as well as mitochondria. Lysosomal accumulation occurs by pH trapping, that is, diffusion of the amine in unprotonated form into the acidic interior of the organelle, where the amine is protonated, preventing its efflux, so that it impairs phospholipid degradation. Mitochondrial accumulation takes place electrophoretically. The amine is protonated in the intermembrane space and then sucked into the matrix space by the strong negative potential (–220 mV), where it may impair β-oxidation and oxidative phosphorylation.

Reversible Intracellular Binding—Chemicals such as organic and inorganic cations and polycyclic aromatic hydrocarbons accumulate in melanin-containing cells by binding to melanin.

Mechanisms Opposing Distribution to a Target

Binding to Plasma Proteins—Most xenobiotics must dissociate from proteins in order to leave the blood and enter cells. Therefore, strong binding to plasma proteins delays and prolongs the effects and elimination of toxicants.

Specialized Barriers—Brain capillaries lack fenestrae and are joined by extremely tight junctions, preventing the access of hydrophilic chemicals to the brain except by active transport. The spermatogenic cells are surrounded by Sertoli cells that are tightly joined to form the blood–testis barrier. Transfer of hydrophilic toxicants across the placenta is also restricted. However, none of these barriers are effective against lipophilic substances.

Distribution to Storage Sites—Some chemicals accumulate in tissues (i.e., storage sites) where they do not exert significant effects. Such storage decreases toxicant availability for their target sites.

Association with Intracellular Binding Proteins—Binding to nontarget intracellular sites, such as metallothionein, temporarily reduces the concentration of toxicants at the target site.

Export from Cells—Intracellular toxicants may be transported back into the extracellular space. The ATP-dependent membrane transporter family that is known as the multidrug-resistance (mdr) proteins extrudes chemicals from cells.

Excretion versus Reabsorption

Excretion—Excretion is the removal of xenobiotics from blood and their return to the external environment. Excretion is a physical mechanism, whereas biotransformation is a chemical mechanism for eliminating the toxicant.

The route and speed of excretion depend largely on the physicochemical properties of the toxicant. The major excretory organs—the kidney and the liver—efficiently remove highly hydrophilic chemicals such as organic acids and bases.

There are no efficient elimination mechanisms for nonvolatile, highly lipophilic chemicals. If resistant to biotransforma-

tion, such chemicals are eliminated very slowly and tend to accumulate in the body on repeated exposure. Three rather inefficient processes are available for the elimination of such chemicals: (1) excretion from the mammary gland in breast milk, (2) excretion in bile, and (3) excretion into the intestinal lumen from blood. Volatile, nonreactive toxicants such as gases and volatile liquids diffuse from pulmonary capillaries into the alveoli and are exhaled.

Reabsorption—Toxicants delivered into the renal tubules may diffuse back across the tubular cells into the peritubular capillaries. This tubular fluid reabsorption increases the intratubular concentration as well as the residence time of the chemical by slowing urine flow. Reabsorption by diffusion is dependent on the lipid solubility of the chemical and inversely related to the extent of ionization, because the nonionized molecule is more lipid soluble.

Toxicants delivered to the GI tract by biliary, gastric, and intestinal excretion and secretion by salivary glands and exocrine pancreas may be reabsorbed by diffusion across the intestinal mucosa. Reabsorption of compounds excreted into bile is possible only if they are sufficiently lipophilic or are converted to more lipid-soluble forms in the intestinal lumen.

Toxication versus Detoxication

Toxication—Biotransformation to harmful products is called *toxication* or *metabolic activation*. With some xenobiotics, toxication confers physicochemical properties that adversely alter the microenvironment of biological processes or structures. Occasionally, chemicals acquire structural features and reactivity by biotransformation that allows for a more efficient interaction with specific receptors or enzymes. Most often toxication renders xenobiotics and occasionally other molecules in the body, such as nitric oxide, indiscriminately reactive toward endogenous molecules with susceptible functional groups. This increased reactivity may be due to conversion into (1) electrophiles, (2) free radicals, (3) nucleophiles, or (4) redox-active reactants. The most reactive metabolites are electron-deficient molecules and molecular fragments such as electrophiles and neutral or cationic free radicals. Some nucleophiles are reactive (e.g., HCN and CO).

Detoxication—Biotransformations that eliminate the ultimate toxicant or prevent its formation are called *detoxications*. In some cases, detoxication may compete with toxication.

Detoxication of Toxicants with No Functional Groups—In general, chemicals without functional groups, such as benzene and toluene, are detoxicated in two phases. Initially, a functional group such as hydroxyl or carboxyl is introduced into the molecule, and then, an endogenous acid such as glucuronic acid, sulfuric acid, or an amino acid is added to the functional group by a transferase. With some exceptions, the final products are inactive, highly hydrophilic organic acids that are readily excreted.

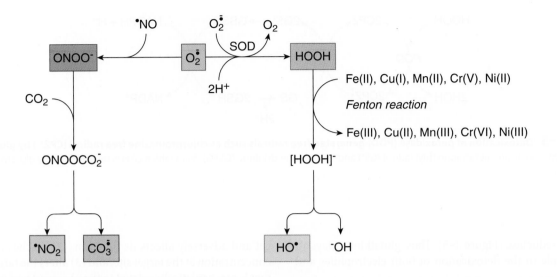

FIGURE 3-3 **Two pathways for toxication of superoxide anion radical ($O_2^{•-}$) via nonradical products (ONOO$^-$ and HOOH) to radical products ($^•NO_2$, $CO_3^{•-}$, and HO$^•$).** In one pathway, conversion of ($O_2^{•-}$) to HOOH is spontaneous or is catalyzed by SOD. Homolytic cleavage of HOOH to hydroxyl radical and hydroxyl ion is called the Fenton reaction and is catalyzed by the transition metal ions shown. Hydroxyl radical formation is the ultimate toxication for xenobiotics that form $O_2^{•-}$ or for HOOH, the transition metal ions listed, and some chemicals that form complexes with these transition metal ions. In the other pathway, $O_2^{•-}$ reacts avidly with nitric oxide ($^•NO$), the product of $^•NO$ synthase (NOS), forming peroxynitrite (ONOO$^-$). Spontaneous reaction of ONOO$^-$ with carbon dioxide (CO_2) yields nitrosoperoxy carbonate ($ONOOCO_2^-$) that is homolytically cleaved to nitrogen dioxide ($^•NO_2$) and carbonate anion radical ($CO_3^{•-}$). All three radical products indicated in this figure are oxidants, whereas $^•NO_2$ is also a nitrating agent.

Detoxication of Nucleophiles—Nucleophiles generally are detoxicated by conjugation at the nucleophilic functional group, preventing peroxidase-catalyzed conversion of the nucleophiles to free radicals and biotransformation of phenols, aminophenols, catechols, and hydroquinones to electrophilic quinines and quinoneimines.

Detoxication of Electrophiles—Generally, detoxication of electrophilic toxicants involves conjugation with the nucleophile glutathione. This reaction may occur spontaneously or can be facilitated by glutathione S-transferases. Covalent binding of electrophiles to proteins can be regarded as detoxification, provided that the protein has no critical function and does not become a neoantigen or otherwise harmful.

Detoxication of Free Radicals—Because $O_2^{•-}$ can be converted into much more reactive compounds (Figure 3–3), its elimination is an important detoxication mechanism. Superoxide dismutases (SODs), located in the cytosol (Cu, Zn-SOD) and the mitochondria (Mn-SOD), convert $O_2^{•-}$ to HOOH (Figure 3–4). Subsequently, HOOH is reduced to water by cytosolic glutathione peroxidase or peroxisomal catalase (Figure 3–4).

No enzyme eliminates HO$^•$ owing to its extremely short half-life (10^{-9} s). The only effective protection against HO$^•$ is to prevent its formation by converting its precursor, HOOH, to water (Figure 3–4).

Peroxynitrite (ONOO$^-$), which is not a free radical oxidant, is significantly more stable than HO$^•$, and rapidly reacts with

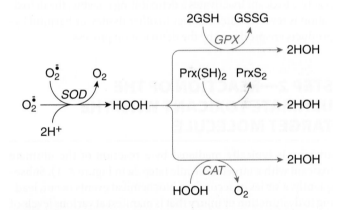

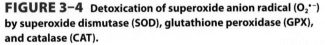

FIGURE 3-4 Detoxication of superoxide anion radical ($O_2^{•-}$) by superoxide dismutase (SOD), glutathione peroxidase (GPX), and catalase (CAT).

CO_2 to form reactive free radicals (Figure 3–3). Glutathione peroxidase can reduce ONOO$^-$ to nitrite (ONO$^-$). In addition, ONOO$^-$ reacts with oxyhemoglobin, heme-containing peroxidases, and albumin, all of which could be important sinks for ONOO$^-$. Furthermore, elimination of the two ONOO$^-$ precursors—that is, $^•NO$ by reaction with oxyhemoglobin and $O_2^{•-}$ by SODs—is a significant mechanism in preventing ONOO$^-$ buildup.

Peroxidase-generated free radicals are eliminated by electron transfer from glutathione. This results in the oxidation of glutathione, which is reversed by NADPH-dependent

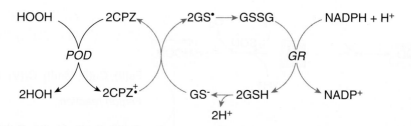

FIGURE 3–5 **Detoxication of peroxidase (POD)-generated free radicals such as chlorpromazine free radical (CPZ•+) by glutathione (GSH).** The byproducts are glutathione thiyl radical (GS•) and glutathione disulfide (GSSG), from which GSH is regenerated by glutathione reductase (GR).

glutathione reductase (Figure 3–5). Thus, glutathione plays an important role in the detoxication of both electrophiles and free radicals.

Detoxication of Protein Toxins—Extra- and intracellular proteases are involved in the inactivation of toxic polypeptides. Venom toxins, such as α- and β-bungaratoxin, erabutoxin, and phospholipase, lose their activity when thioredoxin reduces their essential disulfide bond.

When Detoxication Fails—Detoxication may be insufficient because the toxicant overwhelms the detoxication processes, a reactive toxicant inactivates a detoxicating enzyme, the detoxication is reversed after transfer to other tissues, or harmful byproducts are produced by the detoxication process.

STEP 2—REACTION OF THE ULTIMATE TOXICANT WITH THE TARGET MOLECULE

Toxicity is typically mediated by a reaction of the ultimate toxicant with a target molecule (step 2a in Figure 3–1). Subsequently, a series of secondary biochemical events occur, leading to dysfunction or injury that is manifest at various levels of biological organization, such as at the target molecule itself, cell organelles, cells, tissues and organs, and even the whole organism.

Attributes of Target Molecules

Practically all endogenous compounds are potential targets for toxicants. The most prevalent and toxicologically relevant targets are nucleic acids (especially DNA), proteins, and membranes. The first target for reactive metabolites is often the enzyme responsible for their production or the adjacent intracellular structures. Not all targets for chemicals contribute harmful effects. Covalent binding to proteins without adverse consequences may even represent a form of detoxication by sparing toxicologically relevant targets. To conclusively identify a target molecule as being responsible for toxicity, it should be demonstrated that the ultimate toxicant (1) reacts with the target and adversely affects its function, (2) reaches an effective concentration at the target site, and (3) alters the target in a way that is mechanistically related to the observed toxicity.

Types of Reactions

The ultimate toxicant may bind to the target molecules noncovalently or covalently and may alter it by hydrogen abstraction, electron transfer, or enzymatically.

Noncovalent Binding—Apolar interactions or the formation of hydrogen and ionic bonds is typically involved in the interaction of toxicants with targets such as membrane receptors, intracellular receptors, ion channels, and some enzymes. Noncovalent binding usually is reversible because of the comparatively low bonding energy.

Covalent Binding—Being practically irreversible, covalent binding permanently alters endogenous molecules. Covalent adduct formation is common with electrophilic toxicants such as nonionic and cationic electrophiles and radical cations. These toxicants react with nucleophilic atoms that are abundant in biological macromolecules, such as proteins and nucleic acids. Neutral free radicals such as $HO•$, $•NO_2$, and $Cl_3C•$ also can bind covalently to biomolecules.

Hydrogen Abstraction—Neutral free radicals can readily abstract H atoms from endogenous compounds, converting those compounds into radicals. Radicals can also remove hydrogen from CH_2 groups of free amino acids or from amino acid residues in proteins and convert them to carbonyls, forming cross-links with DNA or other proteins.

Electron Transfer—Chemicals can exchange electrons to oxidize or reduce other molecules, leading to formation of harmful byproducts. For example, chemicals can oxidize Fe(II) in hemoglobin to Fe(III), producing methemoglobinemia.

Enzymatic Reactions—A few toxins act enzymatically on specific target proteins. For example, diphtheria toxin blocks the function of elongation factor 2 in protein synthesis and cholera toxin activates a G protein through such a mechanism.

In summary, most ultimate toxicants act on endogenous molecules on the basis of their chemical reactivity. Those with more than one type of reactivity may react by different mechanisms with various target molecules.

Effects of Toxicants on Target Molecules

Dysfunction of Target Molecules—Some toxicants activate protein target molecules, mimicking endogenous ligands. More commonly, chemicals inhibit the function of target molecules, by blocking neurotransmitter receptors or ion channels, inhibiting enzymes, and interfering with cytoskeleton dynamics.

Protein function is impaired when conformation or structure is altered by interaction with the toxicant. Many proteins possess critical moieties that are essential for catalytic activity or assembly to macromolecular complexes. Covalent and/or oxidative modification of these moieties by xenobiotics can cause aberrant signal transduction and/or impaired maintenance of the cell's energy and metabolic homeostasis. Toxicants may also interfere with the template function of DNA. The covalent binding of chemicals to DNA causes nucleotide mispairing during replication.

Destruction of Target Molecules—In addition to adduct formation, toxicants alter the primary structure of endogenous molecules by means of cross-linking and fragmentation. Cross-linking imposes both structural and functional constraints on the linked molecules.

Other target molecules are susceptible to spontaneous degradation after chemical attack. Free radicals such as $Cl_3COO^\bullet$ and $HO^\bullet$ can initiate peroxidative degradation of lipids by hydrogen abstraction from fatty acids, thereby destroying lipids in cellular membranes and also generating endogenous lipid radicals and electrophiles, which can harm the structure of DNA. Several forms of DNA fragmentation are caused by toxicants, for example, multiple hydroxyl radical attacks on a short length of DNA, which occur after ionizing radiation, causing double-strand breaks that are typically lethal to the affected cell.

Neoantigen Formation—Covalent binding of xenobiotics or their metabolites to protein may evoke an immune response. Some chemicals (e.g., dinitrochlorobenzene, penicillin, and nickel) bind to proteins spontaneously. Others may obtain reactivity by autoxidation to quinones (e.g., urushiols, the allergens in poison ivy) or by enzymatic biotransformation.

Toxicity Not Initiated by Reaction with Target Molecules

Some xenobiotics alter the biological microenvironment (see step 2b in Figure 3–1) leading to a toxic response. Included here are (1) chemicals that alter H^+ ion concentrations in the aqueous biophase, (2) solvents and detergents that physicochemically alter the lipid phase of cell membranes and destroy transmembrane solute gradients, and (3) xenobiotics that cause harm merely by occupying a site or space.

STEP 3—CELLULAR DYSFUNCTION AND RESULTANT TOXICITIES

Reaction of toxicants with a target molecule may result in impaired cellular function as the third step in the development of toxicity (Figures 3–1 and 3–6). Each cell in a multicellular organism carries out defined programs, some of which determine whether cells undergo division, differentiation, or apoptosis. Other programs control the ongoing (momentary) activity of differentiated cells. For regulation of these cellular programs, cells possess signaling networks that can be activated and inactivated by external signaling molecules.

As outlined in Figure 3–6, the nature of the primary cellular dysfunction caused by toxicants, but not necessarily the ultimate outcome, depends on the role of the target molecule affected. The reaction of a toxicant with targets serving external functions can influence the operation of other cells and integrated organ systems. However, if the target molecule is involved predominantly in the cell's internal maintenance, the resultant dysfunction can ultimately compromise survival of the cell.

Toxicant-induced Cellular Dysregulation

Cells are regulated by signaling molecules that activate specific cellular receptors linked to signal-transducing networks that transmit the signals to the regulatory regions of genes and/or functional proteins. Receptor activation may ultimately lead to altered gene expression and/or a chemical modification of specific proteins, typically by phosphorylation. Programs controlling the destiny of cells primarily affect gene expression, whereas those regulating the ongoing activities primarily influence the activity of functional proteins. However, one signal often evokes both responses because of branching and interconnection of signaling networks.

Dysregulation of Gene Expression—Dysregulation of gene expression may occur at elements that are directly responsible for transcription, at components of the intracellular signal-transduction pathway, and at the synthesis, storage, or release of the extracellular signaling molecules.

Dysregulation of Transcription—Transcription of genetic information from DNA to mRNA is controlled largely by interplay between transcription factors (TFs) and the regulatory or promoter region of genes. Xenobiotics may interact with the promoter region of the gene, the TFs, or other components of the transcription initiation complex. However, altered activation of TFs appears to be the most common modality.

Many natural compounds, such as hormones and vitamins, influence gene expression by binding to and activating TFs. Whereas xenobiotics may mimic the natural ligands, both may cause toxicity when administered at extreme doses or at critical periods during ontogenesis. Other compounds that act on TFs can also change the pattern of cell differentiation by overexpressing various genes.

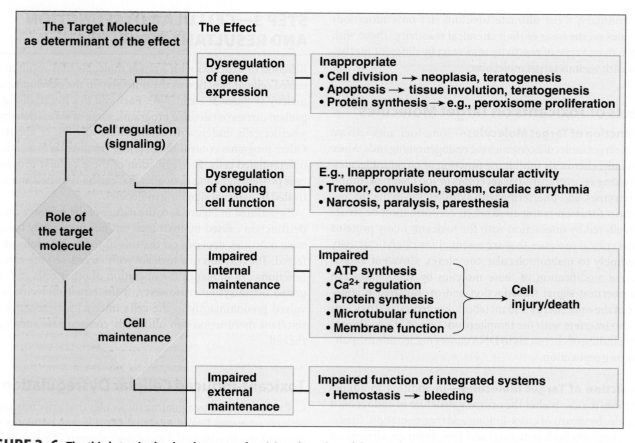

FIGURE 3–6 The third step in the development of toxicity: alteration of the regulatory or maintenance function of the cell.

Xenobiotics may also dysregulate transcription by altering the regulatory gene regions and promoter methylation.

Dysregulation of Signal Transduction—Extracellular signaling molecules, such as growth factors, cytokines, hormones, and neurotransmitters, can ultimately activate TFs utilizing cell surface receptors and intracellular signal-transducing networks. Figure 3–7 depicts such networks and identifies some important signal-activated TFs that control transcriptional activity of genes that influence cell cycle progression and thus determine the fate of cells. An example is the c-Myc protein, which, on dimerizing with Max protein and binding to its cognate nucleotide sequence, transactivates cyclin D and E genes. The cyclins, in turn, accelerate the cell-division cycle by activating cyclin-dependent protein kinases, which are involved in regulating the cell cycle. Mitogenic signaling molecules thus induce cellular proliferation.

The signal from the cell surface receptors to the TFs is relayed by successive protein–protein interactions and protein phosphorylations, that is, a signal molecule phosphorylates another protein like mitogen-activated kinase (MAPK), which activates that protein to phosphorylate and activate another. For example, ligands induce growth factor receptors (item 6 in Figure 3–7) on the surface of all cells to self-phosphorylate, and these phosphorylated receptors then bind to adapter proteins through which they activate Ras. The active Ras initiates the MAPK cascade, involving serial phosphorylations of protein kinases, which finally reaches the TFs. These signal transducers are typically but not always activated by phosphorylation catalyzed by protein kinases and are usually inactivated by dephosphorylation carried out by protein phosphatases.

Chemicals may cause aberrant signal transduction most often by altering protein phosphorylation, and occasionally by interfering with the GTPase activity of G proteins, disrupting normal protein–protein interactions, or establishing abnormal ones, or by altering the synthesis or degradation of signaling proteins. Such interventions may ultimately influence cell cycle progression.

Chemically Altered Signal Transduction with Proliferative Effect: Xenobiotics that facilitate phosphorylation of signal transducers often promote mitosis and tumor formation. The phorbol esters and fumonisin B activate protein kinase C (PKC) mimicking diacylglycerol (DAG), one of the physiologic activators of PKC (Figure 3–7). The other physiologic PKC activator, Ca^{2+}, is mimicked by Pb^{2+}. Activated PKC promotes mitogenic signaling by starting a cascade that activates other kinases and allows certain TFs to bind to DNA. Protein kinases may also be activated by interacting proteins that had been altered by a xenobiotic.

Aberrant phosphorylation of proteins may result from decreased dephosphorylation by phosphatases. Inhibition of phosphatases appears to be the underlying mechanism of the

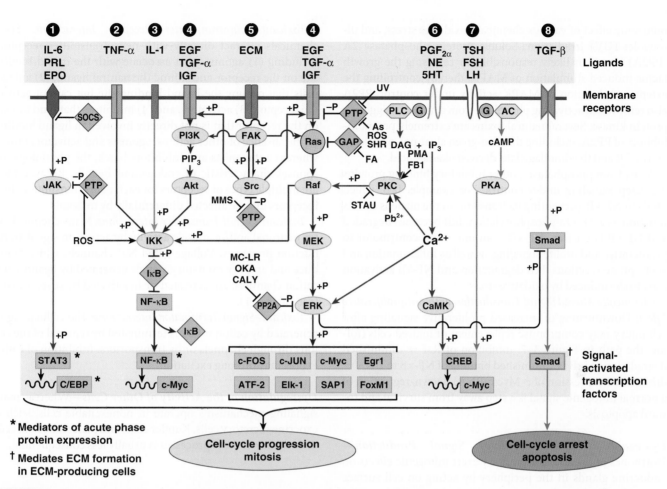

FIGURE 3–7 **Signal-transduction pathways from cell membrane receptors to signal-activated nuclear transcription factors that influence transcription of genes involved in cell-cycle regulation.** The symbols of cell membrane receptors are numbered 1 to 8 and some of their activating ligands are indicated. Circles represent G proteins, oval symbols protein kinases, rectangles transcription factors, wavy lines genes, and diamond symbols inhibitory proteins, such as protein phosphatases (PTP and PP2A), the GTPase-activating protein GAP, and the inhibitory binding protein IκB. Arrowheads indicate stimulation or formation of second messengers (e.g., DAG, IP$_3$, cAMP, and Ca^{2+}), whereas blunt arrows indicate inhibition. Phosphorylation and dephosphorylation are indicated by +P and –P, respectively. Abbreviations for interfering chemicals are printed in black (As = arsenite; CALY = calyculin A; FA = fatty acids; FB1 = fumonisin B; MC-LR = microcystin-LR; OKA = okadaic acid; MMS = methylmethane sulfonate; PMA = phorbol miristate acetate; ROS = reactive oxygen species; SHR = SH-reactive chemicals, such as iodoacetamide; STAU = staurosporin).

In the center of the depicted networks is the pathway activated by growth factors, such as EGF, that acts on a tyrosine kinase receptor (#6), which uses adaptor proteins (Shc, Grb2, and SOS; not shown) to convert the inactive GDP-bound Ras to active GTP-bound form, which in turn activates the MAP-kinase phosphorylation cascade (Raf, MAPKK, and MAPK). The phosphorylated MAPK moves into the nucleus and phosphorylates transcription factors, thereby enabling them to bind to cognate sequences in the promoter regions of genes to facilitate transcription. There are numerous interconnections between the signal-transduction pathways. Some of these connections permit the use of the growth factor receptor (#6)–MAPK "highway" for other receptors (e.g., 4, 5, and 7) to send mitogenic signals. For example, receptor (#4) joins in via its G protein β/γ subunits and tyrosine kinase Src; the integrin receptor (#5), whose ligands are constituents of the extracellular matrix (ECM), possibly connects via G-protein Rho (not shown) and focal adhesion kinase (FAK); and the G-protein-coupled receptor (#7) via phospholipase C (PLC)-catalyzed formation of second messengers and activation of protein kinase C (PKC). The mitogenic stimulus relayed along the growth factor receptor (#6)–MAPK axis can be amplified by, for example, the Raf-catalyzed phosphorylation of IκB, which unleashes NF-κB from this inhibitory protein, and by the MAPK-catalyzed inhibitory phosphorylation of Smad that blocks the cell-cycle arrest signal from the TGF-β receptor (#9). Activation of protein kinases (PKC, CaMK, and MAPK) by Ca^{2+} can also trigger mitogenic signaling. Several xenobiotics that are indicated in the figure may dysregulate the signaling network. Some may induce cell proliferation by either activating mitogenic protein kinases (e.g., PKC) or inhibiting inactivating proteins, such as protein phosphatases (PTP and PP2A), GAP, or IκB. Others, for example, inhibitors of PKC, oppose mitosis and facilitate apoptosis.

This scheme is oversimplified and tentative in several details. Virtually all components of the signaling network (e.g., G proteins, PKCs, and MAPKs) are present in multiple, functionally different forms whose distribution may be cell specific. The pathways depicted are not equally relevant for all cells. In addition, these pathways regulating gene expression not only determine the fate of cells, but also control certain aspects of the ongoing cellular activity.

mitogenic effect of various chemicals, oxidative stress, and ultraviolet (UV) irradiation. Soluble protein phosphatase 2A (PP2A) in cells is likely responsible for reversing the growth factor-induced stimulation of MAPK, thereby controlling the extent and duration of MAPK activity under control. PP2A also removes an activating phosphate from a mitosis-triggering protein kinase. Several natural toxins are extremely potent inhibitors of PP2A, including the blue-green algae poison microcystin-LR and the dinoflagellate-derived okadaic acid.

Apart from phosphatases, other inhibitory binding proteins can keep signaling under control. For example, IκB, which binds to NF-κB, preventing its transfer into the nucleus and its function as a TF. On phosphorylation, IκB becomes degraded and NF-κB is set free. NF-κB is an important contributor to proliferative and prolife signaling, as well as inflammation and acute-phase reactions. IκB degradation and NF-κB activation can also be induced by oxidative stress.

Chemically Altered Signal Transduction with Antiproliferative Effect: Downturning of increased proliferative signaling after cell injury may compromise replacement of injured cells (follow the path in Figure 3–7: inhibition of Raf → diminished degradation of IκB → diminished binding of NF-κB to DNA → diminished expression of c-Myc mRNA). Down-regulation of a normal mitogenic signal is a step away from survival and toward apoptosis.

Dysregulation of Extracellular Signal Production—Hormones of the anterior pituitary exert mitogenic effects on endocrine glands in the periphery by acting on cell surface receptors. Pituitary hormone production is under negative feedback control by hormones of the peripheral glands. Perturbation of this circuit adversely affects pituitary hormone secretion and, in turn, the peripheral glands. Decreased secretion of pituitary hormone produces apoptosis followed by involution of the peripheral target gland.

Dysregulation of Ongoing Cellular Activity—Toxicants can adversely affect ongoing cellular activity in specialized cells by disrupting any step in signal coupling.

Dysregulation of Electrically Excitable Cells—Many xenobiotics influence cellular activity in excitable cells, such as neurons, skeletal, cardiac, and smooth muscle cells. Release of neurotransmitters and muscle contraction are controlled by transmitters and modulators synthesized and released by adjacent neurons. Chemicals that interfere with these mechanisms are listed in Table 3–1.

Perturbation of ongoing cellular activity by chemicals may be due to an alteration in (1) the concentration of neurotransmitters, (2) receptor function, (3) intracellular signal transduction, or (4) the signal-terminating processes.

Alteration in Neurotransmitter Levels: Chemicals may alter synaptic levels of neurotransmitters by interfering with their synthesis, storage, release, or removal from the vicinity of the receptor.

Toxicant–Neurotransmitter Receptor Interactions: Some chemicals interact directly with neurotransmitter receptors, including (1) agonists that associate with the ligand-binding site on the receptor and mimic the natural ligand, (2) antagonists that occupy the ligand-binding site but cannot activate the receptor, (3) activators, and (4) inhibitors that bind to a site on the receptor that is not directly involved in ligand binding. In the absence of other actions, agonists and activators mimic, whereas antagonists and inhibitors block, the physiologic responses characteristic of endogenous ligands. Because there are multiple types of receptors for each neurotransmitter, these receptors may be affected differentially by toxicants.

Toxicant–Signal Transducer Interactions: Many chemicals alter neuronal and/or muscle activity by acting on signal-transduction processes. Voltage-gated Na+ channels, which transduce and amplify excitatory signals generated by ligand-gated cation channels, are activated or inactivated by several toxins (see Table 3–1).

Toxicant–Signal Terminator Interactions: The cellular signal generated by cation influx is terminated by removal of the cations through channels or by transporters. Inhibition of cation export may prolong excitation.

Dysregulation of the Activity of Other Cells—Whereas many signaling mechanisms operate in nonexcitable cells, such as exocrine secretory cells, Kupffer cells, and pancreatic beta cells, disturbance of these processes is usually less consequential.

Impairment of Internal Cellular Maintenance: Mechanisms of Toxic Cell Death

For survival, all cells must synthesize endogenous molecules, assemble macromolecular complexes, membranes, and cell organelles, maintain the intracellular environment, and produce energy for operation. Agents that disrupt these functions jeopardize survival. There are three critical biochemical disorders that chemicals inflicting cell death may initiate, namely, ATP depletion, sustained rise in intracellular Ca^{2+}, and overproduction of ROS and RNS.

Depletion of ATP—ATP plays a central role in cellular maintenance both as a chemical for biosynthesis and as the major source of energy. ATP is utilized in numerous biosynthetic reactions, and is incorporated into cofactors as well as nucleic acids. It is required for muscle contraction and polymerization of the cytoskeleton, fueling cellular motility, cell division, vesicular transport, and the maintenance of cell morphology. ATP drives ion transporters (e.g., Na+,K+-ATPase) that maintain conditions essential for various cell functions.

Chemical energy is released by hydrolysis of ATP to ADP or AMP. The ADP is rephosphorylated in the mitochondria by ATP synthase (Figure 3–8) via a process that couples oxidation of hydrogen to water and is termed *oxidative phosphorylation*.

TABLE 3–1 Agents acting on signaling systems for neurotransmitters and causing dysregulation of the momentary activity of electrically excitable cells such as neurons and muscle cells.[1]

Receptor/Channel/Pump		Agonist/Activator		Antagonist/Inhibitor	
Name	**Location**	**Agent**	**Effect**	**Agent**	**Effect**
1. Acetylcholine nicotinic receptor	Skeletal muscle	Nicotine	Muscle fibrillation, then paralysis	Tubocurarine, lophotoxin	Muscle paralysis
		Anatoxin-a Cytisine *Ind*: ChE inhibitors		α-Bungarotoxin α-Cobrotoxin α-Conotoxin Erabutoxin b *Ind*: botulinum toxin	
	Neurons	See above	Neuronal activation	Pb^{2+}, general anesthetics	Neuronal inhibition
2. Glutamate receptor	CNS neurons	*N*-Methyl-D-aspartate	Neuronal activation → convulsion, neuronal injury ("excitotoxicity")	Phencyclidine	Neuronal inhibition → anesthesia
		Kainate, domoate Quinolinate Quisqualate *Ind*: hypoxia, HCN → glutamate release		Ketamine General anesthetics	Protection against "excitotoxicity"
3. GABA_A receptor	CNS neurons	Muscimol, avermectins sedatives (barbiturates, benzodiazepines) General anesthetics (halothane) Alcohols (ethanol)	Neuronal inhibition → sedation, general anesthesia, coma, depression of vital centers	Bicuculline Picrotoxin Pentylenetetrazole Cyclodiene insecticides Lindane, TCAD *Ind*: isoniazid	Neuronal activation → tremor, convulsion
4. Glycine receptor	CNS neurons, motor neurons	Avermectins (?) General anesthetics	Inhibition of motor neurons → paralysis	Strychnine *Ind*: tetanus toxin	Disinhibition of motor neurons → tetanic convulsion
5. Acetylcholine M_2 muscarinic receptor	Cardiac muscle	*Ind*: ChE inhibitors	Decreased heart rate and contractility	Belladonna alkaloids (e.g., atropine) Atropine-like drugs (e.g., TCAD)	Increased heart rate
6. Opioid receptor	CNS neurons, visceral neurons	Morphine and congeners (e.g., heroin, meperidine) *Ind*: clonidine	Neuronal inhibition → analgesia, central respiratory depression, constipation, urine retention	Naloxone	Antidotal effects in opiate intoxication
7. Voltage-gated Na^+ channel	Neurons, muscle cells, etc.	Aconitine, veratridine Grayanotoxin Batrachotoxin Scorpion toxins Ciguatoxin DDT, pyrethroids	Neuronal activation → convulsion	Tetrodotoxin, saxitoxin μ-Conotoxin Local anesthetics Phenytoin Quinidine	Neuronal inhibition → paralysis, anesthesia Anticonvulsive action

(continued)

TABLE 3-1 Agents acting on signaling systems for neurotransmitters and causing dysregulation of the momentary activity of electrically excitable cells such as neurons and muscle cells. (Continued)

Receptor/Channel/Pump		Agonist/Activator		Antagonist/Inhibitor	
Name	**Location**	**Agent**	**Effect**	**Agent**	**Effect**
8. Voltage-gated Ca^{2+} channel	Neurons, muscle cell, etc.	Maitotoxin (?) Atrotoxin (?) Latrotoxin (?)	Neuronal/muscular activation, cell injury	ω-Conotoxin Pb^{2+}	Neuronal inhibition → paralysis
9. Voltage/Ca^{2+}-activated K$^+$ channel	Neurons, smooth and skeletal muscle, cardiac muscle	Pb^{2+}	Neuronal/muscular inhibition	Ba^{2+}; apamin (bee venom), dendrotoxin, 20-HETE; hERG inhibitors (e.g., cisapride, terfenadine)	Neuronal/muscular activation → convulsion/spasm vasoconstriction PMV tachycardia (torsade de pointes)
10. Na$^+$,K$^+$-ATPase	Universal			Digitalis glycosides Oleandrin Chlordecone	Increased cardiac contractility, excitability Increased neuronal excitability → tremor
11. Acetylcholine M$_3$ muscarinic receptor	Smooth muscle, glands	*Ind*: ChE inhibitors	Smooth muscle spasm	Belladonna alkaloids (e.g., atropine)	Smooth muscle relaxation → intestinal paralysis, decreased salivation, decreased perspiration
Acetylcholine M$_1$ muscarinic receptor	CNS neurons	Oxotremorine *Ind*: ChE inhibitors	Salivation, lacrimation Neuronal activation → convulsion	Atropine-like drugs (e.g., TCAD) See above	
12. Adrenergic alpha$_1$ receptor	Vascular smooth muscle	(Nor)epinephrine *Ind*: cocaine, tyramine amphetamine, TCAD	Vasoconstriction → ischemia, hypertension	Prazosin	Antidotal effects in intoxication with alpha$_1$-receptor agonists
13. 5-HT$_2$ receptor	Smooth muscle	Ergot alkaloids (ergotamine, ergonovine)	Vasoconstriction → ischemia, hypertension	Ketanserine	Antidotal effects in ergot intoxication
14. Adrenergic beta$_1$ receptor	Cardiac muscle	(Nor)epinephrine *Ind*: cocaine, tyramine amphetamine, TCAD	Increased cardiac contractility and excitability	Atenolol, metoprolol	Antidotal effects in intoxication with beta$_1$-receptor agonists

[1]Numbering of the signaling elements in this table corresponds to the numbering of their symbols in Figure 3–12. This tabulation is simplified and incomplete. Virtually all receptors and channels listed occur in multiple forms with different sensitivity to the agents. The reader should consult the pertinent literature for more detailed information. CNS = central nervous system; ChE = cholinesterase; *Ind* = indirectly acting (i.e., by altering neurotransmitter level); 20-HETE = 20-hydroxy-5,8,11,14-eicosatetraenoic acid; PMV = polymorphic ventricular; TCAD = tricyclic antidepressant.
The ? indicates there is some uncertainty regarding this action.

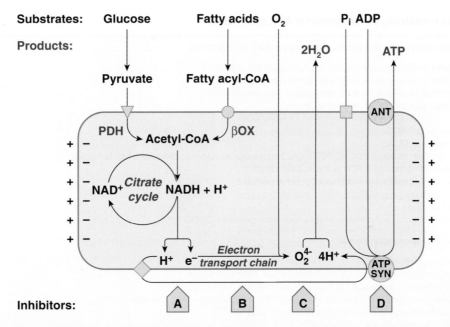

FIGURE 3–8 **ATP synthesis (oxidative phosphorylation) in mitochondria.** Arrows with letters A-D point to the ultimate sites of action of four categories of agents that interfere with oxidative phosphorylation (Table 3–2). For simplicity, this scheme does not indicate the outer mitochondrial membrane and that protons are extruded from the matrix space along the electron transport chain at three sites. βOX = beta-oxidation of fatty acids; e^- = electron; P_i = inorganic phosphate; ANT = adenine nucleotide translocator; ATP SYN = ATP synthase (F_oF_1ATPase).

Oxidative phosphorylation also requires several steps, each of which can be interfered with by toxins, as described in Table 3–2. Impairment of oxidative phosphorylation is detrimental to cells because failure of ADP rephosphorylation results in the accumulation of ADP and its breakdown products, as well as depletion of ATP.

Substances in class A interfere with the delivery of hydrogen to the electron transport chain. Class B chemicals inhibit the transfer of electrons along the electron transport chain to oxygen. Class C agents interfere with oxygen delivery to the terminal electron transporter, cytochrome oxidase. Chemicals in class D inhibit oxidative phosphorylation by: (1) direct inhibition of ATP synthase, (2) interference with ADP delivery, (3) interference with inorganic phosphate delivery, and (4) deprivation of ATP synthase from its driving force, the controlled influx of protons into the matrix space. Finally, chemicals causing mitochondrial DNA injury, thereby impairing synthesis of specific proteins encoded by the mitochondrial genome, are listed in group E.

Sustained Rise of Intracellular Ca²⁺—Intracellular Ca^{2+} levels are highly regulated and maintained by the impermeability of the plasma membrane to Ca^{2+} and by transport mechanisms that remove Ca^{2+} from the cytoplasm. Ca^{2+} is actively pumped from the cytosol across the plasma membrane and is sequestered in the endoplasmic reticulum and mitochondria (Figure 3–8).

Toxicants induce elevation of cytoplasmic Ca^{2+} levels by promoting Ca^{2+} influx into or inhibiting Ca^{2+} efflux from the cytoplasm (Table 3–3). Opening of the ligand- or voltage-gated Ca^{2+} channels or damage to the plasma membrane causes Ca^{2+} to move down its concentration gradient from extracellular fluid to the cytoplasm. Toxicants also may increase cytosolic Ca^{2+} inducing its leakage from the mitochondria or the endoplasmic reticulum. They also may diminish Ca^{2+} efflux through inhibition of Ca^{2+} transporters or depletion of their driving forces. Sustained elevation of intracellular Ca^{2+} is harmful because it can result in (1) depletion of energy reserves by inhibiting the ATPase used in oxidative phosphorylation, (2) dysfunction of microfilaments, (3) activation of hydrolytic enzymes, and (4) generation of ROS and RNS.

There are at least three mechanisms by which sustained elevations in intracellular Ca^{2+} levels influence the cellular energy balance. First, high cytoplasmic Ca^{2+} levels cause increased mitochondrial Ca^{2+} uptake by the Ca^{2+} "uniporter," which, like ATP synthase, utilizes the inside negative mitochondrial membrane potential as the driving force. Consequently, mitochondrial Ca^{2+} uptake dissipates the membrane potential and inhibits the synthesis of ATP. Moreover, agents that oxidize mitochondrial NADH activate a transporter that extrudes Ca^{2+} from the matrix space. The ensuing continuous Ca^{2+} uptake and export ("Ca^{2+} cycling") by the mitochondria further compromise oxidative phosphorylation.

Second, an uncontrolled rise in cytoplasmic Ca^{2+} causes cell injury by microfilamental dissociation. An increase of cytoplasmic Ca^{2+} causes dissociation of actin filaments from proteins that promote anchoring of the filament to the plasma membrane, predisposing the membrane to rupture.

TABLE 3–2 Agents impairing mitochondrial ATP synthesis.[1]

A. Inhibitors of hydrogen delivery to the electron transport chain acting on/as

1. Glycolysis (critical in neurons): hypoglycemia, iodoacetate, and NO^+ at GAPDH
2. Gluconeogenesis (critical in renal tubular cells): coenzyme A depletors (see below)
3. Fatty acid oxidation (critical in cardiac muscle): hypoglycin, 4-pentenoic acid
4. Pyruvate dehydrogenase: arsenite, DCVC, p-benzoquinone
5. Citrate cycle
    (a) Aconitase: fluoroacetate, $ONOO^-$
    (b) Isocitrate dehydrogenase: DCVC
    (c) Succinate dehydrogenase: malonate, DCVC, PCBD-cys, 2-bromohydroquinone, cis-crotonalide fungicides
6. Depletors of TPP (inhibit TPP-dependent PDH and α-KGDH): ethanol
7. Depletors of coenzyme A: 4-(dimethylamino)phenol, p-benzoquinone
8. Depletors of NADH
    (a) See group A.V.i in Table 3-3
    (b) Activators of poly(ADP-ribose) polymerase, MNNG, hydrogen peroxide, $ONOO^-$

B. Inhibitors of electron transport acting on/as

1. Inhibitors of electron transport complexes
    (a) NADH–coenzyme Q reductase (complex I): rotenone, amytal, MPP^+, paraquat
    (b) Cytochrome Q–cytochrome c reductase (complex III): antimycin-A, myxothiazole
    (c) Cytochrome oxidase (complex IV): cyanide, hydrogen sulfide, azide, formate, •NO, phosphine (PH_3)
    (d) Multisite inhibitors: dinitroaniline and diphenylether herbicides, $ONOO^-$
2. Electron acceptors: CCl_4, doxorubicin, menadione, MPP^+

C. Inhibitors of oxygen delivery to the electron transport chain

1. Chemicals causing respiratory paralysis: CNS depressants (e.g., opioids), convulsants
2. Chemicals impairing pulmonary gas exchange: CO_2, NO_2, phosgene, perfluoroisobutene
3. Chemicals inhibiting oxygenation of Hb: carbon monoxide, methemoglobin-forming chemicals
4. Chemicals causing ischemia: ergot alkaloids, cocaine

D. Inhibitors of ADP phosphorylation acting on/as

1. ATP synthase: oligomycin, cyhexatin, DDT, chlordecone
2. Adenine nucleotide translocator: atractyloside, DDT, free fatty acids, lysophospholipids
3. Phosphate transporter: N-ethylmaleimide, mersalyl, p-benzoquinone
4. Chemicals dissipating the mitochondrial membrane potential (uncouplers)
    (a) Cationophores: pentachlorophenol, dinitrophenol-, benzonitrile-, thiadiazole herbicides, salicylate, amiodarone, perhexiline, valinomycin, gramicidin, calcimycin (A23187)
    (b) Chemicals permeabilizing the mitochondrial inner membrane: PCBD-cys, chlordecone

E. Chemicals causing mitochondrial DNA damage and/or impaired transcription of key mitochondrial proteins

1. Antiviral drugs: zidovudine, zalcitabine, didanosine, fialuridine
2. Chloramphenicol (when overdosed)
3. Ethanol (when chronically consumed)

[1]The ultimate sites of action of these agents are indicated in Figure 3–8. DCVC = dichlorovinyl-cysteine; GAPDH = glyceraldehyde 3-phosphate dehydrogenase; α-KGDH = α-ketoglutarate dehydrogenase; MNNG = N-methyl-N'-nitro-N-nitrosoguanidine; MPP^+ = 1-methyl-4-phenylpyridinium; PCBD-cys = pentachlorobutadienylcysteine; PDH = pyruvate dehydrogenase; TPP = thyamine pyrophosphate.

Third, high Ca^{2+} levels may lead to activation of hydrolytic enzymes that degrade proteins, phospholipids, and nucleic acids. Many integral membrane proteins are targets for Ca^{2+}-activated neutral proteases, or calpains. Indiscriminate activation of phospholipases by Ca^{2+} causes membrane breakdown directly and by the generation of detergents. Activation of a Ca^{2+}–Mg^{2+}-dependent endonuclease causes fragmentation of chromatin.

Overproduction of ROS and RNS—A number of xenobiotics can directly generate ROS and RNS, such as the redox cyclers and transition metals (Figure 3–3). Overproduction of ROS and RNS can be secondary to intracellular hypercalcemia, as Ca^{2+} helps generate ROS and/or RNS by activating dehydro-genases in the citric acid cycle leading to increased activity in the electron transport chain and increased formation of $O_2^{•-}$ and HOOH, and by activating nitric oxide synthase, which leads to formation of $ONOO^-$.

Interplay between the Primary Metabolic Disorders Spells Cellular Disaster—The primary derailments in cellular biochemistry discussed above may interact and amplify each other in a number of ways:

1. Depletion of cellular ATP reserves deprives the endoplasmic and plasma membrane Ca^{2+} pumps of fuel, causing elevation of Ca^{2+} in the cytoplasm. With the influx of Ca^{2+} into the mitochondria, the mitochondrial membrane potential declines, hindering ATP synthase.

TABLE 3–3 Agents causing sustained elevation of cytosolic Ca²⁺.

A. Chemicals inducing Ca²⁺ influx into the cytoplasm

I.   Via ligand-gated channels in neurons
   1. Glutamate receptor agonists ("excitotoxins"): glutamate, kainate, domoate
   2. TRPV1 receptor (capsaicin receptor) agonists: capsaicin, resiniferatoxin
II. Via voltage-gated channels: maitotoxin (?), HO•
III. Via "newly formed pores": maitotoxin, amphotericin B, chlordecone, methylmercury, alkyltins
IV. Across disrupted cell membrane
   1. Detergents: exogenous detergents, lysophospholipids, free fatty acids
   2. Hydrolytic enzymes: phospholipases in snake venoms, endogenous phospholipase A₂
   3. Lipid peroxidants: carbon tetrachloride
   4. Cytoskeletal toxins (by inducing membrane blebbing): cytochalasins, phalloidin
V.   From mitochondria
   1. Oxidants of intramitochondrial NADH: alloxan, t-BHP, NAPBQI, divicine, fatty acid hydroperoxides, menadione, MPP⁺
   2. Others: phenylarsine oxide, gliotoxin, •NO, ONOO⁻
VI. From the endoplasmic reticulum
   1. IP₃ receptor activators: γ-HCH (lindan), IP₃ formed during "excitotoxicity"
   2. Ryanodine receptor activators: δ-HCH

B. Chemicals inhibiting Ca²⁺ export from the cytoplasm (inhibitors of Ca²⁺-ATPase in cell membrane and/or endoplasmic reticulum)

I.   Covalent binders: acetaminophen, bromobenzene, CCl₄, chloroform, DCE
II. Thiol oxidants: cystamine (mixed disulfide formation), diamide, t-BHP, O₂•⁻, and HOOH generators (e.g., menadione, diquat)
III. Others: vanadate, Cd²⁺
IV. Chemicals impairing mitochondrial ATP synthesis (see Table 3–3)

Key: DCE = 1,1-dichloroethylene; t-BHP = t-butyl hydroperoxide; HCH = hexachlorocyclohexane; MPP⁺ = 1-methyl-4-phenylpyridinium; NAPBQI = N-acetyl-p-benzoquinoneimine. The ? indicates there is some uncertainty regarding this action.

2. Intracellular hypercalcemia facilitates formation of ROS and RNS, which oxidatively inactivates the Ca²⁺ pump, aggravating the hypercalcemia.

3. ROS and RNS can also drain the ATP reserves. •NO is a reversible inhibitor of cytochrome oxidase, NO⁺ (nitrosonium cation, a product of •NO) inactivates glyceraldehyde 3-phosphate dehydrogenase and impairs glycolysis, whereas ONOO⁻ irreversibly inactivates several components of the electron transport chain, inhibiting cellular ATP synthesis.

4. Furthermore, ONOO⁻ can induce DNA single-strand breaks, which activate poly(ADP-ribose) polymerase (PARP). As part of the repair strategy, activated PARP transfers multiple ADP-ribose moieties from NAD⁺ to nuclear proteins and PARP itself. Because consumption of NAD⁺ severely compromises ATP synthesis (see Figure 3–8) and resynthesis of NAD⁺ consumes ATP, a cellular energy deficit occurs as a major consequence of DNA damage by ONOO⁻.

Mitochondrial Permeability Transition (MPT) and the Worst Outcome: Necrosis—Mitochrondrial Ca²⁺ uptake, decreased mitochondrial membrane potential, generation of ROS and RNS, depletion of ATP, and consequences of the primary metabolic disorders (e.g., accumulation of inorganic phosphate, free fatty acids, and lysophosphatides) are all considered as causative factors of an abrupt increase in the mitochondrial inner-membrane permeability, termed MPT. This is believed to be caused by the opening of a proteinaceous pore that spans both mitochondrial membranes and is permeable to solutes of 1500 Da. This opening permits free influx into the matrix space of protons, causing rapid and complete dissipation of the membrane potential, cessation of ATP synthesis, and the osmotic influx of water causing mitochondrial swelling. Ca²⁺ accumulated in the matrix space effluxes through the pore, flooding the cytoplasm. Such mitochondria are not only incapable of synthesizing ATP, but also even waste the remaining sources because depolarization of the inner membrane forces the ATP synthase to operate in the reverse mode, as an ATPase, hydrolyzing ATP. Then glycolysis may become compromised by the insufficient ATP supply to the glycolytic enzymes that require ATP (hexokinase and phosphofructokinase). A complete bioenergetic catastrophe ensues in the cell if the metabolic disorders evoked by the toxicant (such as those listed in Tables 3–2 and 3–3) are so extensive that most or all mitochondria undergo MPT, causing depletion of cellular ATP, and culminating in cell lysis or necrosis (see Figure 3–9).

An Alternative Outcome of MPT: Apoptosis—Chemicals that adversely affect cellular energy metabolism, Ca²⁺ homeostasis, and redox state and ultimately cause necrosis may also induce apoptosis. While the necrotic cell swells and lyses, the apoptotic cell shrinks; its nuclear and cytoplasmic materials condense, and then it breaks into membrane-bound fragments (apoptotic bodies) that are phagocytosed.

In contrast to the random sequence of multiple metabolic defects that a cell suffers on its way to necrosis, the routes to apoptosis are ordered, involving cascade-like activation of catabolic processes that finally disassemble the cell. Many details of the apoptotic pathways are presented schematically in Figure 3–10. It appears that most, if not all, chemical-induced cell deaths will involve the mitochondria, and that MPT is a

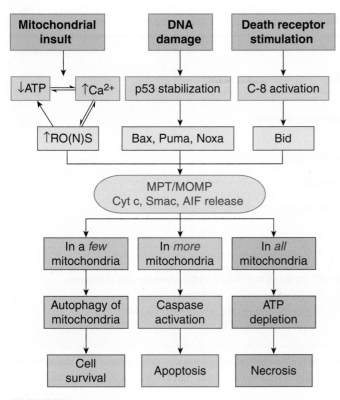

FIGURE 3–9 "Decision plan" on the fate of injured cell. See the text for details. MOMP = mitochondrial outer membrane permeabilization; MPT = mitochondrial permeability transition; Puma = p53-upregulated modulator of apoptosis; RO(N)S = reactive oxygen or nitrogen species.

crucial event. Another related event is release into the cytoplasm of cytochrome c (cyt c), a small hemeprotein that normally resides in the mitochondrial intermembrane space attached to the surface of inner membrane.

As cyt c is the penultimate link in the mitochondrial electron transport chain, its loss will block ATP synthesis, increase formation of $O_2^{\bullet-}$, and potentially thrust the cell toward necrosis. Simultaneously, the unleashed cyt c represents a signal or an initial link in the chain of events directing the cell to the apoptotic path (Figure 3–10). On binding, together with ATP, to an adapter protein, cyt c can induce proteolytic cleavage of proteins called caspases or cysteine proteases that cleave cytoplasmic proteins into fragments, beginning apoptosis. Some caspases (e.g., 2, 8, and 9) activate procaspases. These signaling caspases carry the activation wave to the so-called effector caspases (e.g., 3, 6, and 7), which activate or inactivate specific cellular proteins.

The decisive mitochondrial events of cell death are controlled by the Bcl-2 family of proteins, which includes members that facilitate (e.g., Bax, Bad, and Bid) and those that inhibit (e.g., Bcl-2 and Bcl-XL) these processes. Death-promoting members can oligomerize and form pores in the mitochondrial outer membrane, thereby facilitating release of cyt c and other intermembrane proapoptotic proteins via MPT induced by toxic insult of the mitochondria; however, mitochondrial outer membrane permeabilization (MOMP) alone by Bax and its congeners

is sufficient to evoke egress of cyt c from the mitochondria. The relative amount of these antagonistic proteins functions as a regulatory switch between cell survival and death.

The proapoptotic Bax and Bid proteins also represent links whereby death programs, initiated by DNA damage in the nucleus or by stimulation of certain receptors called Fas receptors at the cell surface, can trigger the mitochondria into the apoptotic process (Figure 3–10). DNA damage induces stabilization and activation of p53 protein, which increases expression of Bax protein, a member of the Bcl-2 family. DNA damage is potentially mutagenic and carcinogenic and apoptosis of cells with damaged DNA is an important self-defense against oncogenesis. Stimulation of Fas receptors can directly activate caspases, and can engage the mitochondria into the death program via caspase-mediated activation of Bid, another member of the Bcl-2 family (Figure 3–10). Thus, apoptosis can be executed via multiple pathways; the preferred route will depend on the initial insult as well as on the type and state of the cell.

ATP Availability Determines the Form of Cell Death— Many xenobiotics can cause both apoptosis and necrosis. Toxicants tend to induce apoptosis at low exposure levels or early after exposure at high levels, whereas they cause necrosis later at high exposure levels. Recent findings suggest that the availability of ATP is critical in determining the form of cell death. When only a few mitochondria develop MPT, they, and with them the proapoptotic signals (e.g., externalized cyt c), are removed by lysosomal autophagy. When MPT involves more mitochondria, the autophagic mechanism becomes overwhelmed and the released cyt c initiates caspase activation and apoptosis (Figure 3–10). When MPT involves virtually all mitochondria, ATP becomes severely depleted, preventing execution of the ATP-requiring apoptotic program and cytolysis occurs.

STEP 4—REPAIR OR DYSREPAIR

The fourth step in the development of toxicity is inappropriate repair (Figure 3–1). Many toxicants alter macromolecules, which, if not repaired, cause damage at higher levels of the biological hierarchy in the organism and influence the progression of toxicity.

Molecular Repair

Damaged molecules may be repaired in different ways. Some chemical alterations, such as oxidation of protein thiols and methylation of DNA, are simply reversed. Hydrolytic removal of the molecule's damaged unit or units and insertion of a newly synthesized unit or units often occur with chemically altered DNA and peroxidized lipids. In some instances, the damaged molecule is totally degraded and resynthesized.

Repair of Proteins—Thiol groups are essential for the function of numerous proteins. Oxidation of protein thiols can be reversed by enzymatic reduction that is catalyzed by thioredoxin and glutaredoxin. Once oxidized, the catalytic thiol groups in these proteins are recycled by reduction with NADPH.

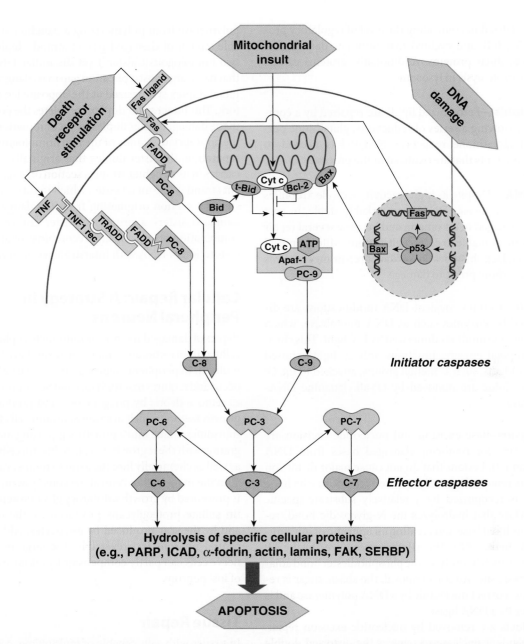

FIGURE 3–10 Apoptotic pathways initiated by mitochondrial insult, nuclear DNA insult, and Fas or TNF receptor-1 stimulation. The figure is a simplified scheme of three pathways to apoptosis. (1) Mitochondrial insult (see text) ultimately opens the permeability transition pore spanning both mitochondrial membranes and/or causes release of cytochrome c (cyt c) from the mitochondria. Cyt c release is facilitated by Bax or Bid proteins and opposed by Bcl-2 protein. (2) DNA insult, especially double-strand breaks, activates p53 protein, which increases the expression of Bax (that mediates cyt c release) and the membrane receptor protein Fas. (3) Fas ligand or tumor necrosis factor binds to and activates their respective receptor, Fas and TNF1 receptor. These ligand-bound receptors and the released cyt c interact with specific adapter proteins (i.e., FADD, RAIDD, and Apaf-1) through which they proteolytically activate procaspases (PC) to active caspases (C). The latter in turn cleave and activate other proteins (e.g., the precursor of Bid, P-Bid) and PC-3, a main effector procaspase. The active effector caspase-3 activates other effector procaspases (PC-6 and PC-7). Finally, C-3, C-6, and C-7 clip specific cellular proteins, whereby apoptosis occurs. These pathways are not equally relevant in all types of cells and other pathways, such as those employing TGF-β as an extracellular signaling molecule, and ceramide as an intracellular signaling molecule, also exist. DFF = DNA fragmentation factor; FAK = focal adhesion kinase; PARP = poly(ADP-ribose) polymerase; SREBP = sterol regulatory element binding protein.

Repair of oxidized hemoglobin (methemoglobin) occurs by means of electron transfer from cytochrome b_5, which is then regenerated by a NADH-dependent cytochrome b_5 reductase. Molecular chaperones such as the heat-shock proteins are syn-

thesized in large quantities in response to protein denaturation. Damaged proteins can either be refolded with the help of chaperone proteins or degraded, following ubiquitination in proteasomes. Also, the ATP/ubiquitin-dependent proteolytic system is specialized in controlling the level of regulatory proteins (e.g., p53, IκB, and cyclins) that eliminate damaged or mutated intracellular proteins. Additionally, proteins can be eliminated by proteolysis in lysosomes.

Repair of Lipids—Peroxidized lipids are repaired by a complex process involving a series of reductants, glutathione peroxidase, and glutathione reductase. NADPH is needed to recycle the reductants that are oxidized in the process.

Repair of DNA—Despite its high reactivity with electrophiles and free radicals, nuclear DNA is remarkably stable, in part because it is packaged in chromatin and because several repair mechanisms are available to correct alterations. Mitochondrial DNA, however, lacks histones and efficient repair mechanisms and therefore is more prone to damage.

Direct Repair—Certain covalent DNA modifications are directly reversed by enzymes such as DNA photolyase, which cleaves adjacent pyrimidines dimerized by UV light. This chromophore-equipped enzyme functions only in light-exposed cells. Minor adducts, such as methyl groups, attached to the O^6 position of guanine are removed by O^6-alkylguanine-DNA-alkyltransferase.

Excision Repair—Base excision and nucleotide excision are two mechanisms for removing damaged bases from DNA (Chapters 8 and 9). Lesions that do not cause major distortion of the helix are removed typically by base excision, in which the altered base is recognized by a relatively substrate-specific DNA-glycosylase that hydrolyzes the *N*-glycosidic bond, releasing the modified base and creating an apurinic or apyrimidinic (AP) site in the DNA. The AP site is recognized by the AP endonuclease, which hydrolyzes the phosphodiester bond adjacent to the abasic site. After its removal, the abasic sugar is replaced with the correct nucleotide by a DNA polymerase and is sealed in place by a DNA ligase.

Bulky adducts are removed by nucleotide-excision repair. An ATP-dependent nuclease recognizes the distorted double helix and excises a number of intact nucleotides on both sides of the lesion together with the one containing the adduct. The excised section of the strand is restored by insertion of nucleotides into the gap by DNA polymerase and ligase, using the complementary strand as a template.

PARP appears to be an important contributor in excision repair. On base damage or single-strand break, PARP binds to the injured DNA and becomes activated. The active PARP cleaves NAD⁺ to use the ADP-ribose moiety of this cofactor for attaching long chains of polymeric ADP-ribose to nuclear proteins. This causes the DNA to unwind, giving access to the repair enzymes and allowing the broken DNA to be fixed.

Recombinational (or Postreplication) Repair—Recombinational repair occurs when the excision of a bulky adduct or an intrastrand pyrimidine dimer fails to occur before DNA replication begins. At replication, such a lesion prevents DNA

polymerase from polymerizing a daughter strand along a sizable stretch of damaged parent strand. Replication results in two homologous ("sister") yet dissimilar DNA duplexes: one that has a large postreplication gap in its daughter strand and an intact duplex synthesized at the opposite leg of the replication fork. This intact sister duplex completes the postreplication gap in the damaged sister duplex by recombination ("crossover") of the appropriate strands of the two homologous duplexes. After separation, the sister duplex that originally contained the gap carries in its daughter strand a section originating from the parent strand of the intact sister, which in turn carries in its parent strand a section originating from the daughter strand of the damaged sister—a process of sister chromatid exchange. A combination of excision and recombinational repairs occurs in restoration of DNA with interstrand cross-links.

Cellular Repair: A Strategy in Peripheral Neurons

Repair of damaged neurons is minimally applied in overcoming cellular injuries because mature neurons have lost their ability to multiply. In peripheral neurons with axonal damage, repair does occur and requires macrophages and Schwann cells. Macrophages remove debris by phagocytosis and produce cytokines and growth factors, which activate Schwann cells to proliferate and transdifferentiate into a growth-supporting mode. While comigrating with the regrowing axon, Schwann cells physically guide as well as chemically lure the axon to reinnervate the target cell.

In the mammalian central nervous system, axonal regrowth is prevented by growth inhibitory glycoproteins and chondroitin sulfate proteoglycans produced by the oligodendrocytes and by the scar produced by astrocytes. Although damage to central neurons is irreversible, the large number of reserve nerve cells can partly compensate by taking over the functions of lost neurons.

Tissue Repair

In tissues with cells capable of multiplying, damage is reversed by apoptosis or necrosis of the injured cells and regeneration of the tissue by proliferation.

Apoptosis: An Active Deletion of Damaged Cells— Apoptosis initiated by cell injury can be regarded as tissue repair. A cell undergoing apoptosis shrinks as its nuclear and cytoplasmic materials condense, and then it breaks into membrane-bound fragments (apoptotic bodies) that are phagocytosed without inflammation. Also, apoptosis may intercept the process leading to neoplasia by eliminating the cells with potentially mutagenic DNA damage.

Apoptosis of damaged cells has a full value as a tissue repair process only for tissues that are made up of constantly renewing cells (e.g., the bone marrow, the respiratory and GI epithelium, and the epidermis of the skin), or of conditionally dividing cells (e.g., hepatic and renal parenchymal cells), because the apoptotic cells are readily replaced. The value of apoptosis as a tissue repair strategy is markedly lessened in organs containing non-replicating and nonreplaceable cells, such as the neurons, cardiac muscle cells, and female germ cells.

Proliferation: Regeneration of Tissue—Tissues are composed of various cells and the extracellular matrix. Cadherins allow adjacent cells to adhere to one other, whereas connexins connect neighboring cells internally by association of these proteins into gap junctions. Integrins link cells to the extracellular matrix. Therefore, repair of injured tissues involves both regeneration of lost cells and the extracellular matrix and reintegration of the newly formed elements into tissues and organs.

Replacement of Lost Cells by Mitosis—Soon after injury, cells adjacent to the damaged area enter the cell-division cycle. Quiescent cells residing in G_0 enter G_1 and progress to mitosis (M).

Sequential changes in gene expression occur in the cells that are destined to divide. Early after injury, intracellular signaling turns on, and expression of numerous genes is increased. Among these so-called immediate-early genes are those that code for TFs that amplify the initial gene-activation process by stimulating other genes directly or through cell surface receptors and the coupled transducing networks. A few hours later, the so-called delayed-early genes are expressed whose products regulate the cell-division cycle. Genes for the cell cycle accelerator proteins and also genes whose products decelerate the cell cycle become temporarily overexpressed, suggesting that this duality keeps tissue regeneration precisely regulated. Thus, genetic expression is reprogrammed so that DNA synthesis and mitosis gain priority over specialized cellular activities.

The regenerative process is probably initiated by the release of chemical mediators from damaged cells. Nonparenchymal cells, such as resident macrophages and endothelial cells, are receptive to these chemical signals and produce a host of signaling molecules that promote and propagate the regenerative process. The cytokines TNF-α and interleukin=6 (IL-6) purportedly promote transition of the quiescent cells into cell cycle ("priming"), whereas the growth factors, especially the hepatocyte growth factor (HGF) and transforming growth factor-α (TGF-α), initiate the progression of the "primed" cells in the cycle toward mitosis.

Besides mitosis, cell migration also significantly contributes to restitution of certain tissues. In the mucosa of the GI tract, cells of the residual epithelium rapidly migrate to the site of injury as well as elongate and thin to reestablish the continuity of the surface even before this could be achieved by cell replication. Mucosal repair is dictated by growth factors and cytokines operative in tissue repair elsewhere and also by specific peptides associated with the mucous layer of the GI tract that become overexpressed at sites of mucosal injury.

Replacement of the Extracellular Matrix—The extracellular matrix is composed of proteins, glycosaminoglycans, and the glycoprotein and proteoglycans. Activation of resting stellate cells is mediated chiefly by two growth factors, platelet-derived growth factor (PDGF) and transforming growth factor-β (TGF-β), that may be released from platelets accumulating and degranulating at sites of injury and later from the activated stellate cells themselves. Proliferation of stellate cells is induced by the potent mitogen PDGF, whereas TGF-β acts on the stellate cells to stimulate the synthesis of extracellular matrix components, including collagens, fibronectin, tenascin, and proteoglycans. TGF-β also plays a central role in extracellular matrix formation in other tissues.

Side Reactions to Tissue Injury—In addition to mediators that aid in the replacement of lost cells and the extracellular matrix, resident macrophages and endothelial cells activated by cell injury also produce inflammation, altered production of acute-phase protein, and generalized reactions such as fever.

Inflammation

Cells and Mediators: Alteration of the microcirculation and accumulation of inflammatory cells are largely initiated by resident macrophages secreting cytokines such as TNF-α and IL-1 in response to tissue damage. These cytokines, in turn, stimulate neighboring stromal cells, such as the endothelial cells and fibroblasts, to release mediators that induce dilation of the local microvasculature and cause permeabilization of capillaries. Activated endothelial cells also facilitate the egress of circulating leukocytes into the injured tissue by releasing chemoattractants and expressing cell-adhesion molecules. Subsequently a stronger interaction (adhesion) is established between the endothelial cells and leukocytes with participation of intercellular adhesion molecules (e.g., ICAM-1) and leukocytes are able to enter the tissues by crossing the endothelial layer. This is facilitated by gradients of chemoattractants, including chemotactic cytokines, platelet-activating factor (PAF) and leukotriene B4, that induce expression of leukocyte integrins.

Inflammation Produces Reactive Oxygen and Nitrogen Species: Macrophages as well as leukocytes recruited to a site of injury undergo a respiratory burst, producing free radicals and activated enzymes. Membrane-bound NAD(P)H oxidase, activated in both macrophages and granulocytes, produces superoxide anion radical ($O_2^{\bullet-}$) from molecular oxygen. The $O_2^{\bullet-}$ can give rise to the hydroxyl radical ($HO^{\bullet}$).

Macrophages, but not granulocytes, generate another cytotoxic free radical, nitric oxide ($^{\bullet}NO$), from arginine by nitric oxide synthase:

$$\text{L-Arginine} + O_2 \rightarrow \text{L-Citrulline} + {}^{\bullet}NO$$

Subsequently, $O_2^{\bullet-}$ and $^{\bullet}NO$, both of which are products of activated macrophages, can react with each other, yielding peroxynitrite anion; on reaction with carbon dioxide, this decays into two radicals, nitrogen dioxide and carbonate anion radical:

$$O_2^{\bullet-} + {}^{\bullet}NO \rightarrow ONOO^-$$
$$ONOO^- + CO_2 \rightarrow ONOOCO_2^-$$
$$ONOOCO_2^- \rightarrow {}^{\bullet}NO_2 + CO_3^{\bullet-}$$

Granulocytes discharge the lysosomal enzyme myeloperoxidase into engulfed extracellular spaces, the phagocytic vacuoles.

Myeloperoxidase catalyzes the formation of hypochlorous acid (HOCl) from hydrogen peroxide (HOOH) and chloride ion:

$$HOOH + H^+ + Cl^- \rightarrow HOH + HOCl$$

HOCl can form $HO^\bullet$ as a result of electron transfer from Fe^{2+} or from $O_2^{\bullet-}$ to HOCl:

$$HOCl + O_2^{\bullet-} \rightarrow O_2 + Cl^- + HO^\bullet$$

All the above reactive chemicals, as well as the discharged lysosomal proteases, are destructive products of inflammatory cells. Although these chemicals exert antimicrobial activity at the site of microbial invasion, they can damage adjacent healthy tissues at the site of toxic injury and contribute to propagation of tissue injury.

Altered Protein Synthesis: Acute-phase Proteins—Cytokines released from macrophages and endothelial cells of injured tissues, IL-6, IL-1, and TNF, act on cell surface receptors to increase or decrease the transcriptional activity of genes encoding certain proteins called positive and negative acute-phase proteins.

Positive acute-phase proteins may play roles in minimizing tissue injury and facilitating repair. For example, many of them inhibit lysosomal proteases released from the injured cells and recruited leukocytes.

Because negative acute-phase proteins play important roles in the toxication and detoxication of xenobiotics, the disposition and toxicity of chemicals may be altered markedly during the acute phase of tissue injury.

Generalized Reactions—Cytokines released from activated macrophages and endothelial cells at the site of injury also may evoke neurohormonal responses. Thus, IL-1, TNF, and IL-6 alter the temperature set point of the hypothalamus, triggering fever. In addition, IL-1 and IL-6 act on the pituitary to induce the release of ACTH, which in turn stimulates the secretion of cortisol from the adrenals. This represents a negative feedback loop because corticosteroids inhibit cytokine gene expression.

Mechanisms of Adaptation

Adaptation involves responses acting to preserve or regain the biological homeostasis in the face of increased harm from a noxious stimulus. Adaptation of toxicity may result from biological changes causing (1) diminished delivery of the toxicant to the target, (2) decreased size or susceptibility of the target, (3) increased capacity of the organism to repair itself, and (4) strengthened mechanisms to compensate the toxicant-inflicted dysfunction. Adaptation involves sensing the noxious chemical and/or the initial damage or dysfunction, and a response that typically occurs through altered gene expression.

Certain chemicals induce adaptive changes that lessen their delivery by diminishing the absorption, increasing their sequestration by intracellular binding proteins, enhancing their detoxication, or promoting their cellular export. For example, the amount of iron or cadmium in the diet influences the expression of a divalent metal transporter in enterocytes and the expression of binding proteins ferritin and metallothionein. Another example involves the cellular response to electrophiles. Figure 3–11 illustrates many genes that code for (1) enzymes that detoxify xenobiotics, (2) enzymes that eliminate ROS, (3) proteins that detoxify heme, (4) enzymes involved in glutathione homeostasis, and (5) transporters that pump xenobiotics and their metabolites out of cells. Those interested in additional examples should consult the 7th edition of *Casarett & Doull's Toxicology: The Basic Science of Poisons*.

When Repair Fails

Repair mechanisms often fail to protect against injury because the fidelity of the repair mechanisms is not absolute, making it possible for some lesions to be overlooked. Repair fails most typically when the damage overwhelms the repair mechanisms as when necessary enzymes or cofactors are consumed. Sometimes the toxicant-induced injury adversely affects the repair process itself. Finally, some types of toxic injuries cannot be repaired effectively, as occurs when xenobiotics are covalently bound to proteins.

It is also possible that repair contributes to toxicity, as when excessive amounts of NAD^+ are cleaved by PARP when this enzyme assists in repairing broken DNA strands, or when too much NAD(P)H is consumed for the repair of oxidized proteins and endogenous reductants. Either event can compromise oxidative phosphorylation, which is also dependent on the supply of reduced cofactors (see Figure 3–8), thus causing or aggravating ATP depletion that contributes to cell injury. However, repair also may play an active role in toxicity. This is observed after chronic tissue injury, when the repair process goes astray and leads to uncontrolled proliferation instead of tissue remodeling. Such proliferation of cells may yield neoplasia, whereas overproduction of extracellular matrix results in fibrosis.

Toxicity Resulting from Dysrepair

Dysrepair occurs at the molecular, cellular, and tissue levels. Some toxicities involve dysrepair at an isolated level, such as a specific enzyme or process, or at different levels, such as tissue necrosis, fibrosis, and chemical carcinogenesis.

Tissue Necrosis—Several mechanisms that may lead to cell death may involve molecular damage that is potentially reversible by repair mechanisms. Cell injury progresses toward cell necrosis if molecular repair mechanisms are inefficient or the molecular damage is not readily reversible.

Progression of cell injury to tissue necrosis can be intercepted by two repair mechanisms working in concert: apoptosis and cell proliferation. Injured cells can initiate apoptosis, which counteracts the progression of the toxic injury by preventing necrosis of injured cells and the consequent inflammatory response.

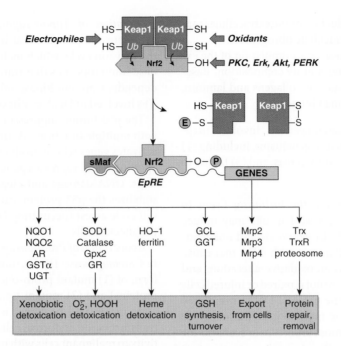

FIGURE 3–11 **Signaling by Keap1/Nrf2 mediates the electrophile response.** Normally NF-E2-related factor 2 (Nrf2) is kept inactive and at a low intracellular level by interacting with Keap1, which promotes its proteosomal degradation by ubiquitination. Electrophiles covalently bind to, whereas oxidants oxidize, the reactive thiol groups of Keap1, causing Keap1 to release Nrf2. Alternatively, Nrf2 release may follow phosphorylation of Keap1 by protein kinases. After being released from Keap1, the active Nrf2 accumulates in the cell, translocates into the nucleus, and forms a heterodimer with small Maf proteins to activate genes that contain electrophile response element (EpRE) in their promoter region. These include enzymes, binding proteins, and transporters functioning in detoxication and elimination of xenobiotics, ROS, and endogenous reactive chemicals, as well as some proteins that can repair or eliminate oxidized proteins. Induction of such proteins represents an electrophile–stress response that provides protection against a wide range of toxicants. *Abbreviations*: AR = aldose reductase; G6PDH = glucose 6-phosphate dehydrogenase; GCL = glutamate-cysteine ligase; GGT = gamma-glutamyltranspeptidase; GPX2 = glutathione peroxidase 2; GR = glutathione reductase; GSTα = glutathione S-transferase α subunit; HO-1 = heme oxygenase 1; NQO1 = NAD(P)H:quinone oxidoreductase; NQO2 = NRH:quinone oxidoreductase; 2; Mrp2, Mrp3, and Mrp4 = multidrug-resistance protein 2, 3, and 4; SOD1 = superoxide dismutase 1; UGT = UDP-glucuronosyltransferase; Trx = thioredoxin; TrxR = thioredoxin reductase.

Another important repair process that can halt the propagation of toxic injury is proliferation of cells adjacent to the injured cells. Initiated soon after cellular injury, this early cell division is thought to be instrumental in the rapid and complete restoration of the injured tissue and the prevention of necrosis. The sensitivity of a tissue to injury and the capacity of the tissue for repair are apparently two independent variables, both influencing whether tissue restitution ensues with survival or tissue necrosis occurs with death.

The efficiency of repair is also an important determinant of the dose–response relationship for toxicants that cause tissue necrosis. Tissue necrosis is caused by a certain dose of a toxicant not only because that dose ensures sufficient concentration of the ultimate toxicant at the target site to initiate injury, but also because that quantity of toxicant causes a degree of damage sufficient to compromise repair, allowing for progression of the injury. Tissue necrosis occurs because the injury overwhelms and disables the repair mechanisms, including (1) repair of damaged molecules, (2) elimination of damaged cells by apoptosis, and (3) replacement of lost cells by cell division.

Fibrosis—Fibrosis, a pathologic condition characterized by excessive deposition of an extracellular matrix of abnormal composition, is a specific manifestation of dysrepair of the injured tissue. As discussed above, cellular injury initiates a surge in cellular proliferation and extracellular matrix production, which normally ceases when the injured tissue is remodeled. If increased production of extracellular matrix is not halted, fibrosis develops.

TGF-β appears to be a major mediator of fibrogenesis. The increased expression of TGF-β is a common response mediating regeneration of the extracellular matrix after an acute injury. Normally, TGF-β production ceases when repair is complete. Failure to halt TGF-β overproduction, which leads to fibrosis, could be caused by continuous injury or a defect in the regulation of TGF-β.

The fibrotic action of TGF-β is due to (1) stimulation of the synthesis of individual matrix components by specific target cells and (2) inhibition of matrix degradation. Interestingly, TGF-β induces transcription of its own gene in target cells, suggesting that the TGF-β produced by these cells can amplify in an autocrine manner the production of the extracellular matrix. This positive feedback may facilitate fibrogenesis.

Fibrosis involves not only excessive accumulation of the extracellular matrix, but also changes in its composition. Basement membrane components, such as collagens and laminin, increase disproportionately during fibrogenesis.

Carcinogenesis—Chemical carcinogenesis involves inappropriate function of various repair mechanisms, including (1) failure of DNA repair, (2) failure of apoptosis, and (3) failure to terminate cell proliferation.

Failure of DNA Repair: Mutation, the Initiating Event in Carcinogenesis—Chemical and physical insults may induce neoplastic transformation of cells by genotoxic and nongenotoxic mechanisms. Chemicals that react with DNA may cause damage such as adduct formation, oxidative alteration, and strand breakage. If these lesions are not repaired or injured cells are not eliminated, a lesion in the parental DNA strand may induce a heritable alteration, or mutation, in the daughter strand during replication. The most unfortunate scenario for the organism occurs when the altered genes express mutant proteins that reprogram cells for multiplication. When such cells undergo mitosis, their descendants also have a similar propensity for proliferation. Moreover, because enhanced cell division increases the likelihood of mutations, these cells eventually acquire additional mutations that may further increase their growth advantage over their normal counterparts. The final outcome of this process is a tumor consisting of transformed, rapidly proliferating cells.

Mutation of Proto-oncogenes: Proto-oncogenes are highly conserved genes encoding proteins that stimulate progression of cells through the cell cycle. The products of proto-oncogenes include (1) growth factors; (2) growth factor receptors; (3) intracellular signal transducers such as G proteins, protein kinases, cyclins, and cyclin-dependent protein kinases; and (4) nuclear TFs. Transient increases in the production or activity of proto-oncogene proteins are required for regulated growth, as during embryogenesis, tissue regeneration, and stimulation of cells by growth factors or hormones. In contrast, permanent activation and/or overexpression of these proteins favors neoplastic transformation. One mechanism whereby genotoxic carcinogens induce neoplastic cell transformation is by producing an activating mutation of a proto-oncogene. The altered gene (called an *oncogene*) encodes a permanently active protein that forces the cell into the division cycle.

An example of mutational activation of an oncogene protein is that of the Ras proteins. Ras proteins are localized on the inner surface of the plasma membrane and function as crucial mediators in responses initiated by growth factors (see Figure 3–7). Ras serves as a molecular switch, being active in the GTP-bound form and inactive in the GDP-bound form. Some mutations of the Ras gene dramatically lower the GTPase activity of the protein, which in turn locks Ras in the permanently active GTP-bound form. Continual rather than signal-dependent activation of Ras can lead eventually to uncontrolled proliferation and transformation.

Mutation of Tumor-suppressor Genes: Tumor-suppressor genes encode proteins that inhibit the progression of cells in the division cycle, which include cyclin-dependent protein kinase inhibitors, TFs that transactivate genes encoding cyclin-dependent protein kinase inhibitors, and proteins that block TFs involved in DNA synthesis and cell division (Figure 3–12).

The p53 tumor-suppressor gene encodes a 53-kDa protein with multiple functions. Acting as a TF, the p53 protein transactivates genes whose products arrest the cell cycle or promote apoptosis, and represses genes that encode antiapoptotic proteins. DNA damage and illegitimate expression of oncogenes stabilizes the p53 protein, causing its accumulation, inducing cell cycle arrest (permitting DNA repair) or even apoptosis of the affected cells.

Cooperation of Proto-oncogenes and Tumor-suppressor Genes in Carcinogenesis: The accumulation of genetic damage in the form of (1) mutant proto-oncogenes (which encode activated proteins) and (2) mutant tumor-suppressor genes (which encode inactivated proteins) is the main driving force in the transformation of normal cells with controlled proliferative activity to malignant cells with uncontrolled proliferative activity. Because the number of cells in a tissue is regulated by a balance between mitosis and apoptosis, uncontrolled proliferation results from perturbation of this balance.

Failure of Apoptosis: Promotion of Mutation and Clonal Growth—Preneoplastic cells, or cells with mutations, have much higher apoptotic activity than do normal cells. Therefore, apoptosis counteracts clonal expansion of the initiated cells and tumor cells. Facilitation of apoptosis can induce tumor regression, whereas inhibition of apoptosis is detrimental because mutations and clonal expansion of preneoplastic cells are facilitated.

Failure to Terminate Proliferation: Promotion of Mutation, Proto-oncogene Expression, and Clonal Growth—Enhanced mitotic activity promotes carcinogenesis for a number of reasons:

1. Enhanced mitotic activity increases the probability of mutations. With activation of the cell-division cycle, a substantial shortening of the G1 phase occurs, and less time is available for the repair of injured DNA before replication.
2. Overproduced proto-oncogene proteins may cooperate with oncogene proteins to facilitate the neoplastic transformation of cells, thereby allowing less time for DNA methylation, which decreases gene transcription by inhibiting the interaction of TFs with the promoter region. Nonexpressed genes are fully methylated.
3. Cell-to-cell communication through gap junctions and intercellular adhesion through cadherins are temporarily disrupted during proliferation, which contributes to the invasiveness of tumor cells.

Nongenotoxic Carcinogens: Promoters of Mitosis and Inhibitors of Apoptosis—Many chemicals do not alter DNA or induce mutations yet induce cancer after chronic administration. Designated *nongenotoxic* or *epigenetic* carcinogens, these chemicals cause cancer by promoting carcinogenesis initiated

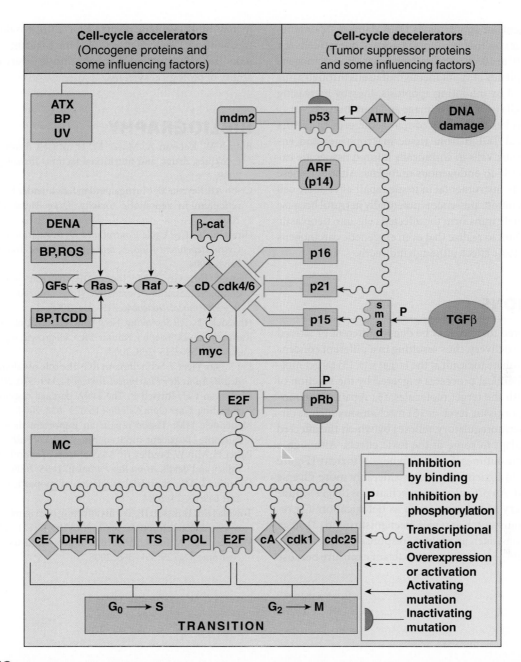

FIGURE 3–12 Key regulatory proteins controlling the cell-division cycle with some signaling pathways and xenobiotics affecting them. Proteins on the left, represented by blue symbols, accelerate the cell cycle and are oncogenic if permanently active or expressed at high level. In contrast, proteins on the right, represented by salmon symbols, decelerate or arrest the cell cycle and thus suppress oncogenesis, unless they are inactivated (e.g., by mutation).

Cyclin D (cD) activates cyclin-dependent protein kinases 4 and 6 (cdk4/6), which in turn phosphorylate the retinoblastoma protein (pRb) causing dissociation of pRb from transcription factor E2F. The unleashed E2F binds to and transactivates genes whose products are essential for DNA synthesis (e.g., dihydrofolate reductase [DHFR], thymidine kinase [TK], thymidylate synthetase [TS], and DNA polymerase [POL]) or are regulatory proteins (e.g., cyclin E [cE], cyclin A [cA], and cyclin-dependent protein kinase 1 [cdk1]) that promote further progression of the cell cycle. Expression of cD is increased, for example, by signals evoked by growth factors (GFs) via Ras proteins and by transcription factors, such as myc and β-catenin (β-cat). Benzpyrene (BP), reactive oxygen species (ROS), and diethylnitrosamine (DENA) may cause mutation of the Ras or Raf gene that results in permanently active mutant Ras protein, but BP and TCDD may also induce simple overexpression of normal Ras protein.

Cell cycle progression is counteracted by pRb (which inhibits the function of E2F), cyclin-dependent protein kinase inhibitors (such as p15, p16, and p21), p53 (that transactivates the p21 gene), and ARF (also called p14 that binds to mdm2, thereby neutralizing the antagonistic effect of mdm2 on p53). Signals evoked by DNA damage and TGF-β will ultimately result in accumulation of p53 and p15 proteins, respectively, and deceleration of the cell cycle. In contrast, mutations that disable the tumor-suppressor proteins facilitate cell-cycle progression and neoplastic conversion and are common in human tumors. Aflatoxin B1 (ATX), BP, and UV light cause such mutations of the p53 gene.

by genotoxic agents or spontaneous DNA damage. Spontaneous DNA damage commonly occurs in normal human cells at a rate of 1 out of 10^8 to 10^{10} base pairs. Nongenotoxic carcinogens increase the frequency of spontaneous mutations through a mitogenic effect and by inhibiting apoptosis, thereby increasing the number of cells with DNA damage and mutations.

Cell injury evokes the release of mitogenic growth factors such as HGF and TGF-α from tissue macrophages and endothelial cells. Thus, cells in chronically injured tissues are exposed continuously to endogenous mitogens. Although these growth factors are instrumental in tissue repair after acute cell injury, their continuous presence is potentially harmful because they may ultimately transform the affected cells into neoplastic cells. It is important to realize that even epigenetic carcinogens can exert a genotoxic effect, although indirectly.

CONCLUSIONS

Selective or altered toxicity may be due to different or altered (1) exposure; (2) delivery, thus resulting in a different concentration of the ultimate toxicant at the target site; (3) target molecules; (4) biochemical processes triggered by the reaction of the chemical with the target molecules; (5) repair at the molecular, cellular, or tissue level; or (6) mechanisms such as circulatory and thermoregulatory reflexes by which the affected organism can adapt to some of the toxic effects. Although a simplified scheme outlines the development of toxicity (Figure 3–1), the route to toxicity can be considerably more diverse and complicated. An organism has mechanisms that (1) counteract the delivery of toxicants, such as detoxication; (2) reverse the toxic injury, such as repair mechanisms; and (3) offset some dysfunctions, such as adaptive responses. Thus, toxicity is not an inevitable consequence of toxicant exposure because it may be prevented, reversed, or compensated for by such mechanisms. Toxicity develops if the toxicant exhausts or impairs the protective mechanisms and/or overrides the adaptability of biological systems.

BIBLIOGRAPHY

Bursch W, Karwan A, Mayer M, et al: Cell death and autophagy: cytokines, drugs, and nutritional factors. *Toxicology* 254:147–157, 2008.

Cribb AE, Peyrou M, Muruganandan S, Schneider L: The endoplasmic reticulum in xenobiotic toxicity. *Drug Metab Rev* 37:405–442, 2005.

Giordano A: *Cell Cycle Control and Dysregulation Protocols: Cyclins, Cyclin-dependent Kinases, and Other Factors.* Totowa, NJ: Humana Press, 2004.

Hansen JM, Go Y-M, Jones DP: Nuclear and mitochondrial compartmentation of oxidative stress and redox signaling. *Annu Rev Pharmacol Toxicol* 46:215–234, 2006.

Hancock JT: *Cell Signalling.* New York: Oxford University Press, 2005.

Karunagaran D, Joseph J, Kumar TR: Cell growth regulation. *Adv Exp Med Biol* 595:245–268, 2007.

Liu X, Van Fleet T, Schnellmann RG: The role of calpain in oncotic cell death. *Annu Rev Pharmacol Toxicol* 44:349–370, 2004.

McGowan CH, Russell P: The DNA damage response: sensing and signaling. *Curr Opin Cell Biol* 16:629–633, 2004.

Mehendele HM: Tissue repair: an important determinant of final outcome of toxicant-induced injury. *Toxicol Pathol* 33:41–51, 2005.

Pober JS, Min W, Bradley JR: Mechanisms of endothelial dysfunction, injury and death. *Annu Rev Pathol* 4:71–95, 2009.

Orrenius S: Mitochondrial regulation of apoptotic cell death. *Toxicol Lett* 149:19–23, 2004.

Toivola DM, Eriksson JE: Toxins affecting cell signalling and alteration of cytoskeletal structure. *Toxicol In Vitro* 13:521–530, 1999.

Wallace KB: Mitochondrial off targets of drug therapy. *Trends Pharmacol Sci* 29:361–366, 2008.

QUESTIONS

1. The severity of a toxin depends, in large part, on the concentration of the toxin at its site of action. Which of the following will decrease the amount of toxin reaching its site of action?
   a. absorption across the skin.
   b. excretion via the kidneys.
   c. toxication.
   d. reabsorption across the intestinal mucosa.
   e. discontinuous endothelial cells of hepatic sinusoids.

2. Toxication (or metabolic activation) is the biotransformation of a toxin to a more toxic and reactive species. Which of the following is not a reactive chemical species commonly formed by toxication?
   a. electrophiles.
   b. nucleophiles.
   c. superoxide anions.
   d. hydroxy radicals.
   e. hydrophilic organic acids.

3. Which of the following is not an important step in detoxication of chemicals?
   a. formation of redox-active reactants.
   b. reduction of hydrogen peroxide by glutathione peroxidase.
   c. formation of hydrogen peroxide by superoxide dismutase.
   d. reduction of glutathione disulfide (GSSG) by glutathione reductase (GR).
   e. conversion of hydrogen peroxide to water and molecular oxygen by catalase.

4. Regarding the interaction of the ultimate toxicant with its target molecule, which of the following is false?
   a. Toxins often oxidize or reduce their target molecules, resulting in the formation of a harmful byproduct.
   b. The covalent binding of a toxin with its target molecule permanently alters the target's function.
   c. The noncovalent binding of a toxin to an ion channel irreversibly inhibits ion flux through the channel.
   d. Abstraction of hydrogen atoms from endogenous compounds by free radicals can result in the formation of DNA adducts.
   e. Several toxins can act enzymatically on their specific target proteins.

5. All of the following are common effects of toxicants on target molecules EXCEPT:
   a. blockage of neurotransmitter receptors.
   b. interference with DNA replication due to adduct formation.
   c. cross-linking of endogenous molecules.
   d. opening of ion channels.
   e. mounting of an immune response.

6. Which of the following proteins functions to prevent the progression of the cell cycle?
   a. NF-κB.
   b. MAPK.
   c. CREB.
   d. c-Myc.
   e. IκB.

7. Which of the following would have the largest negative impact on intracellular ATP levels?
   a. moderately decreased caloric intake.
   b. interference with electron delivery to the electron transport chain.
   c. inability to harvest ATP from glycolysis.
   d. increased synthesis of biomolecules.
   e. active cell division.

8. What happens when a toxin induces elevation of cytoplasmic calcium levels?
   a. Mitochondrial uptake of calcium dissipates the electrochemical gradient needed to synthesize ATP.
   b. Formation of actin filaments increases the strength and integrity of the cytoskeleton.
   c. It decreases the activity of intracellular proteases, nucleases, and phospholipases.
   d. The cell becomes dormant until the calcium is actively pumped from the cell.
   e. The generation of reactive oxygen species slows because of calcium-induced decrease in activity of the TCA cycle.

9. Cytochrome *c* is an important molecule in initiating apoptosis in cells. All of the following regarding cytochrome *c* are true EXCEPT:
   a. The release of cytochrome *c* into the cytoplasm is an important step in apoptosis initiation.
   b. The loss of cytochrome *c* from the electron transport chain blocks ATP synthesis by oxidative phosphorylation.
   c. Loss of cytochrome *c* from the inner mitochondrial membrane results in increased formation of reactive oxygen species.
   d. Bax proteins mediate cytochrome *c* release.
   e. Caspases are proteases that increase cytoplasmic levels of cytochrome *c*.

10. All of the following regarding DNA repair are true EXCEPT:

    a. In a lesion that does not cause a major distortion of the double helix, the incorrect base is cleaved and the correct base is inserted in its place.

    b. Base excision repair and nucleotide excision repair are both dependent on a DNA polymerase and a DNA ligase.

    c. In nucleotide excision repair, only the adduct is cleaved, and the gap is then filled by DNA polymerase.

    d. Pyrimidine dimers can be cleaved and repaired directly by DNA photolyase.

    e. Recombinational repair requires that a sister strand serve as a template to fill in missing nucleotides.

11. Apoptosis can serve as a tissue repair process in a number of cell types. In which of the following cell types would this be a plausible mechanism of tissue repair?

    a. female germ cells.

    b. gastrointestinal epithelium.

    c. neurons.

    d. retinal ganglion cells.

    e. cardiac muscle cells.

12. Which of the following is NOT associated with carcinogenesis?

    a. mutation.

    b. normal p53 function.

    c. Ras activation.

    d. inhibition of apoptosis.

    e. DNA repair failure.

Risk Assessment

Elaine M. Faustman and Gilbert S. Omenn

KEY POINTS

- *Risk assessment* is the systematic scientific characterization of potential adverse health effects resulting from human exposures to hazardous agents or situations.
- *Risk* is defined as the probability of an adverse outcome under specified conditions.

- *Risk management* refers to the process by which policy actions are chosen to control hazards.

INTRODUCTION AND HISTORICAL CONTEXT

Toxicologic research and toxicity testing conducted and interpreted by toxicologists constitute the scientific core of an important activity known as *risk assessment* for chemical exposures. The National Research Council detailed the steps of hazard identification, dose–response assessment, exposure analysis, and characterization of risks in *Risk Assessment in the*

Federal Government: Managing the Process (widely known as *The Red Book*). The scheme shown in Figure 4–1 provides a consistent framework for risk assessment across agencies with bidirectional arrows showing an ideal situation where mechanistic research feeds directly into risk assessments and critical data uncertainty drives research. Often, public policy objectives require extrapolations that go far beyond the observation of actual effects and reflect different tolerances for risks, generating controversy.

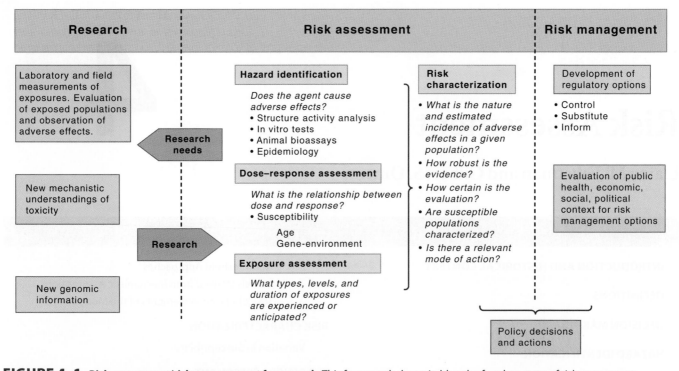

FIGURE 4–1   Risk assessment/risk management framework. This framework shows in blue the four key steps of risk assessment: hazard identification, dose–response assessment, exposure assessment, and risk characterization. It shows an interactive, two-way process where research needs from the risk assessment process drive new research, and new research findings modify risk assessment outcomes. (Adapted from NRC, *Risk Assessment in the Federal Government: Managing the Process,* Washington, DC: National Academies Press, 1993, reprinted with permission from the National Academies Press, National Academy of Sciences.)

The Presidential/Congressional Commission on Risk Assessment and Risk Management formulated a comprehensive framework that applies two crucial concepts: (1) putting each environmental problem or issue into public health and/or ecological context and (2) proactively engaging the relevant stakeholders, affected or potentially affected community groups, from the very beginning of the six-stage process shown in Figure 4–2. Particular exposures and potential health effects must be evaluated across sources and exposure pathways and in light of multiple endpoints, and not the current general approach of evaluating one chemical in one environmental medium (air, water, soil, food, and products) for one health effect at a time.

DEFINITIONS

Risk assessment is the systematic scientific characterization of potential adverse health effects resulting from human exposures to hazardous agents or situations. *Risk* is defined as the probability of an adverse outcome based on the exposure and potency of the hazardous agent(s). The term *hazard* is used in the United States and Canada to refer to intrinsic toxic properties, whereas internationally this term is defined as the probability of an adverse outcome. Risk assessment requires qualitative information about the strength of the evidence and the nature of the outcomes—as well as quantitative assessment of the exposures, host susceptibility factors, and potential

magnitude of the risk—and then a description of the uncertainties in the estimates and conclusions. The objectives of risk assessment are outlined in Table 4–1.

The phrase *characterization of risk* reflects the combination of qualitative and quantitative analyses. Unfortunately, many users tend to equate risk assessment with quantitative risk assessment, generating a number for an overly precise risk estimate, while ignoring crucial information about the mechanism of effect across species, inconsistent findings across studies, multiple variable health effects, and means of avoiding or reversing the effects of exposures.

TABLE 4–1   Objectives of risk assessment.

1. Balance risks and benefits
• Drugs
• Pesticides
2. Set target levels of risk
• Food contaminants
• Water pollutants
3. Set priorities for program activities
• Regulatory agencies
• Manufacturers
• Environmental/consumer organizations
4. Estimate residual risks and extent of risk reduction after steps are taken to reduce risks

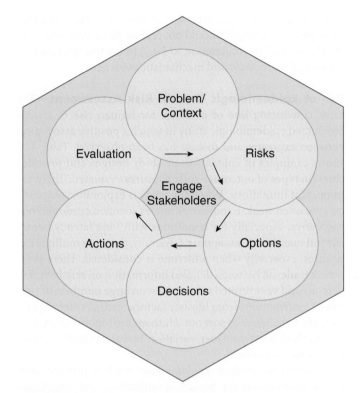

FIGURE 4-2 **Risk management framework for environmental health from the U.S. Commission on Risk Assessment and Risk Management, "Omenn Commission."** The framework comprises six stages: (1) formulating the problem in a broad public health context; (2) analyzing risks; (3) defining options; (4) making risk-reduction decisions; (5) implementing those actions; and (6) evaluating the effectiveness of the taken actions. Interactions with stakeholders are critical and thus have been put at the center of the framework.

Risk management refers to the process by which policy actions are chosen to control hazards identified in the risk assessment/risk characterization stage of the six-stage framework (Figure 4–2). Risk managers consider scientific evidence and risk estimates—along with statutory, engineering, economic, social, and political factors—in evaluating alternative options and choosing among those options.

Risk communication is the challenging process of making risk assessment and risk management information comprehensible to community groups, lawyers, local elected officials, judges, business people, labor, and environmentalists. A crucial, too-often neglected requirement for communication is listening to the fears, perceptions, priorities, and proposed remedies of these "stakeholders."

DECISION MAKING

Risk management decisions are reached under diverse statutes in the United States and many other countries. Some statutes specify reliance on risk alone, whereas others require a balancing of risks and benefits of the product or activity (Table 4–1).

Risk assessments provide a valuable framework for priority setting within regulatory and health agencies, in the chemical development process within companies, and in resource allocation by environmental organizations. Currently, there are significant efforts toward the harmonization of testing protocols and the assessment of risks and standards.

A major challenge for risk assessment, risk communication, and risk management is to work across disciplines to demonstrate the biological plausibility and clinical significance of the conclusions from studies of chemicals thought to have potential adverse effects. Biomarkers of exposure, effect, or individual susceptibility can link the presence of a chemical in various environmental compartments to specific sites of action in target organs and to host responses. Individual behavioral and social risk factors may be critically important to both the risk and the reduction of risk. Finally, public and media attitudes toward local polluters, other responsible parties, and relevant government agencies can greatly influence the communication process and the choices for risk management.

HAZARD IDENTIFICATION

Assessing Toxicity of Chemicals—Methods

Structure/Activity Relationships—Given the cost of $2 to $4 million and the 3 to 5 years required for testing a single chemical in a lifetime rodent carcinogenicity bioassay, initial decisions on whether to continue development of a chemical, submit a premanufacturing notice, or require additional testing may be based largely on structure/activity relationships and limited short-term assays. A chemical's structure, solubility, stability, pH sensitivity, electrophilicity, volatility, and chemical reactivity can be important information for hazard identification.

Structure–activity relationships have been used for assessment of complex mixtures. However, it is difficult to predict activity across chemical classes and especially across multiple toxic endpoints using a single biological response. Computerized SAR methods have given limited results, whereas three-dimensional (3D) molecular modeling, which utilizes pharmacophore mapping, 3D searching and molecular design, and establishment of 3D quantitative structure–activity relationships, has been more successful.

In Vitro and Short-term Tests—The next approach for hazard identification comprises tests ranging from in vitro bacterial mutation assays to more elaborate short-term tests such as skin-painting studies in mice or altered rat liver-foci assays conducted in vivo. Other assays evaluate development, reproduction, neurotoxicity, and immunotoxicity. New assay methods from molecular and developmental biology for developmental toxicity risk assessment should accelerate use of a broader range of model organisms and assay approaches for noncancer risk assessments. Short-term assay validation and application is particularly important to risk assessment because such assays can provide information about mechanisms of effects while being faster and less expensive than lifetime bioassays.

Animal Bioassays—Animal bioassay data are key components of the hazard identification process. A basic premise of risk assessment is that chemicals that cause tumors in animals can cause tumors in humans. All human carcinogens that have been adequately tested in animals produce positive results in at least one animal model. Although this association cannot establish that all agents and mixtures that cause cancer in experimental animals also cause cancer in humans, nevertheless, in the absence of adequate data on humans, it is biologically plausible and prudent to regard agents and mixtures for which there is sufficient evidence of carcinogenicity in experimental animals as if they presented a carcinogenic risk to humans—a reflection of the "precautionary principle." The USEPA assumes relevance of animal bioassays unless lack of relevance for human assessment is specifically determined. In general, the most appropriate rodent bioassays are those that test exposure pathways of most relevance to predicted or known human exposure pathways. Bioassays for reproductive and developmental toxicity and other noncancer endpoints have a similar rationale.

Consistent features in the design of standard cancer bioassays include testing in two species and both sexes, with 50 animals per dose group and near lifetime exposure. Important choices include the strains of rats and mice, the number of doses, and dose levels (typically 90, 50, and 10 to 25 percent of the maximally tolerated dose [MTD]), and the details of the required histopathology (number of organs to be examined, choice of interim sacrifice pathology, etc.). Positive evidence of chemical carcinogenicity can include increases in number of tumors at a particular organ site, induction of rare tumors, earlier induction (shorter latency) of commonly observed tumors, and/or increases in the total number of observed tumors.

Critical problems exist in using the hazard identification data from rodent bioassays for quantitative risk assessments. This is because of the limited dose–response data available from these rodent bioassays and nonexistent response information for environmentally relevant exposures. Results thus have traditionally been extrapolated from a dose–response curve in the 10 to 100 percent biologically observable tumor response range down to 10^{-6} risk estimates (upper confidence limit) or to a benchmark or reference dose-related risk.

Addition of mechanistic investigations and assessment of multiple noncancer endpoints into the bioassay design represent important enhancements of lifetime bioassays. It is feasible and desirable to tie these bioassays together with mechanistically oriented short-term tests and biomarker and genetic studies in lower doses than those leading to frank tumor development and help address the issues of extrapolation over multiple orders of magnitude to predict response at environmentally relevant doses.

In an attempt to improve the prediction of cancer risk to humans, transgenic mouse models have been developed as possible alternatives to the standard 2-year cancer bioassay. By using mice that incorporate or eliminate a gene that is linked to human cancer, these transgenic models have the power to improve the characterization of key cellular processes and the mode of action of toxicological responses. It is suggested that these models currently should not replace the 2-year assay, but should be used in conjunction to assist in the interpretation of additional toxicologic and mechanistic evidence.

Use of Epidemiologic Data in Risk Assessment—The most convincing line of evidence for human risk is a well-conducted epidemiologic study in which a positive association between exposure and disease has been observed. Table 4–2 shows examples of epidemiologic study designs and provides clues on types of outcomes and exposures evaluated. There are important limitations. When the study is exploratory, hypotheses are often weak. Exposure estimates are often crude and retrospective, especially for conditions with long latency before clinical manifestations appear. Generally, there are multiple exposures, especially when a lifetime is considered. There is always a trade-off between detailed information on relatively few persons and very limited information on large numbers of persons. Contributions from lifestyle factors, such as smoking and diet, are a challenge to sort out. Humans are highly outbred, so the method must consider variation in susceptibility among those who are exposed.

Nevertheless, human epidemiology studies provide very useful information for hazard identification and sometimes quantitative information for data characterization. Three major types of epidemiology study designs are available: cross-sectional studies, cohort studies, and case–control studies (Table 4–2). Cross-sectional studies survey groups of humans to identify risk factors (exposure) and disease but are not useful for establishing cause and effect. Cohort studies evaluate individuals selected on the basis of their exposure to an agent under study. These prospective studies monitor over time individuals who initially are disease-free to determine the rates at which they develop disease. In case–control studies, subjects are selected on the basis of disease status: disease cases and matched cases of disease-free individuals. Exposure histories of the two groups are compared to determine key consistent features in their exposure histories. All case–control studies are retrospective studies.

Epidemiologic findings are judged by the following criteria: strength of association, consistency of observations (reproducibility in time and space), specificity (uniqueness in quality or quantity of response), appropriateness of temporal relationship (did the exposure precede responses?), dose–responsiveness, biological plausibility and coherence, verification, and analogy (biological extrapolation). In addition, epidemiologic study designs should be evaluated for their power of detection, appropriateness of outcomes, verification of exposure assessments, completeness of assessing confounding factors, and general applicability of the outcomes to other populations at risk. Power of detection is calculated using study size, variability, accepted detection limits for endpoints under study, and a specified significance level.

Recent advances from the human genome project, increased sophistication of molecular biomarkers, and improved mechanistic bases for epidemiologic hypotheses have allowed epidemiologists to expand our understanding of biological

TABLE 4-2 Example of three types of epidemiologic study designs.

Methodological Attributes	Type of Study		
	Cohort	Case–Control	Cross-sectional
Initial classification	Exposure–nonexposure	Disease–nondisease	Either one
Time sequence	Prospective	Retrospective	Present time
Sample composition	Nondiseased individuals	Cases and controls	Survivors
Comparison	Proportion of exposed with disease	Proportion of cases with exposure	Either one
Rates	Incidence	Fractional (percent)	Prevalence
Risk index	Relative risk–attributable risk	Relative odds	Prevalence
Advantages	Lack of bias in exposure, yields rates of incidence and risk	Inexpensive, small number of subjects, rapid results, suitable for rare diseases, no attrition	Quick results
Disadvantages	Large number of subjects required, long follow-up, attrition, change in time of criteria and methods, costly, inadequate for rare diseases	Incomplete information, biased recall, problem in selecting control and matching, yields only relative risk—cannot establish causation, population of survivors	Cannot establish causation (antecedent consequence), population of survivors, inadequate for rare diseases

plausibility and clinical relevance. "Molecular epidemiology" with improved molecular biomarkers of exposure, effect, and susceptibility has allowed investigators to more effectively link molecular events in the causative disease pathway. The range of biomarkers has grown dramatically and includes identification of single nucleotide polymorphisms, genomic profiling, transcriptome analysis, and proteomic analysis.

DOSE–RESPONSE ASSESSMENT

Integrating Quantitative Aspects of Risk Assessment

Quantitative considerations in risk assessment include dose–response assessment, exposure assessment, variation in susceptibility, and characterization of uncertainty.

The fundamental basis of the quantitative relationships between exposure to an agent and the incidence of an adverse response is the dose–response assessment. Analysis of dose–response relationships must start with the determination of the critical effects to be quantitatively evaluated. It is usual practice to choose the data sets with adverse effects occurring at the lowest levels of exposure; the "critical" adverse effect is defined as the significant adverse biological effect that occurs at the lowest exposure level.

Threshold Approaches—Threshold dose–response relationships characterization includes identification of "no or lowest observed adverse effect levels" (NOAELs or LOAELs). On the dose–response curve illustrated in Figure 4–3, the threshold, indicated as T, represents the dose below which no

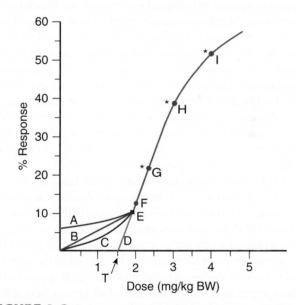

FIGURE 4-3 Dose–response curve. This figure is designed to illustrate a typical dose–response curve with points E to I indicating the biologically determined responses. Statistical significance of these responses is indicated with a "*" symbol. The threshold is shown by T, a dose below which no change in biological response occurs. Point E represents the point of departure (POD), the dose near the lower end of the observed dose–response range, below which extrapolation to lower doses is necessary. Point F is the highest nonstatistical significant response point; hence, it is the "no observed adverse effect level" (NOAEL) for this example. Point G is the "lowest observed adverse effect level" (LOAEL) for this example. Curves A to D show some options for extrapolating the dose–response relationship below the range of biologically observed data points, POD, point E.

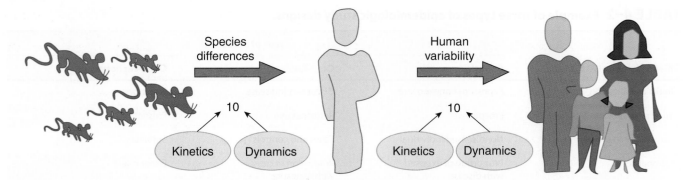

FIGURE 4–4 **Toxicokinetic (TK) and toxicodynamic (TD) considerations inherent in interspecies and interindividual extrapolations.** *Toxicokinetics* refers to the processes of absorption, distribution, elimination, and metabolism of a toxicant. *Toxicodynamics* refers to the actions and interactions of the toxicant within the organism and describes processes at organ, tissue, cellular, and molecular levels. This figure shows how uncertainty in extrapolation both across and within species can be considered as being due to two key factors: a kinetic component and a dynamic component. Refer to the text for detailed explanations.

additional increase in response is observed. The NOAEL is identified as the highest nonstatistically significant dose tested; in this example it is point F, at 2 mg/kg body weight. Point G is the LOAEL (2.5 mg/kg body weight), as it is the lowest dose tested with a statistically significant effect.

In general, animal bioassays are constructed with sufficient numbers of animals to biological responses at the 10 percent response range. *Significance* usually refers to both biological and statistical criteria and is dependent on the number of dose levels tested, the number of animals tested at each dose, and background incidence of the adverse response in the nonexposed control groups. The NOAEL should not be perceived as risk-free.

As described in Chapter 2, approaches for characterizing dose–response relationships include identification of effect levels such as LD_{50} (dose producing 50 percent lethality), LC_{50} (concentration producing 50 percent lethality), ED_{10} (dose producing 10 percent response), as well as NOAELs.

NOAELs have traditionally served as the basis for risk assessment calculations, such as reference doses or acceptable daily intake (ADI) values. References doses (RfDs) or concentrations (RfCs) are estimates of a daily exposure to an agent that is assumed to be without adverse health impact on the human population. ADI values may be defined as the daily intake of chemical during an entire lifetime, which appears to be without appreciable risk on the basis of all known facts at that time. Reference doses and ADI values typically are calculated from NOAEL values by dividing by uncertainty (UF) and/or modifying factors (MF):

$$RfD = \frac{NOAEL}{UF \times MF}$$

$$ADI = \frac{NOAEL}{UF \times MF}$$

Tolerable daily intakes (TDI) can be used to describe intakes for chemicals that are not "acceptable" but are "tolerable" as

they are below levels thought to cause adverse health effects. These are calculated in a manner similar to ADI. In principle, dividing by these factors allows for interspecies (animal-to-human) and intraspecies (human-to-human) variability with default values of 10 each. An additional UF can be used to account for experimental inadequacies—for example, to extrapolate from short-exposure-duration studies to a situation more relevant for chronic study or to account for inadequate numbers of animals or other experimental limitations. If only a LOAEL value is available, then an additional 10-fold factor commonly is used to arrive at a value more comparable to a NOAEL. Traditionally, a safety factor of 100 would be used for RfD calculations to extrapolate from a well-conducted animal bioassay (10-fold factor animal-to-human) and to account for human variability in response (10-fold factor human-to-human variability).

MF can be used to adjust the UF if data on mechanisms, pharmacokinetics, or relevance of the animal response to human risk justify such modification.

Recent efforts have focused on using data-derived factors to replace the 10-fold UF traditionally used in calculating RfDs and ADIs. Such efforts have included reviewing the human pharmacologic literature from published clinical trials and developing human variability databases for a large range of exposures and clinical conditions. Intra- and interspecies UF have two components: toxicokinetic and toxicodynamic aspects. Figure 4–4 shows these distinctions. This approach provides a structure for incorporating scientific information on specific aspects of the overall toxicologic process into the reference dose calculations; thus, relevant data can replace a portion of the overall "uncertainty" surrounding these extrapolations.

The NOAEL approach has been criticized on several points, including that (1) the NOAEL must, by definition, be one of the experimental doses tested; and (2) once this is identified, the rest of the dose–response curve is ignored. Because of these limitations, an alternative to the NOAEL approach, the benchmark dose (BMD) method, was proposed. In this approach, the dose–response is modeled and the lower confidence bound for a dose at a specified response level (benchmark response [BMR]) is calculated. The BMR is usually specified at 1, 5, or 10 percent. The BMD_x (with x representing the percent BMR) is used as an alternative to the NOAEL value for reference dose calculations. Thus, the RfD would be:

$$RfD = \frac{BMD_x}{UF \times MF}$$

The proposed values to be used for the UF and MF for BMDs can range from the same factors as for the NOAEL to lower values due to increased confidence in the response level and increased recognition of experimental variability owing to use of a lower confidence bound on dose.

Advantages of the BMD approach can include (1) the ability to take into account the full dose–response curve; (2) the inclusion of a measure of variability (confidence limit); and (3) the use of a consistent BMR level for RfD calculations across studies. Obviously, limitations in the animal bioassays in regard to minimal test doses for evaluation, shallow dose–responses, and use of study designs with widely spaced test doses will limit the utility of these assays for any type of quantitative assessments, whether NOAEL- or BMD-based approaches.

Nonthreshold Approaches—As Figure 4–3 shows, numerous dose–response curves can be proposed in the low-dose region of the dose–response curve if a threshold assumption is not made. Because the risk assessor generally needs to extrapolate beyond the region of the dose–response curve for which experimentally observed data are available, the choice of models to generate curves in this region has received lots of attention. For nonthreshold responses, methods for dose–response assessments have also utilized models for extrapolation to de minimus (10^{-4} to 10^{-6}) risk levels at very low doses, far below the biologically observed response range and far below the effect levels evaluated for threshold responses. Two general types of dose–response models exist: statistical (or probability distribution models) and mechanistic models.

The distribution models are based on the assumption that each individual has a tolerance level for a test agent and that this response level is a variable following a specific probability distribution function. These responses can be modeled using a cumulative dose–response function. However, extrapolation of the experimental data from 50 percent response levels to a "safe," "acceptable," or "de minimus" level of exposure—for example, one in a million risk above background—illustrates the huge gap between scientific observations and highly protective risk limits (sometimes called *virtually safe doses,* or those corresponding to a 95 percent upper confidence limit on adverse response rates).

Models Derived from Mechanistic Assumptions—This modeling approach designs a mathematical equation to describe dose–response relationships that are consistent with postulated biological mechanisms of response. These models are based on the idea that a response (toxic effect) in a particular biological unit (animal or human) is the result of the random occurrence of one or more biological events (stochastic events).

A series of "hit models" exist for cancer modeling, where a hit is defined as a critical cellular event that must occur before a toxic effect is produced. The simplest mechanistic model is the one-hit (one-stage) linear model in which only one hit or critical cellular interaction is required for a cell to be altered. As theories of cancer have grown in complexity, multihit models have been developed that can describe hypothesized single-target multihit events, as well as multitarget, multihit events in carcinogenesis.

Toxicologic Enhancements of the Models—Three exemplary areas of research that have improved the models used in risk extrapolation are time to tumor information, physiologically based toxicokinetic modeling (described in Chapter 7), and biologically based dose–response (BBDR) modeling. The BBDR model aims to make the generalized mechanistic models discussed in the previous section more clearly reflect specific biological processes. Measured rates are incorporated into the mechanistic equations to replace default or computer-generated values.

Development of BBDR models for endpoints other than cancer is limited; however, several approaches have been explored in developmental toxicity utilizing cell cycle kinetics, enzyme activity, litter effects, and cytotoxicity as critical endpoints. Approaches have been proposed that link pregnancy-specific toxicokinetic models with temporally sensitive toxicodynamic models for developmental impacts. Unfortunately, the lack of specific, quantitative biological information for most toxicants and for most endpoints limits study and utilization of these models.

RISK CHARACTERIZATION

Variation in Susceptibility

Toxicology has been slow to recognize the marked variation among humans. Generally, assay results and toxicokinetic modeling utilize means and standard deviations to measure variation, or even standard errors of the mean, thereby ignoring variability in response due to differences in age, sex, health status, and genetics.

One key challenge for risk assessment will be interpretation and linking of observations from highly sensitive molecular and genome-based methods with the overall process of toxicity. Biomarkers of early effects, like frank clinical pathology, arise as a function of exposure, response, and time. Early, subtle, and possibly reversible effects can generally be distinguished from irreversible disease states.

The challenge for interpretation of early and highly sensitive response biomarkers is made clear in the analysis of data from gene expression arrays. Because our relatively routine ability to monitor gene responses has grown exponentially in the last decade, the need for toxicologists to interpret such observations for risk assessment and the overall process of toxicity has increased with equal or greater intensity.

Microarray analysis for risk assessment requires sophisticated analyses to arrive at a functional interpretation and linkage to a conventional toxicologic endpoint. Because of the vast number of measured responses with gene expression arrays, pattern analysis techniques are being used. The extensive databases across chemical classes, pathological conditions, and stages of disease progression that are essential for these analyses are being developed.

EXPOSURE ASSESSMENT

The primary objectives of exposure assessment are to determine source, type, magnitude, and duration of contact with the agent of interest. Obviously a key element of the risk assessment process, hazard does not occur in the absence of exposure. However, exposure data are frequently identified as the key area of uncertainty in overall risk determination. The primary goal of using exposure information in quantitative risk assessment is not only to determine the type and amount of total exposure, but also to find out specifically how much may be reaching target tissues. A key step in making an exposure assessment is determining what exposure pathways are relevant for the risk scenario under development. The subsequent steps entail quantitation of each pathway identified as a potentially relevant exposure and then summarizing these pathway-specific exposures for calculation of overall exposure.

Additional considerations for exposure assessments include how time and duration of exposures are evaluated in risk assessments. In general, estimates for cancer risk use averages over a lifetime. In a few cases, short-term exposure limits (STELs) are required and characterization of brief but high levels of exposure is required. In these cases exposures are not averaged over the lifetime and the effects of high, short-term doses are estimated. With developmental toxicity, a single exposure can be sufficient to produce an adverse developmental effect; thus, daily doses are used, rather than lifetime weighted averages.

INFORMATION RESOURCES

The Toxicology Data Network (TOXNET) from the National Library of Medicine (http://sis.nlm.nih.gov/) provides access to databases on toxicology, hazardous chemicals, and related areas. These information sources vary in the included level of assessment, ranging from just listings of scientific references without comment to extensive peer-reviewed risk assessment information.

The World Health Organization (http://www.who.int/) provides chemical-specific information through the International Programme on Chemical Safety (http://www.who.int/pcs/

IPCS/index.htm) criteria documents and health and safety documents. The International Agency for Research on Cancer (IARC) provides data on specific classes of carcinogens as well as individual agents. The National Institutes for Environmental Health Sciences (NIEHS) National Toxicology Program provides technical reports on the compounds tested as a part of this national program (http://ehis.niehs.nih.gov/roc/toc9.html).

RISK PERCEPTION AND COMPARATIVE ANALYSES OF RISK

Individuals respond very differently to information about hazardous situations and products, as do communities and whole societies. Understanding these behavioral responses is critical in stimulating constructive risk communication and evaluating potential risk management options. In a classic study, students, League of Women Voters members, active club members, and scientific experts were asked to rank 30 activities or agents in order of their annual contribution to deaths. Club members ranked pesticides, spray cans, and nuclear power as safer than did other lay persons. Students ranked contraceptives and food preservatives as riskier and mountain climbing as safer than did others. Experts ranked electric power, surgery, swimming, and X-rays as more risky and nuclear power and police work as less risky than did lay persons. There are also group differences in perceptions of risk from chemicals among toxicologists, correlated with their employment in industry, academia, or government.

Psychological factors such as dread, perceived uncontrollability, and involuntary exposure interact with factors that represent the extent to which a hazard is familiar, observable, and "essential" for daily living. Figure 4–5 presents a grid on the parameters controllable/uncontrollable and observable/not observable for a large number of risky activities; for each of the two paired main factors, highly correlated factors are described in the boxes.

Public demand for government regulations often focuses on involuntary exposures (especially in the food supply, drinking water, and air) and unfamiliar hazards, such as radioactive waste, electromagnetic fields, asbestos insulation, and genetically modified crops and foods. Many people respond very negatively when they perceive that information about hazards or even about new technologies without reported hazards has been withheld by the manufacturers (genetically modified foods) or by government agencies (HIV-contaminated blood transfusions in the 1980s; extent of hazardous chemical or radioactive wastes).

Most people regularly compare risks of alternative activities—on the job, in recreational pursuits, in interpersonal interactions, and in investments. Determining how best to conduct comparative risk analyses has proved difficult due to the great variety of health and environmental benefits, the gross uncertainties of dollar estimates of benefits and costs, and the different distributions of benefits and costs across the population.

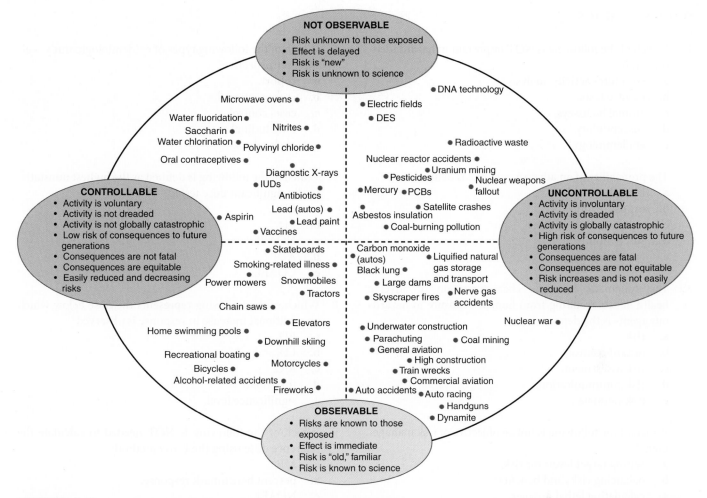

FIGURE 4-5 **Perceptions of risk illustrated using a "risk space" axis diagram.** Risk space has axes that correspond roughly to a hazard's perceived "dreadedness" and to the degree to which it is familiar or observable. Risks in the upper right quadrant of this space are most likely to provoke calls for government regulation.

SUMMARY

The objectives of risk assessments vary with the issues, risk management needs, and statutory requirements. However, the National Research Council and Risk Commission frameworks are sufficiently flexible to address these various objectives, accommodate new knowledge, and provide guidance for priority setting in industry, environmental organizations, and government regulatory and public health agencies. Toxicology, epidemiology, exposure assessment, and clinical observations can be linked with biomarkers, cross-species investigations of mechanisms of effects, and systematic approaches to risk assessment, risk communication, and risk management. Advances in toxicology are certain to improve the quality of risk assessments for a broad array of health endpoints as scientific findings substitute data for assumptions and help to describe and model uncertainty more credibly.

BIBLIOGRAPHY

Cote ML: Study designs in genetic epidemiology. *Methods Mol Biol* 520:247–257, 2009.

EPA: *Guidelines for Carcinogen Risk Assessment (Cancer Guidelines)*. Federal Register Notice, 2005. http://cfpub.epa.gov/ncea/raf/recordisplay.cfm?deid=116283.

Hsieh A: A nation's genes for a cure to cancer: evolving ethical, social and legal issues regarding population genetic databases. *Columbia J Law Soc Probl* 37:259–411, 2004.

Maines MD, Costa LG, Reed DJ, et al (eds): *Current Protocols in Toxicology*. New York: Wiley, 2000.

NRC: *Scientific Frontiers in Developmental Toxicology and Risk Assessment*. Washington, DC: National Research Council, 2000.

Ricci PF: *Environmental and Health Risk Assessment and Management: Principles and Practices*. Dordrecht: Springer, 2006.

Robson M, Toscano W: *Risk Assessment for Environmental Health*. San Francisco: Jossey-Bass, 2007.

Slovic P, Peters E, Finucane ML, Macgregor DG: Affect, risk, and decision making. *Health Psychol* 24:S35–S40, 2005.

QUESTIONS

1. Which of the following is NOT important in hazard identification?
   a. structure–activity analysis.
   b. in vitro tests.
   c. animal bioassays.
   d. susceptibility.
   e. epidemiology.

2. The probability of an adverse outcome is defined as:
   a. hazard.
   b. exposure ratio.
   c. risk.
   d. susceptibility.
   e. epidemiology.

3. The systematic scientific characterization of adverse health effects resulting from human exposure to hazardous agents is the definition of:
   a. risk.
   b. hazard control.
   c. risk assessment.
   d. risk communication.
   e. risk estimate.

4. Which of the following is not an objective of risk management?
   a. setting target levels for risk.
   b. balancing risks and benefits.
   c. calculating lethal dosages.
   d. setting priorities for manufacturers.
   e. estimating residual risks.

5. Which of the following is NOT a feature in the design of standard cancer bioassays?
   a. more than one species.
   b. both sexes.
   c. near lifetime exposure.
   d. approximately 50 animals per dose group.
   e. same dose level for all groups.

6. Which of the following types of epidemiologic study is always retrospective?
   a. cohort.
   b. cross-sectional.
   c. case–control.
   d. longitudinal.
   e. exploratory.

7. Which of the following is defined as the highest nonstatistically significant dose tested?
   a. ED_{50}.
   b. ED_{100}.
   c. NOAEL.
   d. ADI.
   e. COAEL.

8. Which of the following represents the dose below which no additional increase in response is observed?
   a. ED_{10}.
   b. LD_{10}.
   c. RfC.
   d. threshold.
   e. significance level.

9. Which of the following is NOT needed to calculate the reference dose using the BMD method?
   a. MF.
   b. percent benchmark response.
   c. NOAEL.
   d. UF.
   e. benchmark dose.

10. Virtually safe doses are described at which confidence level?
    a. 90 percent.
    b. 95 percent.
    c. 99 percent.
    d. 99.9 percent.
    e. 99.99 percent.

C H A P T E R

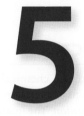

Absorption, Distribution, and Excretion of Toxicants

Lois D. Lehman-McKeeman

INTRODUCTION

The disposition of a chemical or *xenobiotic* is defined as the composite actions of its *absorption, distribution, biotransformation,* and *elimination.* The quantitative characterization of xenobiotic disposition is termed *pharmacokinetics* or *toxicokinetics* (see Chapter 7).

The toxicity of a substance depends on the dose. The concentration of a chemical at the site of action is usually proportional to the dose, but the same dose of two or more chemicals may lead to vastly different concentrations in a particular target organ of toxicity owing to differences in the disposition of the chemicals. Various factors affecting disposition are depicted in Figure 5–1. For example, (1) if the fraction absorbed or the rate of absorption

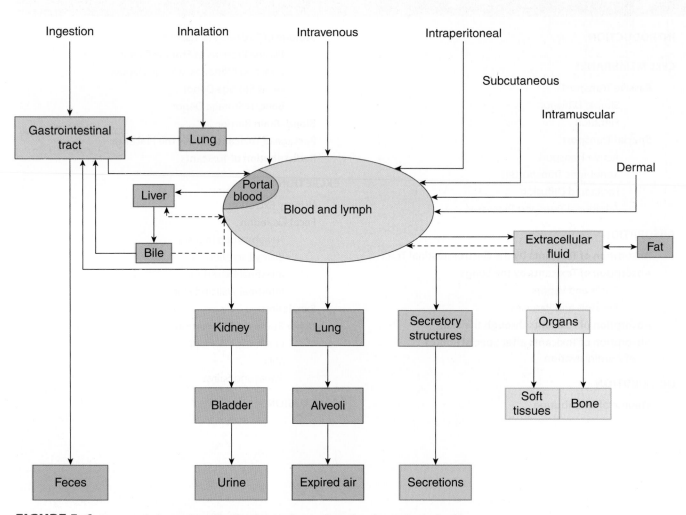

FIGURE 5–1 Routes of absorption, distribution, and excretion of toxicants in the body.

is low, a chemical may never attain a sufficiently high concentration at a potential site of action to cause toxicity, (2) the distribution of a toxicant may be such that it is concentrated in a tissue other than the target organ, thus decreasing toxicity, (3) biotransformation of a chemical may result in the formation of less toxic or more toxic metabolites at a fast or slow rate with obvious consequences for the concentration and thus the toxicity at the target site, and (4) the more rapidly a chemical is eliminated from an organism, the lower will be its concentration and hence its toxicity in target tissues. If a chemical is distributed to and stored in fat, its elimination is likely to be slow because very low plasma levels preclude rapid renal clearance or other clearances.

The skin, lungs, and alimentary canal are the main barriers that separate higher organisms from an environment containing a large number of chemicals. Exceptions are caustic and corrosive agents (acids, bases, salts, and oxidizers) that act topically. A chemical absorbed into the bloodstream through any of these three barriers is distributed throughout the body, including the site where it produces damage, the *target organ* or *target tissue*. A chemical may have one or several target organs. Because several factors other than the concentration influence the susceptibility of organs to toxicants, the organ or tissue with the highest concentration of a toxicant is not necessarily the site of toxicity.

CELL MEMBRANES

Toxicants usually pass through the membranes of a number of cells, such as the stratified epithelium of skin, the thin cell layers of lungs or gastrointestinal tract, the capillary endothelium, and the cells of the target organ or tissue. Proteins are inserted in the bilayer, and some proteins even cross it, allowing the formation of aqueous pores. A toxicant may pass through a membrane by either: (1) passive transport, in which the cell expends no energy, or (2) specialized transport, in which the cell provides energy to translocate the toxicant across its membrane.

Passive Transport

Simple Diffusion—Most toxicants cross membranes by simple diffusion. Small hydrophilic molecules (up to a molecular weight of about 600) permeate membranes through aqueous pores, in a process termed *paracellular diffusion*, whereas hydrophobic molecules diffuse across the lipid domain of membranes. The majority of toxicants are larger organic molecules of differing lipid solubility. Their rate of transport across membranes correlates with their lipid solubility. The log of the octanol/water partition coefficient is an informative physicochemical parameter relative to assessing potential membrane permeability, with positive values associated with high lipid solubility.

The ionized form of weak organic acids or bases usually has low lipid solubility and does not permeate readily through the lipid domain of a membrane. In contrast, the nonionized form is more lipid soluble and diffuses across membranes at a rate that is proportional to its lipid solubility. The pH at which a weak organic acid or base is 50 percent ionized is called its pK_a or pK_b. Like pH, both pK_a and pK_b are defined as the negative logarithm

of the ionization constant of a weak organic acid or base. With the equation $pK_a = 14 - pK_b$, pK_a can also be calculated for weak organic bases. An organic acid with a low pK_a is a relatively strong acid, and one with a high pK_a is a weak acid. The opposite is true for bases. Knowledge of the chemical structure is required to distinguish between organic acids and bases, as the numerical value of pK_a does not indicate this characteristic.

The degree of ionization of a chemical depends on its pK_a and on the pH of the solution. The relationship between pK_a and pH is described by the Henderson–Hasselbalch equations:

$$\text{For acids: } pK_a - pH = \log \frac{[\text{nonionized}]}{[\text{ionized}]}$$

$$\text{For bases: } pK_a - pH = \log \frac{[\text{ionized}]}{[\text{nonionized}]}$$

Filtration—When water flows in bulk across a porous membrane, any solute small enough to pass through the pores flows with it. Passage through these channels is called *filtration*. One of the main differences between various membranes is the size of these channels. In the renal glomeruli, a primary site of filtration, these pores allow molecules smaller than albumin (approximately 60 kDa) to pass through. The channels in most cells are much smaller, permitting substantial passage of molecules with molecular weights of no more than a few hundred daltons.

Special Transport

Active Transport—Active transport is characterized by: (1) movement of chemicals against electrochemical or concentration gradients, (2) saturability at high substrate concentrations, thus exhibiting a transport maximum (T_m), (3) selectivity for certain structural features of chemicals, (4) competitive inhibition by chemical antagonists or compounds that are carried by the same transporter, and (5) requirement for expenditure of energy, so that metabolic inhibitors block the transport process.

Xenobiotic Transporters—Around 5 percent of all human genes are transporter related, indicating the importance of transport function in normal biological and toxicologic outcomes. Xenobiotic transporters can be divided into two categories: (1) active, energy-dependent transporters of the large superfamily known as ATP-binding cassette (ABC) transporters and (2) solute carriers (SLCs) that predominantly function through facilitative diffusion (Table 5–1).

The multidrug-resistant (mdr) proteins/p-glycoproteins and the multiresistant drug proteins (mrp) both exude chemicals out of cells; however, phase II metabolites (glucuronides and glutathione conjugates) appear to be their preferred substrates. The name *organic-anion transporting peptide (oatp) family* is a misnomer because this transporter family transports not only acids, but also bases and neutral compounds, and is important in the hepatic uptake of xenobiotics. In contrast, the organic-anion transporter (oat) family is especially important in the renal uptake of anions, whereas the organic-cation transporter

TABLE 5-1 **Major transporters involved in xenobiotic disposition.**

Abbreviation	Name	Function
Active transporters (ABC family)		
mdr1/P-gp	Multidrug-resistant protein/P-glycoprotein	Efflux from gut, brain, and placenta; biliary excretion
bsep	Bile salt export pump	Bile salt transport
mrp	Multidrug resistance-associated proteins	Multidrug resistance in many tissues, organic-anion efflux, glucuronide, and glutathione conjugates, nucleoside transport
BCRP	Breast cancer resistance protein	Organic-anion efflux, mainly sulfate conjugates
Facilitated transporters (SLC family)		
oatp	Organic-anion transporting polypeptide	Transport of organic anions, cations, and neutral compounds (Na^+ independent)
oat	Organic-anion transporter	Transport of organic anions, predominantly in kidney
oct	Organic-cation transporter	Transport of organic cations, predominantly in kidney and liver
pept	Peptide transporter	Transport of di- and tripeptides, some xenobiotics

(oct) family is important in both the renal and hepatic uptake of xenobiotics. The nucleotide transporter (nt) family, the divalent-metal ion transporter (dmt), and the peptide transporter (pept) aid in gastrointestinal absorption of nucleotides, metals, and di- and tripeptides.

Facilitated Diffusion—Facilitated diffusion is carrier-mediated transport that exhibits the properties of active transport except that the substrate is not moved against an electrochemical or concentration gradient and the transport process does not require the input of energy. As noted earlier, octs, which function in the uptake of organic cations in the liver and kidney, mediate movement by facilitated diffusion.

Additional Transport Processes—Other forms of specialized transport, including phagocytosis and pinocytosis, are proposed mechanisms for cell membranes flowing around and engulfing particles.

ABSORPTION

The process by which toxicants cross body membranes and enter the bloodstream is referred to as *absorption*. The main sites of absorption are the GI tract, lungs, and skin. Enteral administration includes all routes pertaining to the alimentary canal (sublingual, oral, and rectal), whereas parenteral administration involves all other routes (intravenous, intraperitoneal, intramuscular, subcutaneous, etc.).

Absorption of Toxicants by the Gastrointestinal Tract

The GI tract is one of the most important sites of toxicant absorption. Many environmental toxicants enter the food chain and are absorbed together with food from the GI tract.

The GI tract may be viewed as a tube traversing the body. Although within the body, GI contents can be considered exterior to the body. Unless a noxious agent has caustic or irritating properties, poisons in the GI tract usually do not produce systemic injury to an individual until they are absorbed.

Absorption of toxicants can take place along the entire GI tract, even in the mouth and rectum. If a toxicant is an organic acid or base, it tends to be absorbed by simple diffusion in the part of the GI tract in which it exists in the most lipid-soluble (nonionized) form. Factors such as the mass action law, surface area, and blood flow rate also influence the absorption of weak organic acids or bases.

The mammalian GI tract has specialized transport systems (carrier mediated) for the absorption of nutrients and electrolytes (Table 5–2). The GI tract also has at least one active transport system that decreases the absorption of xenobiotics. The mdr (also termed p-glycoprotein) is localized in enterocytes. When chemicals that are substrates for mdr enter the enterocyte, they are exuded back into the intestinal lumen.

The number of toxicants actively absorbed by the GI tract is low; most enter the body by simple diffusion. Lipid-soluble substances are absorbed by this process more rapidly and extensively than are water-soluble substances.

TABLE 5–2 Site distribution of specialized transport systems in the intestine of man and animals.

Substrates	Location of Absorptive Capacity in Small Intestine			
	Upper	Middle	Lower	Colon
Sugar (glucose, galactose, etc.)	++	+++	++	0
Neutral amino acids	++	+++	++	0
Basic amino acids	++	++	++	?
Gamma globulin (newborn animals)	+	++	+++	?
Pyrimidines (thymine and uracil)	+	+	?	?
Triglycerides	++	++	+	?
Fatty acid absorption and conversion to triglyceride	+++	++	+	0
Bile salts	0	+	+++	
Vitamin B_{12}	0	+	+++	0
Na^+	+++	++	+++	+++
H^+ (and/or HCO_3^- secretion)	0	+	++	++
Ca^{2+}	+++	++	+	?
Fe^{2+}	+++	++	+	?
Cl^-	+++	++	+	0

Particulate matter can also be absorbed by the GI epithelium. In this case, particle size determines absorption rate and lipid solubility and ionization characteristics are less important. Particle size is inversely related to absorption rate.

The resistance or lack of resistance of chemicals to alteration by the acidic pH of the stomach, enzymes of the stomach or intestine, or the intestinal flora is of extreme importance. Simple diffusion is proportional not only to surface area of villi and microvilli and permeability, but also to residency time in various segments of the alimentary canal. Therefore, the rate of absorption of a toxicant remaining for longer periods in the intestine increases, whereas that with a shorter residency time decreases. The residency time of a chemical in the intestine depends on intestinal motility.

Experiments have shown that the oral toxicity of some chemicals is increased by diluting the dose. This phenomenon may be explained by more rapid stomach emptying induced by increased dosage volume, which in turn leads to more rapid absorption in the duodenum because of the larger surface area there.

The absorption of a toxicant from the GI tract also depends on the physical properties of a compound, such as lipid solubility, and the dissolution rate. An increase in lipid solubility typically increases the absorption of chemicals and the dissolution rate is inversely proportional to particle size.

The amount of a chemical entering the systemic circulation after oral administration depends on the amount absorbed into the GI cells, biotransformation by the GI cells, and extraction by the liver into bile. Transporters can influence this amount by affecting the uptake or efflux from the cells. This phenomenon of the removal of chemicals before entrance into the systemic circulation is referred to as *presystemic elimination,* or *first-pass effect.*

Absorptive differences between species may be due to differences in absorptive capabilities among animals because absorption sometimes depends on previous biotransformation by GI bacteria. Anatomical considerations such as relative surface area of the GI tract, differences in gastrointestinal flora, and pH differences can help explain the between-species variability.

Absorption of Toxicants by the Lungs

Toxicants absorbed by the lungs are usually gases, vapors of volatile or volatilizable liquids, and aerosols.

Gases and Vapors—The absorption of inhaled gases takes place mainly in the lungs. However, before a gas reaches the lungs, it passes through the nose, with its turbinates, which increase the surface area. Because the mucosa of the nose is covered by a film of fluid, gas molecules can be retained by the nose and not reach the lungs if they are very water soluble or react with cell surface components. Therefore, the nose acts as a "scrubber" for water-soluble gases and highly reactive gases.

When a gas is inhaled into the lungs, gas molecules diffuse from the alveolar space into the blood and then dissolve until gas molecules in blood are in equilibrium with gas molecules in the alveolar space. At equilibrium, the ratio of the concentration of chemical in the blood and chemical in the gas phase is constant. This solubility ratio is called the *blood-to-gas partition coefficient*. This constant is unique for each gas. When equilibrium is reached, the rate of transfer of gas molecules from the alveolar space to blood equals the rate of removal by blood from the alveolar space.

The rate of absorption of gases in the lungs is variable and depends on a toxicant's solubility ratio (concentration in blood/concentration in gas phase before or at saturation) at equilibrium. For gases with a very low solubility ratio, the rate of transfer depends mainly on blood flow through the lungs (perfusion-limited), whereas for gases with a high solubility ratio, it is primarily a function of the rate and depth of respiration (ventilation-limited).

The blood carries dissolved gas molecules to the rest of the body. In each tissue, gas molecules are transferred from the blood to the tissue until equilibrium is reached. After releasing part of the gas to tissues, blood returns to the lungs to take up more of the gas. The process continues until a gas reaches equilibrium between blood and each tissue. At this time, no net absorption of gas takes place as long as the exposure concentration remains constant, because a steady state has been reached. Of course, if biotransformation and excretion occur, alveolar absorption will continue until a corresponding steady state is established. The lung can also potentially contribute to the biotransformation or elimination of chemicals before their entrance into the systemic circulation.

Aerosols and Particles—The major characteristics that affect absorption after exposure to aerosols are the aerosol size and water solubility of any chemical present in the aerosol. The site of deposition of aerosols depends largely on the size of the particles. In general, the smaller the particle, the further into the respiratory tree the particle will deposit. Particles 5 μm or larger usually are deposited in the nasopharyngeal region (Figure 5–2) and are removed by nose wiping, blowing, or sneezing. The mucous blanket of the ciliated nasal surface propels insoluble particles by the movement of the cilia. These particles and particles inhaled through the mouth are swallowed within minutes. Soluble particles may dissolve in the mucus and be carried to the pharynx or may be absorbed through the nasal epithelium into blood.

Particles approximately 2.5 μm are deposited mainly in the tracheobronchiolar regions of the lungs, from which they are cleared by retrograde movement of the mucus layer in the ciliated portions of the respiratory tract. Particles eventually may be swallowed and absorbed from the GI tract. Toxicants or viral infections that damage cilia may impair the efficiency of this process.

Particles 1 μm and smaller penetrate to the alveolar sacs of the lungs. They may be absorbed into blood or cleared through the lymphatics after being scavenged by alveolar macrophages.

As particle size decreases, the number of potential particles in a unit of space increases along with the total surface area of

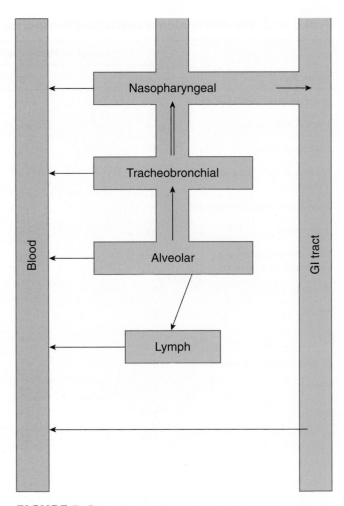

FIGURE 5–2 **Schematic diagram of the absorption and translocation of chemicals by lungs.**

the particles. This relationship indicates that nanoparticles have the propensity to deliver a high amount of particulate to the lungs. If the particulate is toxic, the severity of response could be related to particle size.

Removal or absorption of particulate matter from the alveoli appears to occur by three major mechanisms. First, particles may be removed from the alveoli by a physical process. It is thought that particles deposited on the fluid layer of the alveoli are aspirated onto the mucociliary escalator of the tracheobronchial region. From there, they are transported to the mouth and may be swallowed. Second, particles from the alveoli may be removed via phagocytosis by the alveolar macrophages. These cells are found in large numbers in normal lungs and contain many phagocytized particles of both exogenous and endogenous origin. They migrate to the distal end of the mucociliary escalator and are cleared and eventually swallowed. Third, removal may occur via the lymphatics, although particulates may remain in lymphatic tissue for long time periods.

The overall removal of particles from the alveoli is relatively inefficient; on the first day only about 20 percent of particles are cleared, and the portion remaining longer than 24 h is

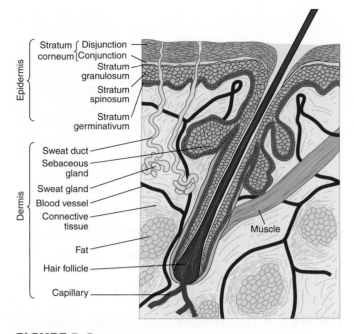

FIGURE 5–3 Diagram of a cross-section of human skin.

cleared very slowly. The rate of clearance by the lungs can be predicted by a compound's solubility in lung fluids. The lower the solubility, the lower is the removal rate.

Absorption of Toxicants through the Skin

Human skin comes into contact with many toxic agents. Fortunately, the skin is not very permeable and therefore is a relatively good barrier for separating organisms from their environment. However, some chemicals can be absorbed by the skin in sufficient quantities to produce systemic effects.

To be absorbed through the skin, a toxicant must pass through the epidermis or the appendages (sweat and sebaceous glands and hair follicles). Chemicals that are absorbed through the skin have to pass through seven cell layers before entering the blood and lymph capillaries in the dermis (Figure 5–3). The rate-determining barrier in the dermal absorption of chemicals is the stratum corneum, the uppermost layer of the epidermis with densely packed keratinized cells that have lost their nuclei and thus are biologically inactive.

All toxicants move across the stratum corneum by passive diffusion. Polar substances appear to diffuse through the outer surface of protein filaments of the hydrated stratum corneum, whereas nonpolar molecules dissolve in and diffuse through the lipid matrix between the protein filaments. The permeability of the skin depends on both the diffusivity and the thickness of the stratum corneum. For example, the stratum corneum is much thicker on the palms and soles (400 to 600 μm in callous areas) than on the arms, back, legs, and abdomen (8 to 15 μm).

Percutaneous absorption also consists of diffusion of the toxicant through the lower layers of the epidermis (stratum granulosum, spinosum, and germinativum) and the dermis.

These cell layers, which are far inferior to the stratum corneum as a barrier, contain a porous, nonselective, aqueous diffusion medium. Toxicants pass through this area by diffusion and enter the systemic circulation through the numerous venous and lymphatic capillaries in the dermis.

Several factors that can increase the absorption of toxicants through the skin include (1) compromised stratum corneum integrity, (2) increased stratum corneum hydration, (3) increased temperature, which increases dermal blood flow, (4) low solubility of toxicant in the vehicle, and (5) small size. The small size of nanoparticles will potentially increase penetration and systemic exposures to these small molecules.

Absorption of Toxicants after Special Routes of Administration

Besides absorption through the skin, lungs, or GI tract, chemical agents can be administered to laboratory animals by special routes, including (1) intraperitoneal, (2) subcutaneous, (3) intramuscular, and (4) intravenous. The intravenous route introduces the toxicant directly into the bloodstream, eliminating the process of absorption. Intraperitoneal injection results in rapid absorption of xenobiotics because of the rich blood supply and the relatively large surface area of the peritoneal cavity. Intraperitoneally administered compounds are absorbed primarily through the portal circulation and therefore must pass through the liver before reaching other organs by way of systemic circulation. Subcutaneously and intramuscularly administered toxicants are usually absorbed at slower rates but enter directly into the general circulation.

The toxicity of a chemical may or may not depend on the route of administration. If a toxicant is injected intraperitoneally, the compound may be completely extracted and biotransformed by the liver with subsequent excretion into the bile without gaining access to the systemic circulation. Any toxicant displaying the first-pass effect with selective toxicity for an organ other than the liver and GI tract is expected to be less toxic when administered intraperitoneally than when injected intravenously, intramuscularly, or subcutaneously because of extraction in the liver.

DISTRIBUTION

After entering the blood, a toxicant may distribute throughout the body. The rate of distribution to organs or tissues is determined primarily by blood flow and the rate of diffusion out of the capillary bed into the cells of a particular organ or tissue. The final distribution depends largely on the affinity of a xenobiotic for various tissues.

Volume of Distribution

Total body water may be divided into three distinct compartments: (1) plasma water, (2) interstitial water, and (3) intracellular water. Extracellular water is made up of plasma water plus interstitial water. The concentration of a toxicant in blood depends largely on its volume of distribution (Vd). Vd is the volume in which the amount of drug would need to be uniformly dissolved in order to produce the observed blood concentration. A high concentration would be observed in the plasma if the chemical were distributed into plasma water only, and a much lower concentration would be reached if it were distributed into a large pool, such as total body water.

Distribution of toxicants is usually complex, and binding to and/or dissolution in various storage sites of the body, such as fat, liver, and bone, are critical factors in determining the distribution of chemicals.

Some toxicants do not readily cross cell membranes and therefore have restricted distribution, whereas other toxicants rapidly pass through cell membranes and are distributed throughout the body. Some toxicants accumulate in certain parts of the body as a result of protein binding, active transport, or high solubility in fat. The site of accumulation of a toxicant may also be its site of major toxic action, but more often it is not. If a toxicant accumulates at a site other than the target organ or tissue, the accumulation may be viewed as a protective process in that plasma levels and consequently the concentration of a toxicant at the site of action are diminished. However, because any chemical in a storage depot is in equilibrium with the free fraction of toxicant in plasma, it is released into the circulation as the unbound fraction of toxicant is eliminated.

Storage of Toxicants in Tissues

Since only the free fraction of a chemical is in equilibrium throughout the body, binding to or dissolving in certain body constituents greatly alters the distribution of a xenobiotic. Toxicants are often concentrated in a specific tissue, which may or may not be their site of toxic action. As a chemical is biotransformed or excreted from the body, more is released from the storage site. As a result, the biological half-life of stored compounds can be very long.

Plasma Proteins as Storage Depot—Several plasma proteins bind xenobiotics as well as some physiologic constituents of the body. As depicted in Figure 5–4, albumin, transferrin, globulins, and lipoproteins can bind a large number of different compounds.

Protein–ligand interactions occur primarily as a result of hydrophobic forces, hydrogen bonding, and van der Waals forces. Because of their high molecular weight, plasma proteins and the toxicants bound to them cannot cross capillary walls. Consequently, the fraction of toxicant bound to plasma proteins is not immediately available for distribution into the extravascular space or filtration by the kidneys. However, the interaction of a chemical with plasma proteins is a reversible process. As unbound chemical diffuses out of capillaries, bound chemical dissociates from the protein until the free fraction reaches equilibrium between the vascular space and the extravascular space. In turn, diffusion in the extravascular space to sites more distant from the capillaries continues, and the resulting

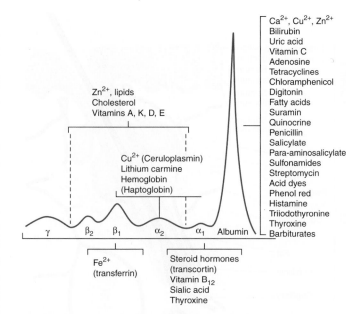

FIGURE 5–4 Ligand interactions with plasma proteins.

concentration gradient causes continued dissociation of the bound fraction in plasma.

Toxicity is typically manifested by the amount of a xenobiotic that is unbound. Severe toxic reactions can occur if a toxicant is displaced from plasma proteins by another agent, increasing the free fraction of the toxicant in plasma. This will result in an increased equilibrium concentration of the toxicant in the target organ, with the potential for toxicity. Xenobiotics can also compete with and displace endogenous compounds that are bound to plasma proteins.

Liver and Kidney as Storage Depots—The liver and kidney have a high capacity for binding a multitude of chemicals. These two organs probably concentrate more toxicants than do all the other organs combined. Proteins such as ligandin and metallothionein have a high affinity for many organic compounds and metals, respectively.

Fat as Storage Depot—Many highly lipophilic toxicants with a high lipid/water partition coefficient are distributed and concentrated in body fat. Storage lowers the concentration of the toxicant in the target organ; therefore, the toxicity of such a compound can be expected to be less severe in an obese person than in a lean individual. However, the possibility of a sudden increase in the concentration of a chemical in the blood and thus in the target organ of toxicity when rapid mobilization of fat occurs must be considered. Several studies have shown that signs of intoxication can be produced by short-term starvation of experimental animals that were previously exposed to persistent organochlorine insecticides.

Bone as Storage Depot—Skeletal uptake of xenobiotics is essentially a surface chemistry phenomenon, with exchange taking place between the bone surface of hydroxyapatite crystals and the extracellular fluid in contact with it. Deposition and reversible storage of toxicants in bone is dynamic and may or may not be detrimental. Lead is not toxic to bone, but the chronic effects of fluoride deposition (skeletal fluorosis) and radioactive strontium (osteosarcoma and other neoplasms) are well documented.

Blood–Brain Barrier

The blood–brain barrier (BBB), though not an absolute barrier to the passage of toxic agents into the CNS, is less permeable than most other areas of the body. There are four major anatomical and physiologic reasons why some toxicants do not readily enter the CNS. First, the capillary endothelial cells of the CNS are tightly joined, leaving few or no pores between the cells. Second, the brain capillary endothelial cells contain an ATP-dependent mdr protein that exudes some chemicals back into the blood. Third, the capillaries in the CNS are to a large extent surrounded by glial cell processes (astrocytes). Fourth, the protein concentration in the interstitial fluid of the CNS is much lower than that in other body fluids, limiting the movement of water-insoluble compounds by paracellular transport, which is possible in a largely aqueous medium only when such compounds are bound to proteins.

In general, only the free unbound toxicant equilibrates rapidly with the brain. Lipid solubility and the degree of ionization are important determinants of the rate of entry of a compound into the CNS. Increased lipid solubility enhances the rate of penetration of toxicants into the CNS, whereas ionization greatly diminishes it. A few xenobiotics appear to enter the brain by carrier-mediated processes.

Active transport processes decrease the concentration of xenobiotics in the brain. Endothelial cells of the brain contain several members of the active and facilitated transporter families (P-gp, BCRP, mrp1, and mrp2) that are responsible for transporting some chemicals from endothelial cells back into the blood (Table 5–1). Some lipophilic compounds may enter the brain, but are so efficiently removed by these transporters that they never reach appreciable concentrations.

The BBB is not fully developed at birth, and this is one reason why some chemicals are more toxic to newborns than to adults.

Passage of Toxicants across the Placenta

Many foreign substances can cross the placenta. In addition to chemicals, viruses (e.g., rubella virus), cellular pathogens (e.g., syphilis spirochetes), and globulin antibodies can traverse the placenta. In this regard, the placental barrier is not as precise an anatomical unit as the BBB. Anatomically, the placental barrier consists of a number of cell layers—at most six—interposed between the fetal and maternal circulations. The placenta contains active transport systems and biotransformation enzymes. These help protect the fetus from some xenobiotics while regulating the movement of essential nutrients.

Among the substances that cross the placenta by passive diffusion, more lipid-soluble substances attain a maternal–fetal equilibrium more rapidly. Under steady-state conditions, the concentrations of a toxic compound in the plasma of the mother and fetus are usually the same. The concentration in the various tissues of the fetus depends on the ability of fetal tissue to concentrate a toxicant. Differential body composition between mother and fetus may be another reason for an apparent placental barrier. For example, fetuses have very little fat; hence, they do not accumulate highly lipophilic chemicals.

Redistribution of Toxicants

The most critical factors that affect the distribution of xenobiotics are the organ blood flow and its affinity for a xenobiotic. The initial phase of distribution is determined primarily by blood flow to the various parts of the body. Therefore, a well-perfused organ such as the liver may attain high initial concentrations of a xenobiotic. However, chemicals may have a high affinity for a binding site (e.g., intracellular protein or bone matrix) or to a cellular constituent (e.g., fat), and, with time, will redistribute to these high-affinity sites.

EXCRETION

Toxicants are eliminated from the body by several routes. Many xenobiotics, though, have to be biotransformed to more water-soluble products before they can be excreted into urine (Chapter 6). All body secretions appear to have the ability to excrete chemicals; toxicants have been found in sweat, saliva, tears, and milk.

Urinary Excretion

Toxic compounds are excreted into urine by the same mechanisms the kidney uses to remove end products of intermediary metabolism from the body: glomerular filtration, tubular excretion by passive diffusion, and active tubular secretion. Compounds up to a molecular weight of about 60 kDa are filtered at the glomeruli. The degree of plasma protein binding affects the rate of filtration, because protein–xenobiotic complexes are too large to pass through the pores of the glomeruli.

A toxicant filtered at the glomeruli may remain in the tubular lumen and be excreted with urine or may be reabsorbed across the tubular cells of the nephron back into the bloodstream. Toxicants with a high lipid/water partition coefficient are reabsorbed efficiently, whereas polar compounds and ions are excreted with urine.

Xenobiotics can also be excreted into urine by active secretion. Figure 5–5 illustrates the various families of transporters in the kidney. The oat family is localized on the basolateral membranes of the proximal tubule. The oct family is responsible for the renal uptake of some cations. Once xenobiotics are in the tubular cell, they are exuded into the lumen by mdr protein and by mrp. In contrast, the octn2 and PEP2 reabsorb chemicals from the tubular lumen. Some less polar xenobiotics may diffuse into the lumen. In contrast to filtration, protein-bound toxicants are available to active transport. Uric acid is secreted by a unique oat, URAT1, in the renal tubules.

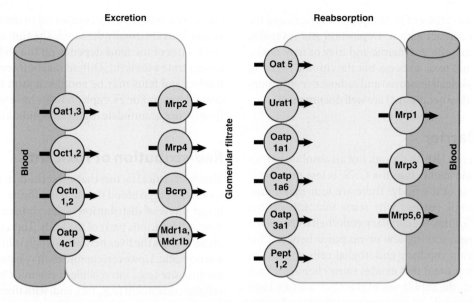

FIGURE 5–5 **Schematic model showing the transport systems in the proximal tubule of the kidney.** The families of transporters are organic-anion transporters (oat), organic-cation transporters (oct), multidrug-resistant protein (mdr), multiresistant drug protein (mrp), peptide transporters (PEP), and urate transporter (URAT).

Because many functions of the kidney are incompletely developed at birth, some xenobiotics are eliminated more slowly in newborns than in adults and therefore may be more toxic to newborns. For example, the clearance of penicillin by premature infants is only 20 percent of that observed in older children. The development of this organic acid transport system in newborns can be stimulated by the administration of substances normally excreted by this transporter.

The renal proximal tubule reabsorbs small plasma proteins that are filtered at the glomerulus. A toxicant binding those small proteins can be carried into the proximal tubule cells and exert toxicity.

Fecal Excretion

Fecal excretion is the other major pathway for the elimination of xenobiotics from the body.

Nonabsorbed Ingesta—In addition to indigestible material, varying proportions of nutrients and xenobiotics that are present in food or are ingested voluntarily (drugs) pass through the alimentary canal unabsorbed, contributing to fecal excretion.

Biliary Excretion—The biliary route of elimination is perhaps the most important contributing source to the fecal excretion of xenobiotics and their metabolites. The liver removes toxic agents from blood after absorption from the GI tract, because blood from the GI tract passes through the liver before reaching the general circulation. Thus, the liver can extract compounds from blood and prevent their distribution to other parts of the body. Furthermore, the liver is the main site of biotransformation of toxicants, and the metabolites thus formed may be excreted directly into bile. Xenobiotics and/or their metabolites entering

the intestine with bile may be excreted with feces or undergo an enterohepatic circulation.

Figure 5–6 illustrates the many transporters localized on hepatic parenchymal cells that move foreign substances from plasma into liver and from liver into bile. Biliary excretion is regulated predominantly by xenobiotic transporters present on the canalicular membrane. Sodium-dependent taurocholate peptide (ntcp) present on the sinusoidal side of the parenchymal cell transports bile acids such as taurocholate into the liver, whereas the bile salt excretory protein (bsep) transports bile acids out of the liver cell into the bile canaliculi. The sinusoidal membrane of the hepatocyte has a number of transporters including organic-anion transporting polypeptide (oatp) 1 and 2, and oct that move xenobiotics into the liver. Once inside the hepatocyte, the xenobiotic itself can be transported into the blood or bile, or be biotransformed by phase I and II drug-metabolizing enzymes to more water-soluble products that are then transported into the bile or back into the blood. Multidrug-resistant protein one (mdr1) and multiresistant drug protein two (mrp2) are responsible for transporting xenobiotics into bile, whereas mrp3 and mrp6 transport xenobiotics back into the blood.

An important concept relating to biliary excretion is the phenomenon of enterohepatic circulation. Once a compound is excreted into bile and enters the intestine, it can be reabsorbed or eliminated with feces. Many organic compounds are conjugated before excretion into bile. Such polar metabolites are not sufficiently lipid soluble to be reabsorbed. However, intestinal microflora may hydrolyze glucuronide and sulfate conjugates, making them sufficiently lipophilic for reabsorption and enterohepatic cycling. This principle has been utilized in the treatment of dimethylmercury poisoning; ingestion of a polythiol resin binds the mercury and thus prevents its reabsorption and cycling.

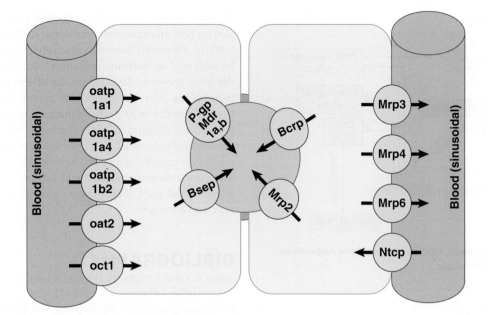

FIGURE 5–6   Schematic model showing the transport systems in the liver. oatp = organic-anion transporting polypeptide, oct = organic-cation transporter, bsep = bile salt excretory protein, mdr = multidrug-resistant protein, mrp = multiresistant drug protein, BCRP = breast cancer resistance protein, and ntcp = sodium-dependent taurocholate peptide.

Intestinal Excretion—Many chemicals in feces directly transfer from blood into the intestinal contents by passive diffusion. In some instances, rapid exfoliation of intestinal cells may contribute to the fecal excretion of some compounds. Intestinal excretion is a relatively slow process that is a major pathway of elimination only for compounds that have low rates of biotransformation and/or low renal or biliary clearance.

Intestinal Wall and Flora—Mucosal biotransformation and reexcretion into the intestinal lumen occur with many compounds. It has been estimated that 30 to 42 percent of fecal dry matter originates from bacteria. Moreover, a considerable proportion of fecally excreted xenobiotic is associated with excreted bacteria. However, chemicals may be profoundly altered by bacteria before excretion with feces. It seems that biotransformation by intestinal flora favors reabsorption rather than excretion. Nevertheless, there is evidence that in many instances xenobiotics found in feces derive from bacterial biotransformation.

Exhalation

Substances that exist predominantly in the gas phase at body temperature and volatile liquids are eliminated mainly by the lungs. A practical application of this principle is seen in the breath analyzer test for determining the amount of ethanol in the body.

No specialized transport systems have been described for the excretion of toxic substances by the lungs. Some xenobiotic transporters, including mrp1 and P-gp, have been identified in the lung, but overall, compounds seem to be eliminated by simple

diffusion. Elimination of gases is roughly inversely proportional to the rate of their absorption. The rate of elimination of a gas with low solubility in blood is perfusion-limited, whereas that of a gas with high solubility in blood is ventilation-limited.

Other Routes of Elimination

Cerebrospinal Fluid—All compounds can leave the CNS with the bulk flow of cerebrospinal fluid (CSF). In addition, lipid-soluble toxicants also can exit at the site of the BBB. Active transport using the transport systems present in the blood–CSF barrier can also remove toxicants.

Milk—The secretion of toxic compounds into milk is extremely important because (1) a toxicant may be passed with milk from the mother to the nursing offspring and (2) compounds can be passed from cows to humans by way of dairy products. Toxic agents are excreted into milk by simple diffusion. Because milk is more acidic (pH ≈ 6.5) than plasma, basic compounds may be concentrated in milk, whereas acidic compounds may attain lower concentrations in milk than in plasma. Whereas about 3 to 4 percent of milk consists of lipids, and the lipid content of colostrum after parturition is even higher, lipid-soluble xenobiotics diffuse along with fats from plasma into the mammary gland and are excreted with milk during lactation.

Sweat and Saliva—The excretion of toxic agents in sweat and saliva is quantitatively of minor importance. Toxic compounds excreted into sweat may produce dermatitis. Substances excreted in saliva enter the mouth, where they are usually swallowed and thus are available for GI absorption.

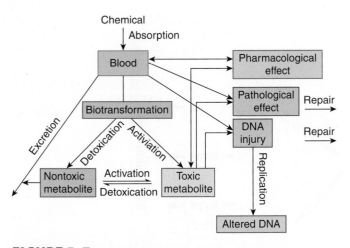

FIGURE 5-7 **Schematic representation of the disposition and toxic effects of chemicals.**

CONCLUSION

Humans are in continuous contact with toxic agents. Depending on their physical and chemical properties, toxicants may be absorbed by the GI tract, the lungs, and/or the skin. The body has the ability to biotransform and excrete these compounds into urine, feces, and air. However, when the rate of absorption exceeds the rate of elimination, toxic compounds may accumulate, reaching a critical concentration at a target site, and toxicity may ensue (Figure 5–7). Whether a chemical elicits toxicity depends not only on its inherent potency and site specificity, but also on how an organism can dispose of that toxicant.

Many chemicals have very low inherent toxicity but have to be activated by biotransformation into toxic metabolites and the toxic response depends on the rate of production of toxic metabolites. Alternatively, a very potent toxicant may be detoxified rapidly by biotransformation. Toxic effects are related to the concentration of "toxic chemical" at the site of action (in the target organ), whether a chemical is administered or generated by biotransformation in the target tissue or at a distant site. Thus, the toxic response exerted by chemicals is critically influenced by the rates of absorption, distribution, biotransformation, and excretion.

BIBLIOGRAPHY

Anzai N, Kanai Y, Endou H: Organic anion transporter family: current knowledge. *J Pharmacol Sci* 100:411–426, 2006.

Goodman J: *Goodman and Gilman's The Pharmacological Basis of Therapeutics,* 11th ed. New York: McGraw-Hill, 2005.

Lin JH: Tissue distribution and pharmacodynamics: a complicated relationship. *Curr Drug Metab* 7:39–65, 2006.

Mizuno N, Niwa T, Yotsumoto Y, Sugiyama Y: Impact of drug transporter studies on drug discovery and development. *Pharmacol Rev* 55:425–461, 2003.

Myllynen P, Pasanen M, Pelkonen O: Human placenta: a human organ for developmental toxicology research and biomonitoring. *Placenta* 26:361–371, 2005

Zhai H, Wilhelm KP, Maibach HI (eds): *Marzulli and Maibach's Dermatotoxicology* 7th edn. Boca Raton: CRC Press, 2008.

QUESTIONS

1. Biotransformation is vital in removing toxins from the circulation. All of the following statements regarding biotransformation are true EXCEPT:
   a. Many toxins must be biotransformed into a more lipid-soluble form before they can be excreted from the body.
   b. The liver is the most active organ in the biotransformation of toxins.
   c. Water solubility is required in order for many toxins to be excreted by the kidney.
   d. The kidney plays a major role in eliminating toxicants from the body.
   e. The lungs play a minor role in ridding the body of certain types of toxins.

2. Which of the following statements about active transport across cell membranes is FALSE?
   a. Unlike simple or facilitated diffusion, active transport pumps chemicals against an electrochemical or concentration gradient.
   b. Unlike simple diffusion, there is a rate at which active transport becomes saturated and cannot move chemicals any faster.
   c. Active transport requires the expenditure of ATP in order to move chemicals against electrochemical or concentration gradients.
   d. Active transport exhibits a high level of specificity for the compounds that are being moved.
   e. Metabolic inhibitors do not affect the ability to perform active transport.

3. Which of the following might increase the toxicity of a toxin administered orally?
   a. increased activity of the mdr transporter (p-glycoprotein).
   b. increased biotransformation of the toxin by gastrointestinal cells.
   c. increased excretion of the toxin by the liver into bile.
   d. increased dilution of the toxin dose.
   e. increased intestinal motility.

4. Which of the following most correctly describes the first-pass effect?
   a. The body is most sensitive to a toxin the first time that it passes through the circulation.
   b. Orally administered toxins are partially removed by the GI tract before they reach the systemic circulation.
   c. It only results from increased absorption of toxin by GI cells.
   d. It is often referred to as "postsystemic elimination."
   e. A majority of the toxin is excreted after the first time the blood is filtered by the kidneys.

5. Which of the following is an important mechanism of removing particulate matter from the alveoli?
   a. coughing.
   b. sneezing.
   c. blowing one's nose.
   d. absorption into the bloodstream, followed by excretion via the kidneys.
   e. swallowing.

6. For a toxin to be absorbed through the skin, it must past through multiple layers in order to reach the systemic circulation. Which of the following layers is the most important in slowing the rate of toxin absorption through the skin?
   a. stratum granulosum.
   b. stratum spinosum.
   c. stratum corneum.
   d. stratum basale.
   e. dermis.

7. A toxin is selectively toxic to the lungs. Which of the following modes of toxin delivery would most likely cause the LEAST damage to the lungs?
   a. intravenous.
   b. intramuscular.
   c. intraperitoneal.
   d. subcutaneous.
   e. inhalation.

8. Which of the following is NOT an important site of toxicant storage in the body?
    a. adipose tissue.
    b. bone.
    c. plasma proteins.
    d. muscle.
    e. liver.

9. Which of the following regarding the blood–brain barrier is TRUE:
    a. The brains of adults and newborns are equally susceptible to harmful blood-borne chemicals.
    b. The degree of lipid solubility is a primary determinant in whether or not a substance can cross the blood–brain barrier.
    c. Astrocytes play a role in increasing the permeability of the blood–brain barrier.
    d. Active transport processes increase the concentration of xenobiotics in the brain.
    e. The capillary endothelial cells of the CNS possess large fenestrations in their basement membranes.

10. Which of the following will result in DECREASED excretion of toxic compounds by the kidneys?
    a. a toxic compound with a molecular weight of 25,000 Da.
    b. increased activity of the multidrug-resistance (mdr) protein.
    c. increased activity of the multiresistant drug protein (mrp).
    d. increased activity of the organic cation transporter.
    e. increased hydrophilicity of the toxic compound.

Biotransformation of Xenobiotics

Andrew Parkinson and Brian W. Ogilvie

KEY POINTS

- *Biotransformation* is the metabolic conversion of endogenous and xenobiotic chemicals to more water-soluble compounds.
- Xenobiotic biotransformation is accomplished by a limited number of enzymes with broad substrate specificities.
- Phase I reactions involve hydrolysis, reduction, and oxidation. These reactions expose or introduce a functional group (—OH, —NH$_2$, —SH, or —COOH), and usually result in only a small increase in hydrophilicity.

- Phase II biotransformation reactions include glucuronidation, sulfonation (more commonly called sulfation), acetylation, methylation, and conjugation with glutathione (mercapturic acid synthesis), which usually result in increased hydrophilicity and elimination.

Biotransformation is the metabolic conversion of endogenous and xenobiotic chemicals to more water-soluble compounds. Generally, the physical properties of a xenobiotic are changed from those favoring absorption (lipophilicity) to those favoring excretion in urine or feces (hydrophilicity). An exception to this general rule is the elimination of volatile compounds by exhalation.

Chemical modification of a xenobiotic by biotransformation may alter its biological effects. Some drugs undergo biotransformation to active metabolites that exert their pharmacodynamic or toxic effect. In most cases, however, biotransformation terminates the pharmacologic effects of a drug and lessens the toxicity of xenobiotics. Enzymes catalyzing biotransformation reactions often determine the intensity and duration of action of drugs and play a key role in chemical toxicity and chemical tumorigenesis.

GENERAL PRINCIPLES

Basic Properties of Xenobiotic Biotransforming Enzymes

Xenobiotic biotransformation is accomplished by a limited number of enzymes with broad substrate specificities. The synthesis of some of these enzymes is triggered by the xenobiotic (by the process of enzyme induction), but in most cases the enzymes are expressed constitutively (i.e., they are synthesized in the absence of a discernible external stimulus). Although the synthesis of steroid hormones is catalyzed by cytochrome P450 enzymes in steroidogenic tissues, this family of enzymes in the liver converts steroid hormones into water-soluble metabolites to be excreted.

The structure (i.e., amino acid sequence) of a given biotransforming enzyme may differ among individuals, which can give rise to differences in rates of xenobiotic biotransformation. The study of the causes, prevalence, and impact of heritable differences in xenobiotic biotransforming enzymes is known as *pharmacogenetics.*

Biotransformation versus Metabolism

The terms *biotransformation* and *metabolism* are often used synonymously, particularly when applied to drugs. The term *metabolism* is often used to describe the total fate of a xenobiotic, which includes absorption, distribution, biotransformation, and elimination. However, *metabolism* is commonly used to mean biotransformation, which is understandable from the standpoint that the products of xenobiotic biotransformation are known as *metabolites.* Furthermore, individuals with a genetic enzyme deficiency resulting in impaired xenobiotic biotransformation are described as *poor metabolizers* rather than poor biotransformers.

Stereochemical Aspects of Biotransformation

Stereochemical properties influence the interaction between a xenobiotic and its biotransforming enzyme. Many xenobiotics,

especially drugs, contain one or more chiral centers and can exist in two mirror-image stereoisomers or enantiomers. The biotransformation of some chiral xenobiotics occurs stereoselectively, which means that one enantiomer (stereoisomer) is biotransformed faster than its antipode.

Categories of Xenobiotic Biotransforming Enzymes

The reactions catalyzed by xenobiotic biotransforming enzymes are generally divided into four categories: (1) hydrolysis, (2) reduction, (3) oxidation, and (4) conjugation (Table 6–1). Hydrolysis, reduction, and oxidation reactions expose or introduce a functional group (—OH, —NH$_2$, —SH, or —COOH), and usually result in only a small increase in hydrophilicity. Conjugation biotransformation reactions include glucuronidation, sulfonation (more commonly called sulfation), acetylation, methylation, conjugation with glutathione (mercapturic acid synthesis), and conjugation with amino acids (such as glycine, taurine, and glutamic acid). Most result in a large increase in xenobiotic hydrophilicity; hence, they greatly promote the excretion of foreign chemicals.

Distribution of Xenobiotic Biotransforming Enzymes

Xenobiotic biotransforming enzymes are widely distributed throughout the body and are present in several subcellular compartments. In vertebrates, the liver is the richest source of enzymes catalyzing biotransformation reactions. These enzymes are also located in the skin, lung, nasal mucosa, kidney, eye, gastrointestinal tract, as well as numerous other tissues. Intestinal microflora play an important role in the biotransformation of certain xenobiotics. Biotransformation enzymes are located primarily in the endoplasmic reticulum (microsomes) or the soluble fraction of the cytoplasm (cytosol), with lesser amounts in mitochondria, nuclei, and lysosomes (see Table 6–1).

HYDROLYSIS, REDUCTION, AND OXIDATION

Hydrolysis

Carboxylesterases, Cholinesterases, and Paraoxonase—
The hydrolysis of carboxylic acid esters, amides, and thioesters is largely catalyzed by carboxylesterases and by two cholinesterases: true acetylcholinesterase in erythrocyte membranes and pseudocholinesterase, which is also known as butyrylcholinesterase and is located in serum. Phosphoric acid esters are hydrolyzed by paraoxonase, a serum enzyme also known as aryldialkylphosphatase. Phosphoric acid anhydrides are hydrolyzed by a related organophosphatase.

Carboxylesterases in serum and tissues and serum cholinesterase collectively determine the duration and site of action

TABLE 6–1 General pathways of xenobiotic biotransformation and their major subcellular location.

Reaction	Enzyme or Specific Reaction	Localization
Hydrolysis	Carboxylesterase	Microsomes, cytosol, lysosomes, blood
	Alkaline phosphatase	Plasma membrane
	Peptidase	Blood, lysosomes
	Epoxide hydrolase	Microsomes, cytosol
Reduction	Azo- and nitro-reduction	Microflora
	Carbonyl (aldo-keto) reduction	Cytosol, microsomes, blood
	Disulfide reduction	Cytosol
	Sulfoxide reduction	Cytosol
	Quinone reduction	Cytosol, microsomes
	Dihydropyrimidine dehydrogenase	Cytosol
	Reductive dehalogenation	Microsomes
	Dehydroxylation (cytochrome b_5)	Microsomes
	Dehydroxylation (aldehyde oxidase)	Cytosol
Oxidation	Alcohol dehydrogenase	Cytosol
	Aldehyde dehydrogenase	Mitochondria, cytosol
	Aldehyde oxidase	Cytosol
	Xanthine oxidase	Cytosol
	Monoamine oxidase	Mitochondria
	Diamine oxidase	Cytosol
	Peroxidase	Microsomes, lysosomes, saliva
	Flavin-monooxygenases	Microsomes
	Cytochrome P450	Microsomes
Conjugation	UDP-glucuronosyltransferase	Microsomes
	Sulfotransferase	Cytosol
	Glutathione transferase	Cytosol, microsomes, mitochondria
	Amino acid transferase	Mitochondria, microsomes
	N-Acetyltransferase	Mitochondria, cytosol
	Methyltransferase	Cytosol, microsomes, blood

of certain drugs. In general, enzymatic hydrolysis of amides occurs more slowly than that of esters. The hydrolysis of xenobiotic esters and amides in humans is largely catalyzed by just two carboxylesterases called hCE1 and hCE2.

Carboxylesterases are glycoproteins that are present in serum and most tissues. Carboxylesterases hydrolyze numerous endogenous lipid compounds and generate pharmacologically active metabolites from several ester or amide prodrugs.

In addition, carboxylesterases may convert xenobiotics to toxic and tumorigenic metabolites.

Cholinesterases play an important role in limiting the toxicity of organophosphates, which inhibit acetylcholinesterase and thus the termination of acetylcholine action. Factors that decrease esterase activity potentiate the toxic effects of organophosphates, whereas factors that increase serine esterase activity have a protective effect.

Paraoxonases, calcium-dependent enzymes containing a critical sulfhydryl group, catalyze the hydrolysis of a broad range of organic compounds, including lactones. Thus, "lactonase" is a more encompassing name for this group of enzymes.

Prodrugs and Alkaline Phosphatase—Many prodrugs are designed to be hydrolyzed by hydrolytic enzymes such as carboxylesterases, cholinesterases, and alkaline phosphatase. Thus, these enzymes may be used to activate prodrugs in vivo and thereby generate potent anticancer agents in highly selected target sites, releasing the drug in the vicinity of the tumor cells.

Peptidases—Numerous human peptides and several recombinant peptide hormones, growth factors, cytokines, soluble receptors, and monoclonal antibodies are used therapeutically. These peptides are hydrolyzed in the blood and tissues by a variety of peptidases, which cleave the amide linkage between adjacent amino acids.

Epoxide Hydrolase—Epoxide hydrolase catalyzes the *trans*-addition of water to alkene epoxides and arene oxides, and is present in virtually all tissues. It plays an important role in detoxifying electrophilic epoxides that might otherwise bind to proteins and nucleic acids and cause cellular toxicity and genetic mutations. There are five distinct forms of epoxide hydrolase in mammals: microsomal epoxide hydrolase (mEH), soluble epoxide hydrolase (sEH), cholesterol epoxide hydrolase, LTA4 hydrolase, and hepoxilin hydrolase. The latter three enzymes appear to hydrolyze endogenous epoxides exclusively and have virtually no capacity to detoxify xenobiotic oxides.

In contrast to the high degree of substrate specificity displayed by the cholesterol, LTA4, and hepoxilin epoxide hydrolases, the mEH and sEH hydrolyze many alkene epoxides and arene oxides. Generally, these two forms of epoxide hydrolases and cytochrome P450 enzymes, which are often responsible for producing the toxic epoxides, have a similar cellular localization that presumably ensures the rapid detoxication of alkene epoxides and arene oxides generated during the oxidative biotransformation of xenobiotics.

Epoxide hydrolase is one of the several inducible enzymes in liver microsomes. Induction of epoxide hydrolase is invariably associated with the induction of cytochrome P450.

Reduction

Certain metals and xenobiotics containing an aldehyde, ketone, disulfide, sulfoxide, quinone, N-oxide, alkene, azo, or nitro group are often reduced in vivo. The reaction may proceed enzymatically or nonenzymatically by interaction with reducing agents, such as the reduced forms of glutathione, FAD, FMN, and NADP. Likewise, enzymes, such as alcohol dehydrogenase (ADH), aldehyde oxidase, and cytochrome P450, can catalyze both reductive and oxidative reactions depending on the substrate and conditions.

Azo- and Nitro-reduction—Azo- and nitro-reduction are catalyzed by intestinal microflora and under certain conditions (i.e., low oxygen tension), by two liver enzymes: cytochrome P450 and NADPH-quinone oxidoreductase (also known as DT-diaphorase). The reactions require NADPH and are inhibited by oxygen. The anaerobic environment of the lower gastrointestinal tract is well suited for azo- and nitro-reduction.

Carbonyl Reduction—The reduction of certain aldehydes to primary alcohols and of ketones to secondary alcohols is catalyzed by NAD(P)H-dependent reductases belonging to one of the two superfamilies, the aldo-keto reductases (AKRs) and the short-chain dehydrogenases/reductases (SDRs). AKRs are members of a superfamily of cytosolic enzymes that reduce both xenobiotic and endobiotic compounds. SDR carbonyl reductases are monomeric enzymes, present in blood and the cytosolic fraction of various tissues. Hepatic carbonyl reductase activity is present mainly in the cytosolic fraction, with a different carbonyl reductase present in the microsomes.

Disulfide Reduction—Disulfide reduction by glutathione is a three-step process, the last step of which is catalyzed by glutathione reductase. The first steps can be catalyzed by glutathione S-transferase, or they can occur nonenzymatically.

Sulfoxide and N-Oxide Reduction—Thioredoxin-dependent enzymes in liver and kidney cytosol can reduce sulfoxides, which were formed by cytochrome P450. Under reduced oxygen tension, the NADPH-dependent reduction of N-oxides in liver microsomes may be catalyzed by cytochrome P450 or NADPH–cytochrome P450 reductase.

Quinone Reduction—Quinones can be reduced to hydroquinones by two cytosolic flavoproteins, NQO1 and NQO2, without oxygen consumption. NADPH-quinone oxidoreductase-1 (DT-diaphorase) and NADPH-quinone oxidoreductase-2 have different substrate specificities. The two-electron reduction of quinones also can be catalyzed by carbonyl reductase. This pathway of quinone reduction is essentially nontoxic and is not associated with oxidative stress.

The second pathway of quinone reduction catalyzed by microsomal NADPH–cytochrome P450 reductase results in the formation of a semiquinone free radical by a one-electron reduction of the quinone. The oxidative stress associated with autooxidation of a semiquinone free radical, which produces superoxide anion, hydrogen peroxide, and other active oxygen species, can be extremely cytotoxic.

The properties of the hydroquinone determine whether, during the metabolism of quinine-containing xenobiotics, NQO functions as a protective antioxidant or a prooxidant activator leading to the formation of reactive oxygen species and reactive semiquinone free radicals.

Dehalogenation—There are three major mechanisms for removing halogens (F, Cl, Br, and I) from aliphatic xenobiotics: (1) *reductive dehalogenation* involves replacement of a halogen with hydrogen; (2) *oxidative dehalogenation* replaces a halogen and hydrogen on the same carbon atom with oxygen; and

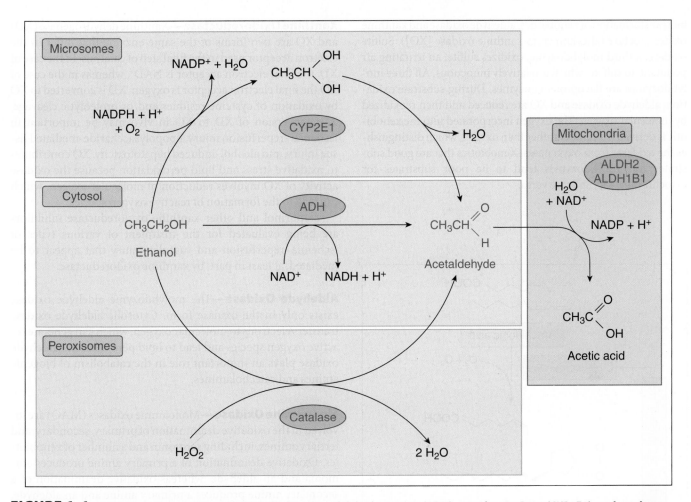

FIGURE 6–1 Oxidation of ethanol to acetaldehyde by ethanol dehydrogenase (ADH), cytochrome P450 (CYP2E1), and catalase. Note the oxidation of ethanol to acetic acid involves multiple organelles.

(3) *double dehalogenation* involves the elimination of two halogens on adjacent carbon atoms to form a carbon–carbon double bond. A variation of this third mechanism is *dehydrohalogenation,* in which a halogen and hydrogen on adjacent carbon atoms are eliminated to form a carbon–carbon double bond.

Oxidation

Alcohol Dehydrogenase—ADH is a cytosolic enzyme present in several tissues including the liver, which has the highest levels, the kidney, the lung, and the gastric mucosa. There are five major classes of ADH. The class I ADH isozymes (α-ADH, β-ADH, and γ-ADH) are responsible for the oxidation of ethanol and other small aliphatic alcohols. Class II ADH (π-ADH) is primarily expressed in liver where it preferentially oxidizes larger aliphatic and aromatic alcohols. Long-chain alcohols (pentanol and larger) and aromatic alcohols are preferred substrates for class III ADH (χ-ADH). Class IV ADH (σ- or μ-ADH), which is not expressed in liver, is the most active of the medium-chain ADHs in oxidizing retinol. Class V ADH has no subunit designation.

Aldehyde Dehydrogenase—Aldehyde dehydrogenase (ALDH) oxidizes aldehydes to carboxylic acids with NAD$^+$ as the cofactor. The enzymes also have esterase activity. The 19 identified ALDHs differ in their primary amino acid sequences and in the quaternary structure. In contrast to ALDH1A1 and ALDH2, which specifically reduce NAD$^+$, ALDH3A1 reduces both NAD$^+$ and NADP$^+$.

As shown in Figure 6–1, ALDH2 is a mitochondrial enzyme that, by virtue of its high affinity, is primarily responsible for oxidizing simple aldehydes, such as acetaldehyde. Genetic deficiencies in other ALDHs impair the metabolism of other aldehydes.

Dihydrodiol Dehydrogenase—The AKR superfamily includes several forms of dihydrodiol dehydrogenases, which are cytosolic, NADPH-requiring oxidoreductases that oxidize various polycyclic aromatic hydrocarbons to potentially toxic metabolites.

Molybdenum Hydroxylases—Two major molybdenum hydroxylases or molybdozymes participate in the biotransformation of xenobiotics: aldehyde oxidase and xanthine oxidoreductase (also known as xanthine oxidase [XO]). Sulfite oxidase, a third molybdozyme, oxidizes sulfite, an irritating air pollutant, to sulfate, which is relatively innocuous. All three molybdozymes are flavoprotein enzymes. During substrate oxidation, aldehyde oxidase and XO are reduced and then reoxidized by molecular oxygen. The oxygen incorporated into the xenobiotic is derived from water rather than oxygen, which distinguishes the oxidases from oxygenases. Xenobiotics that are good substrates for molybdozymes tend to be poor substrates for cytochrome P450, and vice versa.

Xanthine Oxidoreductase—Xanthine dehydrogenase (XD) and XO are two forms of the same enzyme that differ in the electron acceptor used in the final step of catalysis. In the case of XD, the final electron acceptor is NAD$^+$, whereas in the case of XO the final electron acceptor is oxygen. XD is converted to XO by oxidation of cysteine residues and/or proteolytic cleavage. The conversion of XD to XO in vivo may be important in ischemia–reperfusion injury, lipopolysaccharide-mediated tissue injury, and alcohol-induced hepatotoxicity. XO contributes to oxidative stress and lipid peroxidation because the oxidase activity of XO involves reduction of molecular oxygen, which can lead to the formation of reactive oxygen species.

Allopurinol and other xanthine oxidoreductase inhibitors are being evaluated for the treatment of various types of ischemia–reperfusion and vascular injury that appear to be mediated, at least in part, by xanthine oxidoreductase.

Aldehyde Oxidase—The molybdozyme aldehyde oxidase exists only in the oxidase form. Cytosolic aldehyde oxidase transfers electrons to molecular oxygen, which can generate reactive oxygen species and lead to lipid peroxidation. Aldehyde oxidase plays an important role in the catabolism of biogenic amines and catecholamines.

Monoamine Oxidase—Monoamine oxidases (MAO) are involved in the oxidative deamination of primary, secondary, and tertiary amines, including serotonin and a number of xenobiotics. Oxidative deamination of a primary amine produces ammonia and an aldehyde, whereas oxidative deamination of a secondary amine produces a primary amine and an aldehyde.

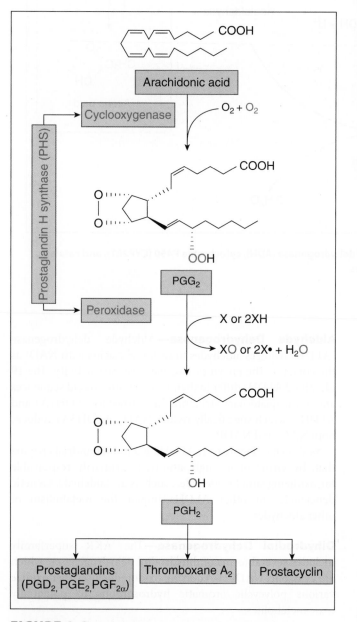

FIGURE 6–2 **Cooxidation of xenobiotics (X) during the conversion of arachidonic acid to PGH$_2$ by prostaglandin H synthase.**

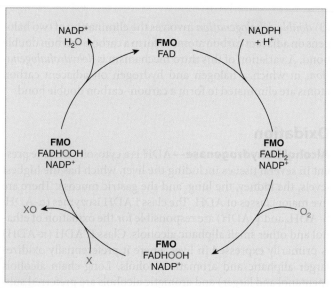

FIGURE 6–3 **Catalytic cycle of flavin monooxygenase (FMO).** X and XO are the xenobiotic substrate and oxygenated product, respectively. The 4a-hydroperoxyflavin and 4a-hydroxyflavin of FAD are depicted as FADHOOH and FADHOH, respectively.

The aldehydes formed by MAO are usually oxidized further by other enzymes to the corresponding carboxylic acids. MAO is located throughout the brain and in the outer membrane of mitochondria of the liver, kidney, intestine, and blood platelets.

The substrate is oxidized by MAO, which itself is reduced using FAD. The oxygen incorporated into the substrate is derived from water, not molecular oxygen. The catalytic cycle is completed by reoxidation of the reduced enzyme ($FADH_2 \rightarrow FAD$) by oxygen, which generates hydrogen peroxide.

Semicarbazide-sensitive amine oxidase (SSAO) is a copper-containing enzyme that catalyzes fundamentally the same reaction as MAO. It can be distinguished from MAO by its sensitivity to inhibitors and presence in plasma and various cell surfaces, whereas MAO is found in mitochondria.

Peroxidase-dependent Cooxidation—Oxidative biotransformation of xenobiotics by peroxidases couples the reduction of hydrogen peroxide and lipid hydroperoxides to the oxidation of other substrates via a process known as *cooxidation*. An important peroxidase is prostaglandin H synthetase (PHS), which possesses two catalytic activities: a *cyclooxygenase* that converts arachidonic acid to prostaglandins and a *peroxidase* that converts the hydroperoxide to the corresponding alcohol PGH_2. PSH has two forms (PSH1 and PSH2) that are better known as two forms of cyclooxygenase, namely, COX1 and COX2. PSH peroxidases are important in the activation of xenobiotics to toxic or tumorigenic metabolites, particularly in extrahepatic tissues that contain low levels of cytochrome P450. Oxidation of xenobiotics by peroxidases

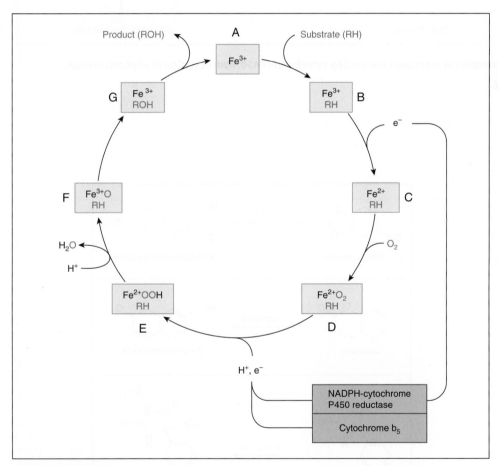

Other reactions

One-electron reduction	**C** (Fe^{2+} RH)	$\longrightarrow$	**A** (Fe^{3+}) + RH $\overline{\cdot}$
Superoxide anion production	**D** (Fe^{2+} O_2RH)	$\longrightarrow$	**B** (Fe^{3+} RH) + O_2 $\overline{\cdot}$
Hydrogen peroxide production	**E** (Fe^{2+} OOH RH) + H^+	$\longrightarrow$	**B** (Fe^{3+} RH) + H_2O_2
Peroxide shunt	**B** (Fe^{3+} RH) + XOOH	$\longrightarrow$	**F** $(FeO)^{3+}$ RH + XOH

FIGURE 6–4 Catalytic cycle of cytochrome P450.

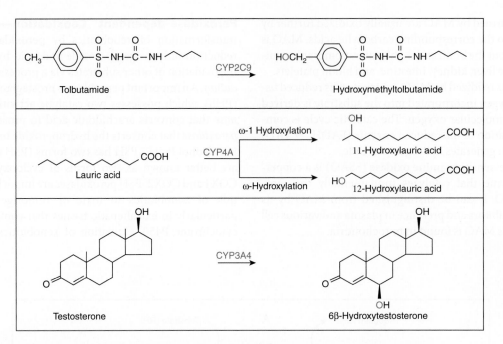

FIGURE 6–5 Examples of reactions catalyzed by cytochrome P450: hydroxylation of aliphatic carbon.

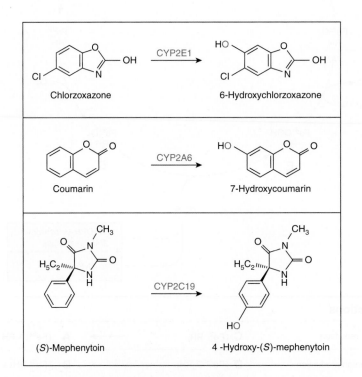

FIGURE 6–6 Examples of reactions catalyzed by cytochrome P450: hydroxylation of aromatic carbon.

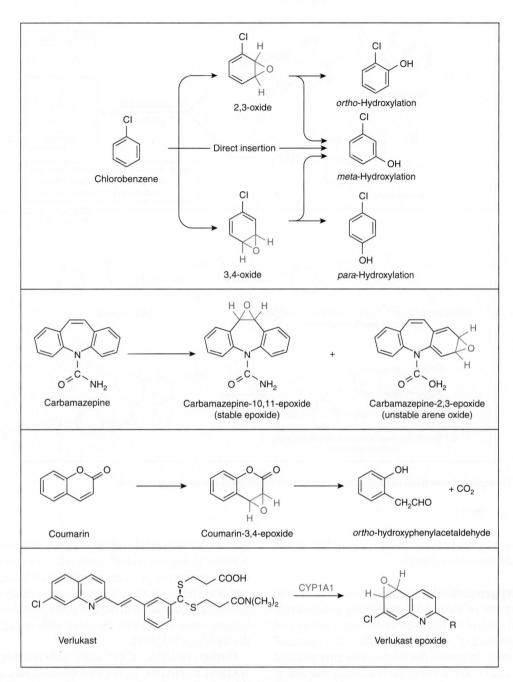

FIGURE 6–7 **Examples of reactions catalyzed by cytochrome P450: epoxidation.**

involves direct transfer of the peroxide oxygen to the xenobiotic, as shown in Figure 6–2 for the conversion of substrate X to product XO.

Xenobiotics that serve as electron donors, such as amines and phenols, can also be oxidized to free radicals during the reduction of a hydroperoxide by peroxidases. In this case, the hydroperoxide is still converted to the corresponding alcohol, but the peroxide oxygen is reduced to water instead of being incorporated into the xenobiotic. For each molecule of hydroperoxide reduced (which is a two-electron process), two molecules of xenobiotic can be oxidized (each by a one-electron

process). Many of the metabolites produced are reactive electrophiles that can cause tissue damage.

PSH2 may play at least two distinct roles in tumor formation: it may convert certain xenobiotics to DNA-reactive metabolites and *initiate* tumor formation, and it may *promote* subsequent tumor growth, perhaps through formation of growth-promoting eicosanoids.

PHS is unique among peroxidases because it can both generate hydroperoxides and catalyze peroxidase-dependent reactions, as shown in Figure 6–2. Xenobiotic biotransformation by PHS is controlled by the availability of arachidonic acid,

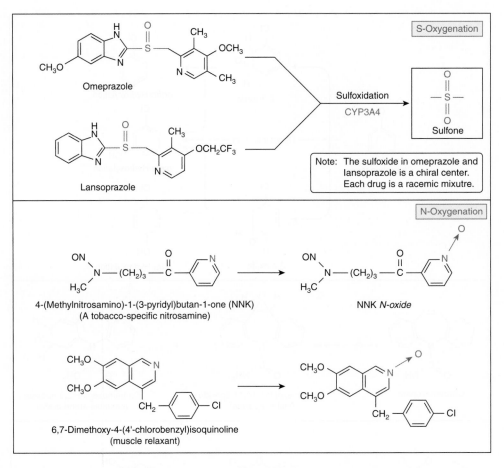

FIGURE 6-8 Examples of reactions catalyzed by cytochrome P450: heteroatom oxygenation.

whereas conversion by other peroxidases is controlled by the availability of hydroperoxide substrates.

Flavin Monooxygenases—Liver, kidney, intestine, brain, and lung contain one or more FAD-containing monooxygenases (FMO) that oxidize the nucleophilic nitrogen, sulfur, and phosphorus heteroatom of various xenobiotics. The mammalian FMO gene family comprises five microsomal enzymes that require NADPH and O_2, and many of the reactions catalyzed by FMO can also be catalyzed by cytochrome P450.

The mechanism of catalysis by FMO is depicted in Figure 6–3. After the FAD moiety is reduced to $FADH_2$ by NADPH, the oxidized cofactor $NADP^+$ remains bound to the enzyme. $FADH_2$ then binds oxygen to produce a relatively stable peroxide. During the oxygenation of xenobiotics, the flavin peroxide oxygen is transferred to the substrate (depicted as X → XO in Figure 6–3). The final step in the catalytic cycle involves restoration of FAD to its oxidized state and release of $NADP^+$. This final step is rate-limiting, and it occurs after substrate oxygenation.

Cytochrome P450—The cytochrome P450 (CYP) system ranks first in terms of catalytic versatility and the sheer number of xenobiotics it detoxifies or activates. The highest concentra-

tion of CYP enzymes involved in xenobiotic biotransformation is found in hepatic endoplasmic reticulum (microsomes), but CYP enzymes are present in virtually all tissues. All CYP enzymes are heme-containing proteins that catalyze the monooxygenation of one atom of oxygen into a substrate, and the other oxygen atom is reduced to water with reducing equivalents derived from NADPH.

During catalysis, CYP does not interact directly with NADPH or NADH. In the endoplasmic reticulum, electrons are relayed from NADPH to cytochrome P450 via a flavoprotein called NADPH–cytochrome P450 reductase. In mitochondria, electrons are transferred from NADPH to CYP via ferredoxin and ferredoxin reductase.

There are notable exceptions to the principle that cytochrome P450 requires a second enzyme (i.e., a flavoprotein) for catalytic activity. One exception applies to thromboxane A synthase (CYP5A1) and prostaglandin I_2 synthase (prostacyclin synthase or CYP8A1), which are involved in the conversion of arachidonic acid to eicosanoids. In both cases, cytochrome P450 functions as an isomerase and catalyzes a rearrangement of the oxygen atoms introduced into arachidonic acid by cyclooxygenase. The second exception involves two CYP enzymes expressed in the bacterium *Bacillus megaterium*. These CYP enzymes are considerably larger than most CYP enzymes

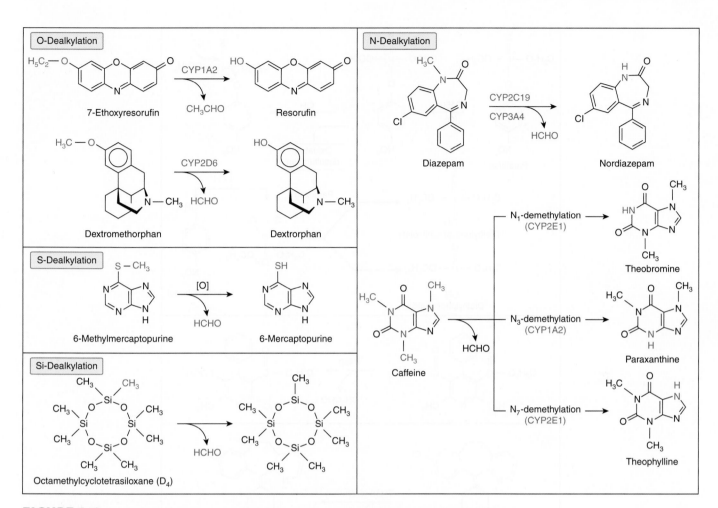

FIGURE 6–9 Examples of reactions catalyzed by cytochrome P450: heteroatom dealkylation.

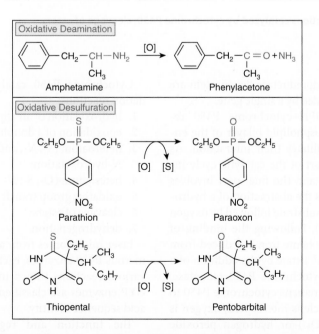

FIGURE 6–10 Examples of reactions catalyzed by cytochrome P450: oxidative group transfer.

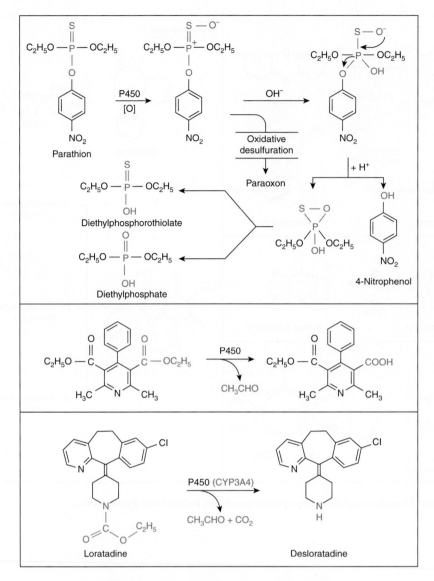

FIGURE 6–11 **Examples of reactions catalyzed by cytochrome P450: cleavage of esters.**

because the P450 moiety and oxidoreductase flavoprotein are expressed in a single protein encoded by a single gene.

Cytochrome P450 and NADPH–cytochrome P450 reductase are embedded in the phospholipid bilayer of the endoplasmic reticulum, which facilitates their interaction. As shown in Figure 6–4, the first part of the catalytic cycle involves the activation of oxygen, and the final part involves substrate oxidation, which entails the abstraction of a hydrogen atom or an electron from the substrate followed by oxygen rebound (radical recombination). Following the binding of substrate to the CYP enzyme, the heme iron is reduced from the ferric (Fe^{3+}) to the ferrous (Fe^{2+}) state by the addition of a single electron from NADPH–cytochrome P450 reductase. Release of the oxidized substrate returns cytochrome P450 to its initial state. If the catalytic cycle is interrupted, oxygen is released as superoxide anion (O_2^-) or hydrogen peroxide (H_2O_2).

Cytochrome P450 catalyzes the following types of oxidation reactions:

1. hydroxylation of an aliphatic or aromatic carbon;
2. epoxidation of a double bond;
3. heteroatom (S-, N-, and I-) oxygenation and N-hydroxylation;
4. heteroatom (O-, S-, N-, and Si-) dealkylation;
5. oxidative group transfer;
6. cleavage of esters;
7. dehydrogenation.

Liver microsomes from all mammalian species contain numerous P450 enzymes, each with the potential to catalyze the various reactions shown in Figures 6–5 to 6–12. In general, CYP enzymes are classified into subfamilies based on amino acid sequence identity.

The function and regulation of CYP1A1, CYP1A2, CYP1B1, CYP2E1, CYP2R1, CYP2S1, CYP2U1, and

TABLE 6–2 Examples of clinically relevant substrates, inhibitors, and inducers of the major human liver microsomal P450 enzymes involved in xenobiotic biotransformation. (Continued)

	CYP2AD6	CYP3A4
Substrates	Atomoxetine, Amitriptyline, Aripiprazole, Brofaromine, (±)-Bufuralol, (S)-Chlorpheniramine, Chlorpromazine, Clomipramine, Codeine, Debrisoquine, Desipramine, Dextromethorphan, Dolasetron, Duloxetine, Fentanyl, Haloperidol (reduced), Imipramine, Loperamide, (R)-Metoprolol, Methylphenidate, Mexiletine, Morphine, Nortriptyline, Ondansetron, Paroxetine, Perhexiline, Pimozide, Propafenone, (+)-Propranolol, Sparteine, Tamoxifen, Thioridazine, Timolol, Tramadol, (R)-Venlafaxine	Alfentanil, Alfuzosin, Alprazolam, Amlodipine, Amprenavir, Aprepitant, Artemether, Astemizole, Atazanavir, Atorvastatin, Azithromycin, Barnidipine, Bexarotene, Bortezomib, Brotizolam, Budesonide, Buspirone, Capravirine, Carbamazepine, Cibenzoline, Cilastazol, Cisapride, Clarithromycin, Clindamycin, Clopidogrel, Cyclosporine, Depsipeptide, Dexamethasone, Dextromethorphan, Diergotamine, α-Dihydroergocriptine, Disopyramide, Docetaxel, Domperidone, Dutasteride, Ebastine, Eletriptan, Eplerenone, Ergotamine, Erlotinib, Erythromycin, Eplerenone, Ethosuximide, Etoperidone, Everolimus, Ethinyl estradiol, Etoricoxib, Felodipine, Fentanyl, Fluticasone, Gallopamil, Gefitinib, Gepirone, Granisetron, Gestodene, Halofantrine, Laquinimod, Imatinib, Indinavir, Isradipine, Itraconazole, Karenitecin, Ketamine, Levomethadyl, Lonafarnib, Lopinavir, Loperamide, Lumefantrine, Lovastatin, Medroxyprogesterone, Methylprednisolone, Mexazolam, Midazolam, Mifepristone, Mosapride, Nicardipine, Nifedipine, Nimoldipine, Nisoldipine, Nitrendipine, Norethindrone, Oxatomide, Oxybutynin, Perospirone, Pimozide, Pranidipine, Praziquantel, Quetiapine, Quinidine, Quinine, Reboxetine, Rifabutin, Ritonavir, Rosuvastatin, Ruboxistaurin, Salmetrol, Saquinavir, Sildenafil, Sibutramine, Simvastatin, Sirolimus, Sunitinib, Tacrolimus, Tadalafil, Telithromycin, Terfenadine, Testosterone, Tiagabine, Tipranavir, Tirilazad, Tofisopam, Triazolam, Trimetrexate, Vardenafil, Vinblastine, Vincristine, Vinorelbine, Ziprasidone, Zonisamide
Inhibitors	Amiodarone, Buproprion, Chlorpheniramine, Cimetidine, Clomipramine, Duloxetine, Haloperidol, Fluoxetine, Methadone, Mibefradil, Paroxetine, Quinidine, Sertraline, Terbinafine	Amiodarone, Amprenavir, Aprepitant, Atazanavir, Azamulin, Bosentan, Cimetidine, Clarithromycin, Diltiazem, Erythromycin, Felbamate, Fluconazole, Fluvoxamine, Fosamprenavir, Gestodene, Grapefruit juice, Ketoconazole, Indinavir, Itraconazole, Mibefradil, Nefazodone, Nelfinavir, Ritonavir, Roxithromycin, Saquinavir, St. John's wort, Telithromycin, Troleandomycin, Verapamil
Inducers	NA	Amprenavir, Avasimibe, Bosentan, Carbamazepine, Clotrimazole, Cyproterone acetate, Dexamethasone, Efavirenz, Etoposide, Guggulsterone, Hyperforin, Lovastatin, Mifepristone, Nelfinavir, Nifedipine, Omeprazole, Paclitaxel, PCBs, Phenobarbital, Phenytoin, Rifabutin, Rifampin, Rifapentine, Ritonavir, Simvastatin, Spironolactone, Sulfinpyrazole, Topotecan, Troglitazone, Troleandomycin, Vitamin E, Vitamin K2, Yin zhi wuang

same individual. Due to their broad substrate specificity, it is possible that two or more CYP enzymes can contribute to the metabolism of a single compound.

The pharmacologic or toxic effects of certain drugs are exaggerated in a significant percentage of the population due to a heritable deficiency in a CYP enzyme. Inasmuch as the biotransformation of a xenobiotic in humans is frequently dominated by a single CYP enzyme, the considerable effort in identifying which CYP enzyme or enzymes are involved in eliminating the drug is known as *reaction phenotyping* or *enzyme mapping*. Four approaches to reaction phenotyping are as follows:

1. *Correlation analysis* involves measuring the rate of xenobiotic metabolism by several samples of human liver microsomes and correlating reaction rates with the variation in the level or activity of the individual P450 enzymes in the same microsomal samples.
2. *Chemical inhibition* evaluates the effects of known CYP enzyme inhibitors on the metabolism of a xenobiotic by human liver microsomes. Inhibitors of cytochrome CYP must be used cautiously because most of them can inhibit more than one CYP enzyme.
3. *Antibody inhibition* determines the effects of inhibitory antibodies against selected CYP enzymes on the biotransformation of a xenobiotic by human liver microsomes. This method alone can potentially establish which human CYP enzyme is responsible for biotransforming a xenobiotic.

4. *Biotransformation by purified or recombinant human CYP enzymes* establishes whether a particular CYP enzyme can or cannot biotransform a xenobiotic, but it does not address whether that CYP enzyme contributes substantially to reactions catalyzed by human liver microsomes.

Examples of substrates, inhibitors, and inducers for each CYP enzyme in human liver microsomes are given in Table 6–2. Because reaction phenotyping in vitro is not always carried out with toxicologically relevant substrate concentrations, the CYP enzyme that appears responsible for biotransforming the drug in vitro may not be the CYP enzyme responsible for biotransforming the drug in vivo.

Activation of Xenobiotics by Cytochrome P450—The role of human CYP enzymes in the activation of procarcinogens and protoxicants and some cytochrome P450-dependent reactions are summarized in Table 6–3. Many of the chemicals listed in Table 6–3 are also detoxified by cytochrome P450 by conversion to less toxic metabolites. In some cases, the same CYP enzyme catalyzes both activation and detoxication reactions. For example, CYP3A4 activates aflatoxin B_1 to the hepatotoxic and tumorigenic 8,9-epoxide, but it also detoxifies aflatoxin B_1 by 3-hydroxylation to aflatoxin Q_1. Complex factors determine the balance between xenobiotic activation and detoxication.

TABLE 6–3　Examples of xenobiotics activated by human P450.

CYP1A2	CYP2D6	CYP2E1
Acetaminophen	NNK	Acetaminophen
2-Acetylaminofluorene		Acrylonitrile
4-Aminobiphenyl	**CYP2F1**	Benzene
2-Aminofluorene		Carbon tetrachloride
2-Naphthylamine	3-Methylindole	Chloroform
NNK	Acetaminophen	Dichloromethane
Amino acid pyrolysis products (DiMeQx,	Valproic acid	1,2-Dichloropropane
MeIQ, MeIQx, Glu P-2, IQ, PhIP, Trp P-1,		Ethylene dibromide
Trp P-2)	**CYP1A1 and 1B1**	Ethylene dichloride
Tacrine		Ethyl carbamate
	Benzo[a]pyrene and other polycyclic	Halothane
	aromatic hydrocarbons	N-Nitrosodimethylamine
CYP2A6 and 2A13		Styrene
	CYP3A4	Trichloroethylene
NNK and bulky nitrosamines		Vinyl chloride
N-Nitrosodiethylamine	Acetaminophen	
Aflatoxin B1	Aflatoxin B_1 and G_1	
	6-Aminochrysene	**CYP4B1**
CYP2B6	Benzo[a]pyrene 7,8-dihydrodiol	
	Cyclophosphamide	Ipomeanol
6-Aminochrysene	Ifosfamide	3-Methylindole
Cyclophosphamide	1-Nitropyrene	2-Aminofluorene
Ifosfamide	Sterigmatocystin	
	Senecionine	
CYP2C8, 9, 18, 19	Tris(2,3-dibromopropyl) phosphate	
Tienilic acid		
Phenytoin		
Valproic acid		

NNK = 4-(methylnitrosamino)-1-(3-pyridyl)-1-butanone, a tobacco-specific nitrosamine.
Data adapted from Guengerich FP, Shimada T: Oxidation of toxic and carcinogenic chemicals by human cytochrome P-450 enzymes. *Chem Res Toxicol* 4:391–407, 1991.

Inhibition of Cytochrome P450—In addition to predicting the likelihood of some individuals being poor metabolizers due to a genetic deficiency in P450 expression, information on which human CYP enzyme metabolizes a drug can help predict or explain drug interactions. Inhibitory drug interactions generally fall into two categories: direct and metabolism-dependent inhibition. Direct inhibition can be subdivided into two types. The first involves competition between two drugs that are metabolized by the same CYP enzyme. The second is also competitive in nature, but the inhibitor is not a substrate for the affected CYP enzyme. Metabolism-dependent inhibition occurs when cytochrome P450 converts a xenobiotic to a metabolite that is a more potent inhibitor, either reversible or irreversible, than the parent compound.

Induction of Cytochrome P450—Inducers of cytochrome P450 increase the rate of xenobiotic biotransformation. Some of the CYP enzymes in human liver microsomes are inducible

(Table 6–2). As an underlying cause of serious adverse effects, P450 induction lowers blood levels, which compromises the therapeutic goal of drug therapy but does not cause an exaggerated response to the drug.

Although induction of cytochrome P450 may increase the activation of procarcinogens to DNA-reactive metabolites, there is little evidence from either human epidemiologic studies or animal experimentation that P450 induction enhances the incidence or multiplicity of tumors caused by known chemical carcinogens. In fact, most evidence points to a protective role of enzyme induction against chemical-induced neoplasia. Cytochrome P450 induction can cause pharmacokinetic tolerance whereby larger drug doses must be administered to achieve therapeutic blood levels due to increased drug biotransformation.

P450 Knockout Mice—Transgenic mice that lack one or more CYP enzymes may be used to evaluate the role of specific

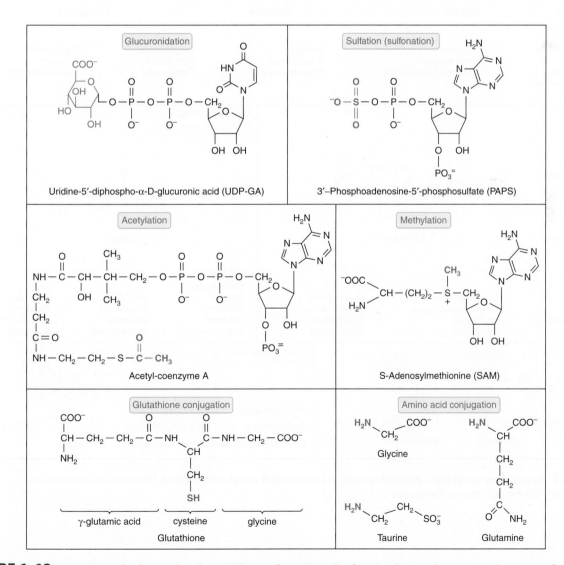

FIGURE 6–13 **Structures of cofactors for phase II biotransformation.** The functional group that reacts with or is transferred to the xenobiotic is shown in blue.

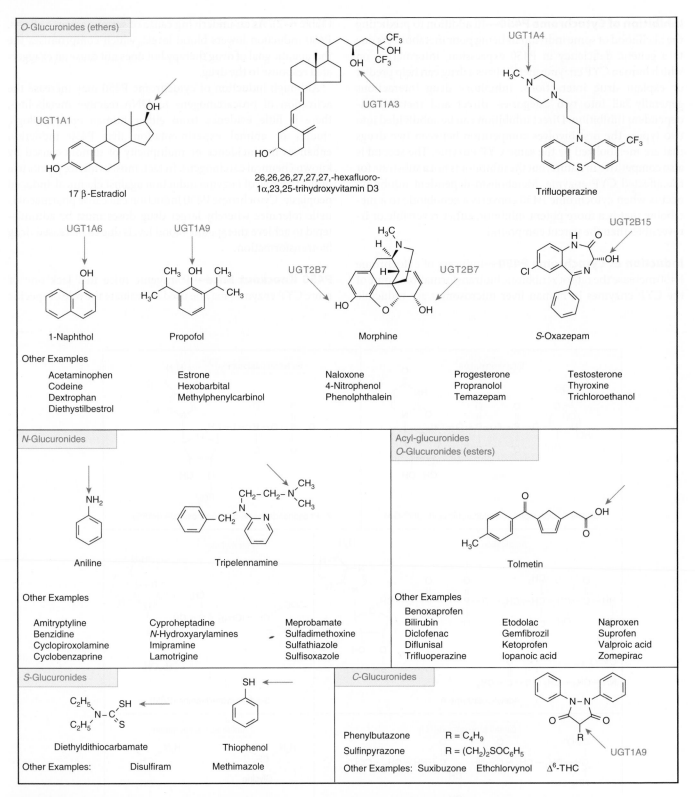

FIGURE 6–14 Examples of xenobiotics and endogenous substrates that are glucuronidated. The arrow indicates the site of glucuronidation, with the UGT enzyme if selective.

CYP enzymes in xenobiotic activation. Studies in knockout mice are relevant to humans because their counterpart can be found in those individuals who lack certain CYP enzymes or other xenobiotic biotransforming enzymes. Experiments in knockout mice underscore how genetic polymorphisms in the human population are risk modifiers for the development of chemically induced disease.

CONJUGATION

Conjugation reactions include glucuronidation, sulfonation (more commonly called sulfation), acetylation, methylation, conjugation with glutathione (mercapturic acid synthesis), and conjugation with amino acids (such as glycine, taurine, and glutamic acid). The cosubstrates for these reactions, which are shown in Figure 6–13, react with functional groups that are either present on the xenobiotic or are introduced or exposed during oxidation, reduction, or hydrolysis. With the exception of methylation and acetylation, conjugations result in a large increase in xenobiotic hydrophilicity, which greatly facilitates excretion of foreign chemicals. Glucuronidation, sulfation, acetylation, and methylation involve reactions with activated or "high-energy" cosubstrates, whereas conjugation with amino acids or glutathione involves reactions with activated xenobiotics. Except for the glucuronosyltransferases, most conjugation enzymes are mainly located in the cytosol (Table 6–1).

Glucuronidation

Glucuronidation requires the cosubstrate uridine diphosphate-glucuronic acid (UDP-glucuronic acid), and the reaction is catalyzed by UDP-glucuronosyltransferases (UGTs). Examples of xenobiotics that are glucuronidated are shown in Figure 6–14. The site of glucuronidation is generally an electron-rich nucleophilic heteroatom (O, N, or S) as found in aliphatic alcohols and phenols, carboxylic acids, primary and secondary aromatic and aliphatic amines, and free sulfhydryl groups. Endogenous substrates for glucuronidation include bilirubin, steroid hormones, and thyroid hormones.

Glucuronide conjugates of xenobiotics and endogenous compounds are polar, water-soluble metabolites. Whether glucuronides are excreted from the body in bile or urine depends on the size of the aglycone (parent compound or unconjugated metabolite). The carboxylic acid moiety of glucuronic acid, which is ionized at physiologic pH, promotes excretion because (1) it increases the aqueous solubility of the xenobiotic and (2) it is recognized by the biliary and renal organic anion transport systems, which enables glucuronides to be secreted into urine and bile. Glucuronides of xenobiotics are substrates for β-glucuronidase present in the intestinal microflora. The intestinal enzyme can release the aglycone, which undergoes *enterohepatic circulation* delaying elimination of the xenobiotic.

Cofactor availability can limit the rate of glucuronidation of drugs that are administered in high doses and are conjugated extensively, such as aspirin and acetaminophen.

TABLE 6–4 **Examples of xenobiotics and endogenous compounds that undergo sulfate conjugation .**

Functional Group	Example
Primary alcohol	Chloramphenicol, ethanol, hydroxymethyl polycyclic aromatic hydrocarbons, polyethylene glycols
Secondary alcohol	Bile acids, 2-butanol, cholesterol, dehydroepiandrosterone, doxaminol
Phenol	Acetaminophen, estrone, ethinylestradiol, naphthol, pentachlorophenol, phenol, picenadol, salicylamide, trimetrexate
Catechol	Dopamine, ellagic acid, α-methyl-DOPA
N-Oxide	Minoxidil
Aliphatic amine	2-Amino-3,8-dimethylimidazo[4,5,-f]-quinoxaline (MeIQx)[1]
	2-Amino-3-methylinidazo-[4,5-f]-quinoline (IQ)[1]
	2-Cyanoethyl-*N*-hydroxythioacetamide, despramine
Aromatic amine	2-Aminonaphthalene, aniline
Aromatic hydroxylamine	*N*-Hydroxy-2-aminonaphthalene
Aromatic hydroxyamide	*N*-Hydroxy-2-acetylaminofluorene

[1]Amino acid pyrolysis products.

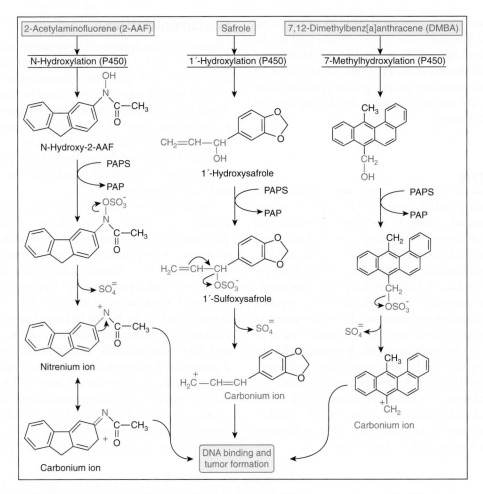

FIGURE 6–15 Role of sulfation in the generation of tumorigenic metabolites (nitrenium or carbonium ions) of 2-acetylaminofluorene, safrole, and 7,12-dimethylbenz[*a*]anthracene (DMBA).

UGTs expressed in rat liver microsomes belong to two gene families, UGT1 and UGT2, each containing several subfamilies with many similar members. Members of gene family 2 are composed of six exons that are not shared between members with the exception of UGT2A2 and UGT2A1. In contrast, members of family 1 are formed from a single gene with multiple copies of the first exon, each of which can be connected in cassette fashion with a common set of exons.

Sulfonation

Many xenobiotics and endogenous substrates undergo sulfonation. Sulfate conjugation is catalyzed by sulfotransferases, a multigene family of enzymes that generally produces a highly water-soluble sulfuric acid ester. The cosubstrate for the reaction is 3′-phosphoadenosine-5′-phosphosulfate (PAPS; see Figure 6–13).

Sulfate conjugation involves the transfer of sulfonate, not sulfate (i.e., SO_3^-, not SO_4^-) from PAPS to the xenobiotic. (The commonly used terms *sulfation* and *sulfate conjugation* are used here, even though *sulfonation* and *sulfonate conjugation*

are more appropriate descriptors.) Table 6–4 lists examples of xenobiotics and endogenous compounds that are sulfonated without prior biotransformation by oxidation enzymes. An even greater number of xenobiotics are sulfated after a hydroxyl group is exposed or introduced during oxidative or hydrolytic biotransformation.

Sulfate conjugates of xenobiotics are excreted mainly in urine. Sulfatases present in the endoplasmic reticulum and lysosomes primarily hydrolyze sulfates of endogenous compounds. Some sulfate conjugates are substrates for further biotransformation.

PAPS is synthesized from inorganic sulfate (SO_4^{2-}) and ATP in a two-step reaction. The major source of sulfate required for the synthesis of PAPS appears to be derived from cysteine through a complex oxidation sequence. The low cellular concentration of PAPS (~75 μM versus ~350 μM UDP-glucuronic acid and ~10 mM glutathione) limits the capacity for xenobiotic sulfation.

Multiple sulfotransferases have been identified in all mammalian species examined. There are two major enzyme classes: membrane-bound enzymes are found in the Golgi apparatus and soluble enzymes are located in the cytoplasm.

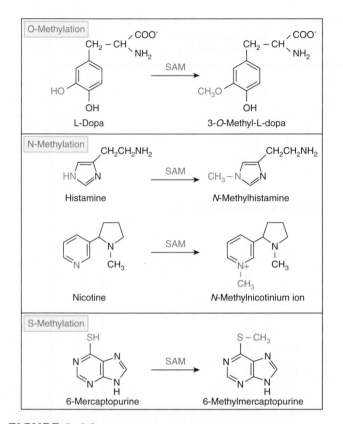

FIGURE 6–16 **Examples of compounds that undergo O-, N-, or S-methylation.**

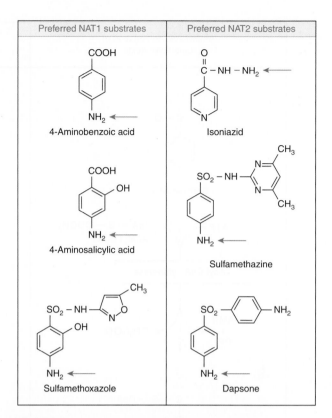

FIGURE 6–17 **Examples of substrates for human N-acetyltransferases, NAT1, and the highly polymorphic NAT2.**

Sulfotransferases are arranged into gene families (SULT1 to SULT5) that share at least 45 percent amino acid sequence identity, and are further subdivided into several subfamilies. Each family appears to work on a specific functional group (i.e., phenols, alcohols, and amines).

In general, sulfonation is an effective means of decreasing the pharmacologic and toxicologic activity of xenobiotics. However, as shown in Figure 6–15, sulfonation has a role in the activation of aromatic amines, methyl-substituted polycyclic aromatic hydrocarbons, and safrole to tumorigenic metabolites.

Methylation

Methylation, a minor pathway of biotransformation, generally decreases the water solubility of xenobiotics and masks functional groups that might otherwise be conjugated by other enzymes. Methylation can also lead to increased toxicity. The cosubstrate for methylation is S-adenosylmethionine (SAM) (Figure 6–13). The methyl group bound to the sulfonium ion in SAM is transferred to xenobiotics and endogenous substrates by nucleophilic attack from an electron-rich heteroatom (O, N, or S) leaving S-adenosylhomocysteine. Examples of xenobiotics and endogenous substrates that undergo O-, N-, or S-methylation are shown in Figure 6–16.

The O-methylation of phenols and catechols is catalyzed by two different enzymes known as phenol O-methyltransferase (POMT) in microsomes and catechol-O-methyltransferase (COMT) in cytosol and microsomes. In rats and humans, COMT is encoded by a single gene with two different promoters and transcription initiation sites. Transcription at one site produces a cytosolic form of COMT, whereas transcription from the other site produces a membrane-bound form by adding a 50-amino acid segment that targets COMT to the endoplasmic reticulum. Substrates for COMT include several catecholamine neurotransmitters and catechol drugs, such as L-DOPA and methyldopa.

Several N-methyltransferases have been described in humans and other mammals. Phenylethanolamine N-methyltransferase catalyzes the N-methylation of the neurotransmitter norepinephrine to form epinephrine in the adrenal medulla and in certain regions of the brain, and is of minimal significance in xenobiotic biotransformation. However, histamine and nicotine N-methyltransferases expressed in liver, intestine, and/or kidney do methylate xenobiotics.

S-Methylation is an important pathway in the biotransformation of sulfhydryl-containing xenobiotics. In humans, S-methylation is catalyzed by thiopurine methyltransferase in cytosol and thiol methyltransferase in microsomes.

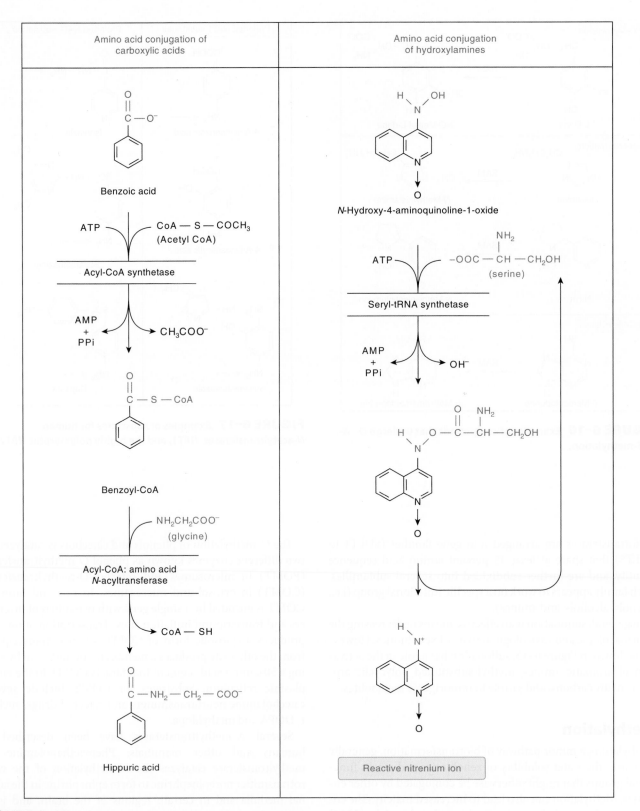

FIGURE 6–18 **Conjugation of xenobiotics with amino acids.**

Acetylation

N-Acetylation is a major route of biotransformation for xenobiotics containing an aromatic amine (R—NH$_2$) or a hydrazine group (R—NH—NH$_2$), which are converted to aromatic amides (R—NH—COCH$_3$) and hydrazides (R—NH—NH—COCH$_3$), respectively. *N*-Acetylation masks an amine with a nonionizable group, so that many *N*-acetylated metabolites are less water soluble than the parent compound. Nevertheless, *N*-acetylation of certain xenobiotics, such as isoniazid, facilitates their urinary excretion.

Xenobiotic *N*-acetylation catalyzed by cytosolic *N*-acetyltransferases requires the cosubstrate acetyl-coenzyme A (acetyl-CoA; Figure 6–13). The two-step reaction involves: (1) transfer of the acetyl group from acetyl-CoA to an active site cysteine residue within the enzyme with release of coenzyme A and (2) subsequent transfer of the acetyl group from the acylated enzyme to the amino group of the substrate with regeneration of the enzyme.

NAT1 and NAT2, the two acetyltransferases existing in humans, are 79 to 95 percent identical in amino acid sequence with an active site cysteine residue in the *N*-terminal region. Although encoded by genes on the same chromosome, NAT1 is expressed in most tissues of the body, whereas NAT2 is mainly expressed only in liver and intestine. Most (but not all) of the tissues that express NAT1 also appear to express low levels of NAT2, at least at the level of mRNA. NAT1 and NAT2 also have different but overlapping substrate specificities. Examples of drugs that are *N*-acetylated by NAT1 and NAT2 are shown in Figure 6–17.

Genetic polymorphisms for *N*-acetylation have been documented in humans, hamsters, rabbits, and mice. Polymorphisms in *NAT2* have a number of pharmacologic and toxicologic consequences: slow NAT2 acetylators are predisposed to drug toxicities, including excessive hypotension from hydralazine, peripheral neuropathy from isoniazid and dapsone, systemic lupus erythematosus from hydralazine and procainamide, and the toxic effects of coadministration of the anticonvulsant phenytoin with isoniazid.

The *N*-acetyltransferases detoxify aromatic amines by converting them to the corresponding amides that are less likely to be activated to DNA-reactive metabolites. However, *N*-acetyltransferases can activate aromatic amines if they are first *N*-hydroxylated by cytochrome P450. The acetoxy esters of *N*-hydroxyaromatic amines, like the corresponding sulfonate esters (Figure 6–15), can break down to form highly reactive nitrenium and carbonium ions that bind to DNA. Whether

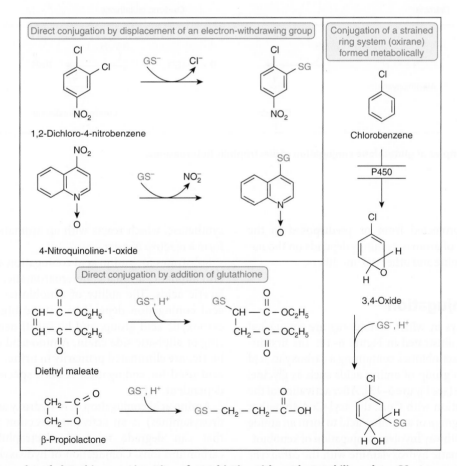

FIGURE 6–19 **Examples of glutathione conjugation of xenobiotics with an electrophilic carbon.** GS⁻ represents the anionic form of glutathione.

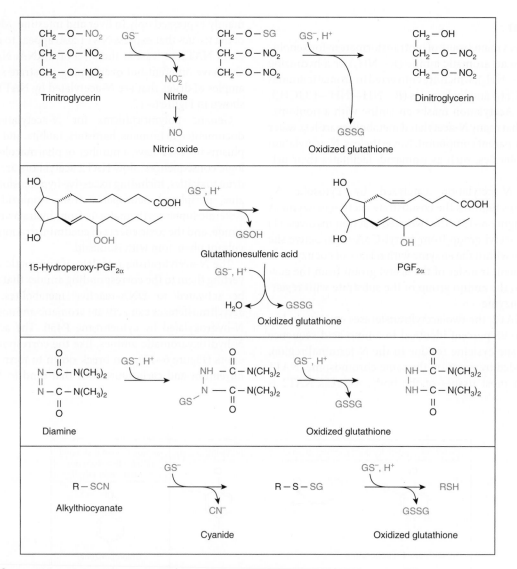

FIGURE 6–20 **Examples of glutathione conjugation of electrophilic heteroatoms.**

fast acetylators are protected from or predisposed to the cancer-causing effects of aromatic amines depends on the nature of the aromatic amine and other risk modifiers.

Amino Acid Conjugation

Two principal pathways by which xenobiotics are conjugated with amino acids are illustrated in Figure 6–18. The first involves conjugation of xenobiotics containing a carboxylic acid group with the amino group of amino acids such as glycine, glutamine, and taurine (see Figure 6–13). After activation of the xenobiotic by conjugation with CoA, the acyl-CoA thioether reacts with the *amino group* of an amino acid to form an amide linkage. The second pathway involves conjugation of xenobiotics containing an aromatic hydroxylamine with the *carboxylic acid group* of such amino acids as serine and proline. This pathway involves activation of an amino acid by aminoacyl-tRNA

synthetase, which reacts with an aromatic hydroxylamine to form a reactive *N*-ester.

Substrates for amino acid conjugation are restricted to certain aliphatic, aromatic, heteroaromatic, cinnamic, and arylacetic acids. The ability of xenobiotics to undergo amino acid conjugation depends on steric hindrance around the carboxylic acid group, and by substituents on the aromatic ring or aliphatic side chain. Amino acid conjugates of xenobiotics are eliminated primarily in urine. The acceptor amino acid used for conjugation is both species- and xenobiotic-dependent.

Amino acid conjugation of *N*-hydroxy aromatic amines (hydroxylamines) is an activation reaction producing *N*-esters that can degrade to form electrophilic nitrenium and carbonium ions. Conjugation of hydroxylamines with amino acids is catalyzed by cytosolic aminoacyl-tRNA synthetases and requires ATP (Figure 6–18).

Glutathione Conjugation

Conjugation of xenobiotics with glutathione includes an enormous array of electrophilic xenobiotics, or xenobiotics that can be biotransformed to electrophiles. The tripeptide glutathione comprises of glycine, cysteine, and glutamic acid (Figure 6–13). Glutathione conjugates are thioethers, which form by nucleophilic attack of glutathione thiolate anion (GS⁻) with an electrophilic carbon, oxygen, nitrogen, or sulfur atom in the xenobiotic. This conjugation reaction is catalyzed by a family of glutathione S-transferases that are present in most tissues, where they are localized in the cytoplasm (>95 percent) and endoplasmic reticulum (<5 percent).

Substrates for glutathione S-transferase are commonly hydrophobic, contain an electrophilic atom, and react nonenzymatically with glutathione at some measurable rate. The mechanism by which glutathione S-transferase increases the rate of glutathione conjugation involves deprotonation of GSH to GS⁻. The concentration of glutathione in liver is extremely high (~5 to 10 mM); hence, the nonenzymatic conjugation of certain xenobiotics with glutathione can be significant. However, some xenobiotics are conjugated with glutathione stereoselectively, indicating that the reaction is largely catalyzed by glutathione S-transferase. Like glutathione, the glutathione S-transferases are themselves abundant cellular components, accounting for up to 10 percent of the total cellular protein. These enzymes bind, store, and/or transport a number of compounds that are not substrates for glutathione conjugation. The cytoplasmic protein formerly known as ligandin, which binds heme, bilirubin, steroids, azo-dyes, polycyclic aromatic hydrocarbons, and thyroid hormones, is an alpha-class GST.

As shown in Figure 6–19, substrates for glutathione conjugation can be divided into two groups: those sufficiently electrophilic to be conjugated directly and those that must first be biotransformed to an electrophilic metabolite prior to conjugation. The conjugation reactions themselves can be divided into two types: *displacement reactions,* in which glutathione displaces an electron-withdrawing group, and *addition reactions,* in which glutathione is added to an activated double bond or strained ring system.

The displacement of an electron-withdrawing group by glutathione typically occurs when the substrate contains halide, sulfate, sulfonate, phosphate, or a nitro group (i.e., good *leaving groups*) attached to an allylic or benzylic carbon atom.

The addition of glutathione to a carbon–carbon double bond is also facilitated by the presence of a nearby electron-withdrawing group; hence, substrates for this reaction typically contain a double bond attached to —CN, —CHO, —COOR, or —COR.

Glutathione can also conjugate xenobiotics with an electrophilic heteroatom (*O, N,* and *S*). In each of the examples shown in Figure 6–20, the initial conjugate formed between glutathione and the heteroatom is cleaved by a second molecule of glutathione to form oxidized glutathione (GSSG). The initial reactions are catalyzed by glutathione S-transferase, whereas the second reaction (which leads to GSSG formation) generally occurs nonenzymatically.

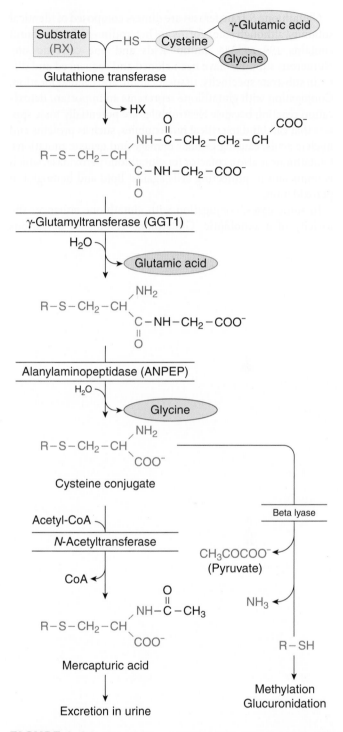

FIGURE 6–21 **Glutathione conjugation and mercapturic acid biosynthesis.**

Glutathione conjugates formed in the liver can be effluxed into bile and blood, and they can be converted to mercapturic acids in the kidney and excreted in urine. As shown in Figure 6–21, the conversion of glutathione conjugates to mercapturic acids involves the sequential cleavage of glutamic acid and glycine from the glutathione moiety, followed by N-acetylation of the resulting cysteine conjugate.

Glutathione *S*-transferases are dimers composed of identical subunits, although some forms are heterodimers. Each subunit contains 199 to 244 amino acids and one catalytic site. Numerous subunits have been cloned and sequenced and differ in substrate specificity, tissue location, and cellular location. Conjugation with glutathione represents an important detoxication reaction because electrophiles are potentially toxic species that can bind to critical nucleophiles, such as proteins and nucleic acids, causing cellular damage and genetic mutations. Glutathione is also a cofactor for glutathione peroxidase, which is important in protecting cells against lipid and hemoglobin peroxidation.

In some cases, conjugation with glutathione enhances the toxicity of a xenobiotic. Glutathione conjugates of various compounds can activate xenobiotics to become toxic by releasing a toxic metabolite, being inherently toxic itself, or being degraded to a toxic metabolite.

BIBLIOGRAPHY

Coleman MD: *Human Drug Metabolism: An Introduction.* Hoboken, NJ: John Wiley, 2005.

Uetrecht JP, Trager W: *Drug Metabolism: Chemical and Enzymatic Aspects.* New York: Informa Healthcare, 2007.

Yan Q: *Pharmacogenomics in Drug Discovery and Development.* Totowa, NJ: Humana Press, 2008.

QUESTIONS

1. Xenobiotic biotransformation is performed by multiple enzymes in multiple subcellular locations. Where would one of these enzymes most likely NOT be located?
   a. cytosol.
   b. Golgi apparatus.
   c. lysosome.
   d. mitochondria.
   e. microsome.

2. All of the following statements regarding hydrolysis, reduction, and oxidation biotransformations are true EXCEPT:
   a. The xenobiotic can be hydrolyzed.
   b. The xenobiotic can be reduced.
   c. There is a large increase in hydrophilicity.
   d. The reactions introduce a functional group to the molecule.
   e. The xenobiotic can be oxidized.

3. Which of the following is often conjugated to xenobiotics during phase II biotransformations?
   a. alcohol group.
   b. sulfhydryl group.
   c. sulfate group.
   d. aldehyde group.
   e. carbonyl group.

4. Which of the following is a true statement about the biotransformation of ethanol?
   a. Alcohol dehydrogenase is only present in the liver.
   b. Ethanol is reduced to acetaldehyde by alcohol dehydrogenase.
   c. Ethanol and hydrogen peroxide combine to form acetaldehyde with the aid of catalase.
   d. In spite of its catalytic versatility, cytochrome P450 does not aid in ethanol oxidation.
   e. Acetaldehyde is oxidized to acetic acid in the mitochondria by aldehyde dehydrogenase.

5. Which of the following enzymes is responsible for the biotransformation and elimination of serotonin?
   a. cytochrome P450.
   b. monoamine oxidase.
   c. flavin monooxygenase.
   d. xanthine oxidase.
   e. paraoxonase.

6. Which of the following reactions would likely NOT be catalyzed by cytochrome P450?
   a. dehydrogenation.
   b. oxidative group transfer.
   c. epoxidation.
   d. reductive dehalogenation.
   e. ester cleavage.

7. All of the following statements regarding cytochrome P450 are true EXCEPT:
   a. Poor metabolism or biotransformation of xenobiotics is often due to a genetic deficiency in cytochrome P450.
   b. Cytochrome P450 can be inhibited by both competitive and noncompetitive inhibitors.
   c. Certain cytochrome P450 enzymes can be induced by one's diet.
   d. Increased activity of cytochrome P450 always slows the rate of xenobiotic activation.
   e. Induction of cytochrome P450 can lead to increased drug tolerance.

8. Which of the following statements regarding phase II biotransformation (conjugation) reactions is true?
   a. Phase II reactions greatly increase the hydrophilicity of the xenobiotic.
   b. Phase II reactions are usually the rate-determining step in the biotransformation and excretion of xenobiotics.
   c. Carboxyl groups are very common additions of phase II reactions.
   d. Most phase II reactions occur spontaneously.
   e. Increased phase II reactions result in increased xenobiotic storage in adipocytes.

9. Where do most phase II biotransformations take place?
   a. mitochondria.
   b. ER.
   c. blood.
   d. nucleus.
   e. cytoplasm.

10. Which of the following is not an important cosubstrate for phase II biotransformation reactions?
   a. UDP-glucuronic acid.
   b. 3'-phosphoadenosine-5'-phosphosulfate (PAPS).
   c. *S*-adenosylmethionine (SAM).
   d. *N*-nitrosodiethylamine.
   e. acetyl CoA.

toxicity. Several factors can greatly alter this systemic availability, including (1) limited absorption after oral dosing, (2) intestinal first-pass effect, (3) hepatic first-pass effect, and (4) mode of formulation, which affects, for example, dissolution rate or incorporation into micelles (for lipid-soluble compounds).

The toxicity of a chemical is in some cases attributed to its biotransformation product(s). Hence, the formation and disposition kinetics of a toxic metabolite is of considerable interest. As expected, the plasma concentration of a metabolite rises as the parent drug is transformed into the metabolite. A biologically active metabolite assumes toxicologic significance when it is the major metabolic product and is cleared much less efficiently than the parent compound.

Saturation Toxicokinetics

As the dose of a compound increases, its volume of distribution or its rate of elimination may change, owing to saturation kinetics. Biotransformation, active transport processes, and protein binding have finite capacities and can be saturated. When the concentration of a chemical in the body is higher than the K_m (chemical concentration at one-half V_{max}, the maximum metabolic capacity), the rate of elimination is no longer proportional to the dose. The transition from first-order to saturation kinetics is important in toxicology because it can lead to prolonged residency time of a compound in the body or increased concentration at the target site of action, which may result in increased toxicity.

Nonlinear toxicokinetics are indicated by the following: (1) the decline in the levels of the chemical in the body is not exponential, (2) AUC_0^∞ is not proportional to the dose, (3) V_d, Cl, k_{el} (or β), or $T_{1/2}$ change with increasing dose, (4) the composition of excretory products changes quantitatively or qualitatively with the dose, (5) competitive inhibition by other chemicals that are biotransformed or actively transported by the same enzyme system occurs, and (6) dose–response curves show a nonproportional change in response with an increasing dose, starting at the dose level at which saturation effects become evident.

The elimination of some chemicals from the body is readily saturated. Important characteristics of zero-order processes are as follows: (1) an arithmetic plot of plasma concentration versus time yields a straight line, (2) the rate or amount of chemical eliminated at any time is constant and is independent of the amount of chemical in the body, and (3) a true $T_{1/2}$ or k_{el} does not exist, but differs depending on dose.

By comparison, the important characteristics of first-order elimination are: (1) the rate at which a chemical is eliminated at any time is directly proportional to the amount of that chemical in the body at that time; (2) a semilogarithmic plot of plasma concentration versus time yields a single straight line; (3) the elimination rate constant (k_{el} or β), apparent volume of distribution (V_d), clearance (Cl), and half-life ($T_{1/2}$) are independent of dose; and (4) the concentration of the chemical in plasma and other tissues decreases similarly by some constant fraction per unit of time, the elimination rate constant (k_{el} or β).

Accumulation during Continuous or Intermittent Exposure

Chronic exposure to a chemical leads to its cumulative intake and accumulation in the body. At a fixed level of continuous exposure, accumulation of a toxicant in the body eventually reaches a point when the intake rate of the toxicant equals its elimination rate, the steady state.

Accumulation can also occur with intermittent exposure. For a chemical with a relatively short half-life compared with the interval between episodes of exposure, little accumulation is expected. In contrast, for a chemical with an elimination half-life approaching or exceeding the between-exposure interval, progressive accumulation is expected over the intervals.

PHYSIOLOGIC TOXICOKINETICS

In classic kinetics, the rate constants are defined by the data and these models are often referred to as *data-based*. In *physiologically based* models, the rate constants represent known or hypothesized biological processes. The advantages of physiologically based models are that (1) these models can provide the time course of distribution of xenobiotics to any organ or tissue, (2) they allow estimation of the effects of changing physiologic parameters on tissue concentrations, (3) the same model can predict the toxicokinetics of chemicals across species by allometric scaling, and (4) complex dosing regimens and saturable processes such as metabolism and binding are easily accommodated.

Basic Model Structure

Physiologic models often look like a number of classic one-compartment models that are linked together. The actual model *structure,* or *how* the compartments are linked together, depends on both the chemical and the organism being studied. It is important to realize that there is no generic physiologic model. Models are simplifications of reality and ideally should contain elements believed to be important in describing a chemical's disposition.

Physiologic modeling has enormous potential predictive power compared with classic compartmental modeling. Because the kinetic constants in physiologic models represent measurable biological or chemical processes, the resultant physiologic models have the potential for extrapolation from observed data to predicted situations.

One of the best illustrations of the predictive power of physiologic models is their ability to extrapolate kinetic behavior from laboratory animals to humans. *Simulations* are the outcomes or results (such as a chemical's concentration in blood or tissue) of numerically integrating model equations over a simulated time period, using a set of initial conditions (such as intravenous dose) and parameter values (such as organ weights and blood flow). Whereas the model structures for the kinetics of chemicals in rodents and humans may be identical, the parameter values, such as organ weight, heart beat rate, respiration rate, etc., for rodents and humans are different. Other

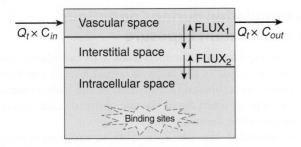

FIGURE 7–3 **Schematic representation of a lumped compartment in a physiologic model.** The blood capillary and cell membranes separating the vascular, interstitial, and intracellular subcompartments are depicted in black. The vascular and interstitial subcompartments are often combined into a single extracellular subcompartment. Q_t is blood flow, C_{in} is chemical concentration into the compartment, and C_{out} is chemical concentration out of the compartment.

parameters, such as solubility in tissues, are similar in the rodent and human models because the composition of tissues in different species is similar. Because the parameters underlying the model structure represent measurable biological and chemical determinants, the appropriate values for those parameters can be chosen for each species, forming the basis for successful interspecies extrapolation. Because physiologic models represent real, measurable values, such as blood flows and ventilation rates, the same model structure can resolve such disparate kinetic behaviors among species.

Compartments

The basic unit of the physiologic model is the lumped compartment (Figure 7–3), which is a single region of the body with a uniform xenobiotic concentration. A compartment may be a particular functional or anatomical portion of an organ, a single blood vessel with surrounding tissue, an entire discrete organ such as the liver or kidney, or a widely distributed tissue type such as fat or skin. Compartments consist of three individual well-mixed phases, or subcompartments. These subcompartments are (1) the *vascular* space through which the compartment is perfused with blood, (2) the *interstitial* space that forms the matrix for the cells, and (3) the *intracellular* space consisting of the cells in the tissue.

As shown in Figure 7–3, the toxicant enters the vascular subcompartment at a certain rate in mass per unit of time (e.g., mg/h). The rate of entry is a product of the blood flow rate to the tissue (Q_t, L/h) and the concentration of the toxicant in the blood entering the tissue (C_{in}, mg/L). Within the compartment, the toxicant moves from the vascular space to the interstitial space at a certain net rate (Flux$_1$) and from the interstitial space to the intracellular space at a different net rate (Flux$_2$). Some toxicants can bind to cell components; thus, within a compartment there may be both free and bound toxicants. The toxicant leaves the vascular space at a certain venous concentration (C_{out}). C_{out} is equal to the concentration of the toxicant in the vascular space.

Parameters

The most common types of parameters, or information required, in physiologic models are *anatomical, physiologic, thermodynamic,* and *transport.*

Anatomical—Anatomical parameters are used to physically describe the various compartments. The size of each of the compartments in the physiologic model must be known. The size is generally specified as a volume (milliliters or liters) because a unit density is assumed even though weights are most frequently obtained experimentally. If a compartment contains subcompartments such as those in Figure 7–3, those volumes also must be known. Volumes of compartments often can be obtained from the literature or from specific toxicokinetic experiments.

Physiologic—Physiologic parameters encompass various processes including blood flow, ventilation, and elimination. The blood flow rate (Q_t, in volume per unit time, such as mL/min or L/h) to individual compartments must be known. Additionally, information on the total blood flow rate or cardiac output (Q_c) is necessary. If inhalation is the route for exposure to the xenobiotic or is a route of elimination, the alveolar ventilation rate (Q_p) also must be known. Blood flow rates and ventilation rates can be taken from the literature or obtained experimentally. Renal clearance rates and parameters to describe rates of biotransformation are required if these processes are important in describing the elimination of a xenobiotic.

Thermodynamic—Thermodynamic parameters relate the *total* concentration of a xenobiotic in a tissue (C_t) to the concentration of *free* xenobiotic in that tissue (C_f). Two important assumptions are that (1) total and free concentrations are in equilibrium with each other and (2) only free xenobiotic can enter and leave the tissue. Whereas total concentration is measured experimentally, it is the free concentration that is available for binding, metabolism, or removal from the tissue by blood. The extent to which a xenobiotic partitions into a tissue is directly dependent on the composition of the tissue and independent of the concentration of the xenobiotic. Thus, the relationship between free and total concentration becomes one of proportionality: total = free × partition coefficient, or $C_t = C_f P_t$. Knowledge of the value of P_t, a *partition* or *distribution* coefficient, permits an indirect calculation of the free concentration of xenobiotic or $C_f = C_t/P_t$.

Table 7–1 compares the partition coefficients for a number of toxic volatile organic chemicals. The larger values for the fat/blood partition coefficients compared with those for other tissues suggest that these chemicals distribute into fat to a greater extent than they distribute into other tissues.

A more complex relationship between the free concentration and the total concentration of a chemical in tissues occurs when the chemical may bind to saturable binding sites on tissue components. In these cases, nonlinear functions relating the free concentration in the tissue to the total concentration are necessary.

TABLE 7–1 Partition coefficients for four volatile organic chemicals in several tissues.

Chemical	Blood/Air	Muscle/Blood	Fat/Blood
Isoprene	3	0.67	24
Benzene	18	0.61	28
Styrene	40	1	50
Methanol	1,350	3	11

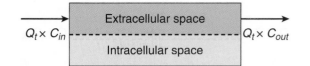

FIGURE 7–4 Schematic representation of a compartment that is blood flow-limited. Rapid exchange between the extracellular space (*salmon*) and intracellular space (*bisque*) maintains the equilibrium between them as symbolized by the dashed line. Q_t is blood flow, C_{in} is chemical concentration into the compartment, and C_{out} is chemical concentration out of the compartment.

Transport—The passage of a chemical across a biological membrane is complex and may occur by passive diffusion, carrier-mediated transport, facilitated transport, or a combination of processes. The simplest of these processes—passive diffusion—is a first-order process. Diffusion of xenobiotics can occur across the blood capillary membrane (Flux$_1$ in Figure 7–3) or across the cell membrane (Flux$_2$ in Figure 7–3). For simple diffusion, the net flux (mg/h) from one side of a membrane to the other is described as Flux = permeability coefficient × driving force, or:

$$\text{Flux} = [PA](C_1 - C_2) = [PA]C_1 - [PA]C_2$$

The permeability coefficient [PA] is often called the *permeability–area cross-product* for the membrane (L/h) and is a product of the cell membrane permeability constant (P, μm/h) for the xenobiotic and the total membrane area (A, μm^2). The permeability constant takes into account the rate of diffusion of the specific xenobiotic and the thickness of the cell membrane. C_1 and C_2 are the *free* concentrations of xenobiotic on each side of the membrane. For any given xenobiotic, thin membranes, large surface areas, and large concentration differences enhance diffusion.

There are two *limiting conditions* for the transport of a xenobiotic across membranes: *perfusion-limited* and *diffusion-limited*.

Perfusion-limited Compartments

A perfusion-limited compartment is also referred to as *blood flow-limited*, or simply *flow-limited*. A flow-limited compartment can be developed if the cell membrane permeability coefficient [PA] for a particular xenobiotic is much greater than the blood flow rate to the tissue (Q_t). In this case, uptake of xenobiotic by tissue subcompartments is limited by the rate at which the blood containing a xenobiotic arrives at the tissue and not by the rate at which the xenobiotic crosses the cell membranes. In most tissues, transport across vascular cell membranes is perfusion-limited. In the generalized tissue compartment in Figure 7–3, this means that transport of the xenobiotic through the loosely knit blood capillary walls of most tissues is rapid compared with delivery of the xenobiotic to the tissue by the blood. As a result, the vascular blood is in equilibrium with the interstitial subcompartment and the two subcompartments are

usually lumped together as a single compartment that is often called the *extracellular space*.

As indicated in Figure 7–3, the cell membrane separates the extracellular compartment from the intracellular compartment. The cell membrane is the most important diffusional barrier in a tissue. Nonetheless, for molecules that are very small (molecular weight <100) or lipophilic, cellular permeability generally does not limit the rate at which a molecule moves across cell membranes. For these molecules, flux across the cell membrane is fast compared with the tissue perfusion rate ([PA] $\gg Q_t$), and the intracellular compartment is in equilibrium with the extracellular compartment, and these tissue subcompartments are usually lumped as a single compartment. This flow-limited tissue compartment is shown in Figure 7–4. Movement into and out of the entire tissue compartment can be described by a single equation:

$$V_t \frac{dC_t}{dt} = Q_t(C_{in} - C_{out})$$

where V_t is the volume of the tissue compartment, C_t the concentration of free xenobiotic in the compartment ($V_t C_t$ equals the amount of xenobiotic in the compartment), $V_t(dC_t/dt)$ the change in the amount of xenobiotic in the compartment with time expressed as mass per unit of time, Q_t the blood flow to the tissue, C_{in} the xenobiotic concentration entering the compartment, and C_{out} the xenobiotic concentration leaving the compartment. These mass balance *differential* equations require that input into one equation must be balanced by outflow from another equation in the physiologic model.

In the perfusion-limited case, C_{out}, or the venous concentration of xenobiotic leaving the tissue, is equal to the free concentration of xenobiotic in the tissue, C_f. As was noted above, C_f (or C_{out}) can be related to the total concentration of xenobiotic in the tissue through a simple linear partition coefficient, $C_{out} = C_f = C_t/P_t$. In this case, the differential equation describing the rate of change in the amount of a xenobiotic in a tissue becomes

$$V_t \frac{dC_t}{dt} = Q_t\left(C_{in} - \frac{C_t}{P_t}\right)$$

In a flow-limited compartment, the assumption is that the concentrations of a xenobiotic in all parts of the tissue are in equilibrium. Additionally, estimates of flux are not required to

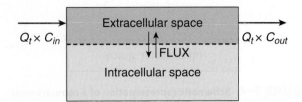

FIGURE 7–5 **Schematic representation of a compartment that is membrane-limited.** Perfusion of blood into and out of the extracellular compartment is depicted by thick arrows. Transmembrane transport (flux) from the extracellular to the intracellular subcompartment is depicted by thin double arrows. Q_t is blood flow, C_{in} is chemical concentration into the compartment, and C_{out} is chemical concentration out of the compartment.

develop the mass balance differential equation for the compartment. Given the information required to estimate flux, this simplifying assumption significantly reduces the number of parameters required in the physiologic model.

Diffusion-limited Compartments

When uptake into a compartment is governed by cell membrane permeability and total membrane area, the model is said to be *diffusion-limited*, or *membrane-limited*. Diffusion-limited transport occurs when the flux of a xenobiotic across cell membranes is slow compared with blood flow to the tissue. In this case, the permeability–area cross-product is small compared with blood flow, or PA << Q_t. Figure 7–5 shows the structure of such a compartment. The xenobiotic concentrations in the interstitial and vascular spaces are in equilibrium and make up the extracellular subcompartment where uptake from the incoming blood is flow-limited. The rate of xenobiotic uptake across the cell membrane (into the intracellular space from the extracellular space) is limited by cell membrane permeability and is thus diffusion-limited. Two mass balance differential equations are necessary to describe this compartment:

1. Extracellular space:

$$V_1 \frac{dC_1}{dt} = Q_t (C_{in} - C_{out}) - [PA]C_1 + [PA]C_2$$

2. Intracellular space:

$$V_2 \frac{dC_2}{dt} = [PA]C_1 - [PA]C_2$$

Here, Q_t is blood flow and C the *free* xenobiotic concentration in entering blood (in), exiting blood (out), extracellular space (1), or intracellular space (2). Both equations contain terms for flux, or transfer across the cell membrane $[PA](C_1 - C_2)$.

Specialized Compartments

Lung—The inclusion of a lung compartment in a physiologic model is an important consideration because inhalation is a common route of exposure to many toxic chemicals. The

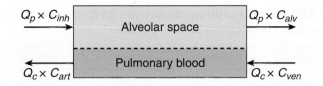

FIGURE 7–6 **Simple model of gas exchange in the alveolar region of the respiratory tract.** Rapid exchange in the lumped lung compartment between the alveolar gas (*blue*) and the pulmonary blood (*salmon*) maintains the equilibrium between them as symbolized by the dashed line. Q_p is alveolar ventilation (L/h); Q_c is cardiac output (L/h); C_{inh} is inhaled vapor concentration (mg/L); C_{art} is concentration of vapor in the arterial blood; C_{ven} is concentration of vapor in the mixed venous blood. The equilibrium relationship between the chemical in the alveolar air (C_{alv}) and the chemical in the arterial blood (C_{art}) is determined by the blood/air partition coefficient P_b, for example, $C_{alv} = C_{art}/P_b$.

assumptions inherent in lung compartment description are: (1) ventilation is continuous, not cyclic; (2) conducting airways function as inert tubes, carrying the vapor to the gas exchange region; (3) diffusion of vapor across the lung cell and capillary walls is perfusion-limited; (4) all xenobiotic disappearing from inspired air appears in arterial blood (i.e., there is no storage of xenobiotic in the lung tissue and insignificant lung mass); and (5) vapor in the alveolar air and arterial blood within the lung compartment are in rapid equilibrium.

In the lung compartment depicted in Figure 7–6, the rate of inhalation of xenobiotic is controlled by the ventilation rate (Q_p) and the inhaled concentration (C_{inh}). The rate of exhalation of a xenobiotic is a product of the ventilation rate and the xenobiotic concentration in the alveoli (C_{alv}). Xenobiotic also can enter the lung compartment via venous blood returning from the heart, represented by the product of cardiac output (Q_c) and the concentration of xenobiotic in venous blood (C_{ven}). Xenobiotic leaving the lungs via the blood is a function of both cardiac output and the concentration of xenobiotic in arterial blood (C_{art}). Putting these four processes together, a mass balance differential equation can be written for the rate of change in the amount of xenobiotic in the lung compartment (L):

$$\frac{dL}{dt} = Q_p (C_{inh} - C_{alv}) + Q_c (C_{ven} - C_{art})$$

Because of these assumptions, at steady state the rate of change in the amount of xenobiotic in the lung compartment becomes equal to zero ($dL/dt = 0$). C_{alv} can be replaced by C_{art}/P_b, and the differential equation can be solved for the arterial blood concentration:

$$C_{art} = \frac{Q_p C_{inh} + Q_c C_{ven}}{Q_c + (Q_p / P_b)}$$

The lung is viewed here as a portal of entry and not as a target organ, and the concentration of a xenobiotic delivered to other organs by the blood, or the arterial concentration of that xenobiotic, is of primary interest.

Liver—The liver is often represented as a compartment in physiologic models because hepatic biotransformation is an important aspect of the toxicokinetics of many xenobiotics. A simple compartmental structure for the liver is assumed to be flow-limited, and this compartment is similar to the general tissue compartment in Figure 7–4, except that the liver compartment contains an additional process for metabolic elimination. One of the simplest expressions for this process is first-order elimination:

$$R = C_f V_l K_f$$

where R is the rate of metabolism (mg/h), C_f the free concentration of xenobiotic in the liver (mg/L), V_l the liver volume (L), and K_f the first-order rate constant for metabolism (h^{-1}).

In physiologic models, the Michaelis–Menten expression for *saturable metabolism*, which employs two parameters, V_{max} and K_M, is written as:

$$R = \frac{V_{max} C_f}{K_M + C_f}$$

where V_{max} is the maximum rate of metabolism (mg/h) and K_M the Michaelis constant, or xenobiotic concentration at one-half the maximum rate of metabolism (mg/L). Because many xenobiotics are metabolized by enzymes that display saturable metabolism, the above equation is a key factor in the success of physiologic models for simulation of chemical disposition across a range of doses.

Other, more complex expressions for metabolism also can be incorporated into physiologic models. Bisubstrate second-order reactions, reactions involving the destruction of enzymes, the inhibition of enzymes, or the depletion of cofactors, have been simulated using physiologic models. Metabolism can be also included in other compartments in much the same way as described for the liver.

CONCLUSION

The field of physiologic modeling is rapidly expanding. Physiologic models of a parent chemical linked in series with one or more active metabolites, models describing biochemical interactions among xenobiotics, and more biologically realistic descriptions of tissues previously viewed as simple lumped compartments are just a few of the most recent applications. Finally, physiologically based *toxicokinetic* models are beginning to be linked to biologically based *toxicodynamic* models to simulate the entire exposure → dose → response paradigm that is basic to the science of toxicology.

BIBLIOGRAPHY

Andersen ME: Toxicokinetic modeling and its applications in chemical risk assessment. *Toxicol Lett* 138:9–27, 2003.

Brown RP, Delp MD, Lindstedt SL, et al: Physiological parameter values for physiologically based pharmacokinetic models. *Toxicol Ind Health* 13(4):407–484, 1997.

Lipscomb JC, Ohanian EV: *Toxicokinetics and Risk Assessment.* New York: Informa Healthcare, 2007.

Tozer TN, Rowland M: *Introduction to Pharmacokinetics and Pharmacodynamics: The Quantitative Basis of Drug Therapy.* Philadelphia: Lippincott Williams & Wilkins, 2006.

QUESTIONS

1. Regarding the two-compartment model of classic toxicokinetics, which of the following is true?
   a. There is rapid equilibration of chemical between central and peripheral compartments.
   b. The logarithm of plasma concentration versus time data yields a linear relationship.
   c. There is more than one dispositional phase.
   d. It is assumed that the concentration of a chemical is the same throughout the body.
   e. It is ineffective in determining effective doses in toxicity studies.

2. When calculating the fraction of a dose remaining in the body over time, which of the following factors need not be taken into consideration?
   a. half-life.
   b. initial concentration.
   c. time.
   d. present concentration.
   e. elimination rate constant.

3. All of the following statements regarding apparent volume of distribution (V_d) are true EXCEPT:
   a. V_d relates the total amount of chemical in the body to the concentration of chemical in the plasma.
   b. V_d is the apparent space into which an amount of chemical is distributed in the body to result in a given plasma concentration.
   c. A chemical that usually remains in the plasma has a low V_d.
   d. V_d will be low for a chemical with high affinity for tissues.
   e. V_d can be used to estimate the amount of chemical in the body if the plasma concentration is known.

4. Chemical clearance:
   a. is independent of V_d.
   b. is unaffected by kidney failure.
   c. is indirectly proportional to V_d.
   d. is performed by multiple organs.
   e. is not appreciable in the GI tract.

5. A chemical with which of the following half-lives ($T_{1/2}$) will remain in the body for the longest period time when given equal dosage of each?
   a. $T_{1/2}$ = 30 min.
   b. $T_{1/2}$ = 1 day.
   c. $T_{1/2}$ = 7 h.
   d. $T_{1/2}$ = 120 s.
   e. $T_{1/2}$ = 1 month.

6. With respect to first-order elimination, which of the following statements is FALSE?
   a. The rate of elimination is directly proportional to the amount of the chemical in the body.
   b. A semilogarithmic plot of plasma concentration versus time shows a linear relationship.
   c. Half-life ($T_{1/2}$) differs depending on the dose.
   d. Clearance is dosage-independent.
   e. The plasma concentration and tissue concentration decrease similarly with respect to the elimination rate constant.

7. The toxicity of a chemical is dependent on the amount of chemical reaching the systemic circulation. Which of the following does NOT *greatly* influence systemic availability?
   a. absorption after oral dosing.
   b. intestinal motility.
   c. hepatic first-pass effect.
   d. intestinal first-pass effect.
   e. incorporation into micelles.

8. Which of the following is NOT an advantage of a physiologically based toxicokinetic model?
   a. Complex dosing regimens are easily accommodated.
   b. The time course of distribution of chemicals to any organ is obtainable.
   c. The effects of changing physiologic parameters on tissue concentrations can be estimated.
   d. The rate constants are obtained from gathered data.
   e. The same model can predict toxicokinetics of chemicals across species.

9. Which of the following will not help to increase the flux of a xenobiotic across a biological membrane?
   a. decreased size.
   b. decreased oil:water partition coefficient.
   c. increased concentration gradient.
   d. increased surface area.
   e. decreased membrane thickness.

10. Which of the following statements is true regarding diffusion-limited compartments?
    a. Xenobiotic transport across the cell membrane is limited by the rate at which blood arrives at the tissue.
    b. Diffusion-limited compartments are also referred to as flow-limited compartments.
    c. Increased membrane thickness can cause diffusion-limited xenobiotic uptake.
    d. Equilibrium between the extracellular and intracellular space is maintained by rapid exchange between the two compartments.
    e. Diffusion of gases across the alveolar septa of a healthy lung is diffusion-limited.

C H A P T E R

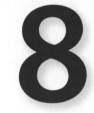

Chemical Carcinogenesis

James E. Klaunig and Lisa M. Kamendulis

KEY POINTS

- The term *cancer* describes a subset of neoplastic lesions.
- A *neoplasm* is defined as a heritably altered, relatively autonomous growth of tissue with abnormal regulation of gene expression.
- *Metastases* are secondary growths of cells from the primary neoplasm.
- A *carcinogen* is an agent whose administration to previously untreated animals leads to a statistically significant increased incidence of neoplasms of one or more histogenetic types as compared with the incidence in appropriate untreated animals.

- *Initiation* requires one or more rounds of cell division for the "fixation" of the DNA damage.
- *Promotion* results from the selective functional enhancement of the initiated cell and its progeny by the continuous exposure to the promoting agent.
- *Progression* is the transition from early progeny of initiated cells to the biologically malignant cell population of the neoplasm.

OVERVIEW

Cancer is a disease of cellular mutation, proliferation, and aberrant cell growth. It ranks as one of the leading causes of death in the world. Multiple causes of cancer have been either firmly established or suggested, including infectious agents, radiation, and chemicals. Estimates suggest that 70 to 90 percent of all human cancers have a linkage to environmental, dietary, and behavioral factors.

Definitions

Table 8–1 lists definitions of terms commonly used in discussing chemical carcinogenesis. For benign neoplasms, the tissue of origin is frequently followed by the suffix "oma"; for example, a benign fibrous neoplasm would be termed *fibroma*, and a benign glandular epithelium termed an *adenoma*. Malignant neoplasms from epithelial origin are called *carcinomas*, whereas those derived from mesenchymal origin are referred to as *sarcoma*. Thus, a malignant neoplasm of fibrous tissue would be a *fibrosarcoma*, whereas that derived from bone would be an *osteosarcoma*.

Carcinogens may be *genotoxic*, meaning that they interact physically with DNA to damage or change its structure. Other carcinogens may change how DNA expresses information without modifying or directly damaging its structure, or may create a situation in a cell or tissue that makes it more susceptible to DNA damage from other sources. Chemicals belonging to this latter category are referred to as *nongenotoxic* carcinogens. Common features of genotoxic and nongenotoxic carcinogens are shown in Table 8–2.

MULTISTAGE CARCINOGENESIS

The carcinogenesis process involves a series of definable and reproducible stages. Operationally, these stages have been defined as initiation, promotion, and progression (Figure 8–1).

TABLE 8–1 Terminology.

Neoplasia	New growth or autonomous growth of tissue
Neoplasm	The lesion resulting from the neoplasia
Benign	Lesions characterized by expansive growth, frequently exhibiting slow rates of proliferation that do not invade surrounding tissues
Malignant	Lesions demonstrating invasive growth, capable of metastases to other tissues and organs
Metastases	Secondary growths derived from a primary malignant neoplasm
Tumor	Lesion characterized by swelling or increase in size, may or may not be neoplastic
Cancer	Malignant neoplasm
Carcinogen	A physical or chemical agent that causes or induces neoplasia
Genotoxic	Carcinogens that interact with DNA resulting in mutation
Nongenotoxic	Carcinogens that modify gene expression but do not damage DNA

TABLE 8–2 Features of genotoxic and nongenotoxic carcinogens.

Genotoxic carcinogens
- Mutagenic
- Can be complete carcinogens
- Tumorigenicity is dose responsive
- No theoretical threshold

Nongenotoxic carcinogens
- Nonmutagenic
- Threshold, reversible
- Tumorigenicity is dose responsive
- May function at tumor promotion stage
- No direct DNA damage
- Species, strain, tissue specificity

chromosomal structure. During carcinogenesis, both hypomethylation and hypermethylation of the genome have been observed. Tumor-suppressor genes have been reported to be hypermethylated in tumors. Hypomethylation has been associated with increased mutation rates because many oncogenes are hypomethylated and their expression is amplified.

Reactive oxygen species have also been shown to modify DNA methylation by interfering with the ability of methyltransferases to interact with DNA; the resulting hypomethylation allow the expression of normally quiescent genes. Also, the abnormal methylation pattern observed in cells transformed by chemical oxidants may contribute to an overall aberrant gene expression and promote tumorigenesis.

Oxidative Stress and Chemical Carcinogenesis—Oxygen radicals can be produced by both endogenous and exogenous sources and are typically counterbalanced by antioxidants. Antioxidant defenses are both enzymatic (e.g., superoxide dismutase, glutathione peroxidase, and catalase) and nonenzymatic (e.g., vitamin E, vitamin C, β-carotene, and glutathione). Endogenous sources of reactive oxygen species include oxidative phosphorylation, P450 metabolism, peroxisomes, and inflammatory cell activation. Through these or other currently unknown mechanisms, a number of chemicals that induce cancer (e.g., chlorinated compounds, radiation, metal ions, barbiturates, and some PPARα agonists) induce reactive oxygen species formation and/or oxidative stress.

Oxidative Damage and Carcinogenesis—Reactive oxygen species left unbalanced by antioxidants can result in damage to cellular macromolecules. In DNA, reactive oxygen species can produce single- or double-stranded DNA breaks, purine, pyrimidine, or deoxyribose modifications, and DNA crosslinks.

Mutations and oxidative damage to mitochondrial DNA have been identified in a number of cancers. Compared with nuclear DNA, mitochondrial genome is relatively susceptible to oxidative base damage due to (1) close proximity to the electron transport system, a major source of reactive oxygen species; (2) mitochondrial DNA is not protected by histones; and (3) DNA repair capacity is limited in the mitochondria.

Oxidative Stress and Cell Growth Regulation—Activation of signaling cascades by reactive oxygen species induced by chemical carcinogens ultimately leads to altered gene expression for a number of genes including those affecting proliferation, differentiation, and apoptosis. Activation of NFκB, a ubiquitously expressed transcription factor, is regulated, in part, by reactive oxygen species and the cellular redox status, and has been observed to occur following a wide variety of extracellular stimuli, including exposure to chemical carcinogens such as PPARα agonists and PCBs.

Gap Junctional Intercellular Communication and Carcinogenesis

Gap junctional intercellular communication appears to play an important role in the regulation of cell growth and cell death, in part through the ability to exchange small molecules (<1 kDa) between cells. If cell communication is blocked between tumor and normal cells, the exchange of growth inhibitory signals from normal cells to initiated cells is prevented thus allowing the potential for unregulated growth and clonal expansion of initiated cell populations.

Polymorphisms in Carcinogen Metabolism and DNA Repair

Genetic polymorphisms arise from human genetic variability. In carcinogenesis, genetic polymorphisms may account for the susceptibility of some individuals to certain cancers. A number of polymorphisms have been described in carcinogen-metabolizing enzymes, with certain alleles linked to altered risk of selective cancers. Glutathione S-transferases (GSTs) are highly polymorphic in humans. The GSTM1 isoform is particularly important in carcinogenesis, because of its high reactivity toward epoxides.

Carcinogenic risk depends on both exposure (dose and duration) as well as genetic susceptibility. For example, if the genetic susceptibility is high, then exposure to a chemical carcinogen will result in a higher risk for cancer development.

Proto-oncogenes and Tumor-suppressor Genes

Proto-oncogenes and tumor-suppressor genes encode a wide array of proteins that function to control cell growth and proliferation. Common characteristics of oncogenes and tumor-suppressor genes are shown in Table 8–5. Mutations in both oncogenes and tumor-suppressor genes contribute to the

TABLE 8–5 Characteristics of proto-oncogenes, cellular oncogenes, and tumor-suppressor genes.

Proto-oncogenes	Oncogenes	Tumor-suppressor Genes
Dominant	Dominant	Recessive
Broad tissue specificity for cancer development	Broad tissue specificity for cancer development	Considerable tissue specificity for cancer development
Germ line inheritance rarely involved in cancer development	Germ line inheritance frequently involved in cancer development	Germ line inheritance frequently involved in cancer development
Analogous to certain viral oncogenes	No known analogs in oncogenic viruses	No known analogs in oncogenic viruses
Somatic mutations activated during all stages of carcinogenesis	Somatic mutations activated during all stages of carcinogenesis	Germ line mutations may initiate, but mutation to neoplasia occurs only during progression stage

progressive development of human cancers. Accumulated damage to multiple oncogenes and/or tumor-suppressor genes can result in altered cell proliferation, differentiation, and/or survival of cancer cells.

Retroviruses—The *Rous sarcoma virus* (RSV) is capable of transforming a normal cell and producing sarcomas. The genome of RSV and other retroviruses consists of two identical copies of mRNA, which is then reverse transcribed into DNA and incorporated into the host-cell genome. Oncogenic transforming viruses like RSV contain the v-*src* gene, a gene required for cancer induction. Normal cells contain a gene closely related to v-*src* in RSV. This discovery showed that cancer may be induced by the action of normal, or nearly normal, genes.

DNA Viruses—Infection by small DNA viruses is lethal to most nonhost animal cells; however, a small proportion integrates the viral DNA into the host-cell genome. The cells that survive infection become permanently transformed due to the presence of one or more oncogenes in the viral DNA. Papilloma viruses can infect and cause tumors in humans. Of the human papilloma viruses, types 16, 18, 31, and 33 are associated with human cervical cancers.

Proto-oncogenes—An oncogene encodes a protein that is capable of transforming cells in culture or inducing cancer in animals. Of the known oncogenes, the majority appear to have been derived from normal genes (i.e., proto-oncogenes), and are involved in cell signaling cascades. Because most proto-oncogenes are essential for maintaining viability, they are highly conserved. Activation of proto-oncogenes to oncogenes arises through mutational events occurring within proto-oncogenes. It has been recognized that a number of chemical carcinogens are capable of inducing mutations in proto-oncogenes. Oncogene products can operate at multiple levels of signaling cascades, including ligand, receptor, and transcription factor stages of transduction.

Tumor-suppressor Genes

Retinoblastoma (Rb) Gene—The proteins encoded by most tumor-suppressor genes act as inhibitors of cell proliferation or cell survival (Table 8–6). The prototype tumor-suppressor

TABLE 8–6 Examples of tumor-suppressor genes and cancer association.

Tumor Suppressor	Disorder	Neoplasm
Rb1	Retinoblastoma	Small-cell lung carcinoma
p53	Li-Fraumeni syndrome	Breast, colon, lung cancers
BRCA1	Unknown	Breast carcinoma
WT-1	Wilm's tumor	Lung cancer
p16	Unknown	Melanoma

gene, *Rb,* was identified by studies of inheritance of retinoblastoma. Loss or mutational inactivation of *Rb* contributes to the development of a wide variety of human cancers. In its unphosphorylated form, Rb binds to the *E2F* transcription factors preventing E2F-mediated transcriptional activation of a number of genes whose products are required for DNA synthesis. Rb becomes phosphorylated during the late G1, causing dissociation from E2F—a process that allows E2F to induce synthesis of DNA replication enzymes, resulting in a commitment to the cell cycle.

p53 Gene—The p53 protein is a tumor-suppressor gene that is essential for checkpoint control and arrests the cell cycle in G1 in cells with damaged DNA. Cells with functional p53 arrest in G1 when exposed to DNA damaging agents, whereas cells lacking functional p53 are unable to block the cell cycle. p53 is activated by a wide array of stressors including ultraviolet light, γ irradiation, heat, and several carcinogens.

In most cells, accumulation of p53 also leads to induction of proteins that promote apoptosis, and therefore would prevent proliferation of cells that are likely to accumulate multiple mutations. When the p53 checkpoint control does not operate properly, damaged DNA can replicate, producing mutations and DNA rearrangements that contribute to the development of transformed cells.

Hormesis and Carcinogenesis

Hormesis is defined as a dose–response curve in which a U-, J-, or inverted U-shaped dose–response is observed; with low-dose exposures often resulting in beneficial rather than harmful effects. Adaptive responses have been proposed to explain the hormetic effects observed by chemical carcinogens. These usually involve actions of the chemical on cellular signaling pathways that lead to changes in gene expression, resulting in enhanced detoxification and excretion of the chemical, as well as preserving the cell cycle and programmed cell death. It has been proposed that following very low doses of chemicals, the upregulation of these mechanisms overcompensates for cell injury such that a reduction in tumor promotion and/or tumor development is seen, and would explain the U- or J-shaped response curves obtained following carcinogen exposure. A common feature of chemical carcinogens for which hormetic effects have been proposed is the formation of reactive oxygen species and the induction of cytochrome P450 isoenzymes.

Chemoprevention

The study of chemicals that prevent, inhibit, or slow down the process of cancer is referred to as *chemoprevention*. A number of chemicals, including drugs, antioxidants, foodstuffs, and vitamins, have been found to inhibit or retard the components of the cancer process in both in vitro and in vivo models. A basic assumption in chemoprevention is that treating early stages of malignant process will halt or delay the progression to neoplasia. Chemopreventive agents may function as inhibitors of carcinogen formation, blocking agents, and/or suppressing agents.

Blocking agents serve to prevent the metabolic activation of genotoxic or nongenotoxic carcinogens by either inhibiting its metabolism or by enhancing the detoxification mechanisms. Suppressing agents induce tissue differentiation, may counteract oncogenes, enhance tumor-suppressor gene activities, inhibit proliferation of premalignant cells, or modify the effect of the carcinogen on the target tissue.

TEST SYSTEMS FOR CARCINOGENICITY ASSESSMENT

Short-term Tests for Mutagenicity

Short-term tests for mutagenicity were developed to identify potentially carcinogenic chemicals based on their ability to induce mutations in DNA either in vivo or in vitro. The majority of these tests measure the mutagenicity of chemicals as a surrogate for carcinogenicity. Although usually very predictive of indirect action and direct action (if a metabolic source is provided), these tests routinely fail to detect nongenotoxic carcinogens.

In Vitro Gene Mutation Assays—The most widely used short-term test is the Ames assay. *Salmonella typhimurium* strains deficient in DNA repair and unable to synthesize histidine are treated with several dose levels of the test compound, after which reversion to the histidine-positive phenotype is ascertained.

The mouse lymphoma assay is a mutagenicity assay used to determine whether a chemical is capable of inducing mutation in eukaryotic cells. The ability of the cell cultures to acquire resistance to trifluorothymidine (the result of forward mutation at the thymidine kinase locus) is quantified. Another mammalian cell mutation assay, the Chinese hamster ovary (CHO) test, is also commonly used to assess the potential mutagenicity of chemicals. This assay uses the hypoxanthine-guanine phosphoribosyltransferase (HGPRT) gene as the endpoint.

In Vivo Gene Mutation Assays—The in vivo tests have advantages over the in vitro test systems in that they take into account the whole animal processes such as absorption, tissue distribution, metabolism, and excretion of chemicals and their metabolites. The commonly used in vivo models include transgenic rodent mutation assay systems based on the genes of the *lac* operon, Muta™Mouse, and Big Blue®.

To detect mutations, following exposure of mice to test chemicals, mutations are analyzed in high molecular weight DNA isolated from the tissue under investigation. The ratio of mutants to the total population will provide a mutation frequency for each chemical and each organ tested. In vivo genotoxicity test systems will fail to identify nongenotoxic/non-DNA reactive compounds.

Chromosomal Alterations—Chromosomal alterations are quite common in malignant neoplasms. Both in vivo and in vitro assays are available to assess chromosomal alterations. To assess induction of chromosomal alterations, cells are harvested in their first mitotic division after the initiation of chemical exposure. Cells are stained with Giemsa and scored for completeness of karyotype (21 ± 2 chromosomes). The classes of aberrations recorded include breaks and terminal deletions, rearrangements and translocations, as well as despiralized chromosomes, and cells containing 10 or more aberrations.

Sister chromatid exchanges (SCEs) are a measure of DNA damage events that are associated with mutation induction and cancer. SCEs are a reflection of an interchange of DNA between different chromatids at homologous loci within a replicating chromosome. Second-division metaphase cells are scored to determine the frequency of SCE/cell for each dose level. Disruption of the DNA replication process or damage to chromosomes by chemicals can alter the genetic material distributed to either of the two daughter nuclei. When this occurs, the genetic material that is not incorporated into a new nucleus may form its own "micronucleus," which is clearly visible with a microscope. For this assay, animals are exposed to chemicals and the frequency of micronucleated cells is determined at some specified time after treatment.

DNA Damage—Primary DNA damage represents possible pre-mutational events that can be detected using mammalian cells in culture or using rodent tissue. Unscheduled DNA synthesis (UDS) is a commonly used assay that measures the ability of a chemical to induce DNA lesions by measuring the increase in DNA repair. Among the available techniques is the measurement of DNA strand breaks both in vivo and in vitro.

Transformation Assays—Various in vitro test systems have been developed to assess the carcinogenic potential of chemicals. The C3H/10T$^{1/2}$ cell line has been widely used in the transformation assays. It was originally derived from fibroblasts taken from the prostate of a C3H mouse embryo. The cells are approximately tetraploid but the chromosome number in the cells varies widely. As such, these cells are chromosomally abnormal and have already passed through some of the stages that might be involved in the production of a cancerous cell. On plating these cells, they will stop growing when their density is sufficiently high (contact growth inhibition). However, the contact inhibition can fail, resulting in cell piling forming a transformed colony. Therefore, following exposure to xenobiotics, this assay assesses carcinogenic potential based on the percentage of colonies that are transformed.

The most frequently used endpoint for cell transformation is morphological transformation of mammalian cell fibroblasts in culture. Transformation assays using Syrian hamster embryo (SHE) cells are available for the assessment of the carcinogenic potential of chemicals. The SHE cell assay measures carcinogenic potential of xenobiotics by assessing transformed colonies based on morphological criteria.

Chronic Testing for Carcinogenicity

Chronic (2-Year) Bioassay—Two-year studies over the lifespan of rodents remain the primary method by which chemicals or physical agents are identified as having the potential to be hazardous to humans. In the chronic bioassay, two or three dose levels (up to the maximum tolerated dose, MTD) of a test chemical and a vehicle control are administered to 50 males and 50 females (mice and rats), beginning at 8 weeks of age, continuing throughout their lifespan. During the study, food consumption and bodyweight gain are monitored, and the animals are observed clinically on a regular basis, and at necropsy the tumor number, location, and pathological diagnosis for each animal is thoroughly assessed.

Organ-specific Bioassays and Multistage Animal Models—Many tissue-specific bioassays have been developed with the underlying goal being to produce a sensitive and reliable assay that could be conducted in a time frame shorter in duration than the 2-year chronic bioassay. These assays are commonly used to detect carcinogenic activity of chemicals in various target organs.

Carcinogenicity Testing in the Liver—The liver represents a major target organ for chemical carcinogens. It has been estimated that nearly half of the chemicals tested in the 2-year chronic bioassay by the National Toxicology Program showed an increased incidence of liver cancer. Liver carcinogenesis assays have been developed to study and distinguish chemicals that affect the initiation or promotion stage of hepatocarcinogenesis. The ability of the test chemical to promote the growth of preneoplastic lesions can be assessed.

Carcinogenicity Testing in the Skin—The mouse skin model has been used to dissect mechanisms of carcinogenesis and also is purported to be a useful intermediate-term cancer bioassay. This model exploits many of the unique properties of the mouse skin, one major advantage being that the development of neoplasia can be followed visually. In addition, the number and relative size of papillomas and carcinomas can be quantified as the tumors progress. Both initiating and promoting activities of chemical carcinogens can be assessed using this model. Grossly, initiated cells of the skin appear identical to normal skin. Because the terminally differentiated cells in the skin are no longer capable of undergoing cell division, only initiated cells retain their proliferative capacity and thus represent the cell populations that give rise to tumors. On repeated application of tumor promoters, selective clonal expansion of initiated keratinocytes occurs, resulting in skin papillomas, which over time can progress to carcinomas.

Carcinogenicity Testing in Other Organs—Test systems to examine the ability of a chemical to promote neoplastic development at organ sites other than liver and skin have also been developed. The available systems include animal models directed at examining carcinogenicity in the lung, kidney, bladder, pancreas, stomach, colon, small intestine, and oral cavity. These models vary in the initiating carcinogen used, and frequency, duration, and site of application, as well as the duration of promoting chemical exposure.

Transgenic Animals in Carcinogenicity Assessment

Animal models with genetic alterations that invoke a susceptibility to carcinogenesis by chemical agents include Tg.AC and rasH2 transgenic mice, and p53$^{+/-}$ and XPA$^{-/-}$ knockout mice. Recently, the feasibility of the use of these animal models as alternative assays for the 2-year chronic bioassay was assessed by the Health and Environmental Sciences Institute (HESI) branch of the International Life Sciences Institute (ILSI). The conclusions drawn from the scientific review suggested that these models appear to have usefulness as screening models for assessment of chemical carcinogenicity; however, they do not provide definitive proof of potential human carcinogenicity. Further, the scientific panel suggested that these models could be used in place of the mouse 2-year bioassay. Coupled with information on genotoxicity, particularly DNA reactivity, structure–activity relationships, results from other bioassays, and the results of other mechanistic investigations including toxicokinetics, metabolism, and mechanistic information, these alternate mouse models for carcinogenicity appear to be useful models for assessing the carcinogenicity of chemical agents.

CHEMICAL CARCINOGENESIS IN HUMANS

Many factors have been implicated in the induction of cancer in humans. Infectious agents, lifestyle, medical treatments, and environmental and occupational exposure account either directly or indirectly for the majority of cancers seen in humans. Of these, the component that contributes the most to human cancer induction and progression is lifestyle: tobacco use, alcohol use, and poor diet (Table 8–7). Tobacco usage either through smoking tobacco, chewing tobacco, or tobacco snuff-type products is estimated to be responsible for 25 to 40 percent of all human cancers. In particular, a strong correlation between tobacco usage and mouth, larynx, lung, esophageal, and bladder cancer exists. It has been estimated that 85 to 90 percent of all lung cancer cases in the United States are a direct result of

TABLE 8–7 Carcinogenic factors associated with lifestyle.

Chemical(s)	Neoplasm(s)
Alcohol beverage	Esophagus, liver, oropharynx, and larynx
Aflatoxins	Liver
Betel chewing	Mouth
Dietary intake (fat, protein, calories)	Breast, colon, endometrium, gallbladder
Tobacco smoking	Mouth, pharynx, larynx, lung, esophagus, bladder

tobacco use. The induction of pancreatic cancer also appears to have a linkage to tobacco use. Alcohol consumption contributes anywhere from 2 to 4 percent of cancers of the esophagus, liver, and larynx.

Poor diets, occupational exposures, and chemotherapeutic therapy account for many human cancers. High-fat and high-calorie diets have been linked to breast, colon, and gallbladder cancer in humans. Diets poor in antioxidants and/or vitamins such as vitamin A and vitamin E probably also contribute to the onset of cancer. The method of cooking may also influence the production of carcinogens produced in the cooking process. Carcinogenic heterocyclic amines and polycyclic aro-

TABLE 8–8 Occupational human carcinogens.

Agent	Industrial Process	Neoplasms
Asbestos	Construction, asbestos mining	Peritoneum, bronchus
Arsenic	Mining and smelting	Skin, bronchus, liver
Alkylating agents (mechloroethamine hydrochloride and bis[chloromethyl] ether)	Chemical manufacturing	Bronchus
Benzene	Chemical manufacturing	Bone marrow
Benzidine, beta-naphthylamine	Dye and textile	Urinary bladder
Chromium and chromates	Tanning, pigment making	Nasal sinus, bronchus
Nickel	Nickel refining	Nasal sinus, bronchus
Polynuclear aromatic hydrocarbons	Steel making, roofing, chimney cleaning	Skin, scrotum, bronchus
Vinyl chloride monomer	Chemical manufacturing	Liver
Wood dust	Cabinet making	Nasal sinus
Beryllium	Aircraft manufacturing, electronics	Bronchus
Cadmium	Smelting	Bronchus
Ethylene oxide	Production of hospital supplies	Bone marrow
Formaldehyde	Plastic, textile, and chemical	Nasal sinus, bronchus
Polychlorinated biphenyls	Electrical-equipment production and maintenance	Liver

TABLE 8–9 Human carcinogenic chemicals associated with medical therapy and diagnosis.

Chemical or Drug	Associated Neoplasms
Alkylating agents (cyclophospamide, melphalan)	Bladder, leukemia
Azathioprine	Lymphoma, reticulum cell sarcoma, skin, Kaposi's sarcoma (?)
Chloramphenicol	Leukemia
Diethylstilbestrol	Vagina (clear cell carcinoma)
Estrogens	Liver cell adenoma, endometrium, skin
Phenacetin	Renal pelvis (carcinoma)
Phenytoin	Lymphoma, neuroblastoma
Thorotrast	Liver (angiosarcoma)

matic hydrocarbons are formed during broiling and grilling of meat. Acrylamide, a suspected human carcinogen, has been found in fried foods at low concentrations. A number of occupations associated with the development of specific cancers are listed in Table 8–8. A number of medical therapeutic and diagnostic tools have also been linked to the induction of human cancer (Table 8–9). Therapeutic immunosuppression given to transplant patients or arising secondary to selective diseases such as acquired immune deficiency syndrome (AIDS) result in an increase in a variety of different neoplasms. These results further support the role of the immune system in identifying and removing early preneoplastic cells from the body.

TABLE 8–10 IARC Classification of the evaluation of carcinogenicity for human beings.

Group	Evidence
1. Agent is carcinogenic to humans	Human data strong Animal data strong
2A. Agent is probably carcinogenic to humans	Human epidemiology data suggestive Animal data positive
2B. Agent is possibly carcinogenic to humans	Human epidemiology data weak Animal data positive
3. Agent is not classifiable as to carcinogenicity to humans	Human and animal data inadequate
4. Agent is probably not carcinogenic to humans	Human and animal data negative

Classification Evaluation of Carcinogenicity in Humans

The assessment and designation of a chemical or a mixture of chemicals as carcinogenic in humans is evaluated by various agencies worldwide. The evaluation usually encompasses both epidemiological and experimental animal and in vitro data utilizing assays as described earlier in this chapter. One of the first devised schemes for the classification of an agent's carcinogenicity was devised by the International Agency for Research on Cancer (IARC) (Table 8–10). The IARC approach assigns the chemical or mixture to one of five groupings based on strength of evidence for the agent's possible, probable, or definite carcinogenicity to humans. Similar classifications exist for the U.S. EPA, the Food & Drug Administration, and the European Community (EC). The classification of agents with regard to human carcinogenicity can be very difficult, in particular when animal data and/or epidemiological data in humans are inconclusive or confounded.

BIBLIOGRAPHY

Shields PG (ed): *Cancer Risk Assessment*. Boca Raton: Taylor & Francis, 2005.
Tannock IF, Hill RP, Bristow RG, Harrington L (eds): *The Basic Science of Oncology*. New York: McGraw-Hill, 2005.
Warshawsky D, Landolph JR (eds): *Molecular Carcinogenesis and the Molecular Biology of Human Cancer*. Boca Raton: CRC/Taylor and Francis, 2006.

QUESTIONS

1. There is evidence that certain dietary components are carcinogenic. Which of the following is NOT tabbed as a dietary carcinogen?
   a. excessive caloric intake.
   b. excessive alcohol consumption.
   c. aflatoxin B1 (a food contaminant).
   d. insufficient caloric intake.
   e. nitrites (found in some lunchmeats).

2. Which of the following statements regarding mechanisms of chemical carcinogenesis is FALSE?
   a. Procarcinogens require metabolism in order to exert their carcinogenic effect.
   b. Free radicals are highly reactive molecules that have a single, unpaired electron.
   c. DNA adducts interfere with the DNA replication machinery.
   d. Mutations in the DNA and failure to repair those mutations can be highly carcinogenic.
   e. Biological reduction of molecular oxygen is the only way free radicals can be formed.

3. In addition to being necessary for transcription to occur, which of the following transcription factors also plays a crucial role in nucleotide excision repair?
   a. TFIIA.
   b. TFIIB.
   c. TFIID.
   d. TFIIF.
   e. TFIIH.

4. Which of the following statements regarding DNA repair is true?
   a. Base excision repair requires the removal of a longer piece of DNA in comparison with nucleotide excision repair.
   b. The repair of double-stranded DNA breaks is more prone to error than is base excision repair.
   c. Dimerization of pyrimidines is repaired via base excision repair.
   d. Mismatch repair can only recognize normal nucleotides that are paired with a noncomplementary nucleotide.
   e. Nucleotide excision and base excision are tolerance mechanisms used to respond to DNA damage.

5. Which of the following statements is a characteristic of the initiation stage of carcinogenesis?
   a. Initiation is reversible in viable cells.
   b. The dose–response exhibits an easily measurable threshold.
   c. Cell division is required for the fixation of the process.
   d. All initiated cells survive over the lifespan of the organism.
   e. Spontaneous initiation of cells is a rare occurrence.

6. Tumor suppressor genes are mutated in a majority of cancers. Which of the following is NOT a characteristic of a tumor suppressor gene?
   a. A mutation in a tumor suppressor gene is dominant.
   b. Germ line inheritance of a mutated tumor suppressor gene is often involved with cancer development.
   c. There is considerable tissue specificity for cancer development.
   d. The *p53* gene is a tumor suppressor gene that also acts as a transcription factor.
   e. Mutations in tumor suppressor genes can result in loss of cell cycle control.

7. Which of the following molecules does NOT play an important role in cell cycle regulation?
   a. p53.
   b. cyclin-D.
   c. MAPK.
   d. MHC.
   e. E2F.

8. Which of the following environmental factors is proportionally responsible for the LEAST amount of cancer deaths?
   a. tobacco.
   b. infection.
   c. diet.
   d. sexual behavior.
   e. alcohol.

9. The evidence of the carcinogenicity of dietary intake is sufficient to include one's diet as associated with neoplasms of all of the following EXCEPT:
   a. colon.
   b. breast.
   c. pancreas.
   d. endometrium.
   e. gallbladder.

10. Which of the following is the correct definition of a complete carcinogen?
    a. a chemical capable only of initiating cells.
    b. a chemical possessing the ability of inducing cancer from normal cells, usually possessing properties of initiating, promoting, and progression agents.
    c. a chemical capable of converting an initiated cell or a cell in the stage of promotion to a potentially malignant cell.
    d. a chemical capable of causing the expansion of initiated cell clones.
    e. a chemical that will cause cancer 100 percent of the time that it is administered.

Genetic Toxicology

R. Julian Preston and George R. Hoffmann

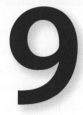

Genetic toxicology assesses the effects of chemical and physical agents on both DNA and on the genetic processes of living cells. This chapter addresses the assays for qualitative and quantitative assessment of cellular changes induced by chemical and physical agents, the underlying molecular mechanisms for these changes, and how such information can be incorporated in risk assessments.

HEALTH IMPACT OF GENETIC ALTERATIONS

Somatic Cells

Oncogenes are genes that stimulate the transformation of normal cells into cancer cells. They originate when genes called proto-oncogenes, involved in normal cellular growth and development, are genetically altered. Mutational alteration of proto-oncogenes can lead to overexpression of their growth-stimulating activity, whereas mutations that inactivate tumor-suppressor genes, which normally restrain cellular proliferation, free cells from their inhibitory influence.

The action of oncogenes is genetically dominant in that a single active oncogene is expressed even though its normal allele is present in the same cell. Among chromosomal alterations that activate proto-oncogenes, translocations are especially prevalent. A translocation can activate a proto-oncogene by moving it to a new chromosomal location with a more active promoter, where its expression is enhanced.

Unlike oncogenes, the cancer-causing alleles that arise from tumor-suppressor genes are typically recessive in that they are not expressed when they are heterozygous. Gene mutations in a tumor-suppressor gene on chromosome 17, called *P53*, occur in many different human cancers, and molecular characterization of *P53* mutations has linked specific human cancers to mutagen exposures.

Six acquired characteristics are essential for the formation of all tumors irrespective of tumor type and species. These include: (1) self-sufficiency in growth signals, (2) insensitivity to antigrowth signals, (3) evasion of apoptosis, (4) limitless replicative potential, (5) sustained angiogenesis, and (6) tissue invasion and metastasis. It seems probable that there is no specific order for obtaining these characteristics.

Gene mutations, chromosome aberrations (morphologic abnormality), and aneuploidy (abnormal number of chromosomes) are all implicated in the development of cancer. Many mutagens and clastogens (chromosome-breaking agents) contribute to carcinogenesis as initiators; however, mutagens, clastogens, and aneugens also may contribute to multiple genetic alterations.

Germ Cells

The relevance of gene mutations to health is evident from the many disorders often caused by base-pair substitutions or small deletions that are inherited as simple Mendelian characteristics. Many genetic disorders (e.g., cystic fibrosis, phenylketonuria, and Tay–Sachs disease) are caused by the expression of recessive mutations. These mutations are mainly inherited from previous generations and are expressed when an individual inherits the mutant gene from both parents.

Besides causing diseases that exhibit Mendelian inheritance, gene mutations undoubtedly contribute to human disease through the genetic component of disorders with a complex etiology such as heart disease, hypertension, and diabetes. Refined cytogenetic methods have led to the discovery of minor variations in chromosome structure that have no apparent effect. Nevertheless, other chromosome aberrations cause fetal death or serious abnormalities. Aneuploidy also contributes to fetal deaths and causes disorders such as Down syndrome. Much of the effect of chromosomal abnormalities occurs prenatally. Among the abnormalities, aneuploidy is the most common, followed by polyploidy. Structural aberrations constitute about 5 percent of the total. Most chromosomal anomalies detected in newborns arise de novo in the germ cells of the parents.

CANCER AND GENETIC RISK ASSESSMENTS

Cancer Risk Assessment

Cancer risk assessment involves investigation of sensitivity of different species and subpopulations to tumor induction by a chemical and development of a dose–response curve of mutations to a chemical.

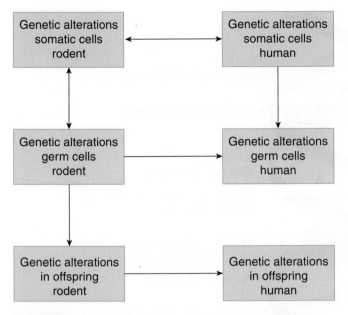

FIGURE 9–1 Parallelogram approach for genetic risk assessment. Data obtained for genetic alterations in rodent somatic and germ cells and human somatic cells are used to estimate the frequency of the same genetic alterations in human germ cells. The final step is to estimate the frequency of these genetic alterations that are transmitted to offspring.

Genetic Risk Assessment

To investigate genetic risk, the frequency of genetic alteration in human germ cells is estimated by extrapolation from data from rodent germ cells and somatic cells. For a complete estimate of genetic risk, it is necessary to obtain an estimate of the frequency of genetic alterations transmitted to the offspring (Figure 9–1).

MECHANISMS OF INDUCTION OF GENETIC ALTERATIONS

DNA Damage

The types of DNA damage range from single- and double-strand breaks in the DNA backbone to cross-links between DNA bases and between DNA bases and proteins and chemical addition to the DNA bases (adducts) (Figure 9–2).

Ionizing Radiations—Ionizing radiations, such as X-rays, gamma rays, and alpha particles, produce DNA single- and double-strand breaks and a broad range of base damages. Multiple damaged sites or cluster lesions appear to be more difficult to repair. These multiple lesions can be formed in DNA from the same radiation energy deposition event. The relative proportions of these different classes of DNA damage vary with type of radiation.

Ultraviolet Light—Ultraviolet light (a nonionizing radiation) induces two predominant lesions, cyclobutane pyrimi-dine dimers and 6,4-photoproducts. These lesions can be quantitated by chemical and immunologic methods.

Chemicals—Chemicals can produce base alterations either directly (DNA-reactive) as adducts or indirectly by intercalation of a chemical between the base pairs. Many electrophilic chemicals react with DNA, forming covalent addition products (adducts). Alkylated bases can also lead to base loss from DNA, which leaves an apurinic or apyrimidinic site, commonly called an AP site. The insertion of incorrect bases into AP sites causes mutations. Bulky DNA adducts are recognized by the cell in a similar way to UV damages and are repaired similarly.

Endogenous Agents—Endogenous agents are responsible for several hundred DNA damages per cell per day. The majority of these damages are altered DNA bases (e.g., 8-oxoguanine and thymine glycol) and AP sites. The cellular processes that can lead to DNA damage are the formation of reactive active oxygen species and deamination of cytosines and S-methylcytosines leading to uracils and thymines, respectively. The process of DNA replication itself is error-prone, and an incorrect base can be added by the polymerase.

DNA Repair

Two processes enable the cell to cope with the DNA damage that it sustains. With extensive damage, the cell can undergo apoptosis. If the damage is less severe, cells have developed a range of repair processes that return the DNA to its undamaged state (error-free repair) or to an improved but still altered state (error-prone repair). The basic principles underlying most repair processes are damage recognition, removal of damage (except for strand breaks or cleavage of pyrimidine dimers), repair DNA synthesis, and ligation.

Base Excision Repair—The major pathways by which DNA base damages are repaired involve removal of the damaged base. The resulting gap can be filled by a DNA polymerase, followed by ligation to the parental DNA. Sites of oxidative damage, either background or induced, are important substrates for base excision repair.

Nucleotide Excision Repair—The nucleotide excision repair (NER) system provides the cell's ability to remove bulky lesions from DNA. NER removes a damage-containing oligonucleotide from DNA by damage recognition, incision, excision, repair synthesis, and ligation. The DNA damage in actively transcribing genes, and specifically the transcribed strand, is preferentially and more rapidly repaired than the DNA damage in the rest of the genome. Thus, the cell protects the integrity of the transcription process.

Double-strand Break Repair—Cell survival is seriously compromised by the presence of broken chromosomes. Unrepaired double-strand breaks trigger one or more DNA damage response systems to either check cell-cycle progression or

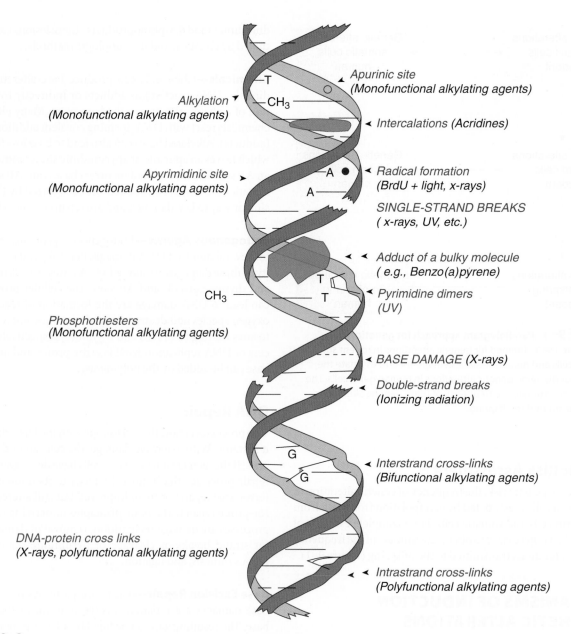

Alkylation
(Monofunctional alkylating agents)

—T

—CH₃

Apurinic site
(Monofunctional alkylating agents)

Intercalations (Acridines)

Apyrimidinic site
(Monofunctional alkylating agents)

—A

A

Radical formation
(BrdU + light, x-rays)

SINGLE-STRAND BREAKS
(x-rays, UV, etc.)

Adduct of a bulky molecule
(e.g., Benzo(a)pyrene)

T

Pyrimidine dimers
(UV)

CH₃—

T

Phosphotriesters
(Monofunctional alkylating agents)

BASE DAMAGE (X-rays)

Double-strand breaks
(Ionizing radiation)

G

Interstrand cross-links
(Bifunctional alkylating agents)

G

DNA-protein cross links
(X-rays, polyfunctional alkylating agents)

Intrastrand cross-links
(Polyfunctional alkylating agents)

FIGURE 9–2 **Spectrum of DNA damage induced by physical and chemical agents.**

induce apoptosis. There are two general pathways for repair of DNA double-strand breaks: homologous recombination and nonhomologous end-joining (NHEJ).

Homologous Recombination—The repair of double-strand breaks (and single-strand gaps) uses the following basic steps. The initial step is the production of a 3′-ended single-stranded tail by exonucleases or helicase activity. Through strand invasion, whereby the single-stranded tail invades an undamaged homologous DNA molecule, together with DNA synthesis, a so-called Holliday junction DNA complex is formed. By cleavage of this junction, two DNA molecules are produced (with or without a structural crossover), neither of which now contain a strand break.

Nonhomologous End-joining—This type of recombination requires the production of double-strand breaks, recombination of DNA pieces, and subsequent religation. A major component of the NHEJ repair complex is a DNA-dependent protein kinase (DNA-PK). This protein probably functions to align the broken DNA ends to facilitate their ligation or to serve as a signal molecule for recruiting other repair proteins.

Mismatch Repair—DNA mismatch repair systems operate to repair mismatched bases. The principal steps are damage recognition by a specific protein that binds to the mismatch, stabilization of the binding by the addition of one or more proteins, cutting the DNA at a distance from the mismatch, excision past the mismatch, resynthesis, and ligation.

O⁶-Methylguanine-DNA Methyltransferase Repair—
The enzyme O⁶-methylguanine-DNA methyltransferase (MGMT) protects cells against the toxic effects of simple alkylating agents by transferring the methyl group from O⁶-methylguanine in DNA to a cysteine residue in MGMT. The adducted base is reverted to a normal one by the enzyme, which is itself inactivated by the reaction.

Formation of Gene Mutations

Somatic Cells—Gene mutations, considered to be small DNA-sequence changes confined to a single gene, are substitutions, small additions, and small deletions. Base substitutions are the replacement of the correct nucleotide by an incorrect one; they can be further subdivided as transitions, where the change is purine for purine or pyrimidine for pyrimidine, and transversions where the change is purine for pyrimidine or vice versa. Frameshift mutations are the addition or deletion of one or a few base pairs (not in multiples of 3) in protein-coding regions.

The great majority of so-called spontaneous (background) mutations arise from *replication* of an altered template. These DNA alterations are either the result of oxidative damage or produced from the deamination of 5-methyl cytosine to thymine at CpG sites resulting in G:C → A:T transitions.

Gene mutations produced by a majority of chemicals and nonionizing radiations are base substitutions, frameshifts, and small deletions. Of these mutations, most are produced by errors of DNA *replication* on a damaged template. The relative mutation frequency will be the outcome of the race between repair and replication, that is, the more repair that takes place prior to replication, the lower the mutation frequency for a given amount of induced DNA damage. Significant regulators of the race are cell-cycle checkpoint genes (e.g., *P53*) because if the cell is checked from entering the S phase at a G_1/S checkpoint, then more repair can take place prior to the cell starting to replicate its DNA.

Germ Cells—The mechanism of production of gene mutations in germ cells is basically the same as in somatic cells. Ionizing radiations produce mainly deletions via errors of DNA repair; the majority of chemicals induce base substitutions, frameshifts, and small deletions by errors of DNA replication.

An important consideration for assessing gene mutations induced by chemicals in germ cells is the relationship between exposure and the timing of DNA replication (i.e., if there is damage, is it able to be repaired before replication?). The spermatogonial stem cell is the major contributor to genetic risk assessment because it is present generally throughout the reproductive lifetime of an individual. Each time a spermatogonial stem cell divides, it produces a differentiating spermatogonium and a stem cell. This stem cell can accumulate genetic damage from chronic exposures.

In oogenesis, the primary oocyte arrests prior to birth, and there is no further S phase until the zygote. For this reason, the oocyte is resistant to the induction of gene mutations by most chemicals.

Formation of Chromosomal Alterations

Somatic Cells

*Structural Chromosome Aberrations—*Sister chromatid exchanges (SCEs; the apparently reciprocal exchange between the sister chromatids of a single chromosome) and gene mutations are common. In particular, damaged DNA serves as the substrate leading to chromosomal aberrations. The DNA repair errors that lead to the formation of chromosome aberrations following ionizing radiation exposure arise from misligation of double-strand breaks or interaction of coincidentally repairing regions during NER of damaged bases. Incorrect rejoining of chromosomal pieces during repair leads to chromosomal exchanges within and between chromosomes. Failure to rejoin double-strand breaks or to complete repair of other types of DNA damage leads to terminal deletions.

The failure to incorporate an acentric fragment into a daughter nucleus at anaphase/telophase, or the failure of a whole chromosome to segregate to the cellular poles at anaphase, can result in the formation of a micronucleus that resides in the cytoplasm. Errors of DNA replication on a damaged template can lead to a variety of chromosomal alterations. The majority of these involve deletion or exchanges of individual chromatids but some can involve both chromatids.

*Numerical Chromosome Changes—*Numerical changes (e.g., monosomies, trisomies, and ploidy changes) can arise from errors in chromosomal segregation due to any of the numerous possible impairments of mitotic control processes. Alteration of various cellular components can result in failure to segregate the sister chromatids to separate daughter cells or in failure to segregate a chromosome to either pole.

*Sister Chromatid Exchange—*SCEs are produced during S phase and are presumed to be a consequence of errors in the replication process.

Germ Cells—The formation of chromosomal alterations in germ cells is basically the same as that for somatic cells, namely, via misrepair for ionizing radiations and radiomimetic chemicals for treatments in G_1 and G_2, and by errors of replication for all radiations and chemicals for DNA damage present during the S phase.

The types of aberrations formed in germ cells are the same as those formed in somatic cells. The specific segregation of chromosomes during meiosis influences the probability of recovery of an aberration, particularly a reciprocal translocation, in the offspring of a treated parent.

ASSAYS FOR DETECTING GENETIC ALTERATIONS

Introduction to Assay Design

Genetic toxicology assays serve two interrelated but distinct purposes in the toxicologic evaluation of chemicals: (1) identifying mutagens for purposes of hazard identification and

TABLE 9–1 Overview of genetic toxicology assays.

I. DNA damage and repair assays
  A. Direct detection of DNA damage
    • Alkaline elution assays for DNA strand breakage
    • Comet assay for DNA strand breakage
    • Assays for chemical adducts in DNA
  B. Bacterial assays for DNA damage
    • Differential killing of repair-deficient and wild-type strains
    • Induction of the SOS system by DNA damage
  C. Assays for repairable DNA damage in mammalian cells
    • Unscheduled DNA synthesis (UDS) in rat hepatocytes
    • UDS in rodent hepatocytes in vivo

II. Prokaryote gene mutation assays
  A. Bacterial reverse mutation assays
    • *Salmonella*/mammalian microsome assay (Ames test)
    • *E. coli* WP2 tryptophan reversion assay
    • *Salmonella* specific base-pair substitution assay (Ames-II assay)
    • *E. coli lacZ* specific reversion assay
  B. Bacterial forward mutation assays
    • *E. coli lacI* assay
    • Resistance to toxic metabolites or analogs in *Salmonella*

III. Assays in nonmammalian eukaryotes
  A. Fungal assays
    • Forward mutations, reversion, and small deletions
    • Mitotic crossing over and gene conversion in yeast
    • Mitotic aneuploidy: chromosome loss or gain in yeast
    • Meiotic nondisjunction in yeast or *Neurospora*
  B. Plant assays
    • Gene mutations affecting chlorophyll in seedlings or *waxy* in pollen
    • Tradescantia stamen hair color mutations
    • Chromosome aberrations or micronuclei in mitotic or meiotic cells
    • Aneuploidy detected by pigmentation or cytogenetics
  C. *Drosophila* assays
    • Sex linked recessive lethal test in germ cells
    • Heritable translocation assays
    • Sex chromosome loss tests for aneuploidy
    • Induction of mitotic recombination in eyes or wings

IV. Mammalian gene mutation assays
  A. In vitro assays for forward mutations
    • *tk* mutations in mouse lymphoma or human cells
    • *hprt* or *xprt* mutations in Chinese hamster or human cells
  B. In vivo assays for gene mutations in somatic cells
    • Mouse spot test (somatic cell specific locus test)
    • *hprt* mutations (6-thioguanine-resistance) in rodent lymphocytes

C. Transgenic assays
    • Mutations in the bacterial *lacI* gene in "Big Blue®" mice and rats
    • Mutations in the bacterial *lacZ* gene in the "Muta™ Mouse"
    • Mutations in the phage *cII* gene in *lacI* or *lacZ* transgenic mice
    • Point mutations and deletions in the *lacZ* plasmid mouse
    • Point mutations and deletions in *delta gpt* mice and rats

V. Mammalian cytogenetic assays
  A. Chromosome aberrations
    • Metaphase analysis in cultured Chinese hamster or human cells
    • Metaphase analysis of rodent bone marrow or lymphocytes in vivo
  B. Micronuclei
    • Cytokinesis-block micronucleus assay in human lymphocytes
    • Micronucleus assay in mammalian cell lines
    • In vivo micronucleus assay in rodent bone marrow or blood
  C. Sister chromatid exchange
    • SCE in human cells or Chinese hamster cells
    • SCE in rodent tissues, especially bone marrow
  D. Aneuploidy in mitotic cells
    • Mitotic disturbance seen by staining spindles and chromosomes
    • Hyperploidy detected by chromosome counting
    • Chromosome gain or loss in cells with intact cytoplasm
    • Micronucleus assay with centromere labeling
    • Hyperploid cells in vivo in mouse bone marrow
    • Mouse bone marrow micronucleus assay with centromere labeling

VI. Germ cell mutagenesis
  A. Measurement of DNA damage
    • Molecular dosimetry based on mutagen adducts
    • UDS in rodent germ cells
    • Alkaline elution assays for DNA strand breaks in rodent testes
  B. Gene mutations
    • Mouse specific-locus test for gene mutations and deletions
    • Mouse electrophoretic specific-locus test
    • Dominant mutations causing mouse skeletal defects or cataracts
    • Mouse tandem-repeat loci analysis
  C. Chromosomal aberrations
    • Cytogenetic analysis in oocytes, spermatogonia, or spermatocytes
    • Micronuclei in mouse spermatids
    • Mouse heritable translocation test
  D. Dominant lethal mutations
    • Mouse or rat dominant lethal assay
  E. Aneuploidy
    • Cytogenetic analysis for aneuploidy arising by nondisjunction
    • Sex chromosome loss test for nondisjunction or breakage
    • Micronucleus assay in spermatids with centromere labeling
    • FISH with probes for specific chromosomes in sperm

(2) characterizing dose–response relationships and mutagenic mechanisms.

Table 9–1 lists many of the assays employed in genetic toxicology. Some assays for gene mutations detect forward mutations, whereas others detect reversion. Forward mutations are genetic alterations in a wild-type gene and are detected by a change in phenotype caused by the alteration or loss of gene function. In contrast, a back mutation or reversion is a mutation that restores gene function in a mutant and thereby brings about a return to the wild-type phenotype. The simplest gene mutation assays rely on selection techniques to detect muta-

tions. By imposing experimental conditions under which only cells or organisms that have undergone mutation can grow, selection techniques greatly facilitate the identification of rare cells that have experienced mutation among the many cells that have not.

Studying mutagenesis in intact animals requires more complex assays, which range from inexpensive short-term tests that can be performed in a few days to complicated assays for mutations in mammalian germ cells. Typically, there remains a gradation in which an increase in relevance for human risk entails more elaborate and costly tests.

Many compounds that are not themselves mutagenic or carcinogenic can be activated into mutagens and carcinogens by mammalian metabolism. Such compounds are called promutagens and procarcinogens. The most widely used metabolic activation system in microbial and cell culture assays is a postmitochondrial supernatant from a rat liver homogenate, along with appropriate buffers and cofactors. Most of the short-term assays in Table 9–1 require exogenous metabolic activation to detect promutagens. Exceptions are those in intact mammals.

Despite their usefulness, in vitro metabolic activation systems cannot mimic mammalian metabolism perfectly. There are differences among tissues in reactions that activate or inactivate foreign compounds, and organisms of the normal flora of the gut can contribute to metabolism in intact mammals.

DNA Damage and Repair Assays

Some assays measure DNA damage itself rather than mutational consequences of DNA damage. They may do so directly, through such indicators as chemical adducts or strand breaks in DNA, or indirectly, through measurement of biological repair processes. Adducts in DNA can be detected by ^{32}P-postlabeling, immunologic methods using antibodies against specific adducts, or fluorometric methods in the case of such fluorescent compounds.

A rapid method of measuring DNA damage is the comet assay. In this assay, cells are incorporated into agarose on slides, lysed so as to liberate their DNA, and subjected to electrophoresis. The DNA is stained with a fluorescent dye for observation and image analysis. Because broken DNA fragments migrate more quickly than larger pieces of DNA, a blur of fragments (a "comet") is observed when the DNA is extensively damaged. The extent of DNA damage can be estimated from the length and other attributes of the comet tail. The comet assay appears to be a sensitive indicator of DNA damage with broad applicability among diverse species, including plants, worms, mollusks, fish, and amphibians.

The occurrence of DNA repair can serve as a readily measured indicator of DNA damage. The most common excision repair assay in mammalian cells is an assay for unscheduled DNA synthesis (UDS). The occurrence of UDS indicates that the DNA had been damaged.

Gene Mutations in Prokaryotes

The most common means of detecting mutations in microorganisms is selecting for reversion in strains that have a specific nutritional requirement differing from wild-type members of the species; such strains are called auxotrophs. In the Ames assay, one measures the frequency of histidine-independent bacteria that arise in a histidine-requiring strain in the presence or absence of the chemical being tested. Auxotrophic (nutrient-deficient) bacteria are treated with the chemical of interest and plated on medium that is deficient in histidine; if the colony survives, it must have a reversion mutation that allows it to survive without exogenous histidine.

The development of specific reversion assays of histidine mutations in *Salmonella* strains and of *lacZ* mutations in *Escherichia coli* has made the identification of specific base-pair substitutions more straightforward.

Genetic Alterations in Nonmammalian Eukaryotes

Gene Mutations and Chromosome Aberrations—The fruit fly, *Drosophila,* has long occupied a prominent place in genetic research because of the sex-linked recessive lethal (SLRL) test. The SLRL test permits the detection of recessive lethal mutations at 600 to 800 different loci on the X chromosome by screening for the presence or absence of wild-type males in the offspring of specifically designed crosses. A significant increase over the frequency of spontaneous SLRLs in the lineages derived from treated males indicates mutagenesis. The SLRL test yields information about mutagenesis in germ cells, which is lacking in microbial and cell culture systems.

Genetic and cytogenetic assays in plants continue to find use in special applications, such as in situ monitoring for mutagens and exploration of the metabolism of promutagens by agricultural plants. In situ monitoring entails looking for evidence of mutagenesis in organisms that are grown in the environment of interest.

Mitotic Recombination—Assays in nonmammalian eukaryotes are important for the study of induced recombination. Recombinogenic effects in yeast have long been used as a general indicator of genetic damage. The best characterized assays for recombinogens are those that detect mitotic crossing over and mitotic gene conversion in the yeast *Saccharomyces cerevisiae*.

Gene Mutations in Mammals

Gene Mutations In Vitro—Mutagenicity assays in cultured mammalian cells have some of the same advantages as microbial assays with respect to speed and cost, and they follow quite similar approaches. The most widely used assays for gene mutations in mammalian cells detect forward mutations that confer resistance to a toxic chemical.

Gene Mutations In Vivo—In vivo assays involve treating intact animals and analyzing genetic effects in appropriate tissues. Mutations may be detected either in somatic cells or in germ cells.

The mouse spot test is a traditional genetic assay for gene mutations in somatic cells. Visible spots of altered phenotype in mice heterozygous for coat color genes indicate mutations in the progenitor cells of the altered regions.

Mutation assays also provide information on mechanisms of mutagenesis. Base-pair substitutions and large deletions can be differentiated through the use of probes for the target gene and Southern blotting, in that base substitutions are too subtle to be detectable on the blots. Gene mutations have been characterized at the molecular level by DNA-sequence analysis both in transgenic rodents and in endogenous mammalian genes.

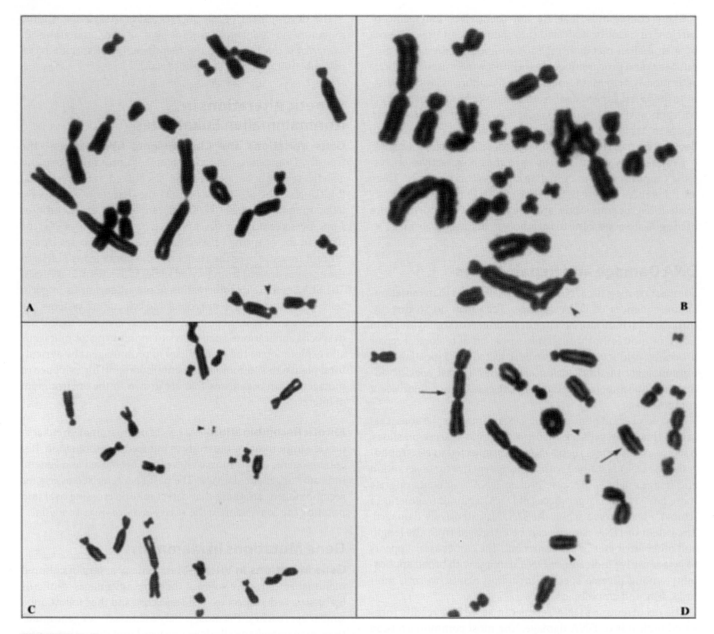

FIGURE 9–3 **Chromosome aberrations induced by x-rays in Chinese hamster ovary (CHO) cells.** *A.* A chromatid deletion (▶). *B.* A chromatid exchange called a triradial (▶). *C.* A small interstitial deletion (▶) that resulted from chromosome breakage. *D.* A metaphase with more than one aberration: a centric ring plus an acentric fragment (▶) and a dicentric chromosome plus an acentric fragment (→).

Transgenic Assays—Transgenic animals are products of DNA technology in which the animal contains foreign DNA sequences that have been added to the genome and are transmitted through the germ line. The foreign DNA is therefore represented in all the somatic cells of the animal.

Mice that carry *lac* genes from *E. coli* use either *lacI* or *lacZ* as a target for mutagenesis. After mutagenic treatment of the transgenic animals, the *lac* genes are recovered from the animal, packaged into phage λ, and transferred to *E. coli* for mutational analysis. Mutant plaques are identified on the basis of phenotype, and mutant frequencies can be calculated for different tissues of the treated animals.

Mammalian Cytogenetic Assays

Chromosome Aberrations—Genetic assays without DNA sequencing are indirect, in that one observes a phenotype and reaches conclusions about genes. In contrast, cytogenetic assays use microscopy for direct observation of the effect of interest. In conventional cytogenetics, metaphase analysis is used to detect chromosomal anomalies. Cells should be treated during a sensitive period of the cell cycle (typically S), and aberrations should be analyzed at the first mitotic division after treatment. Examples of chromosome aberrations are shown in Figure 9–3.

It is essential that sufficient cells be analyzed because a negative result in a small sample is equivocal and inconclusive. Results should be recorded for specific classes of aberrations, not just as an overall index of aberrations per cell.

In interpreting results on the induction of chromosome aberrations in cell cultures, questionable positive results have been found at highly cytotoxic doses, high osmolality, and pH extremes. Although excessively high doses may lead to artifactual positive responses, the failure to test to sufficiently high doses also undermines the utility of a test; therefore, testing should be conducted at an intermediate dose and extended to a dose at which some cytotoxicity is observed.

In vivo assays for chromosome aberrations involve treating intact animals and later collecting cells for cytogenetic analysis. The main advantage of in vivo assays is that they include mammalian metabolism, DNA repair, and pharmacodynamics. The target is a tissue from which large numbers of dividing cells are easily prepared for analysis such as bone marrow.

In interphase cell analysis by fluorescence in situ hybridization (FISH), a nucleic acid probe is hybridized to complementary sequences in chromosomal DNA. The probe is labeled with a fluorescent dye so that the chromosomal location to which it binds is visible by fluorescence microscopy; often, probes are used that cover the whole chromosome, called "chromosome painting."

Chromosome painting facilitates cytogenetic analysis, because aberrations are easily detected by the number of fluorescent regions in a painted metaphase. FISH permits the scoring of stable aberrations, such as translocations and insertions, which are not readily detected in traditional metaphase analysis of unbanded chromosomes.

Micronuclei—Micronuclei are membrane-bounded structures that contain chromosomal fragments, or sometimes whole chromosomes, that were not incorporated into a daughter nucleus at mitosis. Micronuclei usually represent acentric chromosomal fragments, and they are commonly used as simple indicators of chromosomal damage. Micronuclei in a binucleate human lymphocyte are shown in Figure 9–4.

Sister Chromatid Exchange—SCE, in which apparently reciprocal segments have been exchanged between the two chromatids of a chromosome, is visible cytologically through differential staining of chromatids (Figure 9–5). SCE assays are general indicators of mutagen exposure, rather than measures of a mutagenic effect.

Aneuploidy—Assays for aneuploidy include chromosome counting, the detection of micronuclei that contain kinetochores, and the observation of abnormal spindles or spindle–chromosome associations in cells in which spindles and chromosomes have been differentially stained.

The presence of the spindle attachment region of a chromosome (kinetochore) in a micronucleus can indicate that it contains a whole chromosome. Aneuploidy may therefore be detected by means of antikinetochore antibodies with a fluorescent label or FISH with a probe for centromere-specific

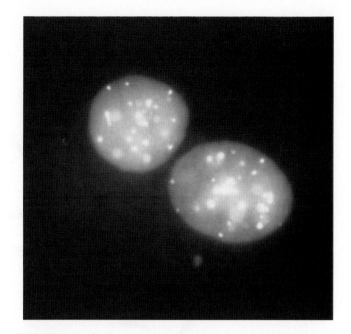

FIGURE 9–4 Micronucleus in a human lymphocyte. The cytochalasin B method was used to inhibit cytokinesis that resulted in a binucleate nucleus. The micronucleus resulted from failure of an acentric chromosome fragment or a whole chromosome being included in a daughter nucleus following cell division. (Image courtesy of James Allen, Jill Barnes, and Barbara Collins.)

DNA. Frequencies of micronuclei ascribable to aneuploidy and to clastogenic effects may therefore be determined concurrently by tabulating micronuclei with and without kinetochores.

Germ Cell Mutagenesis

Gene Mutations—Mammalian germ cell assays provide the best basis for assessing risks to human germ cells. Mammalian assays permit the measurement of mutagenesis at different germ cell stages. Late stages of spermatogenesis are often found to be sensitive to mutagenesis, but spermatocytes, spermatids, and spermatozoa are transitory. Mutagenesis in stem cell spermatogonia and resting oocytes is of special interest in genetic risk assessment because of the persistence of these stages throughout reproductive life.

Chromosomal Alterations—Knowledge of the induction of chromosome aberrations in germ cells is important for assessing risks to future generations. A germ cell micronucleus assay has been developed, in which chromosomal damage induced in meiosis is measured by observation of rodent spermatids. Aneuploidy originating in mammalian germ cells may be detected cytologically through chromosome counting for hyperploidy or genetically in the mouse sex-chromosome loss test.

Besides cytologic observation, indirect evidence for chromosome aberrations is obtained in the mouse heritable translocation assay, which measures reduced fertility in the offspring of treated males. This presumptive evidence of chromosomal rearrangements can be confirmed through cytogenetic analysis.

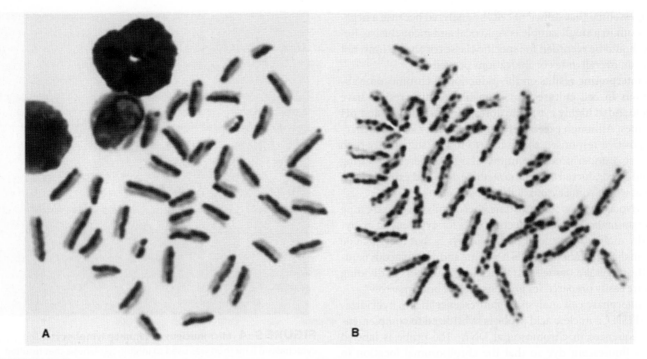

FIGURE 9–5 **Sister chromatid exchanges (SCEs) in human lymphocytes.** *A.* SCEs in untreated cell. *B.* SCEs in cell exposed to ethyl carbamate. The treatment results in a very large increase in the number of SCEs. (Image courtesy of James Allen and Barbara Collins.)

Dominant Lethal Mutations—The mouse or rat dominant lethal assay offers an extensive database on the induction of genetic damage in mammalian germ cells. Commonly, males are treated on an acute or subchronic basis with the agent of interest and then mated with virgin females. The females are killed and necropsied during pregnancy so that embryonic mortality, assumed to be due to chromosomal anomalies, may be characterized and quantified.

Development of Testing Strategies

Concern about adverse effects of mutation on human health, principally carcinogenesis and the induction of transmissible damage in germ cells, has provided the impetus to identify environmental mutagens. Genetic toxicology assays may be used to screen chemicals to detect mutagens and to obtain information on mutagenic mechanisms and dose–responses that contribute to an evaluation of hazards. Besides testing pure chemicals, environmental samples are tested because many mutagens exist in complex mixtures. The analysis of complex mixtures often requires a combination of mutagenicity assays and refined analytical methods.

The first indication that a chemical is a mutagen often lies in chemical structure. Potential electrophilic sites in a molecule are alerts to possible mutagenicity and carcinogenicity, because such sites confer reactivity with nucleophilic sites in DNA.

Assessment of a chemical's genotoxicity requires data from well-characterized genetic assays. Sensitivity refers to the proportion of carcinogens that are positive in the assay, whereas specificity is the proportion of noncarcinogens that are

negative. Sensitivity and specificity both contribute to the predictive reliability of an assay.

Rather than trying to assemble batteries of complementary assays, it is prudent to emphasize mechanistic considerations in choosing assays. Such an approach makes a sensitive assay for gene mutations (e.g., the Ames assay) and an assay for clastogenic effects in mammals pivotal in the evaluation of genotoxicity. Beyond gene mutations, one should evaluate damage at the chromosomal level with a mammalian in vitro or in vivo cytogenetic assay. Other assays offer an extensive database on chemical mutagenesis (*Drosophila* SLRL), a unique genetic endpoint (i.e., aneuploidy; mitotic recombination), applicability to diverse organisms and tissues (i.e., DNA damage assays, such as the comet assay), or special importance in the assessment of genetic risk (i.e., germ cell assays).

HUMAN POPULATION MONITORING

For cancer risk assessment considerations, the human data utilized most frequently, in the absence of epidemiologic data, are those collected from genotoxicity/mutagenicity assessments in human populations. The studies conducted most frequently are for chromosome aberrations, micronuclei, and SCEs in peripheral lymphocytes.

The size of each study group should be sufficiently large to avoid any confounder having undue influence. Certain characteristics should be matched among exposed and unexposed groups. These include age, sex, smoking status, and general dietary features. Study groups of 20 or more individuals can be used as a reasonable substitute for exact matching because confounders will be less influential on chromosome alteration or mutation frequency in larger groups. In some instances, it might be informative to compare exposed groups with a historical control, as well as to a concurrent control.

Reciprocal translocations are transmissible from cell generation to generation, and frequency can be representative of an accumulation over time of exposure. The importance of this is that stable chromosome aberrations observed in peripheral lymphocytes exposed in vivo, but assessed following in vitro culture, are produced in vivo in hematopoietic stem cells or other precursor cells of the peripheral lymphocytes pool.

NEW APPROACHES FOR GENETIC TOXICOLOGY

The ability to manipulate and characterize DNA, RNA, and proteins has been at the root of the advance in our understanding of basic cellular processes and how they can be perturbed. However, the development of sophisticated molecular biology does not in itself imply a corresponding advance in the utility of genetic toxicology and its application to risk assessment. Knowing the types of studies to conduct and knowing how to interpret the data remain as fundamental as always. There is a need for genetic toxicology to avoid the temptation to use more and more sophisticated techniques to address the same questions and in the end make the same mistakes as have been made previously.

Advances in Cytogenetics

Conventional chromosome staining with DNA stains such as Giemsa or the process of chromosome banding requires considerable expenditure of time and a rather high level of expertise. Chromosome banding does allow for the assessment of transmissible aberrations such as reciprocal translocations and inversions with a fairly high degree of accuracy. Stable aberrations are transmissible from parent to daughter cell, and they represent effects of chronic exposures. The more readily analyzed but cell-lethal, nontransmissible aberrations such as dicentrics and deletions reflect only recent exposures and then only when analyzed at the first division after exposure.

Specific chromosomes, specific genes, and chromosome alterations can be detected readily since the development of FISH. In principle, the technique relies on amplification of DNA from particular genomic regions such as whole chromosomes or gene regions and the hybridization of these amplified DNAs to metaphase chromosome preparations or interphase nuclei. Regions of hybridization can be determined by the use of fluorescent antibodies that detect modified DNA bases incorporated during amplification or by incorporating fluorescent bases during amplification. The fluorescently labeled, hybridized regions are detected by fluorescence microscopy. Alterations in tumors can also be detected on a whole-genome basis. Comparative genomic hybridization (CGH) has allowed an accurate and sensitive assessment of chromosomal alterations present in tumors. CGH is adapted for automated screening approaches using biochips.

The types of data collected will affect our understanding of how tumors develop. Data on the dose–response characteristics for a specific chromosomal alteration as a proximate marker of cancer can enhance the cancer risk assessment process by describing effects of low exposures that are below those for which tumor incidence can be reliably assessed. Cytogenetic data can also improve extrapolation of data generated with laboratory animals to humans.

Molecular Analysis of Mutations and Gene Expression

With technological advances, the exact basis of a mutation at the level of the DNA sequence can be established. With hybridization of test DNAs to oligonucleotide arrays, specific genetic alterations or their cellular consequences can be determined rapidly and automatically. cDNA microarray technologies allow the measurement of changes in expression of hundreds or even thousands of genes at one time. The level of expression at the mRNA level is measured by amount of hybridization of isolated cDNAs to oligonucleotide fragments from known genes or expressed sequence tags (EST) on a specifically laid out grid. This technique holds great promise for establishing a cell's response to exposure to chemical or physical agents in the context of normal cellular patterns of gene expression.

CONCLUSION

Genetic toxicology demonstrated that ionizing radiations and chemicals could induce mutations and chromosome alterations in plant, insect, and mammalian cells. Various short-term assays for genetic toxicology identified many mutagens and address the relationship between mutagens and carcinogens. Failure of the assays to be completely predictive resulted in the identification of nongenotoxic carcinogens. Key cellular processes related to mutagenesis have been identified, including multiple pathways of DNA repair, cell-cycle controls, and the role of checkpoints in ensuring that the cell cycle does not proceed until the DNA and specific cellular structures are checked for fidelity. Recent developments in genetic toxicology have improved our understanding of basic cellular processes and alterations that can affect the integrity of the genetic material and its functions. The ability to detect and analyze mutations in mammalian germ cells continues to improve and contribute to a better appreciation for the long-term consequences of mutagenesis in human populations.

BIBLIOGRAPHY

Choy WN: *Genetic Toxicology and Cancer Risk Assessment.* New York: Marcel Dekker, 2001.

Mendrick DL, Mattes WB: *Essential Concepts of Toxicogenomics.* Totowa, NJ: Humana, 2008.

Sahu SC: *Toxicogenomics: A Powerful Tool for Toxicity Assessment.* Oxford: Wiley-Blackwell, 2008.

Semizarov D, Blomme E: *Genomics in Drug Discovery and Development.* Hoboken, NJ: John Wiley, 2009.

QUESTIONS

1. Oncogenes:
   a. maintain normal cellular growth and development.
   b. exert their action in a genetically recessive fashion.
   c. are often formed via translocation to a location with a more active promoter.
   d. can be mutated to form proto-oncogenes.
   e. include growth factors and GTPases, but not transcription factors.

2. Which of the following is NOT one of the more common sources of DNA damage?
   a. ionizing radiation.
   b. UV light.
   c. electrophilic chemicals.
   d. DNA polymerase error.
   e. x-rays.

3. Which of the following pairs of DNA repair mechanisms is most likely to introduce mutations into the genetic composition of an organism?
   a. nonhomologous end-joining (NHEJ) and base excision repair.
   b. nonhomologous end-joining and homologous recombination.
   c. homologous recombination and nucleotide excision repair.
   d. nucleotide excision repair and base excision repair.
   e. homologous recombination and mismatch repair.

4. Which of the following DNA mutations would NOT be considered a frameshift mutation?
   a. insertion of 5 nucleotides.
   b. insertion of 7 nucleotides.
   c. deletion of 18 nucleotides.
   d. deletion of 13 nucleotides.
   e. deletion of 1 nucleotide.

5. Which of the following base pair mutations is properly characterized as a transversion mutation?
   a. $T \rightarrow C$.
   b. $A \rightarrow G$.
   c. $G \rightarrow A$.
   d. $T \rightarrow U$.
   e. $A \rightarrow C$.

6. All of the following statements regarding nondisjunction during meiosis are true EXCEPT:
   a. Nondisjunction events can happen during meiosis I or meiosis II.
   b. All gametes from nondisjunction events have an abnormal chromosome number.
   c. Trisomy 21 (Down syndrome) is a common example of nondisjunction.
   d. In a nondisjunction event in meiosis I, homologous chromosomes fail to separate.
   e. The incorrect formation of spindle fibers is a common cause of nondisjunction during meiosis.

7. Which of the following diseases does NOT have a recessive inheritance pattern?
   a. phenylketonuria.
   b. cystic fibrosis.
   c. Tay–Sachs disease.
   d. sickle cell anemia.
   e. Huntington's disease.

8. What is the purpose of the Ames assay?
   a. to determine the threshold of UV light bacteria can receive before having mutations in their DNA.
   b. to measure the frequency of aneuploidy in bacterial colonies treated with various chemicals.
   c. to determine the frequency of a reversion mutation that allows bacterial colonies to grow in the absence of vital nutrients.
   d. to measure rate of induced recombination in mutagen-treated fungi.
   e. to measure induction of phenotypic changes in *Drosophila*.

9. In mammalian cytogenic assays, chromosomal aberrations are measured after treatment of the cells at which sensitive phase of the cell cycle?
   a. interphase.
   b. M phase.
   c. S phase.
   d. G1.
   e. G2.

10. Which of the following molecules is used to gauge the amount of a specific gene being transcribed to mRNA?
    a. protein.
    b. mRNA.
    c. DNA.
    d. cDNA.
    e. CGH.

Developmental Toxicology

John M. Rogers and Robert J. Kavlock

KEY POINTS

- Developmental toxicology encompasses the study of pharmacokinetics, mechanisms, pathogenesis, and outcome following exposure to agents or conditions leading to abnormal development.
- Developmental toxicology includes teratology, or the study of structural birth defects.
- *Gametogenesis* is the process of forming the haploid germ cells: the egg and the sperm.
- *Organogenesis* is the period during which most bodily structures are established. This period of heightened susceptibility to malformations extends from the third to the eighth week of gestation in humans.

SCOPE OF PROBLEM— THE HUMAN EXPERIENCE

Successful pregnancy outcome in the general population occurs at a surprisingly low frequency. Estimates of adverse outcomes include postimplantation pregnancy loss, 31 percent; major birth defects, 2 to 3 percent at birth and increasing to 6 to 7 percent at 1 year as more manifestations are diagnosed; minor birth defects, 14 percent; low birth weight, 7 percent; infant mortality (prior to 1 year of age), 1.4 percent; and abnormal neurologic function, 16 to 17 percent. Thus, less than half of all human conceptions result in the birth of a completely normal, healthy infant. Many hundreds of chemicals are teratogens; most of them produce birth defects by an unknown mechanism. However, Table 10–1 lists chemicals, chemical classes, or conditions known to alter prenatal development in humans.

Thalidomide

In 1960, a large increase in newborns with rare limb malformations of amelia (absence of the limbs) or various degrees of phocomelia (reduction of the long bones of the limbs) was recorded in West Germany. Congenital heart disease; ocular, intestinal, and renal anomalies; and malformations of the external and inner ears were also involved. Thalidomide, identified as the causative agent, was used throughout much of the world as a sleep aid and to ameliorate nausea and vomiting in pregnancy. It had no apparent toxicity or addictive properties in adult humans or animals at therapeutic exposure levels.

As a result of this catastrophe, regulatory agencies developed requirements for evaluating the effects of drugs on pregnancy outcomes.

Diethylstilbestrol

Diethylstilbestrol (DES) is a synthetic nonsteroidal estrogen widely used from the 1940s to the 1970s in the United States to prevent threatened miscarriage. It was soon linked to clear cell adenocarcinoma of the vagina. Maternal use of DES prior to the 18th week of gestation appeared to be necessary for induction of the genital tract anomalies in offspring; the overall incidence of noncancerous alterations in the vagina and cervix was estimated to be as high as 75 percent. In male offspring of exposed pregnancies, a high incidence of reproductive tract anomalies along with low ejaculated semen volume and poor semen quality were observed. The realization of the latent and devastating manifestations of prenatal DES exposure has broadened the magnitude and scope of potential adverse outcomes of intrauterine exposures. A recent study in mice suggests that the increased susceptibility to abnormalities conferred by DES exposure may be passed on to future generations of exposed mothers.

Ethanol

Although the developmental toxicity of ethanol can be traced to biblical times (e.g., Judges 13:3-4), only since the description of the Fetal Alcohol Syndrome (FAS) in 1971 has a clear acceptance

TABLE 10–1 Human developmental toxicants.

Radiation
- Atomic fallout
- Radioiodine
- Therapeutic

Infections
- Cytomegalovirus
- Herpes simplex virus I and II
- Parvovirus B-19 (erythema infectiosum)
- Rubella virus
- Syphilis
- Toxoplasmosis
- Varicella virus
- Venezuelan equine encephalitis virus

Maternal trauma and metabolic imbalances
- Alcoholism
- Amniocentesis, early
- Chorionic villus sampling (before day 60)
- Cretinism
- Diabetes
- Folic acid deficiency
- Hyperthermia
- Phenylketonuria
- Rheumatic disease and congenital heart block
- Sjogren's syndrome
- Virilizing tumors

Drugs and chemicals
- Aminoglycosides
- Androgenic hormones
- Angiotensin converting enzyme inhibitors: captopril, enalapril
- Angiotensin receptor antagonists: sartans
- Anticonvulsants: diphenylhydantoin, trimethadione, valproic acid, carbamazepine
- Busulfan
- Carbon monoxide
- Chlorambucil
- Cocaine
- Coumarins
- Cyclophosphamide
- Cytarabine
- Diethylstilbestrol
- Danazol
- Ergotamine
- Ethanol
- Ethylene oxide
- Fluconazole
- Folate antagonists: aminopterin, methotrexate
- Iodides
- Lead
- Lithium
- Mercury, organic
- Methimazole
- Methylene blue
- Misoprostal
- Penicillamine
- Polychlorobiphenyls
- Quinine (high dose)
- Retinoids: accutane, isotretinoin, etretinate, acitretin
- Tetracyclines
- Thalidomide
- Tobacco smoke
- Toluene
- Vitamin A (high dose)

of alcohol's developmental toxicity occurred. FAS comprises craniofacial dysmorphism, intrauterine and postnatal growth retardation, retarded psychomotor and intellectual development, and other nonspecific major and minor abnormalities.

In utero exposure to lower levels of ethanol than those that produce full-blown FAS has been associated with a wide range of effects, including isolated components of FAS and milder forms of neurologic and behavioral disorders that have been termed Fetal Alcohol Spectrum Disorder (FASD). Alcohol consumption can affect birth weight in a dose-related fashion.

Tobacco Smoke

Prenatal and early postnatal exposure to tobacco smoke or its constituents may well represent the leading cause of environmentally induced developmental disease and morbidity today. Approximately 25 percent of women in the United States continue to smoke during pregnancy, despite public health programs aimed at curbing this behavior. The consequences of developmental tobacco smoke exposure include spontaneous abortions, perinatal deaths, increased risk of sudden infant death syndrome (SIDS), increased risk of learning, behavioral, and attention disorders, and lower birth weight. One component of tobacco smoke, nicotine, is a known neuroteratogen in experimental animals and can by itself produce many of the adverse developmental outcomes associated with tobacco smoke. Perinatal exposure to tobacco smoke can also affect branching morphogenesis and maturation of the lung, leading to altered physiologic function. Environmental (passive) tobacco smoke also represents a significant risk to the pregnant nonsmoker.

Cocaine

Cocaine is a local anesthetic with vasoconstrictor properties. Effects on the fetus are complicated and controversial and demonstrate the difficulty of monitoring the human population for adverse reproductive outcomes. Accurate exposure ascertainment is difficult, as many confounding factors including socioeconomic status and concurrent use of cigarettes, alcohol, and other drugs of abuse may be involved. In addition, reported effects on the fetus and infant (neurologic and behavioral changes) are difficult to identify and quantify. Nevertheless, adverse effects reliably associated with cocaine exposure in humans include abruptio placentae, premature labor and delivery, microcephaly, altered prosencephalic development, decreased birth weight, SIDS, and a neonatal neurologic syndrome of abnormal sleep, tremor, poor feeding, irritability, and occasional seizures.

Retinoids

Vitamin A (retinol) exposure can cause malformations of the face, limbs, heart, central nervous system, and skeleton. Spontaneous abortion, live-born infants having at least one major malformation, and numerous exposed children having full-scale IQ scores below 85 at age 5 years have been documented.

Angiotensin Converting Enzyme (ACE) Inhibitors and Angiotensin Receptor Antagonists

ACE inhibitors and angiotensin receptor blockers are widely prescribed and, when used in the second half of pregnancy, are known to cause oligohydramnios, fetal growth retardation, pulmonary hypoplasia, joint contractures, hypocalvaria, neonatal renal failure, hypotension, and death. Some studies suggest that exposure in the first trimester should be avoided.

PRINCIPLES OF DEVELOPMENTAL TOXICOLOGY

Some basic principles of teratology put forth by Jim Wilson in 1959 and listed in Table 10–2 are still valid today.

Critical Periods of Susceptibility and Endpoints of Toxicity

Development is characterized by various changes that are orchestrated by a cascade of factors regulating gene transcription throughout development. Intercellular and intracellular signaling pathways essential for normal development rely on transcriptional, translational, and posttranslational controls. The rapid changes occurring during development alter the nature of the embryo/fetus as a target for toxicity. Timing of some key developmental events in humans and experimental animal species is presented in Table 10–3.

Gametogenesis is the process of forming the haploid germ cells: the egg and the sperm. These gametes fuse in the process of *fertilization* to form the diploid *zygote*, or one-celled embryo. Gametogenesis and fertilization are vulnerable to toxicants.

TABLE 10–2 Wilson's general principles of teratology.

I.	Susceptibility to teratogenesis depends on the genotype of the conceptus and the manner in which this interacts with adverse environmental factors
II.	Susceptibility to teratogenesis varies with the developmental stage at the time of exposure to an adverse influence
III.	Teratogenic agents act in specific ways (mechanisms) on developing cells and tissues to initiate sequences of abnormal developmental events (pathogenesis)
IV.	The access of adverse influences to developing tissues depends on the nature of the influence (agent)
V.	The four manifestations of deviant development are death, malformation, growth retardation, and functional deficit
VI.	Manifestations of deviant development increase in frequency and degree as dosage increases, from the no effect to the totally lethal level

Source: Data from Wilson JG: *Environment and Birth Defects.* New York: Academic Press, 1973, pp. 12–30, Elsevier.

TABLE 10-3 Timing of key developmental events in some mammalian species.[1]

	Rat	Rabbit	Monkey	Human
Blastocyst formation	3–5	2.6–6	4–9	4–6
Implantation	5–6	6	9	6–7
Organogenesis	6–17	6–18	20–45	21–56
Primitive streak	9	6.5	18–20	16–18
Neural plate	9.5	—	9–21	18–20
First somite	10	—	—	20–21
First branchial arch	10	—	—	20
First heartbeat	10.2	—	—	22
10 somites	10–11	9	23–24	25–26
Upper limb buds	10.5	10.5	25–26	29–30
Lower limb buds	11.2	11	26–27	31–32
Testes differentiation	14.5	20	—	43
Heart septation	15.5	—	—	46–47
Palate closure	16–17	19–20	45–47	56–58
Urethral groove closed in male	—	—	—	90
Length of gestation	21–22	31–34	166	267

[1]Developmental ages are days of gestation.
Source: Data from Shepard TH: *Catalog of Teratogenic Agents,* 9th ed. Baltimore: The Johns Hopkins University Press, 1998.

Following fertilization, the embryo moves down the fallopian tube and implants in the wall of the uterus. The *preimplantation* period comprises mainly an increase in cell number through a rapid series of cell divisions with little growth in size (*cleavage* of the zygote) and cavitation of the embryo to form a fluid-filled blastocoele. This stage, termed the *blastocyst,* contains cells destined to give rise to the embryo proper and other cells that give rise to extraembryonic membranes and support structures.

Toxicity during preimplantation is generally thought to result in no or slight effect on growth (because of regulative growth) or in death (through overwhelming damage or failure to implant). Patterning of the limbs and lower body may begin at this time. Because of the rapid mitoses occurring during the preimplantation period, chemicals affecting DNA synthesis/integrity or those affecting microtubule assembly would be expected to be particularly toxic if given access to the embryo.

Following implantation the embryo undergoes *gastrulation,* the process of formation of the three primary germ layers—the *ectoderm, mesoderm,* and *endoderm.* As a prelude to organogenesis, the period of gastrulation is quite susceptible to teratogenesis. A number of toxicants administered during gastrulation produce malformations of the eye, brain, and face. These malformations are indicative of damage to the anterior *neural plate,* one of the regions defined by the cellular movements of gastrulation.

The formation of the neural plate in the ectoderm marks the onset of *organogenesis,* during which the rudiments of most bodily structures are established. This period of heightened susceptibility to malformations extends from approximately the third to the eighth week of gestation in humans. The rapid changes of organogenesis require cell proliferation, cell migration, cell–cell interactions, and morphogenetic tissue remodeling. Within organogenesis, there are periods of peak susceptibility for each forming structure. The peak incidence of each malformation coincides with the timing of key developmental events in the affected structure.

The end of organogenesis marks the beginning of the *fetal period,* which is characterized primarily by tissue differentiation, growth, and physiologic maturation. All organs are present and grossly recognizable, although not yet completely developed.

Exposure during the fetal period is most likely to result in effects on growth and functional maturation. Functional anomalies of the central nervous system and reproductive organs—including behavioral, mental, and motor deficits as well as decreases in fertility—are among the possible adverse outcomes.

Dose–Response Patterns and the Threshold Concept

The major effects of prenatal exposure, observed at the time of birth in developmental toxicity studies, are embryo lethality, malformations, and growth retardation. For some agents, these endpoints may represent a continuum of increasing toxicity, with low dosages producing growth retardation and increasing dosages producing malformations and then lethality.

Another key element of the dose–response relationship is the shape of the dose–response curve at low exposure levels. Because of the high restorative growth potential of the mammalian embryo, cellular homeostatic mechanisms, and maternal metabolic defenses, mammalian developmental toxicity has generally been considered a threshold phenomenon. Assumption of a threshold means that there is a maternal dosage below which an adverse response is not elicited because some repair or defense system is able to combat the exposure.

MECHANISMS AND PATHOGENESIS OF DEVELOPMENTAL TOXICITY

The term *mechanisms* refers to cellular-level events that initiate the process leading to abnormal development. *Pathogenesis* comprises the cell-, tissue-, and organ-level sequelae that are ultimately manifest in abnormality. Mechanisms of teratogenesis include mutations, chromosomal breaks, altered mitosis, altered nucleic acid integrity or function, diminished supplies of precursors or substrates, decreased energy supplies, altered membrane characteristics, osmolar imbalance, and enzyme inhibition. Although these cellular insults are not unique to development, they may trigger unique pathogenetic responses in the embryo, such as reduced cell proliferation, cell death, altered cell–cell interactions, reduced biosynthesis, inhibition of morphogenetic movements, or mechanical disruption of developing structures.

Cell death plays a critical role in normal morphogenesis. The term *programmed cell death* refers specifically to *apoptosis*, which is under genetic control in the embryo. Apoptosis is necessary for sculpting the digits from the hand plate and for assuring appropriate functional connectivity between the central nervous system and distal structures. Cell proliferation rates change both spatially and temporally during ontogenesis. There is a delicate balance between cell proliferation, cell differentiation, and apoptosis in the embryo. DNA damage might lead to cell cycle perturbations and cell death.

Damage to DNA can inhibit cell cycle progression at the G_1–S transition, through the S phase, and at the G_2–M transition. If DNA damage is repaired, the cell cycle can return to normal, but if damage is too extensive or cell cycle arrest too long, apoptosis may be triggered. The relationship between DNA damage and repair, cell cycle progression, and apoptosis is depicted in Figure 10–1. From the multiple checkpoints and factors present to regulate the cell cycle and apoptosis, it is clear that different cell populations may respond differently to a similar stimulus, in part because cellular predisposition to apoptosis can vary.

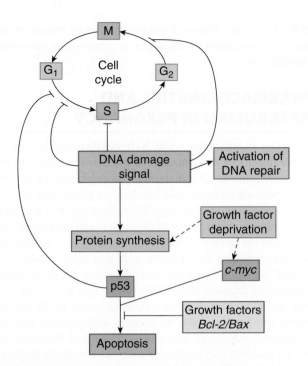

FIGURE 10–1 **Relationships between DNA damage and the induction of cell cycle arrest or apoptosis.** DNA damage can signal inhibition of the cell cycle between G_1 and S, in S phase, or between G_2 and mitosis. The signal(s) can also activate DNA repair mechanisms and synthesis of proteins, including p53, that can initiate apoptosis. Growth factors and products of the proto-oncogene *c-myc* and the *Bcl-2/Bax* gene family, as well as differentiation state and cell cycle phase, are important determinants of the ultimate outcome of embryonal DNA damage.

In addition to affecting proliferation and cell viability, molecular and cellular insults can affect essential processes such as cell migration, cell–cell interactions, differentiation, morphogenesis, and energy metabolism. Although the embryo has compensatory mechanisms to offset such effects, production of a normal or malformed offspring will depend on the balance between damage and repair at each step in the pathogenetic pathway.

Advances in the Molecular Basis of Dysmorphogenesis

Advances in gene targeting and transgenic strategies now allow modification of gene expression at specific points in development and in specific cell types. Conditional knockouts or knockins, inducible gene expression, and other techniques are being used to study the effects of specific gene products on development in great detail. The use of synthetic antisense oligonucleotides allows temporal and spatial restriction of gene ablation by hybridizing to mRNA in the cell, thereby inactivating it. In this way, gene function can be turned off at specific times.

Gain of gene function can also be studied by engineering genetic constructs with an inducible promoter attached to the gene of interest. Ectopic gene expression can be made ubiquitous or site-specific depending on the choice of promoter to drive expression. Transient overexpression of specific genes can be accomplished by adding extra copies using adenoviral transduction.

PHARMACOKINETICS AND METABOLISM IN PREGNANCY

The extent and the form in which chemicals reach the conceptus are important determinants of whether the agent can impact development. The maternal, placental, and embryonic compartments comprise independent yet interacting systems that undergo profound changes throughout the course of pregnancy. Alterations in placental physiology can have significant impact on the uptake, distribution, metabolism, and elimination of xenobiotics. For example, decreases in intestinal motility and increases in gastric emptying time result in longer retention of ingested chemicals in the upper gastrointestinal tract in the mother. Cardiac output increases by 50 percent during the first trimester in humans and remains elevated throughout pregnancy, whereas blood volume increases and plasma proteins and peripheral vascular resistance decrease. The relative increase in blood volume over red cell volume leads to borderline anemia and a generalized edema with a 70 percent elevation of extracellular space. Thus, the volume of distribution of a chemical and the amount bound by plasma proteins may change considerably during pregnancy. Other changes occur in the renal, hepatic, and pulmonary systems as well. Clearly, maternal handling of a chemical influences the extent of embryotoxicity.

The placenta also influences embryonic exposure by helping to regulate blood flow, offering a transport barrier, and metabolizing chemicals. The placenta permits bidirectional transfer of substances between maternal and fetal compartments. It is important to note that virtually any substance present in the maternal plasma will be transported to some extent by the placenta. The passage of most drugs across the placenta seems to occur by simple passive diffusion. Important modifying factors to the rate and extent of transfer include lipid solubility, molecular weight, protein binding, the type of transfer (passive diffusion, and facilitated or active transport), the degree of ionization, and placental metabolism. Blood flow probably constitutes the major rate-limiting step for more lipid-soluble compounds.

Maternal metabolism of xenobiotics is an important and variable determinant of developmental toxicity. As for other health endpoints, the field of pharmacogenomics offers hope for increasing our ability to predict susceptible subpopulations based on empirical relationships between maternal genotype and fetal phenotype.

RELATIONSHIPS BETWEEN MATERNAL AND DEVELOPMENTAL TOXICITY

Although all developmental toxicity must ultimately result from an insult to the conceptus at the cellular level, the insult may occur through a direct effect on the embryo/fetus, indirectly through toxicity of the agent to the mother and/or the placenta, or a combination of direct and indirect effects. Some conditions that may adversely affect the fetus are depicted in Figure 10–2.

The distinction between direct and indirect developmental toxicity is important for interpreting safety assessment results in pregnant animals, as the highest dosage level in these experiments is chosen based on its ability to produce some maternal toxicity (e.g., decreased food or water intake, weight loss, and clinical signs). However, maternal toxicity defined only by such crude manifestations gives little insight to the toxic actions of a xenobiotic. When developmental toxicity is observed only in the presence of maternal toxicity, the developmental effects may be indirect (i.e., caused by an inappropriate growing condition because of an altered maternal environment rather than by a direct interaction of the fetus with the toxin). Greater understanding of the physiologic changes underlying the observed maternal toxicity and elucidation of the association with developmental effects is needed before one can begin to address the relevance of the observations to human safety assessment.

Maternal Factors Affecting Development

Genetics—The genetic makeup of the pregnant female has been well documented as a determinant of developmental outcome. The incidence of cleft lip and/or palate [CL(P)], which occurs more frequently in whites than in blacks, has been investigated in offspring of interracial couples in the United States. Offspring of white mothers had a higher incidence of CL(P) than offspring of black mothers after correcting for paternal race, whereas offspring of white fathers did not have a higher incidence of CL(P) than offspring of black fathers after correcting for maternal race.

Disease—Chronic hypertension in the mother, uncontrolled maternal diabetes mellitus, and certain infections in the mother (i.e., cytomegalovirus and *Toxoplasma gondii*) are leading causes of several types of defects in the fetus. Exposure to hyperthermia (such as febrile illness in the mother) is also implicated in neural defects in the fetus.

Nutrition—A wide spectrum of dietary insufficiencies ranging from protein-calorie malnutrition to deficiencies of vitamins, trace elements, and/or enzyme cofactors is known to adversely affect pregnancy. In fact, folate supplementation by pregnant women can reduce neural tube defect recurrence by over 70 percent.

Stress—Diverse forms of maternal toxicity may have in common the induction of a physiologic stress response. Various forms of physical stress have been applied to pregnant animals in attempts to isolate the developmental effects of stress. Noise stress of pregnant rats or mice throughout gestation can produce developmental toxicity. Restraint stress produces increased fetal death in rats, and malformations of cleft palate, fused and supernumerary ribs, and encephaloceles in mice.

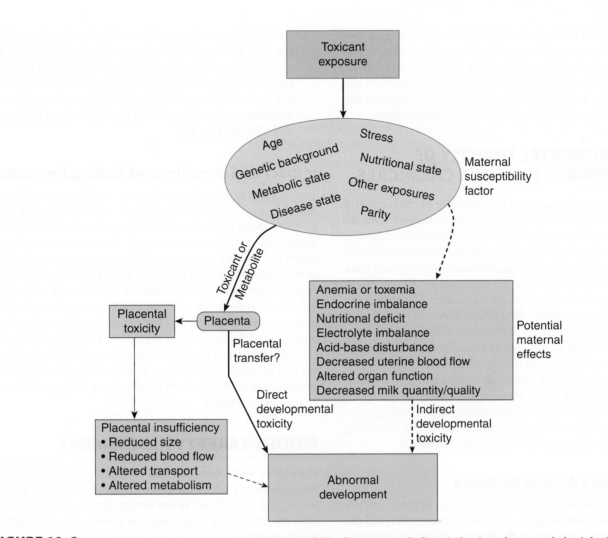

FIGURE 10–2 Interrelationships between maternal susceptibility factors, metabolism, induction of maternal physiologic or functional alterations, placental transfer and toxicity, and developmental toxicity. A developmental toxicant can cause abnormal development through any one or a combination of these pathways. Maternal susceptibility factors determine the predisposition of the mother to respond to a toxic insult, and the maternal effects listed can adversely affect the developing conceptus. Most chemicals traverse the placenta in some form, and the placenta can also be a target for toxicity. In most cases, developmental toxicity is probably mediated through a combination of these pathways.

There is a positive correlation in humans between stress and adverse developmental effects, including low birth weight and congenital malformations.

Placental Toxicity—The placenta is the interface between the mother and the conceptus, providing attachment, nutrition, gas exchange, and waste removal. The placenta also produces hormones critical to the maintenance of pregnancy, and it can metabolize and/or store xenobiotics. Placental toxicity may compromise these functions. Known placental toxicants include cadmium, arsenic or mercury, cigarette smoke, ethanol, cocaine, endotoxin, and sodium salicylate.

Maternal Toxicity—A retrospective analysis of relationships between maternal toxicity and specific types of prenatal effects found species-specific associations between maternal toxicity and

specific adverse developmental effects. Various adverse developmental outcomes include increased intrauterine death, decreased fetal weight, supernumerary ribs, and enlarged renal pelvises.

A number of studies directly relate specific forms of maternal toxicity to developmental toxicity, including those in which the test chemical causes maternal effects that exacerbate the agent's developmental toxicity. However, clear delineation of the relative role(s) of indirect maternal and direct embryo/fetal toxicity is difficult.

Diflunisal, an analgesic and anti-inflammatory drug, causes axial skeletal defects in rabbits. Developmentally toxic dosages resulted in severe maternal anemia and depletion of erythrocyte ATP levels. Teratogenicity, anemia, and ATP depletion were unique to the rabbit. The teratogenicity of diflunisal in the rabbit was probably due to hypoxia resulting from maternal anemia.

Phenytoin, an anticonvulsant, can affect maternal folate metabolism in experimental animals, and these alterations may play a role in the teratogenicity of this drug. A mechanism of teratogenesis was proposed relating depressed maternal heart rate and embryonic hypoxia. Supporting studies have demonstrated that hyperoxia reduces the teratogenicity of phenytoin in mice.

DEVELOPMENTAL TOXICITY OF ENDOCRINE-DISRUPTING CHEMICALS

There is the growing concern that exposure to chemicals that can interact with the endocrine system may pose a serious health hazard. An "endocrine disruptor" has been broadly defined as an exogenous agent that interferes with the production, release, transport, metabolism, binding, action, or elimination of natural hormones responsible for the maintenance of homeostasis and the regulation of developmental processes. Due to the critical role of hormones in directing differentiation in many tissues, the developing organism is particularly vulnerable to fluctuations in the timing or intensity of exposure to chemicals with hormonal or antihormonal activity. Chemicals from a wide variety of chemical classes induce developmental toxicity via at least three modes of action involving the endocrine system: (1) by serving as ligands of steroid receptors; (2) by modifying steroid hormone metabolizing enzymes; and (3) by perturbing hypothalamic-pituitary release of trophic hormones.

Laboratory Animal Evidence

Estrogenic or antiestrogenic developmental toxicants include DES, estradiol, antiestrogenic drugs such as tamoxifen and clomiphene citrate, and some pesticides and industrial chemicals. Female offspring are generally more sensitive to these toxicants than males and altered pubertal development, reduced fertility, and reproductive tract anomalies are common findings.

Antiandrogens represent another major class of endocrine-disrupting chemicals. Principal manifestations of developmental exposure to an antiandrogen are generally restricted to males, and include hypospadias, retained nipples, reduced testes and accessory sex gland weights, and decreased sperm production. Polychlorinated biphenyls (PCBs) may act at several sites to lower thyroid hormone levels during development, and cause body weight and auditory deficits. PCBs also cause learning deficits and alter locomotor activity patterns in rodents and monkeys.

Human Evidence

Whether human health is being adversely impacted from exposures to endocrine disruptors present in the environment is equivocal. Reports in humans are of two types:

1. Observations of adverse effects on reproductive system development and function following exposure to chemicals with known endocrine activities that are present in medicines, contaminated food, or the workplace. These have tended to involve relatively higher exposure to chemicals with known endocrine effects.

2. Epidemiologic evidence of increasing trends in reproductive and developmental adverse outcomes that have an endocrine basis. For example, secular trends have been reported for cryptorchidism, hypospadias, semen quality, and testicular cancer, but due to the lack of exposure assessment, such studies provide limited evidence of a cause and effect relationship.

Impact on Screening and Testing Programs

The findings of altered reproductive development following early life-stage exposures to endocrine-disrupting chemicals helped prompt revision of traditional safety evaluation tests. These now include assessments of female estrous cyclicity, sperm motility and sperm morphology in both parental and F1 generations, the age at puberty in the F1s, histopathology of target organs, anogenital distance in the F2s, and primordial follicular counts in the parental and F1 generations. For the new prenatal developmental toxicity test guidelines, one important modification aimed at improved detection of endocrine disruptors was the expansion of the period of dosing from the end of organogenesis (i.e., palatal closure) to the end of pregnancy in order to include the developmental period of urogenital differentiation.

MODERN SAFETY ASSESSMENT

Experience with chemicals that have the potential to induce developmental toxicity indicates that both laboratory animal testing and surveillance of the human population (i.e., epidemiologic studies) are necessary to provide adequate public health protection.

Regulatory Guidelines for In Vivo Testing

New and internationally accepted testing protocols rely on the investigator to meet the primary goal of detecting and bringing to light any indication of toxicity to reproduction. Key elements of various tests are provided in Table 10–4. The general goal of these studies is to identify the NOAEL, which is the highest dosage level that does not produce a significant increase in adverse effects in the offspring.

Multigeneration Tests

Information pertaining to developmental toxicity can also be obtained from studies in which animals are exposed to the test substance continuously over one or more generations. For additional information on this approach, see Chapter 20.

Children's Health

Infants and children differ both qualitatively and quantitatively from adults in their exposure to pesticide residues in food because of different dietary composition, intake patterns, and different activities, such as crawling on the floor or ground, putting

TABLE 10–4 Summary of in vivo regulatory protocol guidelines for evaluation of developmental toxicity.

Study	Exposure	Endpoints Covered	Comments
Segment I: fertility and general reproduction study	Males: 10 weeks prior to mating Females: 2 weeks prior to mating	Gamete development, fertility, pre- and postimplantation viability, parturition, lactation	Assesses reproductive capabilities of male and female following exposure over one complete spermatogenic cycle or several estrous cycles
Segment II: teratogenicity test	Implantation (or mating) through end of organogenesis (or term)	Viability, weight, and morphology (external, visceral, and skeletal) of conceptuses just prior to birth	Shorter exposure to prevent maternal metabolic adaptation and to provide high exposure to the embryo during gastrulation and organogenesis. Earlier dosing option for bioaccumulative agents or those impacting maternal nutrition. Later dosing option covers male reproductive tract development and fetal growth and maturation
Segment III: perinatal study	Last trimester of pregnancy through lactation	Postnatal survival, growth, and external morphology	Intended to observe effects on development of major organ functional competence during the perinatal period, and thus may be relatively more sensitive to adverse effects at this time
ICH 4.1.1: fertility protocol	Males: 4 weeks prior to mating Females: 2 weeks prior to mating	Males: Reproductive organ weights and histology, sperm counts, and motility Females: viability of conceptuses at midpregnancy or later	Improved assessment of male reproductive endpoints; shorter treatment duration than Segment I
ICH 4.1.2: effects on prenatal and postnatal development, including maternal function	Implantation through end of lactation	Relative toxicity to pregnant versus nonpregnant female; postnatal viability, growth, development, and functional deficits (including behavior, maturation, and reproduction)	
ICH 4.1.3: effects on embryo/fetal development	Implantation through end of organogenesis	Viability and morphology (external, visceral, and skeletal) of fetuses just prior to birth	Similar to Segment II study. Usually conducted in two species (rodent and nonrodent)
OECD 414: prenatal developmental	Implantation (or mating) through day prior to cesarean section	Viability and morphology (external, visceral, and skeletal) of fetuses just prior to birth	Similar to Segment II study. Usually conducted in two species (rodent and nonrodent)

their hands and foreign objects in their mouths, and raising dust and dirt during play. Even the level of their activity (i.e., closer to the ground) can affect their exposure to some toxicants. In addition to exposure differences, children are growing and developing, which makes them more susceptible to some types of insults. Effects of early childhood exposure, including neurobehavioral effects and cancer, may not be apparent until later in life. Debate continues over the approach to be used in risk assessment in consideration of infants and children.

Alternative Testing Strategies

Various alternative test systems have been proposed to refine, reduce, or replace reliance on the standard regulatory mammalian tests for assessing prenatal toxicity (Table 10–5). These can be grouped into assays based on cell cultures, cultures of embryos in vitro (including submammalian species), and short-term in vivo tests. It was initially hoped that the alternative approaches would become generally applicable to all chemicals, and help prioritize full-scale testing. Indeed, given the complexity of embryogenesis and the multiple mechanisms and

target site of potential teratogens, it was perhaps unrealistic to have expected a single test, or even a small battery, to accurately prescreen the activity of chemicals in general.

An exception to the poor acceptance of alternate tests for prescreening for developmental toxicity is the Chernoff/Kavlock in vivo test. In this test, pregnant females are exposed during the period of major organogenesis to a limited number of dosage levels near those inducing maternal toxicity, and offspring are evaluated over a brief neonatal period for external malformations, growth, and viability. It has proven reliable over a large number of chemical agents and classes.

Epidemiology

Reproductive epidemiology studies the associations between specific exposures of the father or pregnant woman and her conceptus and the outcome of pregnancy. The likelihood of linking a particular exposure with a series of case reports increases with the rarity of the defect, the rarity of the exposure in the population, a small source population, a short time span for study, and biological plausibility for the association. In oth-

TABLE 10-5 Brief survey of alternative test methodologies for developmental toxicity.

Assay	Brief Description and Endpoints Evaluated
Mouse ovarian tumor	Labeled mouse ovarian tumor cells added to culture dishes with concanavalin A-coated disks for 20 min. Endpoint is inhibition of attachment of cells to disks
Human embryonic palatal mesenchyme	Human embryonic palatal mesenchyme cell line grown in attached culture. Cell number assessed after 3 days
Micromass culture	Midbrain or limb bud cells dissociated from rat embryos and grown in micromass culture for 5 days. Cell proliferation and biochemical markers of differentiation assessed
Mouse embryonic stem cell (EST) test	Mouse ESTs and 3T3 cells in 96-well plates assessed for viability after 3 and 5 days. ESTs grown for 3 days in hanging drops form embryoid bodies which are plated and examined after 10 days for differentiation into cardiocytes
Chick embryo neural retina cell culture	Neural retinas of day 6.5 chick embryos dissociated and grown in rotating suspension culture for 7 days. Endpoints include cellular aggregation, growth, differentiation, and biochemical markers
Drosophila	Fly larvae grown from egg disposition through hatching of adults. Adult flies examined for specific structural defects (bent bristles and notched wing)
Hydra	*Hydra attenuata* cells are aggregated to form an "artificial embryo" and allowed to regenerate. Dose response compared to that for adult *Hydra toxicity*
FETAX	Midblastula stage *Xenopus* embryos exposed for 96 h and evaluated for viability, growth, morphology
Rodent whole embryo culture	Postimplantation rodent embryos grown in vitro for up to 2 days and evaluated for growth and development
Zebrafish	Zebrafish eggs or blastulae exposed to chemical in water (can be in multiwell plates) for up to 4 days and evaluated for growth, development, and (in some cases) gene expression
Chernoff/Kavlock assay	Pregnant mice or rats exposed during organogenesis and allowed to deliver. Postnatal growth, viability, and gross morphology of litters assessed

er situations, such as occurred with ethanol and valproic acid, associations are sought through either a case–control or a cohort approach. Both approaches require accurate ascertainment of abnormal outcomes and exposures, and a large enough effect and study population to detect an elevated risk. Another challenge to epidemiologists is the high percentage of human pregnancy failures related to a particular exposure that may go undetected in the general population. Furthermore, with the availability of prenatal diagnostic procedures, additional

pregnancies of malformed embryos (particularly neural tube defects) are electively aborted. Thus, the incidence of abnormal outcomes at birth may not reflect the true rate of abnormalities, and the term prevalence, rather than incidence, is preferred when the denominator is the number of live births rather than total pregnancies.

Other issues particularly relevant to reproductive epidemiology include homogeneity, recording proficiency, and confounding. Homogeneity refers to the fact that a particular outcome may be described differently by various recording units and that there can be multiple pathogenetic origins for a given specific outcome. Recording difficulties relate to inconsistencies of definitions and nomenclature, and to difficulties in ascertaining or recalling outcomes as well as exposures. For example, birth weights are usually accurately determined and recalled, but spontaneous abortions and certain malformations may not be. Last, confounding by factors such as maternal age and parity, dietary factors, diseases and drug usage, and social characteristics must be considered in order to control for variables that affect both exposure and outcome.

Epidemiologic studies of abnormal reproductive outcomes are usually undertaken with three objectives in mind: the first is scientific research into the causes of abnormal birth outcomes and usually involves analysis of case reports or clusters; the second aim is prevention and is targeted at broader surveillance of trends by birth defect registries around the world; and the last objective is informing the public and providing assurance. Cohort studies, with their prospective exposure assessment and ability to monitor both adverse and beneficial outcomes, may be the most methodologically robust approach to identifying human developmental toxicants.

Information on differential genetic susceptibility to birth defects continues to accrue. This new knowledge promises to elucidate links between genetics and disease susceptibility. Understanding the genetic basis of vulnerability to environmentally induced birth defects will allow more inclusive risk assessments and a better appreciation of the mechanisms of action of developmental toxicants.

Concordance of Data

Studies of the similarity of responses of laboratory animals and humans for developmental toxicants support the assumption that results from laboratory tests are predictive of potential human effects. Concordance is strongest when there are positive data from more than one test species. Humans tend to be more sensitive to developmental toxicants than is the most sensitive test species.

Elements of Risk Assessment

Extrapolation of animal test data for developmental toxicity follows two basic directions, one for drugs where exposure is voluntary and usually to high dosages and the other for environmental agents where exposure is generally involuntary and to low levels. For drugs, a use-in-pregnancy rating is utilized, wherein the letters A, B, C, D, and X are used to classify the evidence that a chemical poses a risk to the human conceptus. For example, drugs are placed in category A if adequate, well-controlled studies in pregnant humans have failed to demonstrate a risk, and in category X (contraindicated for pregnancy) if studies in animals or humans, or investigational or postmarketing reports, have shown fetal risk that clearly outweighs any possible benefit to the patient. The default category C (risks cannot be ruled out) is assigned when there is a lack of human studies and animal studies are either lacking or are positive for fetal risk, but the benefits may justify the potential risk. Categories B and D represent areas of relatively lesser or greater concern for risk, respectively.

For environmental agents, the purpose of the risk assessment process for developmental toxicity is generally to define the dose, route, timing, and duration of exposure that induces effects at the lowest level in the most relevant laboratory animal model. The exposure associated with this "critical effect" is then subjected to a variety of safety or uncertainty factors in order to derive an exposure level for humans that is presumed to be relatively safe. In the absence of definitive animal test data, certain default assumptions are generally made:

1. An agent that produces an adverse developmental effect in experimental animals will potentially pose a hazard to humans following sufficient exposure during development.
2. All four manifestations of developmental toxicity (death, structural abnormalities, growth alterations, and functional deficits) are of concern.
3. The specific types of developmental effects seen in animal studies are not necessarily the same as those that may be produced in humans.
4. The most appropriate species is used to estimate human risk when data are available (in the absence of such data, the most sensitive species is appropriate).
5. In general, a threshold is assumed for the dose–response curve for agents that produce developmental toxicity.

One troubling and subjective aspect of risk assessment for developmental toxicants is to distinguish between adverse effects that are detrimental to health and lesser effects that are considered not significant to human health. The interpretation of reduced fetal growth in developmental toxicity studies illustrates most of the issues. Whereas we have accepted definitions of low birth weight in humans and understand how intrauterine growth retardation translates to an elevated risk of infant mortality and mental retardation, similar knowledge in rodents is lacking. Further concerns arise from recent epidemiologic evidence suggesting that birth weight in humans is a predictor of adult-onset diseases including hypertension, cardiovascular disease, and diabetes.

PATHWAYS TO THE FUTURE

There are several mechanisms of normal development that are conserved in diverse animals, including the fruit fly, roundworm, zebrafish, frog, chick, and mouse. Seventeen conserved

TABLE 10-6 The 17 intercellular signaling pathways used in development by most metazoans.

Period during Development	Signaling Pathway
Before organogenesis; later for growth and tissue renewal	1. Wingless–Int pathway 2. Transforming growth factor β pathway 3. Hedgehog pathway 4. Receptor tyrosine kinase pathway 5. Notch–Delta pathway 6. Cytokine pathway (STAT pathway)
Organogenesis and cytodifferentiation; later for growth and tissue renewal	7. Interleukin-1-toll nuclear factor-kappa B pathway 8. Nuclear hormone receptor pathway 9. Apoptosis pathway 10. Receptor phosphotyrosine phosphatase pathway
Larval and adult physiology	11. Receptor guanylate cyclase pathway 12. Nitric oxide receptor pathway 13. G-protein-coupled receptor (large G proteins) pathway 14. Integrin pathway 15. Cadherin pathway 16. Gap junction pathway 17. Ligand-gated cation channel pathway

intercellular signaling pathways are described that are used repeatedly at different times and locations during development of these and other animal species, as well as in humans (Table 10-6). The conserved nature of these key pathways provides a strong scientific rationale for using these animal models to advantage for developmental toxicology. These organisms have well-known genetics, embryology, and rapid generation times, and they are also amenable to genetic manipulation to enhance the sensitivity of specific developmental pathways or to incorporate human genes to answer questions of interspecies extrapolation.

Increased understanding of human genetic polymorphisms and their contribution to susceptibility to birth defects, use of sensitized animal models for high- to low-dose extrapolation, use of stress/checkpoint pathways as indicators of developmental toxicity, implementation of bioinformatic systems to improve data archival and retrieval, and increased multidisciplinary education and research on the causes of birth defects will aid assessment of the developmental risk of toxicants.

BIBLIOGRAPHY

Hansen DK, Abbott BD: *Developmental Toxicology.* New York: Informa Healthcare, 2009.

Schardein JL, Macina OT: *Human Developmental Toxicants: Aspects of Toxicology and Chemistry.* Boca Raton, FL: CRC Press, 2007.

QUESTIONS

1. Diethylstilbestrol (DES):
   a. was used to treat morning sickness from the 1940s to the 1970s.
   b. was found to affect only female offspring in exposed pregnancies.
   c. greatly affects the development of the fetal brain.
   d. exposure increases the risk of clear cell adenocarcinoma of the vagina.
   e. is now used to treat leprosy patients.

2. Early (prenatal) exposure to which of the following teratogens is most often characterized by craniofacial dysmorphism?
   a. thalidomide.
   b. retinol.
   c. ethanol.
   d. tobacco smoke.
   e. diethylstilbestrol (DES).

3. The nervous system is derived from which of the following germ layers?
   a. ectoderm.
   b. mesoderm.
   c. epidermal placodes.
   d. paraxial mesoderm.
   e. endoderm.

4. Toxin exposure during which of the following periods is likely to have the LEAST toxic effect on the developing fetus?
   a. gastrulation.
   b. organogenesis.
   c. preimplantation.
   d. third trimester.
   e. first trimester.

5. Regarding prenatal teratogen exposure, which of the following statements is FALSE?
   a. Major effects include growth retardation and malformations.
   b. Exposure to teratogens during critical developmental periods will have more severe effects on the fetus.
   c. There is considered to be a toxin level threshold below which the fetus is capable of repairing itself.
   d. The immune system of the fetus is primitive, so the fetus has little to no ability to fight off chemicals and repair itself.
   e. Embryo lethality becomes more likely as the toxic dose is increased.

6. Which of the following stages of the cell cycle are important in monitoring DNA damage and inhibiting progression of the cell cycle?
   a. G_1–S, anaphase, M–G_1.
   b. G_1–S, S, G_2–M.
   c. S, prophase, G_1.
   d. G_2–M, prophase.
   e. M–G_1, anaphase.

7. Which of the following molecules is NOT important in determining the ultimate outcome of embryonal DNA damage?
   a. p53.
   b. Bax.
   c. Bcl-2.
   d. c-Myc.
   e. NF-κB.

8. Which of the following is NOT a physiologic response to pregnancy?
   a. increased cardiac output.
   b. increased blood volume.
   c. increased peripheral vascular resistance.
   d. decreased plasma proteins.
   e. increased extracellular space.

9. All of the following statements are true EXCEPT:
   a. Offspring of white mothers have a higher incidence of cleft lip or palate than do black mothers, after adjusting for paternal race.
   b. Cytomegalovirus (CMV) is a common viral cause of birth defects.
   c. Folate supplementation during pregnancy decreases the risk of neural tube defects.
   d. Cigarette smoke and ethanol are both toxic to the placenta.
   e. In humans, there is a negative correlation between stress and low birth weight.

10. Which of the following is NOT a mechanism involving the endocrine system by which chemicals induce developmental toxicity?
    a. acting as steroid hormone receptor ligands.
    b. disrupting normal function of steroid hormone metabolizing enzymes.
    c. disturbing the release of hormones from the hypothalamus.
    d. disturbing the release of hormones from the pituitary gland.
    e. elimination of natural hormones.

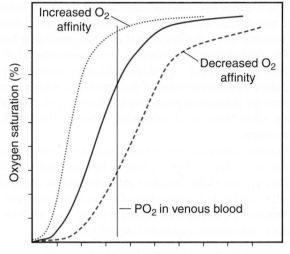

FIGURE 11-2 Hemoglobin-oxygen Dissociation Curves. The normal oxygen dissociation curve (*solid line*) has a sigmoid shape due to the cooperative interaction between the four globin chains in the hemoglobin molecule. Fully deoxygenated hemoglobin has a relatively low affinity for oxygen. Interaction of oxygen with one heme–iron moiety induces a conformational change in that globin chain. Through surface interactions, that conformational change affects the other globin chains, causing a conformational change in all of the globin chains that increases their affinity for oxygen. Homotropic and heterotropic parameters also affect the affinity of hemoglobin for oxygen. An increase in oxygen affinity results in a shift to the left in the oxygen dissociation curve. Such a shift may decrease oxygen delivery to the tissues. A decrease in oxygen affinity results in a shift to the right in the oxygen dissociation curve, facilitating oxygen delivery to the tissues.

TABLE 11-4 Xenobiotics associated with methemoglobinemia.

Therapeutic Agents	Environmental Agents
Aminobenzenes	Nitrobenzenes
Amyl nitrate	Nitroethane
Aniline dyes and aniline derivatives	Nitroglycerin
Benzocaine	Nitrotoluenes
Beta-naphthol disulfonate	*ortho*-Toluidine
Butyl nitrite	Potassium chlorate
Dapsone	Prilocaine
Flutamide	Primaquine
Gasoline additives	Phenacetin
Isobutyl nitrite	Phenazopyridine
Lidocaine	Quinones
Methylene blue	Silver nitrate
Nitrates	Sulfonamide
Nitric oxide	Trinitrotoluene
Nitrites	

delivery of oxygen to tissues, as the oxygen will not be readily released from hemoglobin in the periphery.

The normal erythrocyte has metabolic mechanisms for reducing heme iron back to the ferrous state. Failure of these control mechanisms leads to increased levels of methemoglobin, or *methemoglobinemia*. Various chemicals that cause methemoglobinemia are shown in Table 11–4. Most patients tolerate low levels (<10 percent) of methemoglobin without clinical symptoms. Higher levels lead to tissue hypoxemia that is eventually fatal.

Heterotropic Effects—There are three major heterotropic (extrinsic) effectors of hemoglobin function: pH, erythrocyte 2,3-bisphosphoglycerate (2,3-BPG, formerly designated 2,3-diphosphoglycerate) concentration, and temperature. A decrease in pH (e.g., lactic acid and carbon dioxide) lowers the affinity of hemoglobin for oxygen, that is, it causes a right shift in the oxygen dissociation curve, facilitating the delivery of oxygen to tissues (Figure 11–2). As bicarbonate and carbon dioxide equilibrate in the lung, the hydrogen ion concentration decreases, which results in increased affinity of hemoglobin for oxygen and facilitated oxygen uptake.

Binding of 2,3-BPG to deoxyhemoglobin results in reduced oxygen affinity (a shift to the right of the oxygen dissociation curve). The conformational change induced by binding of oxygen alters the binding site for 2,3-BPG and results in release of 2,3-BPG from hemoglobin. This facilitates uptake of more oxygen for delivery to tissues. The concentration of 2,3-BPG increases whenever there is tissue hypoxemia but may decrease in the presence of acidosis.

The oxygen affinity of hemoglobin decreases as the body temperature increases. This facilitates delivery of oxygen to tissues during periods of extreme exercise and febrile illnesses associated with increased temperature. Correspondingly, oxygen affinity increases and delivery decreases during hypothermia.

The respiratory function of hemoglobin may also be impaired by blocking the ligand binding site with other substances. Carbon monoxide has a relatively low rate of association with deoxyhemoglobin but shows high affinity once bound, and causes a left shift in the oxygen dissociation curve, further compromising oxygen delivery to the tissues. Nitric oxide, an important vasodilator that modulates vascular tone, binds avidly to heme iron. Erythrocytes can influence the availability of nitric oxide in parts of the circulation because the nitric oxide is bound to erythrocyte hemoglobin.

Alterations in Erythrocyte Survival

Erythrocytes normally circulate in blood for about 120 days. Very little protein synthesis occurs during this time, as erythrocytes are anucleate when they enter the circulation and residual mRNA is rapidly lost over the first 1 to 2 days in the circulation. Consequently, senescence occurs over time until the aged erythrocytes are removed by the spleen, where the iron is recovered for reutilization in heme synthesis.

Nonimmune Hemolytic Anemia

Microangiopathic Anemias—Intravascular fragmentation of erythrocytes gives rise to the *microangiopathic hemolytic anemias*. The hallmark of this process is the presence of schistocytes (fragmented RBCs) in peripheral blood. The formation of fibrin strands in the microcirculation is a common mechanism for RBC fragmentation. The erythrocytes are essentially sliced into fragments by the fibrin strands that extend across the vascular lumen and impede the flow of erythrocytes through the vasculature. Excessive fragmentation can also be seen in the presence of abnormal vasculature.

Infectious Diseases—Infectious diseases may be associated with significant hemolysis, by either direct effect on the erythrocyte or an immune-mediated hemolytic process. Erythrocytes are parasitized in malaria and babesiosis, leading to their destruction. Clostridial infections are associated with release of hemolytic toxins that enter the circulation and lyse erythrocytes.

Oxidative Hemolysis—Molecular oxygen is a reactive and potentially toxic chemical species; consequently, the normal respiratory function of erythrocytes generates oxidative stress on a continuous basis. There are several mechanisms that protect against oxidative injury in erythrocytes including NADH-diaphorase, superoxide dismutase, catalase, and the glutathione pathway.

Xenobiotics capable of inducing oxidative injury in erythrocytes are listed in Table 11–5. These agents appear to potentiate the normal redox reactions and are capable of overwhelming the usual protective mechanisms. The interaction between these xenobiotics and hemoglobin leads to the formation of free radicals that denature critical proteins, including hemoglobin, thiol-dependent enzymes, and components of the erythrocyte membrane. Significant oxidative injury usually occurs when the concentration of the xenobiotic is high enough to overcome the normal protective mechanisms, or, more commonly, when there is an underlying defect in the protective mechanisms.

The most common enzyme defect associated with oxidative hemolysis is glucose-6-phosphate dehydrogenase (G-6-PD) deficiency, a sex-linked disorder characterized by diminished G-6-PD activity. It is often clinically asymptomatic until the erythrocytes are exposed to oxidative stress from the host response to infection or exposure to xenobiotics.

Nonoxidative Chemical-induced Hemolysis—Exposure to some xenobiotics is associated with hemolysis without significant oxidative injury. For example, inhalation of gaseous arsenic hydride (arsine) can result in severe hemolysis, with anemia, jaundice, and hemoglobinuria. Lead poisoning is associated with defects in heme synthesis, a shortening of erythrocyte survival, and hemolysis.

Immune Hemolytic Anemia—Immunologic destruction of erythrocytes is mediated by the interaction of IgG or IgM antibodies with antigens expressed on the surface of the erythrocyte. In the case of autoimmune hemolytic anemia, the antigens are intrinsic components of the patient's own erythrocytes.

A number of mechanisms have been implicated in xenobiotic-mediated antibody binding to erythrocytes. Some drugs, of which penicillin is a prototype, appear to bind to the surface of the cell, with the "foreign" drug acting as a *hapten* and eliciting an immune response. The antibodies that arise in this type of response only bind to drug-coated erythrocytes. Other drugs, of which quinidine is a prototype, bind to components of the erythrocyte surface and induce a conformational change in one or more components of the membrane. A third mechanism, for which α-methyldopa is a prototype, results in production of a *drug-induced autoantibody* that cannot be distinguished from the antibodies arising in idiopathic autoimmune hemolytic anemia.

TOXICOLOGY OF THE LEUKON

Components of Blood Leukocytes

The leukon consists of leukocytes, or white blood cells, including granulocytes, which may be subdivided into neutrophils, eosinophils, and basophils; monocytes; and lymphocytes. Granulocytes and monocytes are nucleated ameboid cells that are phagocytic. They play a central role in the inflammatory response and host defense. Unlike the RBC, which resides exclusively within blood, granulocytes and monocytes merely pass through the blood on their way to extravascular tissues, where they reside in large numbers.

TABLE 11–5 Xenobiotics associated with oxidative injury.

Acetanilide	Phenacetin
Aminosalicylic acid	Phenol
Chlorates	Phenylhydrazine
Dapsone	Primaquine
Furazolidone	Phenazopyridine
Hydroxylamine	Sodium sulfoxone
Methylene blue	Sulfamethoxypyridazine
Nalidixic acid	Sulfanilamide
Naphthalene	Sulfasalazine
Nitrofurantoin	Toluidine blue
Nitrobenzene	

Granulocytes are defined by the characteristics of their cytoplasmic granules as they appear on a blood smear. Neutrophils, the largest component of blood leukocytes, are highly specialized in the mediation of inflammation and the ingestion and destruction of pathogenic microorganisms. Eosinophils and basophils modulate inflammation through the release of various mediators.

Evaluation of Granulocytes

In the blood, neutrophils are distributed between *circulating* and *marginated* pools, which are of equal size and in constant equilibrium. A blood neutrophil count assesses only the circulating pool, which remains remarkably constant (1800 to 7500 µL^{-1}) in a healthy adult human. During inflammation, an increased number of immature (nonsegmented) granulocytes may be seen in peripheral blood. In certain conditions, neutrophils may show morphological changes indicative of toxicity.

Toxic Effects on Granulocytes

Effects on Proliferation—The high rate of proliferation of neutrophils makes their progenitor and precursor granulocyte pool particularly susceptible to inhibitors of mitosis. Such effects by cytotoxic drugs are generally nonspecific as they similarly affect cells of the dermis, gastrointestinal tract, and other rapidly dividing tissues. Agents that affect both neutrophils and monocytes pose a greater risk for toxic sequelae, such as infection. Such effects tend to be dose-related, with mononuclear phagocyte recovery preceding neutrophil recovery.

Myelotoxicity is commonly seen with cytoreductive cancer chemotherapy agents, which often act to inhibit DNA synthesis or directly attack its integrity through the formation of DNA adducts or enzyme-mediated breaks. Therefore, nonproliferating cells such as metamyelocytes, bands, and mature neutrophils are relatively resistant. Because stem cells cycle slowly, they are minimally affected by a single administration of a cytotoxic drug. Sustained exposure to drugs affecting stem cells is believed to cause more prolonged myelosuppression.

Effects on Function—Ethanol and glucocorticoids impair phagocytosis and microbe ingestion. Iohexol and ioxaglate, components of radiographic contrast media, have also been reported to inhibit phagocytosis. Superoxide production, required for microbial killing and chemotaxis, is reportedly reduced in patients using parenteral heroin as well as in former opiate abusers on long-term methadone maintenance. Chemotaxis is also impaired following treatment with zinc salts in antiacne preparations.

Idiosyncratic Toxic Neutropenia—Of greater concern are agents that unexpectedly damage neutrophils and granulocyte precursors and induce *agranulocytosis,* which is characterized by a profound depletion in blood neutrophils to less than 500 µL^{-1}. Such injury occurs in specifically conditioned individuals, and is therefore termed *idiosyncratic.*

Idiosyncratic xenobiotic-induced agranulocytosis may involve a sudden depletion of circulating neutrophils concomitant with exposure, which may persist as long as the agent or its metabolites persist in the circulation. Hematopoietic function is usually restored when the agent is detoxified or excreted. Toxicants affecting uncommitted stem cells induce total marrow failure, as seen in aplastic anemia. After agents that affect more differentiated precursors, surviving uncommitted stem cells eventually produce recovery, provided that the risk of infection is successfully managed during the leukopenic episodes.

Mechanisms of Toxic Neutropenia—In *immune-mediated neutropenia,* antigen–antibody reactions lead to destruction of peripheral neutrophils, granulocyte precursors, or both. As with RBCs, an immunogenic xenobiotic can act as a hapten, where the agent must be physically present to cause cell damage, or alternatively, may induce immunogenic cells to produce antineutrophil antibodies that do not require the drug to be present.

Non-immune-mediated toxic neutropenia often shows a genetic predisposition. Direct damage may cause inhibition of granulopoiesis or neutrophil function. Some studies suggest that a buildup of toxic oxidants generated by leukocytes can result in neutrophil damage.

Examples of agents associated with immune and nonimmune neutropenia/agranulocytosis are listed in Table 11–6.

TABLE 11–6 Examples of toxicants that cause immune and nonimmune idiopathic neutropenia.

Drugs Associated with WBC Antibodies	Drugs Not Associated with WBC Antibodies
Aminopyrine	Allopurinol
Ampicillin	Ethambutol
Aprindine	Flurazepam
Azulfidine	Hydrochlorothiazide
Chlorpropamide	Isoniazid
Clozapine	Phenothiazines
CPZ/phenothiazines	Rifampicin
Dicloxacillin	
Gold	
Levamisole	
Lidocaine	
Methimazole	
Metiamide	
Phenytoin	
Procainamide	
Propylthiouracil	
Quinidine	
Tolbutamide	

LEUKEMOGENESIS AS A TOXIC RESPONSE

Human Leukemias

Leukemias are proliferative disorders of hematopoietic tissue that originate from individual bone marrow cells. Historically they have been classified as myeloid or lymphoid, referring to the major lineages for erythrocytes/granulocytes/thrombocytes or lymphocytes, respectively. Poorly differentiated phenotypes have been designated as "acute," including acute lymphoblastic leukemia (ALL) and acute myelogenous leukemia (AML), whereas well-differentiated ones are referred to as "chronic" leukemias, which include chronic lymphocytic leukemia (CLL), chronic myelogenous leukemia (CML), and the myelodysplastic syndromes (MDS).

Mechanisms of Toxic Leukemogenesis

AML is the dominant leukemia associated with drug or chemical exposure, followed by MDS. This represents a continuum of one toxic response that has been linked to cytogenetic abnormalities, particularly the loss of all or part of chromosomes 5 and 7. Remarkably, the frequency of these deletions in patients who develop MDS and/or AML after treatment with alkylating or other antineoplastic agents ranges from 67 to 95 percent, depending on the study. Some of these same changes have been observed in AML patients occupationally exposed to benzene, who also show aneuploidy with a high frequency of involvement of chromosome 7. The relatively low frequency of deletions in chromosomes 5 and 7 in de novo as compared with secondary AML suggests that these cytogenetic markers can be useful in discriminating between toxic exposures and other etiologies of this leukemia.

Leukemogenic Agents

Most *alkylating agents* used in cancer chemotherapy can cause MDS and/or AML. Of the *aromatic hydrocarbons,* only benzene has been proven to be leukemogenic. Treatment with the *topoisomerase II inhibitors,* etoposide and teniposide, can induce AML.

Exposure to *high-dose γ- or x-ray radiation* has long been associated with ALL, AML, and CML, as demonstrated in survivors of the atom bombings of Nagasaki and Hiroshima. Less clear is the association of these diseases with low-dose radiation secondary to fallout or diagnostic radiographs. Other *controversial agents* include 1,3-butadiene, nonionizing radiation (electromagnetic, microwave, infrared, visible, and the high end of the ultraviolet spectrum), cigarette smoking, and formaldehyde.

TOXICOLOGY OF PLATELETS AND HEMOSTASIS

Hemostasis is a multicomponent system responsible for preventing the loss of blood from sites of vascular injury and maintaining circulating blood in a fluid state. Loss of blood is prevented by formation of stable hemostatic plugs. The major constituents of the hemostatic system include circulating platelets, a variety of plasma proteins, and vascular endothelial cells. Alterations in these components or systemic activation of this system can lead to the clinical manifestations of deranged hemostasis, including excessive bleeding and thrombosis. The hemostatic system is a frequent target of therapeutic intervention as well as inadvertent expression of the toxic effect of a variety of xenobiotics.

Toxic Effects on Platelets

The Thrombocyte—Platelets are essential for formation of a stable hemostatic plug in response to vascular injury. Platelets initially adhere to the damaged wall. Activation of a pathway of several factors permits fibrinogen and other multivalent adhesive molecules to form cross-links between nearby platelets, resulting in platelet aggregation. Xenobiotics may interfere with the platelet response by causing thrombocytopenia or interfering with platelet function.

Thrombocytopenia—Like anemia, thrombocytopenia may be due to decreased production or increased destruction. Thrombocytopenia is a common side effect of intensive chemotherapy, due to the predictable effect of antiproliferative agents on hematopoietic precursors. Thrombocytopenia is a clinically significant component of idiosyncratic xenobiotic-induced aplastic anemia. Indeed, the initial manifestation of aplastic anemia may be mucocutaneous bleeding secondary to thrombocytopenia.

Exposure to xenobiotics may cause increased immune-mediated platelet destruction through any one of the several mechanisms. Some drugs, such as penicillin, function as haptens, binding to platelet membrane components and eliciting an immune response specific for the hapten. The responding antibody then binds to the hapten on the platelet surface, leading to removal of the antibody-coated platelet from the circulation.

A second mechanism of immune thrombocytopenia is initiated by a change in a platelet membrane glycoprotein caused by the xenobiotic. This elicits an antibody response, when the responding antibody binds to this altered platelet antigen in the presence of drug, resulting in removal of the platelet from the circulation by the mononuclear phagocytic system.

Thrombocytopenia is an uncommon but serious complication of inhibitors of factors involved in the clot-formation cascade. These inhibitors can change the conformation of these factors, causing exposure of certain peptides (called neoepitopes because they are newly exposed to the immune system) on the factors that react with endogenous antibodies. This leads to phagocytosis of the platelets associated with these factors. Thus, exposure of epitopes that react with naturally occurring antibodies represents a third mechanism of immune-mediated platelet destruction.

Heparin-induced thrombocytopenia (HIT) represents a fourth mechanism of immune-mediated platelet destruction. When heparin (an anticoagulant) binds to certain clotting factors, a neoepitope is exposed, and an immune response is mounted against the neoepitope. This results in platelet aggregation instead of heparin's normal function of preventing clot formation, which can lead to a risk of thrombosis (pieces of clots falling off and lodging in microvasculature, impairing circulation).

Thrombotic thrombocytopenic purpura (TTP) is a syndrome characterized by the sudden onset of thrombocytopenia, a microangiopathic hemolytic anemia, and multisystem organ failure. The syndrome tends to occur following an infectious disease but may also occur following administration of some drugs. The pathogenesis of TTP appears to be related to the ability of a clotting factor called von Willebrand factor (vWF) to activate platelets, even in the absence of significant vascular damage. Acquired TTP is associated with the development of an antibody that inhibits the protease responsible for processing very large vWF multimers into smaller multimers; the large multimers persist in circulation and inappropriately activate the platelets. The organ failure and hemolysis in TTP is due to the formation of platelet-rich microthrombi throughout the circulation. The development of TTP or TTP-like syndromes has been associated with drugs such as ticlopidine, clopidogrel, cocaine, mitomycin, and cyclosporine.

Toxic Effects on Platelet Function—Platelet function is dependent on the coordinated interaction of a number of biochemical response pathways. Major drug groups that affect platelet function include nonsteroidal anti-inflammatory agents, β-lactam-containing antibiotics, cardiovascular drugs, particularly beta blockers, psychotropic drugs, anesthetics, antihistamines, and some chemotherapeutic agents.

Xenobiotics may interfere with platelet function through a variety of mechanisms. Some drugs inhibit the phospholipase A_2/cyclooxygenase pathway and synthesis of thromboxane A_2 (e.g., nonsteroidal anti-inflammatory agents). Other agents appear to interfere with the interaction between platelet agonists and their receptors (e.g., antibiotics, ticlopidine, and clopidogrel). As the platelet response is dependent on rapid increase in cytoplasmic calcium, any agent that interferes with translocation of calcium may inhibit platelet function (e.g., calcium channel blockers). Occasionally, drug-induced antibodies will bind to a critical platelet receptor and inhibit its function.

Toxic Effects on Fibrin Clot Formation

Coagulation—Fibrin clot formation results from sequential activation of a series of serine proteases that culminates in the formation of thrombin. Thrombin is a multifunctional enzyme that converts fibrinogen to fibrin; activates factors V, VIII, XI, XIII, protein C, and platelets; and interacts with a variety of cells (e.g., leukocytes and endothelial cells), activating cellular signaling pathways.

Decreased Synthesis of Coagulation Proteins—Most proteins involved in the coagulation cascade are synthesized in

TABLE 11-7 Conditions associated with abnormal synthesis of vitamin K-dependent coagulation factors.

Warfarin and analogs	Intravenous α-tocopherol
Rodenticides (e.g., brodifacoum)	Dietary deficiency
Broad-spectrum antibiotics	Cholestyramine resin
N-Methyl-thiotetrazole cephalosporins	Malabsorption syndromes

the liver. Therefore, any agent that impairs liver function may cause a decrease in production of coagulation factors. The common tests of the coagulation cascade, the prothrombin time (PT) and activated partial thromboplastin time (aPTT), may be used to screen for liver dysfunction and a decrease in clotting factors.

Factors II, VII, IX, and X are dependent on vitamin K for their complete synthesis. Anything that interferes with absorption of vitamin K from the intestine or with the reduction of vitamin K epoxide may lead to a deficiency of these factors and a bleeding tendency (Table 11-7).

Increased Clearance of Coagulation Factors—Idiosyncratic reactions to xenobiotics include the formation of antibodies that react with coagulation proteins, forming an immune complex that is rapidly cleared from the circulation and resulting in deficiency of the factor. The factors that are most often affected by xenobiotics are listed in Table 11-8. In addition to causing increased clearance from the circulation, these antibodies often inhibit the function of the coagulation factor. Other antibodies have catalytic activity, resulting in proteolysis of the target coagulation factor.

Lupus anticoagulants are antibodies that can potentiate procoagulant mechanisms and interfere with the protein C system, increasing the risk of thrombosis. The development of lupus anticoagulants has been seen in association with chlorpromazine, procainamide, hydralazine, quinidine, phenytoin, and viral infections.

Toxicology of Agents Used to Modulate Hemostasis

Oral Anticoagulants—Oral anticoagulants are readily absorbed from the gastrointestinal tract and bind avidly to albumin in the circulation. The therapeutic window for oral anticoagulants (warfarin) is relatively narrow, and there is considerable interindividual variation in the response to a given dose. A number of factors, including concurrent medications and genetics, affect the individual response. The consequence of insufficient anticoagulant effect is an increased risk of thromboembolism, whereas the consequence of excessive anticoagulation is an increased risk of bleeding. Therapy with these agents must be routinely monitored with the PT, with results expressed in terms of the international normalized ratio (INR).

TABLE 11-8 Relationship between xenobiotics and the development of specific coagulation factor inhibitors.

Coagulation Factor	Xenobiotic
Thrombin	Topical bovine thrombin Fibrin glue
Factor V	Streptomycin Penicillin Gentamicin Cephalosporins Topical bovine thrombin
Factor VIII	Penicillin Ampicillin Chloramphenicol Phenytoin Methyldopa Nitrofurazone Phenylbutazone
Factor XIII	Isoniazid Procainamide Penicillin Phenytoin Practolol
von Willebrand factor	Ciprofloxacin Hydroxyethyl starch Valproic acid Griseofulvin Tetracycline Pesticides

A number of xenobiotics, including foods, have been found to affect the response to oral anticoagulants. Mechanisms for interference with oral anticoagulants include: induction or inhibition of biotransformation; interference with absorption of warfarin from the gastrointestinal tract; displacement of warfarin from albumin in plasma, which temporarily increases the bioavailability of warfarin until equilibrium is reestablished; diminished vitamin K availability; and inhibition of the reduction of vitamin K epoxide, which potentiates the effect of oral anticoagulants. Additionally, administration of oral anticoagulants may affect the activity or the half-lives of other medications.

Oral anticoagulants have been associated with warfarin-induced skin necrosis. Development of microvascular thrombosis in skin occurs most commonly in patients deficient in proteins C or S.

Vitamin K is also necessary for the synthesis of osteocalcin, a major component of bone. Long-term administration of warfarin has been associated with bone demineralization.

Administration of warfarin, particularly during the first 12 weeks of pregnancy, is associated with congenital anomalies in 25 to 30 percent of exposed infants. Many of the anomalies are related to abnormal bone formation. It is thought that warfarin may interfere with synthesis of additional proteins critical for normal structural development.

Heparin—Heparin is widely used for both prophylaxis and therapy of acute venous thromboembolism. The major complication associated with heparin therapy is bleeding. The aPTT is commonly used to monitor therapy with unfractionated heparin. Long-term administration of heparin is associated with an increased risk of clinically significant osteoporosis. Also, heparin administration may cause a transient rise in serum aminotransferases.

Fibrinolytic Agents—Fibrinolytic agents dissolve pathogenic thrombi by converting plasminogen, an inactive zymogen, to plasmin, an active proteolytic enzyme. Plasmin is normally tightly regulated and is not freely present in the circulation. However, administration of fibrinolytic agents regularly results in the generation of free plasmin leading to systemic fibrin(ogen)olysis, which is characterized by prolongation of the PT, aPTT, and thrombin time. All of these effects potentiate the risk of bleeding. Platelet inhibitors and heparin are commonly used in conjunction with fibrinolytic therapy to prevent recurrent thrombosis.

Streptokinase is a protein derived from group C β-hemolytic streptococci and is antigenic in humans. Antibody formation to streptokinase occurs commonly in association with streptococcal infections as well as exposure to streptokinase. Acute allergic reactions may occur in 1 to 5 percent of patients exposed to streptokinase. Allergic reactions also occur with other fibrinolytic agents containing streptokinase (e.g., anisoylated plasminogen–streptokinase complex, alteplase) or streptokinase-derived peptides.

Inhibitors of Fibrinolysis—Inhibitors of fibrinolysis are commonly used to control bleeding in patients with congenital abnormalities of hemostasis, such as von Willebrand disease. Tranexamic acid and ε-aminocaproic acid are small molecules that block the binding of plasminogen and plasmin to fibrin.

Aprotinin is a naturally occurring polypeptide inhibitor of serine proteases that is immunogenic when administered to humans.

RISK ASSESSMENT

Assessing the risk that exposure to new chemical products poses to humans—in terms of significant toxic effects on hematopoiesis and the functional integrity of blood cells and hemostatic mechanisms—is challenging. This is due in part to the complexity of hematopoiesis and the range of important tasks that these components perform. Risk assessment includes preclinical testing of animals and clinical trials in humans. It is hoped that in preclinical trials, the test animals will react similarly to humans on exposure to the xenobiotic, and the animals are examined in detail for signs of toxicity. Subsequent clinical trials are conducted in humans and measure myriad parameters of potential toxicity to determine the relative safety or toxicity of the test substance.

TABLE 11–9 Examples of problem-driven tests used to characterize hematologic observations in preclinical toxicology.

Reticulocyte count
Heinz body preparation
Cell-associated antibody assays (erythrocyte, platelet, neutrophil)
Erythrocyte osmotic fragility test
Erythrokinetic/ferrokinetic analyses
Cytochemical/histochemical staining
Electron microscopy
In vitro hematopoietic clonogenic assays
Platelet aggregation
Plasma fibrinogen concentration
Clotting factor assays
Thrombin time
Bleeding time

Tests used to assess blood and bone marrow in preclinical toxicology studies should provide information on the effects of single- and multiple-dose exposure on erythrocyte parameters (RBC, hemoglobin, PCV, MCV, and MCHC), leukocyte parameters (WBC and absolute differential counts), thrombocyte counts, coagulation tests (PT and aPTT), peripheral blood cell morphology, and bone marrow cytologic and histologic examinations. Additional tests should be employed in a problem-driven fashion as required to better characterize hematotoxicologic potential. Examples of these tests are listed in Table 11–9.

Patient- or population-related risk factors include pharmacogenetic variations in drug metabolism and detoxification that lead to reduced clearance of the agent or production of novel intermediate metabolites, histocompatibility antigens, interaction with drugs or other agents, increased sensitivity of hematopoietic precursors to damage, preexisting disease of the bone marrow, and metabolic defects that predispose to oxidative or other stresses associated with the agent.

A central issue in drug and nontherapeutic chemical development is the *predictive value* of preclinical toxicology data and the expansive but inevitably limited clinical database for the occurrence of significant hematotoxicity on broad exposure to human populations.

BIBLIOGRAPHY

Evans GO: *Animal Hematotoxicology: A Practical Guide for Toxicologists and Biomedical Researchers*. Boca Raton: CRC Press, 2008.

Hillman R, Ault KA, Rinder HM: *Hematology in Clinical Practice: A Guide to Diagnosis and Management*, 4th ed. New York: McGraw-Hill, 2005.

Lichtman MA, Beutler E, Kipps TJ, Seligsohn U, Kaushansky K, Prchal JT (eds): *Williams Hematology*, 7th ed. New York: McGraw-Hill, 2006.

QUESTIONS

1. Which of the following statements is FALSE regarding true anemia?
   a. Alterations of the mean corpuscular volume are characteristic of anemia.
   b. Increased destruction of erythrocytes can lead to anemia.
   c. Decreased production of erythrocytes is not a common cause of anemia because the bone marrow is continuously renewing the red blood cell pool.
   d. Reticulocytes will live for a longer period of time in the peripheral blood when a person is anemic.
   e. The main parameters in diagnosing anemia are RBC count, hemoglobin concentration, and hematocrit.

2. Which of the following types of anemia is properly paired with its cause?
   a. iron deficiency anemia—blood loss.
   b. sideroblastic anemia—vitamin B_{12} deficiency.
   c. megaloblastic anemia—folate supplementation.
   d. aplastic anemia—ethanol.
   e. megaloblastic anemia—lead poisoning.

3. The inability to synthesize the porphyrin ring of hemoglobin will most likely result in which of the following?
   a. iron deficiency anemia.
   b. improper RBC mitosis.
   c. inability to synthesize thymidine.
   d. accumulation of iron within erythroblasts.
   e. bone marrow hypoplasia.

4. Which of the following will cause a right shift in the oxygen dissociation curve?
   a. increased pH.
   b. decreased carbon dioxide concentration.
   c. decreased body temperature.
   d. increased 2,3-BPG concentration.
   e. fetal hemoglobin.

5. All of the following statements regarding erythrocytes are true EXCEPT:
   a. Aged erythrocytes are removed by the liver, where the iron is recycled.
   b. Erythrocytes have a life span of approximately 120 days.
   c. Red blood cells generally lose their nuclei before entering the circulation.
   d. Reticulocytes are immature RBCs that still have a little RNA.
   e. Persons with anemia have a higher than normal reticulocyte:erythrocyte ratio.

6. All of the following statements regarding oxidative hemolysis are true EXCEPT:
   a. Reactive oxygen species are commonly generated by RBC metabolism.
   b. Superoxide dismutase and catalase are enzymes that protect against oxidative damage.
   c. Reduced glutathione (GSH) increases the likelihood of oxidative injuries to RBCs.
   d. Glucose-6-phosphate dehydrogenase deficiency is commonly associated with oxidative hemolysis.
   e. Xenobiotics can cause oxidative injury to RBCs by overcoming the protective mechanisms of the cell.

7. Which of the following sets of leukocytes is properly characterized as granulocytes because of the appearance of cytoplasmic granules on a blood smear?
   a. neutrophils, basophils, and monocytes.
   b. basophils, eosinophils, and lymphocytes.
   c. eosinophils, neutrophils, and lymphocytes.
   d. basophils, eosinophils, and neutrophils.
   e. lymphocytes, neutrophils, and basophils.

8. All of the following statements are true EXCEPT:
   a. Xenobiotics can greatly slow down the proliferation of neutrophils and monocytes, increasing the risk of infection.
   b. Ethanol and cortisol decrease phagocytosis and microbe ingestion by the immune system.
   c. Agranulocytosis is predictable and can be caused by exposure to a number of environmental toxins.
   d. Heroin and methadone abusers have reduced ability to kill microorganisms due to drug-induced reduction in superoxide production.
   e. Toxic neutropenia may be mediated by the immune system.

9. Leukemias:
   a. are often due to cytogenic abnormalities, particularly damage to or loss of chromosomes 8 and 11.
   b. are rarely caused by agents used in cancer chemotherapy.
   c. originate in circulating blood cells.
   d. are characterized as "acute" if their effects are short-lived and severe.
   e. have long been associated with exposure to x-ray radiation.

10. Regarding platelets and thrombocytopenia, which of the following statements is FALSE?
    a. Platelets can be removed from the circulation through a hapten-mediated pathway that is induced by drugs or chemicals.
    b. Cortisol decreases platelet activity by inhibiting thromboxane prostaglandin synthesis.
    c. Toxins can induce a change in a platelet membrane glycoprotein, leading to recognition and removal of the platelet by phagocytes.
    d. Heparin administration can result in platelet aggregation and cause thrombocytopenia.
    e. Thrombotic thrombocytopenic purpura is most commonly caused by infectious disease, but can also be associated with administration of pharmacologic agents.

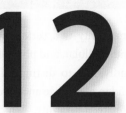

Toxic Responses of the Immune System

Norbert E. Kaminski, Barbara L. Faubert Kaplan,
and Michael P. Holsapple

Immunity is a homeostatic process, a series of delicately balanced, complex, multicellular, and physiologic mechanisms that allow an individual to distinguish foreign material from "self" and to neutralize and/or eliminate the foreign matter. Decreased immunocompetence (immunosuppression) may result in repeated, more severe, or prolonged infections as well as the development of cancer. Immunoenhancement may lead to immune-mediated diseases such as hypersensitivity responses, and if some integral bodily tissue is not identified as self, an autoimmune disease may be the end result.

THE IMMUNE SYSTEM

The immune system comprises numerous lymphoid organs and numerous different cellular populations with a variety of functions. The bone marrow and the thymus support the production of mature T and B lymphocytes and myeloid cells, such as macrophages and polymorphonuclear cells (PMN), and are referred to as primary lymphoid organs.

Within the bone marrow, the cells of the immune system developmentally "commit" to either the lymphoid or myeloid lineages. Cells of the lymphoid lineage make a further commitment to become either T cells or B cells. T-cell precursors are programmed to leave the bone marrow and migrate to the thymus, where they differentiate further.

Mature naive or virgin lymphocytes (those T and B cells that have never undergone antigenic stimulation) are first brought into contact with exogenously derived antigens within the spleen and lymph nodes, otherwise known as the secondary lymphoid organs.

Lymphoid tissues associated with the skin and the mucosal lamina propria of the gut, respiratory tract, and genitourinary tract can be classified as tertiary lymphoid tissues. Tertiary lymphoid tissues are primarily effector sites where memory and effector cells exert immunologic and immunoregulatory functions.

Antigen Recognition

Immunity—Innate immunity is a nonspecific first-line defense response with no associated immunologic memory. The innate immune response to a foreign organism is the same for a secondary or tertiary exposure as it is for the primary exposure. Acquired immunity is characterized by both specificity and memory, resulting in a much greater immune response on secondary challenge.

Antigen—A nonself-molecule, including foreign DNA, RNA, protein, carbohydrates, and even mutated self-proteins, that can be recognized by the immune system is called an antigen. Antigens are usually rearranged for presentation to other immune cells to induce the immunologic response.

Each antigen is recognized by specific antibodies produced by B cells. There are several light-chain genes and several heavy-chain genes coding for antibody protein, and when rearranged in various combinations, contribute to the immense genetic diversity of the produced antibodies.

Innate Immunity

Innate immunity acts as a first line of defense against infectious agents, eliminating most potential pathogens before significant infection occurs. It includes physical and biochemical barriers both inside and outside of the body as well as immune cells designed for specific responses. There is no immunologic memory associated with innate immunity.

Most infectious agents enter the body through the respiratory system, gut, or genitourinary tract, whereas the skin provides an effective barrier. Innate defenses include mucus

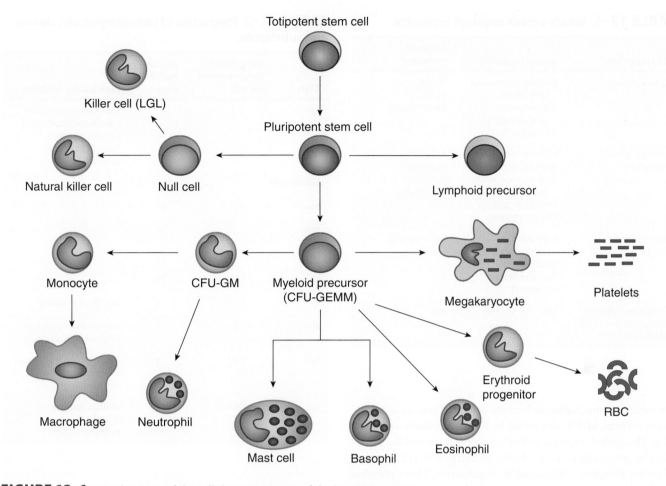

Totipotent stem cell

Killer cell (LGL)

Pluripotent stem cell

Natural killer cell   Null cell

Lymphoid precursor

Monocyte   CFU-GM   Myeloid precursor
(CFU-GEMM)

Megakaryocyte   Platelets

Macrophage   Neutrophil

Erythroid
progenitor

RBC

Mast cell   Basophil   Eosinophil

FIGURE 12–1 **Development of the cellular components of the immune system.**

secreted along the nasopharynx, the presence of lysozyme in most secretions, and cilia lining the trachea and main bronchi. In addition, reflexes such as coughing, sneezing, and elevation in body temperature are also a part of innate immunity. Pathogens that enter the body via the digestive tract are met with severe changes in pH (acid) within the stomach and a host of microorganisms living in the intestines.

Cellular Components: NK, NKT, PMN, and Macrophage—Two general types of cells are involved in nonspecific (innate) host resistance: natural killer (NK) cells and professional phagocytes. NK cells can recognize virally infected and malignant changes on the surface of cells as well as an antibody-coated target cell. The latter recognition is utilized in cell-mediated immunity (CMI). Using surface receptors, the NK cell binds, expels cytolytic granules, and induces apoptosis of the target cell.

NKT cells express surface markers characteristic of both NK and T cells and play a role in innate immunity, as their activation is early and they do not possess immunologic memory. They also produce cytokines and mediate cytolysis of target cells.

Phagocytic cells include PMN (neutrophil) and the monocyte/macrophage, which develop from pluripotent stem cells that

have become committed to the myeloid lineage (Figure 12–1). PMNs are excellent phagocytic cells and can eliminate most microorganisms and induce an inflammatory response.

Macrophages are terminally differentiated monocytes. On exiting the bone marrow, monocytes distribute to the various tissues where they can then differentiate into macrophages. Within different tissues, macrophages have distinct properties and vary in extent of surface receptors, oxidative metabolism, and expression of major histocompatibility complex (MHC) class II, which present the antigen.

Should PMNs be unable to contain an infection, macrophages are then recruited to the site of infection. Macrophages have both phagocytic and bactericidal functions, and can also function as antigen-presenting cells (APCs). They are recruited to sites of inflammation by chemotactic factors, can be activated by cytokines to become more effective killers, and can produce cytokines. Macrophages also play critical roles as scavengers in the daily turnover of senescent tissues such as red cell nuclei from maturing red cells, PMNs, and plasma cells.

Soluble Factors: Acute-phase Proteins and Complement—Soluble components of innate immunity (Table 12–1) are the acute-phase proteins and complement.

TABLE 12–1 Innate versus acquired immunity.

Characteristic	Innate Immunity	Acquired Immunity
Cells involved	Polymorphonuclear cells (PMN) Monocytes/ macrophages NK/NKT cells	T cells B cells Macrophages
Primary soluble mediators	Complement Perforin/granzyme Acute-phase proteins Interferon-α/β Other cytokines	Antibody Cytokines Perforin/ granzyme
Specificity of response	Limited to antigen–receptor binding (TLR, Fc, complement receptors)	Yes (very high specificity)
Response enhanced by repeated antigen challenge	No	Yes

TABLE 12–2 Properties of immunoglobulin classes and subclasses.

Class	Mean Serum Concentration, mg/mL	Human Half-life, days	Biological properties
IgG			Complement fixation (selected subclasses) Crosses placenta Heterocytotropic antibody
Subclasses			
IgG$_1$	9	21	
IgG$_2$	3	20	
IgG$_3$	1	7	
IgG$_4$	1	21	
IgA	3	6	Secretory antibody
IgM	1.5	10	Complement fixation Efficient agglutination
IgD	0.03	3	Possible role in antigen-triggered lymphocyte differentiation
IgE	0.0001	2	Allergic responses (mast-cell degranulation)

On infection, macrophages become activated and secrete various cytokines, which are carried by the bloodstream to distant sites. This global response to foreign agents is termed the *acute-phase response* and consists of fever and large shifts in the types of serum proteins synthesized by hepatocytes. These proteins can bind to bacteria via a process called opsonization and facilitate the binding of complement and the subsequent uptake of the bacteria by phagocytic cells.

The complement system consists of about 30 proteins whose primary functions are the destruction of the membranes of infectious agents and the promotion of an inflammatory response. Complement activation occurs with each component sequentially acting on others to coat the foreign cell and disrupt membrane integrity without harming the host cells. The final components that can enter the membrane and disrupt its integrity are termed the *membrane attack complex* (MAC). The complement-coated material is targeted for elimination by interaction with complement receptors on the surface of circulating immune cells.

Acquired (Adaptive) Immunity

If the primary defenses against infection (innate immunity) are breached, the acquired arm of the immune system is activated and produces a specific immune response to each infectious agent. This branch of immunity can protect the host from future infection by the same agent. Therefore, two key features that distinguish acquired immunity are *specificity* and *memory*. This means that in a normal healthy adult, the speed and magnitude of the immune response to a foreign organism are greater for a secondary challenge than they are for the primary challenge (Table 12–1).

Essential to the development of specific immunity is recognition of antigen and generation of an antibody that can bind to it. An antigen is defined functionally as a substance that can elicit the production of a specific antibody and can be specifically bound by that antibody. Small antigens are termed *haptens* and must be conjugated with carrier molecules (larger antigens) in order to elicit a specific response.

Antibodies, proteins classified as immunoglobulins (Igs), are produced by B cells and are also defined functionally by the antigen with which they react (i.e., anti-sheep red blood cell [anti-sRBC] IgM). There are five types of Ig that are related structurally (Table 12–2): IgM, IgG (and subsets), IgE, IgD, and IgA. All Igs are made up of heavy and light chains and of constant (Fc) and variable regions. It is the variable regions that determine antibody specificity. The variable region interacts with antigen, whereas the Fc region mediates effector functions such as complement fixation and phagocyte binding (via Fc receptors). Antibodies also coat foreign cells to help with opsonization, initiate the complement cascade to lead to cell lysis, bind to viral particles, and bind to antigens on target cells to help NK cells and cytotoxic T lymphocytes (CTL) destroy them.

During an immune response, the cells of the immune system communicate via a vast network of soluble mediators, the cytokines. Nearly all immune cells secrete cytokines, which may have local or systemic effects. Table 12–3 provides a brief summary of the sources and functions of cytokines.

TABLE 12–3 Cytokines: sources and functions in immune regulation.

Cytokine	Source	Physiologic Actions
IL-1	Macrophages B cells Several nonimmune cells	Activation and proliferation of T cells (Th2 > Th1) Proinflammatory Induces fever and acute-phase proteins Induces synthesis of IL-8 and TNF-α
IL-2	T cells	Primary T-cell growth factor Growth factor for B and NK cells Enhances lymphokine production
IL-3	T cells Mast cells	Stimulates the proliferation and differentiation of stromal cells, progenitors of the macrophage, granulocyte, and erythroid lineages
IL-4	T cells Mast cells Stromal cells Basophils CD4$^+$/NK1.1$^+$ cells	Proliferation of activated T cells (Th2 > Th1) and B cells B-cell differentiation and isotype switching may inhibit some macrophage functions Antagonizes IFN-γ Inhibits IL-8 production
IL-5	T cells Mast cells	Proliferation and differentiation of eosinophils Promotes B-cell isotype switching Synergizes with IL-4 to induce secretion of IgE
IL-6	Macrophages Activated T cells B cells Fibroblasts Keratinocytes Endothelial cells Hepatocytes	Enhances B-cell differentiation and immunoglobulin secretion Induction of acute-phase proteins by liver Proinflammatory Proliferation of T cells and increased IL-2 receptor expression Synergizes with IL-4 to induce secretion of IgE
IL-7	Stromal cells Epithelial cells	Proliferation of thymocytes (CD4$^-$/CD8$^-$) Proliferation of pro- and pre-B cells (mice) T-cell growth
IL-8	Macrophages Platelets Fibroblasts NK cells Keratinocytes Hepatocytes Endothelial cells	Activation and chemotaxis of monocytes, neutrophils, basophils, and T cells Proinflammatory
IL-9	Th cells	T-cell growth factor (primarily CD4$^+$ cells) Enhances mast-cell activity Stimulates growth of early erythroid progenitors
IL-10	T cells, Macrophages B cells	Inhibits macrophage cytolytic activity and macrophage activation of T cells General inhibitor of cytokine synthesis by Th1 cells (in presence of APCs) Enhances CD8$^+$ T-cell cytolytic activity Enhances proliferation of activated B cells Mast-cell growth Anti-inflammatory Inhibits endotoxin shock
Interferon-α/β (IFN-α/β) (type 1 IFN)	Leukocytes Epithelial cells Fibroblasts	Induction of class I expression Antiviral activity Stimulation of NK cells
Interferon-γ (IFN-γ)	T cells NK cells Epithelial cells Fibroblasts	Induction of class I and II Activates macrophages (as APC and cytolytic cells) Improves CTL recognition of virally infected cells
Tumor necrosis factor (TNF-α) and lymphotoxin (TNF-β)	Macrophages Lymphocytes Mast cells	Induces inflammatory cytokines Increases vascular permeability Activates macrophages and neutrophils Tumor necrosis (direct action) Primary mediator of septic shock Interferes with lipid metabolism (result is cachexia) Induction of acute-phase proteins

(continued)

TABLE 12–3 Cytokines: sources and functions in immune regulation. (Continued)

Cytokine	Source	Physiologic Actions
Transforming growth factor-β (TGF-β)	Macrophages Megakaryocytes Chondrocytes	Enhances monocyte/macrophage chemotaxis Enhances wound healing: angiogenesis, fibroblast proliferation, deposition of extracellular matrix Inhibits T- and B-cell proliferation Inhibits macrophage cytokine synthesis Inhibits antibody secretion Primary inducer of isotype switch to IgA
GM-CSF	T cells Macrophages Endothelial cells Fibroblasts	Stimulates growth and differentiation of monocytes and granulocytes
Migration inhibitory factor (MIF)	T cells Anterior pituitary cells Monocytes	Inhibits macrophage migration Proinflammatory (induces TNF-α production by macrophages) Appears to play a role in delayed hypersensitivity responses May be a counterregulator of glucocorticoid activity

Cellular Components: APCs, T Cells, and B Cells—In order to elicit a specific immune response to a particular antigen, that antigen must be taken up and processed by accessory cells, called APCs, for presentation to lymphocytes. The macrophage plays a critical role as an APC in acquired immunity. Although thought of more for its ability to produce Ig, the B cell can also serve as an APC.

APCs and lymphocytes interact during the immune response. APCs absorb the antigen, cut it into pieces, and then display a piece of the antigen on its cell surface attached to a complex of proteins called MHC II.

Besides serving as APCs, B lymphocytes are also the effector cells of humoral immunity, producing a number of isotypes of Ig with varying specificities and affinities. On antigen binding to surface Ig, the mature B cell becomes activated and, after proliferation, undergoes differentiation into either a memory B cell or an antibody-forming cell (AFC; plasma cell), actively secreting antigen-specific antibody.

T cells undergo a complex process of maturation wherein only cells that do not recognize self but do bind to MHC II proteins and recognize foreign antigens survive. These become either T-helper cells (which carry a certain protein on their surface called CD4+ and work by facilitating the B-cell response) or T-cytotoxic cells (which carry CD8+ and mediate cell killing).

Humoral and Cell-mediated Immunity—The activation of antigen-specific T cells begins with the interaction of the T-cell receptor (TCR) with MHC class II + peptide. On activation and in the presence of IL-1 secreted by the APC, T cells begin to produce the T-cell growth factor IL-2 and express receptors for them. As T cells begin to proliferate, they secrete numerous lymphokines (Table 12–3), which can influence many aspects of the immune response. The next step in the generation of the humoral response is the interaction of activated T cells with B cells. This may be a direct interaction of the T cell with B cell (antigen-specific) or may simply involve the production of lymphokines, which lead to B-cell growth and differentiation into AFCs or memory B cells. A general diagram of the cellular interactions involved in the humoral immune response is given in Figure 12–2. The production of antigen-specific IgM requires 3 to 5 days after the primary (initial) exposure to antigen (Figure 12–3). On secondary antigen challenge, the B cells undergo isotype switching, producing primarily IgG antibody, which is of higher affinity. In addition, there is a higher serum antibody titer associated with a secondary antibody response.

There are two general forms of CMI, referred to as delayed-type hypersensitivity (DTH) and cell-mediated cytotoxicity. DTH is presented later in this chapter in the section titled "Immune-mediated Disease." In cell-mediated cytotoxicity, the effector cell (CTL or NK) binds in a specific manner to the target cell (Figure 12–4), and the effector cell then releases the contents of its cytolytic granules onto the target cell, causing it to undergo programmed cell death.

Developmental Immunology

Developmental immunotoxicology involves investigation into the effects that xenobiotics have on the ontogeny of the immune system and includes prenatal (in utero), perinatal (<36 h of age), and neonatal periods of exposure. Immune development in humans and other species may be altered after perinatal exposure to immunotoxic chemicals. It has also been suggested that these effects may be more dramatic or persistent than those following exposure during adult life.

The immune system develops initially from a population of pluripotent hematopoietic stem cells that are generated early in gestation from uncommitted mesenchymal stem cells. This early population gives rise to all circulating blood cell lineages.

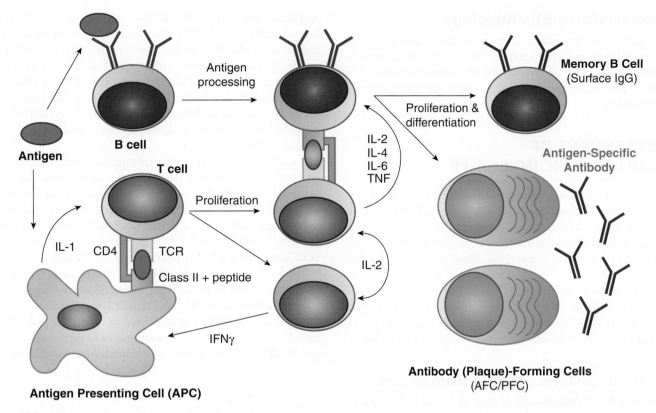

FIGURE 12–2 Cellular interactions in the antibody response.

Immunocompetent cells are produced in the bone marrow and thymus and then leave via the blood to the secondary immune organs: spleen, lymph nodes, and mucosal lymphoid tissue.

As thymic function wanes throughout life and thymocytes are no longer produced here, it is the pool of memory B and T cells that maintains immunocompetence for the life of the individual.

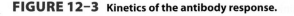

FIGURE 12–3 Kinetics of the antibody response.

1. Identification and engagement of target by effector.

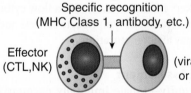

2. Strengthening of interaction and cytoplasmic re-orientation of effector.

3. Degranulation of effector onto target.

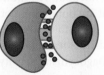

4. Disengagement of effector and death of target.

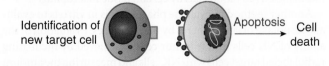

FIGURE 12–4 Cell-mediated cytotoxicity.

Neuroendocrine Immunology

Cytokines, neuropeptides, neurotransmitters, and hormones are an integral and interregulated part of the central nervous system, the endocrine system, and the immune system. The triad of influence these three systems exert over one another is bidirectional.

ASSESSMENT OF IMMUNOLOGIC INTEGRITY

Xenobiotics can have significant effects on the immune system. Among the unique features of immune cells is their ability to be removed from the body and to function in vitro. This unique quality offers the toxicologist an opportunity to comprehensively evaluate the actions of xenobiotics on the immune system.

Many medical devices may have intimate and prolonged contact with the body. Possible immunologic consequences of this contact could be envisioned to include immunosuppression, immune stimulation, inflammation, and sensitization.

Methods to Assess Immunocompetence

General Assessment—All studies of immunocompetence should include toxicologic studies (such as organ weights, serum characteristics, hematologic parameters, and bone marrow function) to investigate the effects of immune modulation on other body organs. Histopathology of lymphoid organs also may provide insight into potential immunotoxicants. Moreover, use of fluorescently labeled monoclonal antibodies to cell surface markers in conjunction with a flow cytometer enables accurate enumeration of lymphocyte subsets and whether the xenobiotic may affect maturation.

Functional Assessment

Innate Immunity—Innate immunity encompasses all those immunologic responses that do not require prior exposure to an antigen and that are nonspecific in nature. These responses include recognition of tumor cells by NK cells, phagocytosis of pathogens by macrophages, and the lytic activity of the complement system.

To evaluate phagocytic activity, macrophages are placed in culture plates and incubated with radiolabeled red blood cells. Those cells that are not bound by the macrophages are removed, as are the cells that are bound but not phagocytized. The macrophages are then lysed to determine the amount of cells that were phagocytized. This test provides information about both the binding and phagocytizing activity of the macrophages and can also be performed in vivo by measuring the uptake of the radiolabeled red blood cells by certain tissue macrophages.

Another method to evaluate phagocytosis in vitro is to evaluate the uptake of latex spheres by macrophages. Evaluation of the ability of NK cells to lyse tumor cells is achieved by incubating radiolabeled target cells with NK cells and measuring the amount of radioactivity released into solution from the target cells.

Acquired Immunity: Humoral—The plaque (antibody)-forming cell (PFC or AFC) assay tests the ability of the host to mount an antibody response to a specific antigen, which requires the coordinated interaction of several different immune cells: macrophages, T cells, and B cells. Therefore, an effect on any of these cells (e.g., antigen processing and presentation, cytokine production, proliferation, or differentiation) can have a profound impact on the ability of B cells to produce antigen-specific antibody.

A standard PFC assay involves immunizing mice with sRBC. The antigen is taken up in the spleen and an antibody response occurs. Four days after immunization, spleens are removed and splenocytes are mixed with RBCs, complement, and agar, the mixture plated, and incubated until the B cells secrete anti-sRBC IgM antibody. This antibody then coats the surrounding sRBCs, and areas of hemolysis (plaques) can be seen.

The PFC assay can be evaluated in vivo using serum from peripheral blood of immunized mice and an enzyme-linked immunosorbent assay (ELISA; Figure 12–5). Serum from mice immunized with sRBCs is incubated in microtiter plates that have been coated with sRBC membranes to serve as the antigen for sRBC-specific IgM or IgG to bind. After incubation, an

1. Bind antigen to plate. Wash.

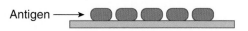

2. Add test sera and incubate. Wash.

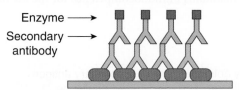

3. Add enzyme-coupled secondary antibody. Wash.

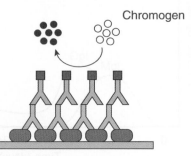

4. Add chromogen and develop color.

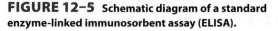

FIGURE 12–5 Schematic diagram of a standard enzyme-linked immunosorbent assay (ELISA).

enzyme-conjugated monoclonal antibody (the secondary antibody) against IgM (or IgG) is added. This antibody recognizes the IgM (or IgG) and binds specifically to that antibody. Then, the enzyme substrate (chromogen) is added. When the substrate comes into contact with the enzyme on the secondary antibody, a color change occurs that can be detected by measuring absorbance with a plate reader.

Acquired Immunity: Cell-mediated—Of numerous assays of CMI, three routinely performed tests are: the CTL assay, the delayed hypersensitivity response (DHR), and the T-cell proliferative responses to antigens.

The CTL assay measures the in vitro ability of splenic T cells to recognize allogeneic or antigenically distinct target cells by evaluating the ability of the CTLs to proliferate and then lyse the target cells. CTLs are incubated with target cells that have been treated so that they cannot themselves proliferate. CTLs recognize the target cells and proliferate until they are harvested. Then, they are incubated with radiolabeled target cells. CTLs that have acquired memory recognize the foreign MHC class I on target cells and lyse them.

The DHR evaluates the ability of memory T cells to recognize foreign antigen, proliferate and migrate to the site of the antigen, and secrete cytokines in vivo. Mice are sensitized by a subcutaneous injection of the chemical. Radiolabeled iodine is allowed to be incorporated into the mouse's mononuclear cells by injecting it into the mouse's bloodstream. Then, some of the sensitizing chemical is injected into the ear, and, after euthanizing the mouse, the ear is evaluated for the presence of radiolabeled mononuclear cells.

Several mechanisms exist to evaluate proliferative capacity of T cells in CMI. The mixed lymphocyte response (MLR) measures the ability of T cells to recognize foreign MHC class I and undergo proliferation.

Flow Cytometric Analysis—Flow cytometry employs light scatter, fluorescence, and absorbance measurements to analyze large numbers of cells on an individual basis. Usually, fluorochrome-conjugated monoclonal antibodies raised against a specific protein are employed for detection. This approach can be used to provide insight into which specific T-cell subsets are targeted after exposure to a xenobiotic, and to identify putative effects on T-cell maturation.

Molecular Biology Approaches to Immunotoxicology— Proteomics (the study of all expressed proteins in a particular cell, and thus the functional expression of the genome) and genomics (the study of all genes encoded by an organism's DNA), combined with bioinformatics, facilitate the evaluation of xenobiotic-induced alterations in the pathways and signaling networks of the immune system.

Mechanistic Approaches to Immunotoxicology—Once an agent has been identified as being an immunotoxicant, it may be necessary to further characterize its mechanism. A general strategy involves the following steps: (1) identifying

the cell type(s) targeted by the agent; (2) determining whether the effects are mediated by the parent compound or by a metabolite of the parent; (3) determining whether the effects are mediated directly or indirectly by the xenobiotic; and (4) elucidating the molecular events responsible for altered leukocyte function.

Regulatory Approaches to the Assessment of Immunotoxicity

The NTP Tier Approach—The National Toxicology Program screens for potential immunotoxic agents using a tier approach. Tier I provides assessment of general toxicity (immunopathology, hematology, and body and organ weights) as well as endline functional assays (proliferative responses, PFC assay, and NK assay). Tier II was designed to further define an immunotoxic effect and includes tests for CMI (CTL and DHR), secondary antibody responses, enumeration of lymphocyte populations, and host resistance models.

Health Effects Test Guidelines—Guidelines for functional immunotoxicity assessments in regulatory studies recommend conduct of three tests. Assessment of immunotoxicity begins by exposure for a minimum of 28 days to the chemical followed by assessment of humoral immunity (PFC assay or anti-sRBC ELISA). If the chemical produces significant suppression of the humoral response, surface marker assessment by flow cytometry may be performed. If the chemical produces no suppression of the humoral response, an assessment of innate immunity (NK assay) may be performed.

Animal Models in Immunotoxicology

Rats and mice have been the animals of choice for studying the actions of xenobiotics on the immune system because: (1) there is a vast database available on the immune system, (2) rodents are less expensive to maintain than larger animals, and (3) a wide variety of reagents (cytokines, antibodies, etc.) are available. Many reagents that are available for studying the human immune system can also be used in rhesus and cynomolgus monkeys. Chicken and fish are being used to evaluate the immunotoxicity of xenobiotics as alternative animal models with heightened environmental consciousness.

The manipulation of the embryonic genome, creating transgenic and knockout mice, may allow complex immune responses to be dissected into their components. In this way, the mechanisms by which immunotoxicants act can be better understood. Severe combined immunodeficient mice (SCID) have been used to study immune regulation, hematopoiesis, hypersensitivity, and autoimmunity.

Evaluation of Mechanisms of Action

Direct effects on the immune system may include chemical effects on immune function, structural alterations in lymphoid organs or on immune cell surfaces, or compositional changes in lymphoid organs or in serum. Xenobiotics may exert an indirect action on the immune system as well. They may be metabolically activated to their toxic metabolites, and may also have effects on other organ systems (e.g., liver damage) that then impact the immune system.

IMMUNOMODULATION BY XENOBIOTICS

Immunosuppression

Immunosuppression can be produced by numerous natural and synthetic chemicals as listed in Table 12–4.

Tobacco Smoke—Pulmonary defenses against inhaled gases and particulates are dependent on both physical and immunologic mechanisms. Immune mechanisms primarily involve the complex interactions between PMNs and alveolar macrophages and their abilities to phagocytize foreign material and produce cytokines.

In humans, the number of alveolar macrophages is increased three- to fivefold in smokers compared with nonsmokers and the macrophages present appear to be in an activated state but have decreased phagocytic and bactericidal activity. Decreased serum Ig levels and decreased NK-cell activity have been reported. Concentration-dependent leukocytosis (increased numbers of T and B cells) is well defined in smokers when compared with nonsmokers. Numerous immunologic studies conducted in animals exposed to cigarette smoke have demonstrated suppression of antibody responses.

Recombinant DNA-derived Proteins—Biologics (e.g., blood or vaccine products) and recombinant DNA-derived

TABLE 12–4 Xenobiotics capable of immunosuppression.

Halogenated aromatic hydrocarbons	**Aromatic hydrocarbons**
Polychlorinated biphenyls Polybrominated biphenyls Polychlorinated dibenzodioxins Polychlorinated dibenzofurans	Carbon tetrachloride Ethylene glycol monomethyl ether 2-Methoxyethanol
Polycyclic aromatic hydrocarbons	**Mycotoxins**
Nitrosamines	Aflatoxin Ochratoxin Tricothecenes Vomitoxin
Pesticides	
Organophosphate pesticides Organochlorine pesticides Organotin pesticides Carbamate pesticides Pyrethroids	**Natural and synthetic hormones**
	Estrogens Androgens Glucocorticoids
Metals	**Therapeutics**
Arsenic Beryllium Cadmium Chromium Cobalt Gold Lead Mercury Nickel Platinum	AIDS therapeutics Biologics Anti-inflammatory agents
	Immunosuppressive drugs
	Azathioprine Cyclophosphamide Cyclosporin A Leflunomide Rapamycin Stavudine (2′,3′-didehydro-2′,3′-dideoxythymidine) Videx (2′,3′-dideoxyinosine; ddI) Zalcitabine (2′,3′-dideoxycytidine; ddC) Zidovudine (3′-azido-3′-deoxythymidine; AZT)
Inhaled substances	
Asbestos Ethylenediamine Formaldehyde Silica Tobacco smoke Urethane	**Drugs of abuse**
	Cannabinoids Cocaine Ethanol Opioids: heroin and morphine
Oxidant gases	
Ozone (O_3) Nitrogen dioxide (NO_2) Sulfur dioxide (SO_2) Phosgene	

proteins may elicit the production of neutralizing antibodies. The effects of neutralizing antibodies may also lead to hypersensitivity reactions.

Ultraviolet Radiation—Ultraviolet radiation (UVR) suppresses DHR in both animals and humans and results in decreased host resistance to infection. Induction of suppressor T cells and alterations in homing patterns have been suggested as possibilities. One plausible explanation is that UVR induces a switch from a predominantly Th1 response (favoring DHR) to a Th2 response (favoring antibody responses).

XENOBIOTIC-INDUCED HYPERSENSITIVITY AND AUTOIMMUNITY

The purpose of the immune system is to protect the individual from disease states, whether infectious, parasitic, or cancerous, through both cellular and humoral mechanisms. In so doing, the ability to distinguish "self" from "nonself" plays a predominant role. However, situations arise in which the individual's immune system responds in a manner producing tissue damage, resulting in a self-induced disease, either (1) hypersensitivity, or allergy, or (2) autoimmunity. Hypersensitivity reactions result from the immune system responding in an exaggerated or inappropriate manner. In the case of autoimmunity, mechanisms of self-recognition break down and Igs and TCRs react with self-antigens, resulting in tissue damage and disease.

Hypersensitivity

Classification of Hypersensitivity Reactions—All four types of hypersensitivity reactions require prior exposure leading to sensitization in order to elicit a reaction on subsequent challenge. Figure 12–6 illustrates the mechanisms of hypersensitivity reactions as classified by Coombs and Gell.

Type I (Immediate Hypersensitivity)—Sensitization occurs as the result of exposure to appropriate antigens through the respiratory tract, dermally, or by exposure through the gastrointestinal tract and is mediated by IgE production. IgE binds to appropriate cells and sensitizes an individual; reexposure to the antigen results in degranulation of the mast cells with the release of preformed mediators and cytokines that promote vasodilatation, bronchial constriction, and inflammation.

Type II (Antibody-dependent Cytotoxic Hypersensitivity)—Type II hypersensitivity is IgG-mediated. Tissue damage may result from the direct action of cytotoxic cells or by antibody activation of the classic complement pathway. Complement activation may result in cell lysis.

Type III (Immune Complex-mediated Hypersensitivity)—Type III hypersensitivity reactions also involve IgG Igs. Ig may form complexes with soluble antigen and the complex may deposit (lodge) in various tissues, causing tissue damage. The most common location is the vascular endothelium in the lung, joints, and kidneys. Macrophages, neutrophils, and platelets attracted to the deposition site contribute to the tissue damage.

Type IV (Cell-mediated Hypersensitivity)—Type IV is a DTH response. Contact hypersensitivity is initiated by topical exposure, and consists of two phases: sensitization and elicitation. Sensitization results in development of activated and memory T cells when the chemical is presented on an APC to T-helper cells in local lymph nodes, leading to generation of memory T cells.

On second contact, antigen-presenting Langerhans–dendritic cells present the processed hapten–carrier complex to memory T cells. These activated T cells then secrete cytokines that bring about further proliferation of T cells and facilitate the movement of inflammatory cells into the skin, resulting in erythema and the formation of papules and vesicles. Cells of the cell-mediated immune response may cause local tissue damage.

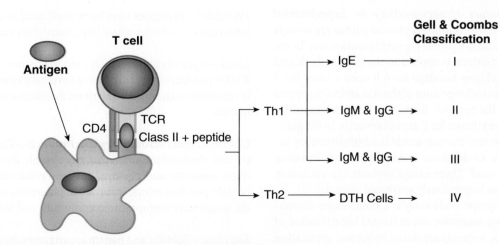

FIGURE 12–6 Schematic of classification of hypersensitivity reactions.

Whereas separation of hypersensitivity responses into types I to IV is helpful in understanding the involved mechanisms, it is important to realize that often pathology is the result of a combination of these mechanisms.

Assessment of Hypersensitivity Responses

Assessment of Respiratory Hypersensitivity in Experimental Animals—Methods for detecting pulmonary hypersensitivity can be divided into two types: (1) those for detecting immunologic sensitization and (2) those for detecting pulmonary sensitization. In the case of types I to III, immunologic sensitization occurs when antigen-specific Ig is produced in response to exposure to an antigen or, in the case of type IV, when a population of sensitized T lymphocytes is produced. Pulmonary sensitization is determined by a change in respiratory function subsequent to the challenge of a sensitized animal.

Guinea pig models have been most frequently used because the lung is the major shock organ for anaphylactic response. Immunologic sensitization may be determined by obtaining sequential blood samples throughout the induction period and measuring antibody titer. Pulmonary sensitization is evaluated by detecting the presence of pulmonary reactivity (either visible respiratory distress or changes in respiratory function) following challenge.

Assessment of IgE-mediated Hypersensitivity Responses in Humans—Two skin tests available for immediate hypersensitivity testing measure a "wheal and flare" reaction. The prick-puncture test introduces very small amounts of antigen under the skin. For test compounds not eliciting a reaction in the less sensitive skin test, the intradermal test using dilute concentrations of antigen may be used, but there is a higher risk of systemic reactions.

In vitro serologic tests, ELISAs, and radioallergosorbent tests (RASTs) may also be used to detect the presence of antigen-specific antibody in the patient's serum.

Bronchial provocation tests may be performed by having the patient inhale an antigen into the bronchial tree and evaluating his or her pulmonary response.

Assessment of Contact Hypersensitivity in Experimental Animals—The two most commonly utilized guinea pig models are the Büehler test and the guinea pig maximization test. In the Büehler test, the test article is applied to the shaven flank and covered with an occlusive bandage for 6 h once a week for 3 weeks. On day 28, a challenge dose of the test article is applied to a shaven area on the opposite flank; the area is evaluated for signs of edema and erythema for 2 days afterwards. In the guinea pig maximization test, the test article is administered by intradermal injection, an adjuvant is employed, and irritating concentrations are used. These assays evaluate the elicitation phase of the response in previously sensitized animals.

The mouse local lymph node assay is a stand-alone alternative to the guinea pig assays for use in hazard identification of chemical sensitizers. Animals are dosed by topical application of the test article to the ears for 3 consecutive days. A few days later, the animals are injected with radiolabeled thymidine, which is incorporated into proliferating lymphocytes. Later, the animals are sacrificed and the local lymph nodes assayed for radiolabeled lymphocytes to see if the test article induced an immune response.

Assessment of Contact Hypersensitivity in Humans—Human testing for contact hypersensitivity reactions is by skin patch testing. Patches containing specified concentrations of the allergen in the appropriate vehicle are applied under an occlusive patch for 48 h. Once the patch is removed, the area is read for signs of erythema, papules, vesicles, and edema. Generally, the test is read again at 72 h and in some cases signs may not appear for up to 1 week or more.

Hypersensitivity Reactions to Xenobiotics—Numerous xenobiotics illicit hypersensitivity reactions. Polyisocyanates, and toluene diisocyanate in particular, used in the production of adhesives and coatings are known to induce the full spectrum of hypersensitivity responses, types I to IV, as well as nonimmune inflammatory and neuroreflex reactions in the lung. Inhaled acid anhydrides, which are used in the manufacturing of paints, varnishes, coating materials, adhesives, and casting and sealing materials, may conjugate with serum albumin or erythrocytes leading to type I, II, or III hypersensitivity reactions on subsequent exposure.

Metals—Metals and metallic substances, including metallic salts, are responsible for producing contact and pulmonary hypersensitivity reactions. Platinum, nickel, chromium, beryllium, and cobalt are commonly implicated.

Drugs—Hypersensitivity responses to drugs are among the major types of unpredictable drug reactions. Drugs are designed to be reactive in the body and multiple treatments are common. This type of exposure is conducive to producing an immunologic reaction. Immunologic mechanisms of hypersensitivity reactions to drugs include types I to IV. Penicillin is the most common agent involved in drug allergy.

Pesticides—Pesticides have been implicated as causal agents in both contact and immediate hypersensitivity reactions.

Latex—Natural rubber latex is used in the manufacture of over 40,000 products from balloons to surgical gloves. Dermatologic reactions to latex include irritant dermatitis and contact dermatitis.

Cosmetics and Personal Hygiene Products—Contact dermatitis and dermatoconjunctivitis may result from exposure to many cosmetic and personal hygiene products. These agents contain paraben esters, sorbic acid, phenolics, organomercurials, quaternary ammonium compounds, and formaldehyde.

Enzymes—Subtilin and papain are enzymes capable of eliciting type I hypersensitivity responses. Subtilin is used in laundry detergents. Both individuals working where the product is made and those using the product may become sensitized. Subsequent exposure may produce signs of rhinitis, conjunctivitis, and asthma. Papain is another enzyme known to induce IgE-mediated disease. It is most commonly used as a meat tenderizer and a clearing agent in beer production.

Formaldehyde—Formaldehyde exposure occurs in the cosmetics and textile industries, and in the furniture, auto upholstery, and resins industries. Occupational exposure to formaldehyde has been associated with the occurrence of asthma.

Autoimmunity

In cases of autoimmunity, self-antigens are the target, and in the case of chemical-induced autoimmunity, the disease state is induced by a modification of host tissues or immune cells by the chemical and not the chemical acting as an antigen/hapten.

Mechanisms of Autoimmunity—Three types of molecules are involved in the process of self-recognition: Igs, TCRs, and the products of MHC. Igs and TCRs are expressed clonally on B and T cells, respectively, whereas MHC molecules are present on all nucleated cells.

The process of negative selection against autoreactive T cells in the thymus is important in the prevention of autoimmune disease. T cells expressing receptors that bind to self-antigens undergo apoptosis (negative selection), whereas those that do not recognize self-proteins proliferate (positive selection) and migrate to the peripheral lymph organs. Some cells that recognize self-molecules do not die, but undergo anergy, where they stay in the body but are inactive.

Several mechanisms may break down self-tolerance, leading to autoimmunity. First, if exposure to antigens is not available in the thymus during embryonic development, such as to myelin, which is not produced until later in development, then antigen-specific T-cell-reactive lymphocytes not subjected to negative selection could induce an autoimmune reaction. Breakdown of self-tolerance to these antigens may be induced by exposure to adjuvants, chemicals used to enhance immunogenicity, or to another antigenically related protein. Second, T-cell anergy can be overcome with chronic lymphocyte stimulation. Third, interference with normal immunoregulation by CD8[+] T-cell suppressor cells may create an environment conducive to the development of autoimmune disease.

As is the case with hypersensitivity reactions, autoimmune disease is often the result of more than one mechanism working simultaneously. Therefore, pathology may be the result of antibody-dependent cytotoxicity, complement-dependent antibody-mediated lysis, or direct or indirect effects of cytotoxic T cells.

Autoimmune Reactions to Xenobiotics—Table 12–5 lists chemicals known to be associated with autoimmunity, showing the proposed self-antigenic determinant or stating adjuvancy

TABLE 12–5 Chemical agents known to be associated with autoimmunity.

Proposed Antigenic Chemical	Clinical Manifestations	Department
Drugs		
Methyldopa	Hemolytic anemia	Rhesus antigens
Hydralazine	SLE-like syndrome	Myeloperoxidase
Isoniazid	SLE-like syndrome	Myeloperoxidase
Procainamide	SLE-like syndrome	DNA
Halothane	Autoimmune hepatitis	Liver microsomal proteins
Nondrug chemicals		
Vinyl chloride	Scleroderma-like syndrome	Abnormal protein synthesized in liver
Mercury	Glomerular neuropathy	Glomerular basement membrane protein
Silica	Scleroderma	Most likely acts as an adjuvant

TABLE 12–6 Chemicals implicated in autoimmunity.

Manifestation	Implicated Chemical
Scleroderma	Solvents (toluene, xylene) Tryptophan Silicones
Systemic lupus erythrematosus	Phenothiazines Penicillamine Propylthiouracil Quinidine L-DOPA Lithium carbonate Trichloroethylene Silicones

as the mechanism of action. Table 12–6 shows chemicals that have been implicated in autoimmune reactions, but in these cases the mechanism of autoimmunity has not been as clearly defined or confirmed.

Multiple Chemical Sensitivity Syndrome—Multiple chemical sensitivity syndrome (MCS) has been associated with hypersensitivity responses to chemicals. The syndrome is characterized by multiple subjective symptoms related to more than one system. The more common symptoms are nasal congestion, headaches, lack of concentration, fatigue, and memory loss. Many mechanisms have been suggested to explain how chemicals cause these symptoms. A major hypothesis is that MCS occurs when chemical exposure sensitizes certain individuals, and, on subsequent exposure to exceedingly small amounts of these or unrelated chemicals, the individual exhibits an adverse response.

NEW FRONTIERS AND CHALLENGES IN IMMUNOTOXICOLOGY

New technology has brought more questions to be answered and new tools to assess these questions. The significant immunotoxicologic challenges needing to be addressed include: (1) how to interpret the significance of minor or moderate immunotoxic effects in animal models in relation to human risk assessment; (2) how to better integrate a consideration of exposure, especially to multiple agents simultaneously, into immunotoxicologic risk assessment; (3) how to design better human studies to assess the impact on the immune system in the species of greatest interest in the context of risk assessment; (4) how to identify and establish sensitive human biomarkers of immunotoxicity; and (5) how to gain a better understanding of the role of genetics in identifying sensitive subpopulations to immune-altering agents.

Systemic hypersensitivity is a frequent cause for withdrawal of drugs that have made it to the market. These findings are generally unexpected in that they were not predicted in preclinical toxicology and immunotoxicology studies. Assays are needed that are more predictive of drug antigenicity, food allergy, or hypersensitivity in humans.

Use of computational toxicology methods to predict potential biological/toxicologic activity of chemicals is growing. The premise is that the structure of a chemical determines the physiochemical properties and reactivities that underlie its biological and toxicologic properties. Being able to predict potential adverse effects will aid the designed development of new chemicals and will potentially reduce the need for animal testing.

Efforts to exploit biomarkers to indicate exposure to a specific chemical, susceptibility to adverse effect, and/or predict disease associated with chemical exposure are ongoing. The most desirable biomarkers are those that indicate *exposure* in the absence of immediate adverse effect. Biomarkers of *effect* would indicate subclinical effects of chemical exposure. Potential biomarkers include cytokine gene expression patterns, cell population quantification using flow cytometry, and serum antibody titers.

Assessments of the use of immunotoxicology data in animals as predictors of risk for human clinical effects have limitations, including the fact that no single immune test has been observed to be highly predictive of altered host resistance. Variability in the virulence of infectious agents in the human population, the complexity of the immune system, and the redundancy (multiple components capable of responding to a foreign challenge) in the immune system may all contribute to the difficulty in quantifying relationships between chemical-induced alterations in immune status and alterations in host resistance in humans.

The balance between immune recognition and destruction of foreign invaders and the proliferation of these microbes and/or cancer cells can be a precarious one. Validated methods to detect xenobiotics that produce adverse effects related to the immune system must be continually improved using the latest knowledge and technologies in order to provide a safe environment.

BIBLIOGRAPHY

Descotes J: *Immunotoxicology of Drugs and Chemicals: An Experimental and Clinical Approach*, 3rd ed. San Diego: Elsevier, 2004.

Hayes AW: *Principles and Methods of Toxicology*, 5th ed. Boca Raton: CRC Press/Taylor and Francis, 2007.

Paul WE (ed): *Fundamental Immunology*, 5th ed. Philadelphia: Lippincott Williams & Wilkins, 2003.

QUESTIONS

1. Which of the following cells or substances is NOT part of the innate immune system?
   a. lysozyme.
   b. monocytes.
   c. complement.
   d. antibodies.
   e. neutrophils.

2. Myeloid precursor stem cells are responsible for the formation of all of the following EXCEPT:
   a. platelets.
   b. lymphocytes.
   c. basophils.
   d. erythrocytes.
   e. monocytes.

3. When an Rh− mother is exposed to the blood of an Rh+ baby during childbirth, the mother will make antibodies against the Rh factor, which can lead to the mother attacking the next Rh+ fetus. This is all possible because of which antibody's ability to cross the placenta?
   a. IgM.
   b. IgE.
   c. IgG.
   d. IgA.
   e. IgD.

4. Which of the following statements is FALSE regarding important cytokine function in regulating the immune system?
   a. IL-1 induces inflammation and fever.
   b. IL-3 is the primary T-cell growth factor.
   c. IL-4 induces B-cell differentiation and isotype switching.
   d. Transforming growth factor-β (TGF-β) enhances monocyte/macrophage chemotaxis.
   e. Interferon gamma (IFN-gamma) activates macrophages.

5. Which of the following is NOT a step performed during an enzyme-linked immunosorbent assay (ELISA)?
   a. A chromogen is added and color is detected.
   b. The antigen of interest is fixed to a microtiter plate.
   c. Radioactively labeled cells are added to the solution.
   d. Enzyme-tagged secondary antibodies are added.
   e. Test sera are added.

6. The delayed hypersensitivity response (DHR) test does NOT:
   a. evaluate memory T-cells' ability to recognize a foreign antigen.
   b. evaluate memory T-cells' ability to secrete cytokines.
   c. evaluate memory T-cells' ability to proliferate.
   d. evaluate memory T-cells' ability to lyse foreign target cells.
   e. evaluate memory T-cells' ability to migrate to the site of foreign antigen.

7. The number of alveolar macrophages in smokers is greatly increased relative to nonsmokers. What is a characteristic of the alveolar macrophages found in smokers?
   a. They are in an inactive state.
   b. They are far larger than normal.
   c. They have increased phagocytic activity.
   d. They are incapable of producing cytokines.
   e. They have decreased bactericidal activity.

8. Which of the following is NOT characteristic of a type I hypersensitivity reaction?
   a. It is mediated by IgE.
   b. It involves immune complex deposition in peripheral tissues.
   c. It involves mast-cell degranulation.
   d. Anaphylaxis is an acute, systemic, and very severe type I hypersensitivity reaction.
   e. It is usually mediated by preformed histamine, prostaglandins, and leukotrienes.

9. Which of the following types of hypersensitivity is NOT mediated by antibodies?
   a. type I.
   b. type II.
   c. type III.
   d. type IV.
   e. type V.

10. Which of the following is NOT a common mechanism of autoimmune disorders?
    a. subjection to positive selection in the thymus.
    b. anergic T cells become activated.
    c. interference with normal immunoregulation by CD8⁺ suppressor T cells.
    d. lack of subjection to negative selection in the thymus.
    e. decreased self-tolerance.

Toxic Responses of the Liver

Hartmut Jaeschke

KEY POINTS

- The liver's strategic location between intestinal tract and the rest of the body facilitates its maintenance of metabolic homeostasis in the body.
- The liver extracts ingested nutrients, vitamins, metals, drugs, environmental toxicants, and waste products of bacteria from the blood for catabolism, storage, and/or excretion into bile.
- Formation of bile is essential for uptake of lipid nutrients from the small intestine, protection of the small intestine from oxidative insults, and excretion of endogenous and xenobiotic compounds.

- Cholestasis is either a decrease in the volume of bile formed or an impaired secretion of specific solutes into bile, which results in elevated serum levels of bile salts and bilirubin.
- Hepatocytes have a rich supply of phase I enzymes that often convert xenobiotics to reactive electrophilic metabolites and of phase II enzymes that add a polar group to a molecule and thereby enhance its removal from the body. The balance between phase I and phase II reactions determines whether a reactive metabolite will initiate liver cell injury or be safely detoxified.

INTRODUCTION

The liver is the main organ where exogenous chemicals are metabolized and eventually excreted. As a consequence, liver cells are exposed to significant concentrations of these chemicals, which can result in liver dysfunction, cell injury, and even organ failure. The liver, with its multiple cell types and numerous functions, can respond in many different ways to acute and chronic insults. To recognize potential liver cell dysfunction and injury, it is necessary to have a general knowledge of basic liver functions, the structural organization of the liver, the processes involved in hepatic excretory functions, and mechanisms of cell and organ injury.

LIVER PHYSIOLOGY

Hepatic Functions

The liver's strategic location between intestinal tract and the rest of the body facilitates the performance of its enormous task of maintaining the metabolic homeostasis of the body. Venous blood from the stomach and intestines flows into the portal vein, through the liver, and then enters the systemic circulation. The liver is the first organ to encounter ingested nutrients, vitamins, metals, drugs, and environmental toxicants as well as waste products of bacteria that enter portal blood. Efficient scavenging or uptake processes extract these absorbed materials from the blood for catabolism, storage, and/or excretion into bile.

All of the major functions of the liver can be detrimentally altered by acute or chronic exposure to toxicants (Table 13–1). When toxicants inhibit or otherwise impede hepatic transport and synthetic processes, dysfunction can occur without appreciable cell damage. Loss of function also occurs when toxicants kill an appreciable number of cells and when chronic insult leads to replacement of cell mass by nonfunctional scar tissue.

Structural Organization

Classically, the liver is divided into hexagonal lobules oriented around terminal hepatic venules (also known as central veins). At the corners of the lobule are the portal triads (or portal tracts), containing a branch of the portal vein, a hepatic arteriole, and a bile duct (Figure 13–1). Blood entering from the portal vein and hepatic artery mixes in the penetrating vessels, enters the sinusoids, percolates along the cords of parenchymal cells (hepatocytes), flows into terminal hepatic venules, and exits the liver via the hepatic vein. The lobule is divided into three regions known as centrolobular, midzonal, and periportal. The preferred concept of a functional hepatic unit is the acinus. The base of the acinus is formed by the terminal branches of the portal vein and hepatic artery, which extend out from the portal tracts. The acinus has three zones: zone 1 is closest to the entry of blood, zone 3 abuts the terminal hepatic vein, and zone 2 is intermediate. The three zones of the acinus roughly coincide with the three regions of the lobule (Figure 13–1).

Acinar zonation is of considerable functional consequence regarding gradients of components both in blood and in hepatocytes. Blood entering the acinus consists of oxygen-depleted blood from the portal vein (60 to 70 percent of hepatic blood flow) plus oxygenated blood from the hepatic artery (30 to 40 percent). En route to the terminal hepatic venule, oxygen rapidly leaves the blood to meet the high metabolic demands of the parenchymal cells. Hepatocytes in zone 3 are exposed to substantially lower concentrations of oxygen than hepatocytes in zone 1. In comparison to other tissues, zone 3 is hypoxic. Well-documented acinar gradients exist for bile salts, bilirubin, and many organic anions.

Heterogeneities in protein levels of hepatocytes along the acinus generate gradients of metabolic functions. Hepatocytes in the mitochondria-rich zone 1 are predominant in fatty acid oxidation, gluconeogenesis, and ammonia detoxification to urea. Gradients of enzymes involved in the bioactivation and detoxification of xenobiotics have been observed along the

TABLE 13–1 **Major functions of liver and consequences of impaired hepatic functions.**

Type of Function	Examples	Consequences of Impaired Functions
Nutrient homeostasis	Glucose storage and synthesis Cholesterol uptake	Hypoglycemia, confusion Hypercholesterolemia
Filtration of particulates	Products of intestinal bacteria (e.g., endotoxin)	Endotoxemia
Protein synthesis	Clotting factors Albumin Transport proteins (e.g., very low-density lipoproteins)	Excess bleeding Hypoalbuminemia, ascites Fatty liver
Bioactivation and detoxification	Bilirubin and ammonia Steroid hormones Xenobiotics	Jaundice, hyperammonemia-related coma Loss of secondary male sex characteristics Diminished drug metabolism Inadequate detoxification
Formation of bile and biliary secretion	Bile acid-dependent uptake of dietary lipids and vitamins Bilirubin and cholesterol Metals (e.g., Cu and Mn) Xenobiotics	Fatty diarrhea, malnutrition, vitamin E deficiency Jaundice, gallstones, hypercholesterolemia Mn-induced neurotoxicity Delayed drug clearance

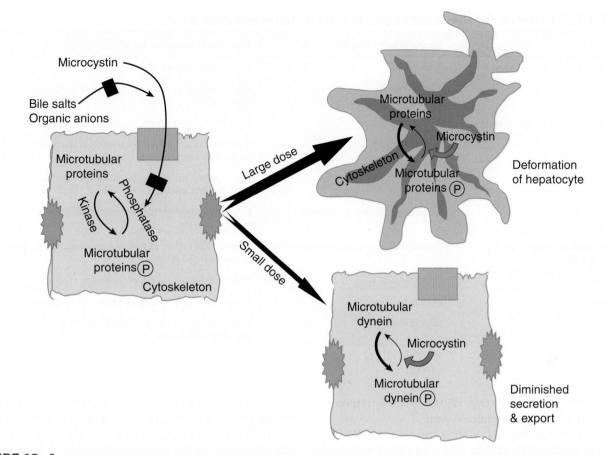

FIGURE 13–4 **Schematic of events in the mechanism by which microcystin damages the structural and functional integrity of hepatocytes.** Microcystin is taken up exclusively into hepatocytes by a sinusoidal transporter in a manner inhibitable by bile salts and organic anions. Then microcystin inhibition of protein phosphatases leads to hyperphosphorylation of cytoskeletal proteins whose dynamic functions are dependent on reversible phosphorylations. Extensive hyperphosphorylation of microtubular proteins leads to a collapse of the microtubular actin filament scaffold into a spiky aggregate that produces a gross deformation of hepatocytes. More subtle changes in microtubule-mediated transport activities have been linked to hyperphosphorylation of dynein, a cytoskeletal motor protein.

Fibrosis and Cirrhosis—Hepatic fibrosis (scarring) is characterized by the accumulation of extensive amounts of collagen fibers, in response to direct injury or to inflammation. With repeated chemical insults, destroyed hepatic cells are replaced by fibrotic scars. With continuing collagen deposition, the architecture of the liver is disrupted by interconnecting fibrous scars. When the fibrous scars subdivide the remaining liver mass into nodules of regenerating hepatocytes, fibrosis has progressed to cirrhosis and the liver has meager residual capacity to perform its essential functions. Cirrhosis is not reversible, has a poor prognosis for survival, and is usually the result of repeated exposure to chemical toxins.

Tumors—Chemically induced neoplasia can involve tumors that are derived from hepatocytes, bile duct cells, or the rare, highly malignant angiosarcomas derived from sinusoidal lining cells. Hepatocellular cancer has been linked to abuse of androgens and a high prevalence of aflatoxin-contaminated diets.

Thorotrast (radioactive thorium dioxide used as a contrast medium for radiology) accumulates in Kupffer cells, the resi-dent macrophage of the sinusoid, and emits radioactivity throughout its very extended half-life, thus increasing the risk for developing gallbladder cancer about 14-fold and over 100-fold for liver cancers. Multiple types of liver tumors are linked to thorium dioxide exposure.

Critical Factors in Toxicant-induced Liver Injury

Why is the liver the target site for so many chemicals of diverse structure? Why do many hepatotoxicants preferentially damage one type of liver cell? Our understanding of these fundamental questions is incomplete. Influences of several factors are of obvious importance (Table 13–3). Location and specialized processes for uptake and biliary secretion produce higher exposure levels in the liver than in other tissues of the body and strikingly high levels within certain types of liver cells. Then the abundant capacity for bioactivation reactions influences the rate of exposure to proximate toxicants. Subsequent events in

TABLE 13-3 **Factors in the site-specific injury of representative hepatotoxicants.**

Site	Representative Toxicants	Potential Explanation for Site Specificity
Zone 1 hepatocytes (versus zone 3)	Fe (overload)	Preferential uptake and high oxygen levels
	Allyl alcohol	Higher oxygen levels for oxygen-dependent bioactivation
Zone 3 hepatocytes (versus zone 1)	CCl$_4$	More P450 isozyme for bioactivation
	Acetaminophen	More P450 isozyme for bioactivation and less GSH for detoxification
	Ethanol	More hypoxic and greater imbalance in bioactivation/detoxification reactions
Bile duct cells	Methylene dianiline, sporidesmin	Exposure to the high concentration of reactive metabolites in bile
Sinusoidal endothelium (versus hepatocytes)	Cyclophosphamide, monocrotaline	Greater vulnerability to toxic metabolites and less ability to maintain glutathione levels
Kupffer cells	Endotoxin, GdCl$_3$	Preferential uptake and then activation
Stellate cells	Vitamin A	Preferential site for storage and then engorgement
	Ethanol (chronic)	Activation and transformation to collagen-synthesizing cell

the pathogenesis appear to be critically influenced by responses of sinusoidal cells and the immune system.

A number of experimental systems are useful for defining factors and mechanisms of liver injury. In vitro systems using the isolated perfused liver, isolated liver cells, and cell fractions allow observations at various levels of complexity without the confounding influences of other systems. Models using cocultures or agents that inactivate a given cell type can document the contributions and interactions between cell types. Whole-animal models are essential for assessment of the progression of injury and responses to chronic insult. Application of gene transfection or repression attenuates some of these interpretive problems. Knockout animals are extremely useful models for studying complex aspects of hepatotoxicity.

Uptake and Concentration—Lipophilic drugs and environmental pollutants readily diffuse into hepatocytes because the fenestrated epithelium of the sinusoid enables close contact between circulating molecules and hepatocytes. The membrane-rich liver concentrates lipophilic compounds. Other toxins are rapidly extracted from blood because they are substrates for sinusoidal transporters. Phalloidin (from a mushroom) and microcystin (from blue-green alga) are illustrative examples of hepatotoxins that target the liver as a consequence of extensive uptake into hepatocytes by sinusoidal transporters. Vitamin A hepatotoxicity initially affects the sinusoidal stellate cells, which actively extract and store this vitamin, and cadmium hepatotoxicity becomes manifest when cells exceed their capacity to complex cadmium with the metal-binding protein metallothionein.

Hepatocytes contribute to the homeostasis of iron by extracting this essential metal from the sinusoid by a receptor-

mediated process and maintaining a reserve of iron within the storage protein ferritin. Acute iron toxicity is most commonly observed in young children who accidently ingest iron tablets. The cytotoxicity of free iron is attributed to its function as an electron donor for the formation of reactive oxygen species, which initiate destructive oxidative stress reactions. Accumulation of excess iron beyond the capacity for its safe storage in ferritin leads to liver damage. Chronic hepatic accumulation of excess iron in cases of hemochromatosis is associated with a spectrum of hepatic disease including liver cancer.

Bioactivation and Detoxification—Hepatocytes have very high constitutive activities of the phase I enzymes that often convert xenobiotics to reactive electrophilic metabolites. Also, hepatocytes have a rich collection of phase II enzymes that add a polar group to a molecule and thereby enhance its removal from the body. Phase II reactions usually yield stable, nonreactive metabolites. In general, the balance between phase I and phase II reactions determines whether a reactive metabolite will initiate liver cell injury or be safely detoxified.

Acetaminophen—One of the most widely used analgesics, acetaminophen (APAP) is a safe drug when used at therapeutically recommended doses. Overdose can cause severe hepatotoxicity, and certain acquired factors (e.g., diet, drugs, diabetes, and obesity) can enhance hepatotoxicity. Typical therapeutic doses of acetaminophen are not hepatotoxic, because most of the acetaminophen gets glucuronidated or sulfated with little drug bioactivation. Injury after large doses of acetaminophen is enhanced by fasting and other conditions that deplete glutathione and is minimized

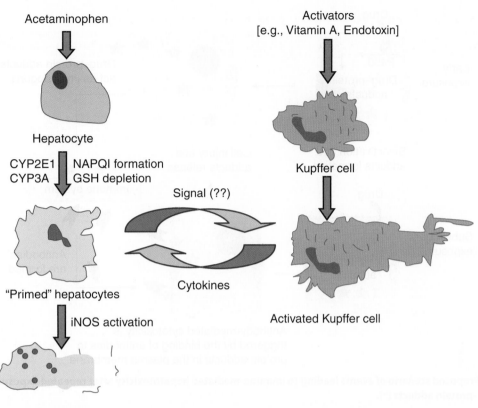

FIGURE 13–5 **Schematic of key events in the bioactivation and hepatotoxicity of acetaminophen.** Bioactivation of acetaminophen by cytochrome P450 isozymes leads to the formation of the reactive intermediate *N*-acetyl-*p*-benzoquinone (NAPQI), which can deplete glutathione or form covalent adducts with hepatic proteins. Experimental observations suggest that such effects "prime" hepatocytes for cytokines released by activated Kupffer cells. Progression to cell death is thought to involve activation of iNOS and other processes that produce reactive nitrogen species and oxidative stress. Agents that activate Kupffer cells exacerbate the toxicity. Exchange of signals between toxicant-primed and activated Kupffer cells is likely a factor in the acute hepatotoxicity produced by many compounds that damage hepatocytes.

by treatments with *N*-acetylcysteine that enhance hepatocyte synthesis of glutathione.

Alcoholics are vulnerable to the hepatotoxic effects of acetaminophen at dosages within the high therapeutic range. This acquired enhancement has widely been attributed to accelerated bioactivation of acetaminophen to the electrophilic *N*-acetyl-*p*-benzoquinone imine (NAPQI) intermediate by ethanol induction of CYP2E1 (Figure 13–5). Inducers of CYP3A including many drugs and dietary chemicals potentially influence acetaminophen toxicity.

An attractive "two hit" type of theory for the hepatotoxicity of acetaminophen suggests that adduction by a reactive drug metabolite "primes" the hepatocytes for destructive insults by reactive nitrogen species (e.g., peroxynitrite) (Figure 13–5).

Ethanol—Genetic conditions of high clinical relevance to the bioactivation/detoxification balance are the polymorphisms in the enzymes that control the two-step metabolism of ethanol. Specifically, ethanol is bioactivated by alcohol dehydrogenase to acetaldehyde, a reactive aldehyde, which is subsequently detoxified to acetate by aldehyde dehydroge-nase. Both enzymes exhibit genetic polymorphisms that result in higher concentrations of acetaldehyde—a "fast" activity isozyme of alcohol dehydrogenase [ALD2*2] and a physiologically very "slow" mitochondrial isozyme of aldehyde dehydrogenase [ALDH2*2]. Approximately 50 percent of Asian populations but virtually no Caucasians have the slow aldehyde dehydrogenase; alcohol consumption by people with this slow polymorphism leads to uncomfortable symptoms of flushing and nausea due to high systemic levels of acetaldehyde.

Cytochrome P450—Cytochrome P450-dependent bioactivation as a mechanism of hepatotoxicity is important even for assumedly *safe* compounds because some P450 isozymes generate reactive oxygen species during biotransformation reactions, which can lead to liver damage. CYP2E1 generation of reactive oxygen species and other free radicals contributes to the etiology of serious, end-stage liver damage.

Besides CYP2E1, the CYP3A isozyme has been linked to the hepatotoxicity caused by the folk medicine plant germander (*Teucrium chamaedrys* L.). Systematic experimental studies

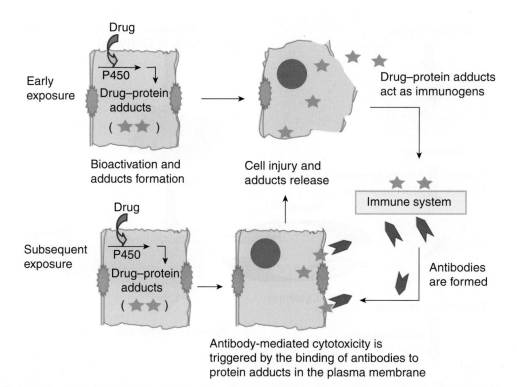

FIGURE 13-6 Proposed scenario of events leading to immune-mediated hepatotoxicity after repeated exposure to a toxicant that produces drug–protein adducts (*).

demonstrated a predominant role for the CYP3A bioactivation of germander constituents to reactive electrophiles.

***Carbon Tetrachloride*—**Cytochrome P450-dependent conversion of CCl_4 to $\bullet CCl_3$ and then to $CCl_3OO\bullet$ is the classic example of xenobiotic bioactivation to a free radical that initiates oxidative damage. Conditions in which cytochrome P450 is depleted lead to decreased liver damage when exposed to CCl_4.

Regeneration—The liver has a high capacity to restore lost tissue and function by regeneration. Loss of hepatocytes due to hepatectomy or cell injury triggers proliferation of all mature liver cells. This process is capable of restoring the original liver mass. However, regeneration is not just a response to cell death, but a process that actively determines the final injury after exposure to hepatotoxic chemicals. Stimulation of repair by exposure to a moderate dose of a hepatotoxicant strongly attenuates tissue damage of a subsequent high dose of the same chemical. Tissue repair follows a dose–response up to a threshold where the injury is too severe and cell proliferation is inhibited.

Inflammation and Immune Responses—Migration of neutrophils, lymphocytes, and other inflammatory cells into regions of damaged liver is a well-recognized feature of the hepatotoxicity produced by many chemicals. In fact, the potentially confusing term *hepatitis* refers to hepatocyte damage by any insult where hepatocyte death is associated with an influx of inflammatory cells.

The influx of inflammatory cells usually facilitates beneficial removal of debris from damaged liver cells. However, detrimental effects are plausible, because activated neutrophils release cytotoxic proteases and reactive oxygen species.

Immune responses are considered factors in the hepatotoxicity occasionally observed after repeated exposure to chemicals, usually drugs. Individuals who develop infrequent, unpredictable responses are considered to be hypersensitive. An immune-mediated response is considered plausible when the problem subsides after therapy is halted and then recurs on drug challenge or restoration of therapy. Although the concept is generally accepted, compelling evidence for immune-mediated responses is available only for ethanol, halothane, and a few other hepatotoxicants. Figure 13–6 depicts key features of the assumed scenario whereby hepatic protein adducts could become antigenic and stimulate the production of antibodies. If on reexposure, more drug–protein adducts are formed, cells with such adducts could be attacked by systemic antibodies.

Apparent immune-mediated injury has been observed in individuals taking the antiarthritic NSAID diclofenac. Hepatic bioactivation of diclofenac leads to the formation of multiple adducts, which may localize to hepatocyte membrane proteins where recognition by antibodies is feasible.

Activation of Sinusoidal Cells—Four kinds of observations, collectively, indicate roles for sinusoidal cell (immune cells present in the liver sinusoids) activation as primary or secondary factors in toxin-induced injury to the liver:

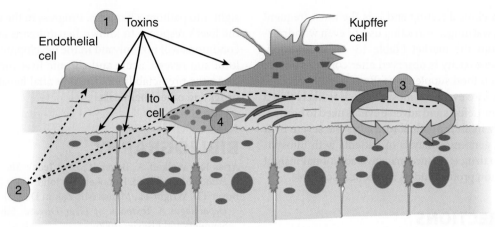

FIGURE 13–7 **Schematic depicting the complex cascade of toxin-evoked interactions between hepatocytes and sinusoidal cells.** Sinusoidal cell responses to toxins can lead to either injury or activation. A scenario could involve (1) toxin injury to hepatocytes, (2) signals from the injured hepatocyte to Kupffer and Ito cells, followed by (3) Kupffer cell release of cytotoxins, and (4) Ito cell secretion of collagen. Activation of Kupffer cells is an important factor in the progression of injury evoked by many toxicants. Stimulation of collagen production by activated Ito cells is a proposed mechanism for toxicant-induced fibrosis.

1. Kupffer and Ito cells exhibit an activated morphology after acute and chronic exposure to hepatotoxicants.
2. Pretreatments that activate or inactivate Kupffer cells appropriately modulate the extent of damage produced by classic toxicants. Kupffer cell activation by vitamin A profoundly enhances the acute toxicity of carbon tetrachloride; this enhancement did not occur when animals were also given an inactivator of Kupffer cells.
3. Activated Kupffer cells secrete appreciable amounts of soluble cytotoxins, including reactive oxygen and nitrogen species.
4. Acute and chronic exposure to alcohol directly or indirectly affects sinusoidal cells.

Figure 13–7 summarizes information presented in this and earlier sections of this chapter about the multiplicity of toxin-induced interactions with and between various liver cells. The effect on a given cell type can be direct or may result from a cascade of signals and responses between cell types.

Mitochondrial Damage—Mitochondrial DNA codes for several proteins in the mitochondrial electron transport chain. Nucleoside analog drugs for the therapy of hepatitis B and AIDS infections cause mitochondrial DNA damage directly, when incorporation of the analog base leads to miscoding or early termination of polypeptides. The severe hepatic mitochondrial injury produced by the nucleoside analog fialuridine is attributed to its higher affinity for the polymerase responsible for mitochondrial DNA synthesis than for the polymerases responsible for nuclear DNA synthesis. Mitochondrial DNA is also more vulnerable to miscoding (mutation) due to its limited capacity for repair.

Alcohol abuse causes mitochondrial injury by shifting the bioactivation/detoxification balance for ethanol, leading to an accumulation of its reactive acetaldehyde metabolite within mitochondria, because mitochondrial aldehyde dehydroge-nase is the major enzymatic process for detoxification of acet-aldehyde. Bioactivation of large amounts of ethanol by alcohol dehydrogenase hampers the detoxification reaction, since the two enzymes require the common, depletable cofactor nicotinamide adenine dinucleotide (NAD). Any type of ethanol-induced change that enhances the leakiness of the mitochondrial transport chain would lead to an increased release of reactive oxygen species capable of attacking nearby mitochondrial constituents.

Idiosyncratic Liver Injury—Idiosyncratic drug hepatotoxicity is a rare but potentially serious adverse event, which is not clearly dose-dependent, is at this point unpredictable, and affects only very few of the patients exposed to a drug or other chemicals. However, idiosyncratic toxicity is a leading cause for

TABLE 13–4 **Examples of drugs with known idiosyncratic hepatotoxicity.**

A. Immune-mediated (allergic) idiosyncratic hepatotoxicity
• Diclofenac (analgesic)
• Halothane (anesthetic)
• Nitrofurantoin (antibiotic)
• Phenytoin (anticonvulsant)
• Tienilic acid (diuretic)
B. Nonimmune-mediated (non-allergic) idiosyncratic hepatotoxicity
• Amiodarone (antiarrhythmic)
• Bromfenac (analgesic)—withdrawn from market
• Diclofenac (analgesic)
• Disulfiram (alcoholism)
• Isoniazid (antituberculosis)
• Ketoconazole (antifungal)
• Rifampicin (antimicrobial)
• Troglitazone (antidiabetes)—withdrawn from market
• Valproate (anticonvulsant)

failure of drugs in clinical testing and it is the most frequent reason for posting warnings, restricting use, or even withdrawal of the drug from the market (Table 13–4). In addition, idiosyncratic hepatotoxicity is observed after consumption of herbal remedies and food supplements. Because idiosyncratic hepatotoxicity is a rare event for most drugs, it is likely that a combination of gene defects and adverse events need to be present simultaneously in an individual to trigger the severe liver injury. A detailed genomic analysis of patients with idiosyncratic responses to drug exposure may give additional insight what gene expression profile renders a patient susceptible.

FUTURE DIRECTIONS

Continued progress in the understanding of drug- and chemical-induced hepatotoxicity will depend on the use of relevant in vivo and in vitro models including human hepatocytes and analysis of human liver tissue. Traditional mechanistic investigations in combination with genomic and proteomic approaches have the greatest potential to yield important new in-

sight into pathomechanisms. Progress in the understanding of the liver's response to known hepatotoxins and other adverse conditions will not only aid in the development of therapies to limit and reverse acute and chronic liver injury, but also improve the predictability of the potential hepatotoxicity of new drugs and other chemicals.

BIBLIOGRAPHY

Arias IM, Wolkoff A, Boyer JL, et al (eds): *The Liver: Biology and Pathobiology*, 5th ed. Hoboken, NJ: John Wiley, 2009.

Boyer TD, Wright TL, Manns MP, Zakim D (eds): *Zakim and Boyer's Hepatology: A Textbook of Liver Disease*, 5th ed. Philadelphia: Saunders and Elsevier, 2006.

Crawford JM: *The Liver and the Biliary Tract*. In Kumar V, Abbas AK, Fausto N, Aster JC (eds): *Robbins and Cotran: Pathologic Basis of Disease*, 8th ed. Philadelphia: Saunders, 2010.

Kaplowitz N, Deleve LD: *Drug-induced Liver Disease*. New York: Marcel Dekker, 2003.

Sahu S: *Hepatotoxicity: from Genomics to In Vitro and In Vivo Models*. Hoboken, NJ: John Wiley, 2008.

QUESTIONS

1. The impairment of hepatic function can have numerous negative consequences. Which of the following is likely NOT caused by impaired hepatic function?
   a. jaundice.
   b. hypercholesterolemia.
   c. hyperammonemia.
   d. hyperglycemia.
   e. hypoalbuminemia.

2. All of the following statements regarding the liver are true EXCEPT:
   a. The major role of the liver is to maintain metabolic homeostasis of the body.
   b. The liver encounters ingested nutrients before the heart does.
   c. Hepatic triads contain a branch of the hepatic portal vein, a branch of the hepatic artery, and a bile ductile.
   d. The liver manufactures and stores bile.
   e. The large fenestrae of hepatic sinusoids facilitate exchange of materials between the sinusoid and the hepatocyte.

3. Activation of which of the following cell types can result in increased secretion of collagen scar tissue, leading to cirrhosis?
   a. hepatocyte.
   b. Ito cell.
   c. Kupffer cell.
   d. endothelial cell.
   e. β-cell.

4. Wilson's disease is a rare genetic disorder characterized by the failure to export which of the following metals into bile?
   a. iron.
   b. zinc.
   c. silver.
   d. lead.
   e. copper.

5. Which of the following is NOT characteristic of apoptosis?
   a. cell swelling.
   b. nuclear fragmentation.
   c. lack of inflammation.
   d. programmed death.
   e. chromatin condensation.

6. A patient suffering from canalicular cholestasis would NOT be expected to exhibit which of the following?
   a. increased bile salt serum levels.
   b. jaundice.
   c. increased bile formation.
   d. dark brown urine.
   e. vitamin A deficiency.

7. Which of the following statements regarding liver injury is FALSE?
   a. Large doses of acetaminophen have been shown to cause a blockade of hepatic sinusoids.
   b. Hydrophilic drugs readily diffuse into hepatocytes because of the large sinusoidal fenestrations.
   c. There are sinusoidal transporters that take toxins up into hepatocytes.
   d. Hepatocellular cancer has been associated with androgen abuse.
   e. In cirrhosis, excess collagen is laid down in response to direct injury or inflammation.

8. The inheritance of a "slow" aldehyde dehydrogenase enzyme would result in which of the following after the ingestion of ethanol?
   a. high ethanol tolerance.
   b. little response to low doses of ethanol.
   c. low serum levels of acetaldehyde.
   d. nausea.
   e. increased levels of blood ethanol compared to an individual with a normal aldehyde dehydrogenase.

9. Which of the following is not a common mechanism of hepatocellular injury?
   a. deformation of the hepatocyte cytoskeleton.
   b. mitochondrial injury.
   c. cholestasis.
   d. interference with vesicular transport.
   e. increased transcytosis between hepatocytes.

10. Ethanol is not known to cause which of the following types of hepatobiliary injury?
    a. fatty liver.
    b. hepatocyte death.
    c. fibrosis.
    d. immune-mediated responses.
    e. canalicular cholestasis.

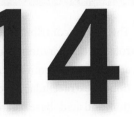

Toxic Responses
of the Kidney

Rick G. Schnellmann

The functional integrity of the mammalian kidney is vital to total body homeostasis, because of its role in the excretion of metabolic wastes, synthesis and release of the hormones renin and erythropoietin, and the regulation of extracellular fluid volume, electrolyte composition, and acid–base balance.

FUNCTIONAL ANATOMY

Gross examination of a sagittal section of the kidney reveals three clearly demarcated anatomical areas: the cortex, medulla, and papilla (Figure 14–1). The cortex receives about 90 percent of blood flow compared with the medulla (~6 to 10 percent) or papilla (1 to 2 percent). Thus, when a blood-born toxicant is delivered to the kidney, a high percentage of the material will be delivered to the cortex and will have a greater opportunity to influence cortical rather than medullary or papillary functions. The functional unit of the kidney, the nephron, may be considered in three portions: the vascular element, the glomerulus, and the tubular element.

Renal Vasculature and Glomerulus

The renal artery branches into afferent arterioles that supply the glomerulus (Figure 14–1). Blood then leaves the glomerular capillaries via the efferent arterioles. Both the afferent and efferent arterioles control glomerular capillary pressure and glomerular plasma flow rate. These arterioles are innervated by the sympathetic nervous system and respond to nerve stimulation, angiotensin II, vasopressin, endothelin, adenosine, and norepinephrine. The efferent arterioles draining the cortical glomeruli branch into a peritubular capillary network, whereas those draining the juxtamedullary glomeruli form a capillary loop, the vasa recta, supplying the medullary structures. These postglomerular capillary loops provide the delivery of nutrients to the postglomerular tubular structures, delivery of wastes to the tubule for excretion, and return of reabsorbed electrolytes, nutrients, and water to the systemic circulation.

The glomerulus is a complex, specialized capillary bed that filters a portion of the blood into an ultrafiltrate that passes into the tubular portion of the nephron. The formation of such an ultrafiltrate is the net result of the balance between transcapillary hydrostatic pressure and colloid oncotic pressure. An additional determinant of ultrafiltration is the effective hydraulic

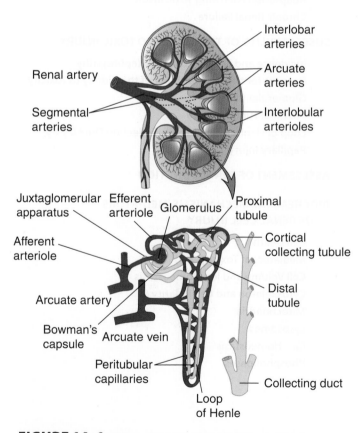

FIGURE 14–1 Schematic of the human kidney showing the major blood vessels and the microcirculation and tubular components of each nephron. (From Guyton AC, Hall JE (11th ed.): *Textbook of Medical Physiology*. Philadelphia: Saunders, 2006, p. 318, with permission from Elsevier.)

permeability of the glomerular capillary wall, in other words, the ultrafiltration coefficient (K_f), which is determined by the total surface area available for filtration and the hydraulic permeability of the capillary wall.

Although the glomerular capillary wall permits a high rate of fluid filtration, it provides a significant barrier to the transglomerular passage of macromolecules; thus, small molecules, such as inulin (MW 5500), are freely filtered, whereas large molecules, such as albumin (MW 56,000 to 70,000), are restricted. Filtration of anionic molecules tends to be restricted compared with that of neutral or cationic molecules of the same size.

Proximal Tubule

The proximal tubule consists of three discrete segments: the S_1 (pars convoluta), S_2 (transition between pars convoluta and pars recta), and S_3 (pars recta) segments. The volume and composition of the glomerular filtrate is progressively altered as fluid passes through each of the different tubular segments. The proximal tubule reabsorbs approximately 60 to 80 percent of solute and water filtered at the glomerulus mostly by numerous transport systems capable of driving concentrative transport of many metabolic substrates. The proximal tubule also reabsorbs virtually all of the filtered low-molecular-weight proteins by specific endocytotic protein reabsorption processes.

Loop of Henle

Approximately 25 percent of the filtered Na^+ and K^+ and 20 percent of the filtered water are reabsorbed by the segments of the loop of Henle. The tubular fluid entering the thin descending limb is iso-osmotic to the renal interstitium; water is freely permeable and solutes, such as electrolytes and urea, may enter from the interstitium. In contrast, the thin ascending limb is relatively impermeable to water and urea, and Na^+ and Cl^- are reabsorbed by passive diffusion. The thick ascending limb is impermeable to water, and electrolytes are reabsorbed by the active $Na^+/K^+/2Cl^-$ cotransport mechanism, with the energy provided by the Na^+,K^+-ATPase.

Distal Tubule and Collecting Duct

The macula densa comprises specialized cells located between the end of the thick ascending limb and the early distal tubule, in close proximity to the afferent arteriole. Under normal physiologic conditions, increased solute delivery or concentration at the macula densa triggers a signal resulting in afferent arteriolar constriction leading to decreases in glomerular filtration rate (GFR) (and hence decreased solute delivery). This regulatory mechanism is a volume-conserving mechanism, designed to decrease GFR and prevent massive losses of fluid/electrolytes due to impaired tubular reabsorption. The renin–angiotensin system and other substances may be involved. The early distal tubule reabsorbs most of the remaining intraluminal Na^+, K^+, and Cl^- but is relatively impermeable to water.

The late distal tubule, cortical collecting tubule, and medullary collecting duct perform the final regulation and fine tuning of urinary volume and composition. The remaining Na^+ is reabsorbed in conjunction with K^+ and H^+ secretion in the late distal tubule and cortical collecting tubule. The combination of medullary and papillary hypertonicity generated by countercurrent multiplication and the action of antidiuretic hormone (vasopressin, ADH) serves to enhance water permeability of the medullary collecting duct.

PATHOPHYSIOLOGIC RESPONSES OF THE KIDNEY

Acute Kidney Injury

One of the most common manifestations of nephrotoxic damage is acute renal failure (ARF), characterized by an abrupt decline in GFR with resulting azotemia, or a buildup of nitrogenous wastes in the blood. Acute kidney injury (AKI) describes the entire spectrum of the disease and is defined as a complex disorder that comprises multiple causative factors with clinical manifestations ranging from minimal elevation in serum creatinine to anuric renal failure. Figure 14–2 illustrates the pathways that lead to diminished GFR following chemical exposure. Table 14–1 provides a partial list of chemicals that produce ARF through different mechanisms.

The maintenance of tubular integrity is dependent on cell-to-cell and cell-to-matrix adhesion (Figure 14–3). It has been hypothesized that after a chemical or hypoxic insult, adhesion of nonlethally damaged, apoptotic, and oncotic cells to the basement membrane is compromised, leading to gaps in the epithelial cell lining, potentially resulting in back-leak of filtrate and diminished GFR. These detached cells may aggregate in the tubular lumen (cell-to-cell adhesion) and/or adhere or reattach to adherent epithelial cells downstream, resulting in tubular obstruction.

Increasing evidence supports the idea that inflammatory cells play a role in ischemia-induced AKI. Injury to the renal vasculature endothelium results in chemokine and proinflammatory cytokine production and neutrophil adhesion, but the specific role of each inflammatory cell remains to be elucidated.

Adaptation Following Toxic Insult

The kidney has a remarkable ability to compensate for a loss in renal functional mass. Following a unilateral nephrectomy, GFR of the remnant kidney increases by approximately 40 to 60 percent. Compensatory increases in single-nephron GFR are accompanied by proportionate increases in proximal tubular water and solute reabsorption; glomerulotubular balance is therefore maintained and overall renal function appears normal by standard clinical tests. Consequently, chemically induced changes in renal function may not be detected until these compensatory mechanisms are overwhelmed by significant nephron loss and/or damage.

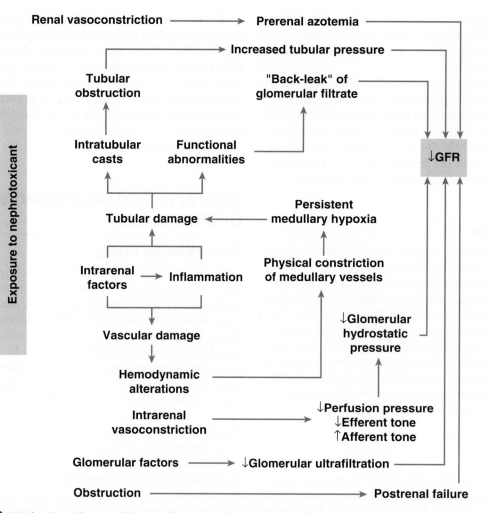

FIGURE 14–2 **Mechanisms that contribute to decreased GFR in acute renal failure.** After exposure to a nephrotoxicant, one or more mechanisms may contribute to a reduction in the GFR. These include renal vasoconstriction resulting in prerenal azotemia and obstruction due to precipitation of a drug or endogenous compound within the kidney. Intrarenal factors include direct tubular obstruction and dysfunction, resulting in tubular back-leak and increased tubular pressure. Alterations in the levels of a variety of vasoactive mediators may result in decreased renal perfusion pressure or efferent arteriolar tone and increased afferent arteriolar tone, leading to decreased glomerular hydrostatic pressure. (Modified from Schnellmann RG, Kelly KJ: *Pathophysiology of Nephrotoxic Acute Renal Failure*. In Schrier RW: *Atlas of Diseases of the Kidney*. Philadelphia: Current Medicine, 1999, p. 15.4, with permission.)

TABLE 14–1 **Mechanisms of chemically induced acute renal failure.**

Prerenal	Vasoconstriction	Crystalluria	Tubular Toxicity	Endothelial Injury	Glomerulopathy	Interstitial Nephritis
Diuretics	Nonsteroidal anti-inflammatory drugs	Sulfonamides	Aminoglycosides	Cyclosporine	Gold	Antibiotics
Angiotensin receptor antagonists	Radiocontrast agents	Methotrexate	Cisplatin	Mitomycin C	Penicillamine	Nonsteroidal anti-inflammatory drugs
Angiotensin converting enzyme inhibitors	Cyclosporine	Acyclovir	Vancomycin	Tacrolimus	Nonsteroidal anti-inflammatory drugs	Diuretics
Antihypertensive agents	Tacrolimus	Triamterene	Pentamidine	Cocaine	drugs	
	Amphotericin B	Ethylene glycol	Radiocontrast agents	Conjugated estrogens		
		Protease inhibitors	Heavy metals	Quinine		
			Haloalkane- and Haloalkene–cysteine conjugates			

endothelial cells. Other enzymes found in lung tissue include epoxide hydrolases, flavin monooxygenases, prostaglandin synthases, glucuronosyltransferases, sulfotransferases, and glutathione S-transferases.

GENERAL PRINCIPLES IN THE PATHOGENESIS OF LUNG DAMAGE CAUSED BY CHEMICALS

Toxic Inhalants, Gases, and Dosimetry

The sites of deposition of toxicants in the respiratory tract define the pattern of their toxicity. Water solubility is the critical factor in determining how deeply a given gas penetrates into the lung. Highly soluble gases such as SO_2 do not penetrate farther than the nose and are therefore relatively nontoxic to animals. Relatively insoluble gases such as ozone and NO_2 penetrate deeply into the lung and reach the smallest airways and the alveoli, where they can elicit toxic responses. Very insoluble gases such as CO and H_2S efficiently pass through the respiratory tract and are taken up by the pulmonary blood supply to be distributed throughout the body.

Particle Deposition and Clearance

Particle size is usually the critical factor that determines the region of the respiratory tract in which a particle or an aerosol will be deposited.

Particle Size

Larger particles are usually distributed to the upper air passages, and smaller particles are transported all the way to the alveoli (Figure 15–4). Patterns of breathing can change the site of deposition of a particle of a given size. Particle shape and density may also play a role in distribution. Inhaled aerosols are most frequently polydisperse in regard to size.

Nanotoxicology

Nanoparticles (diameter <100 nm) are now being used in manufactured products, increasingly released into the environment, and exposed to individuals in great quantities. The toxicologic concerns of nanoparticles reflect three major issues: (1) the enormous surface area relative to mass, with regard to the adsorption of copollutants and the presence of reactive metals on their surface, (2) the possibility that commercially produced nanotubes may be more toxic than spherical nanoparticles, and (3) the concern of whether or not host defenses are effective against particles this small.

Deposition Mechanisms

Deposition of particles occurs primarily by interception, impaction, sedimentation, and diffusion (Brownian movement). Interception occurs when the trajectory of a particle brings it

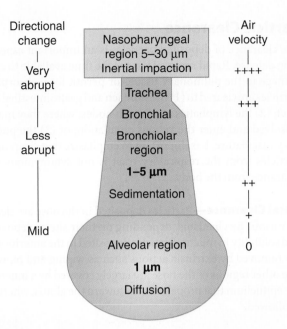

FIGURE 15–4 **Parameters influencing particle deposition.** (From Casarett LJ: *The Vital Sacs: Alveolar Clearance Mechanisms in Inhalation Toxicology*. Volume 3 in Blood FR (ed): *Essays in Toxicology*. New York: Academic Press, 1972, with permission.)

near enough to a surface so that the particle contacts the airway surface. As a result of inertia, particles suspended in air tend to continue to travel along their original path. In a bending airstream, such as at an airway bifurcation, a particle may be impacted on the surface.

Sedimentation brings about deposition in the smaller bronchi, the bronchioles, and the alveolar spaces. As a particle moves downward through air, buoyancy and the resistance of air act on the particle in an upward direction while gravitational force acts on the particle in a downward direction. Eventually, the gravitational force equilibrates with the sum of the buoyancy and the air resistance, and the particle will settle with a constant velocity known as the terminal settling velocity.

Diffusion is important in the deposition of submicrometer particles. A random motion is imparted to these particles by the impact of gas molecules.

An important factor in particle deposition is the pattern of breathing. During quiet breathing, a large proportion of the inhaled particles may be exhaled. During exercise, when larger volumes are inhaled at higher velocities, deposition in airways increases. Breath holding also increases deposition. Factors that modify the diameter of the conducting airways can alter particle deposition. In patients with chronic bronchitis, the mucous layer is greatly thickened and extended peripherally and may partially block the airways in some areas. Jets formed by air flowing through such partially occluded airways have the potential to increase the deposition of particles.

Particle Clearance

The clearance of deposited particles is an important aspect of lung defense. Rapid removal lessens the time available to cause damage to the pulmonary tissues or permit local absorption. Particles are cleared to (1) the stomach and gastrointestinal (GI) tract; (2) the lymphatics and lymph nodes, where they may be dissolved and enter the venous circulation; or (3) the pulmonary vasculature. It is important to emphasize that clearance of particles from the respiratory tract is not synonymous with clearance from the body.

Nasal Clearance—Particles deposited in the nose are cleared by various mechanisms, depending on their site of deposition and solubility in mucus. Particles deposited in the anterior nose are removed by extrinsic actions such as wiping and blowing. The other regions of the nose are largely covered by a mucociliary epithelium that propels mucus toward the glottis, where it is swallowed.

Tracheobronchial Clearance—The mucous layer covering the tracheobronchial tree is moved upward by the beating of the underlying cilia. This mucociliary escalator transports deposited particles and particle-laden macrophages to the oropharynx, where they are swallowed and pass through the GI tract.

Pulmonary Clearance—There are several primary ways by which particulate material is removed from the lower respiratory tract once it has been deposited:

1. Particles may be directly trapped on the lining layer of the conducting airways by impaction and cleared upward, in the tracheobronchial tree via the mucociliary escalator.
2. Particles may be phagocytized by macrophages and cleared via the mucociliary escalator.
3. Particles may be phagocytized by alveolar macrophages and removed via the lymphatic drainage.
4. Materials may dissolve from the surfaces of particles and be removed via the bloodstream or lymphatics.
5. Small particles may directly penetrate epithelial membranes.
6. Insoluble particles, especially long narrow fibers, may be sequestered in the lung for very long periods, often in macrophages located in the interstitium.

ACUTE RESPONSES OF THE LUNG TO INJURY

Mechanisms of Respiratory Tract Injury

Airborne agents can contact cells lining the respiratory tract from the nostrils to the gas-exchanging region. Certain gases and vapors stimulate nerve endings in the nose, particularly those of the trigeminal nerve. The result is holding of the breath or changes in breathing patterns, to avoid or reduce further exposure. If continued exposure cannot be avoided, many acidic or alkaline irritants produce cell necrosis and increased permeability of the alveolar walls. Other inhaled agents can be more insidious; inhalation of high concentrations of HCl, NO_2, NH_3, or phosgene may at first produce very little apparent damage in the respiratory tract. The epithelial barrier in the alveolar zone, after a latency period of several hours, begins to leak, flooding the alveoli and producing a delayed pulmonary edema that is often fatal.

A different pathogenetic mechanism is typical of highly reactive molecules such as ozone. It is unlikely that ozone as such can penetrate beyond the layer of fluid covering the cells of the lung. Instead, ozone lesions are propagated by a cascade of secondary reaction products and by reactive oxygen species arising from free radical reactions.

Metabolism of foreign compounds can be involved in the pathogenesis of lung injury. The lung contains most of the enzymes involved in xenobiotic metabolism that have been identified in other tissues. Microsomal enzymes identified in lung include cytochrome P450s 1A1, 2B1, 2F1, 4B1, and 3A4, as well as NADPH cytochrome P450 reductase, epoxide hydrolase, and flavin-containing monooxygenases. Two important cytosolic enzymes involved in lung xenobiotic metabolism are glutathione S-transferases and glutathione peroxidase.

Oxidative Burden

An undue oxidative burden that often is mediated by free radicals, such as those generated by ozone, NO_2, tobacco smoke, and lung defense cells, contributes to lung damage. Because these oxidant species are potentially cytotoxic, they may mediate or promote the actions of pneumotoxicants such as paraquat and nitrofurantoin. When cellular injury of any type occurs, the release of otherwise contained cellular constituents such as microsomes and flavoproteins into the extracellular space may lead to extracellular generation of deleterious reactive O_2 species.

Neutrophils, monocytes, and macrophages seem particularly adept at converting molecular O_2 to reactive O_2 metabolites; this probably is related to their phagocytosis and antimicrobial activities. As a by-product of this capability, toxic O_2 species are released into surrounding tissues. As most forms of toxic pulmonary edema are accompanied by phagocyte accumulation in the lung microcirculation (pulmonary leukostasis) and parenchyma, oxidative damage may represent a significant component of pneumotoxic lung injury.

Phagocytic production of active oxygen species causes inactivation of proteinase inhibitors and degranulation of mast cells.

The lung can respond with specific defense mechanisms that may be stimulated by constant exposure to airborne microorganisms as well as to low- and high-molecular-weight antigenic materials. The immune system can mount either cellular or humorally mediated responses to these inhaled antigens. Direct immunologic effects occur when inhaled foreign material sensitizes the respiratory system to further exposure to the same material. Bronchoconstriction and chronic pulmonary disease can result from the inhalation of materials that appear to act wholly or partly through an allergic response.

Airway Reactivity

Large airways are surrounded by bronchial smooth muscles, which help maintain airway tone and diameter during expansion and contraction of the lung. Bronchial smooth muscle tone is normally regulated by the autonomic nervous system. Bronchoconstriction can be provoked by cigarette smoke and air pollutants and by cholinergic drugs such as acetylcholine, histamine, various prostaglandins and leukotrienes, substance P, and nitric oxide. Bronchoconstriction causes a decrease in airway diameter and a corresponding increase in resistance to airflow. Characteristic associated symptoms include wheezing, coughing, a sensation of chest tightness, and dyspnea. Exercise potentiates these problems. Because the major component of airway resistance usually is contributed by large bronchi, inhaled chemicals that cause reflex bronchoconstriction are generally irritant gases with moderate solubility.

Pulmonary Edema

Toxic pulmonary edema represents an acute, exudative phase of lung injury that alters ventilation–perfusion relationships and limits diffusive transfer of O_2 and CO_2 even in otherwise structurally normal alveoli.

Cell Proliferation

The effects of toxicants on the lung may be reversible or irreversible. The normal adult lung is an organ for which under normal circumstances very few cells appear to die and need to be replaced. When damaged by a toxic insult, the lung parenchyma is capable of repairing itself. Type I cell damage is followed by proliferation of type II epithelial cells that eventually transform into new type I cells; in the airways, the Clara cells proliferate and divide following injury. The migration of mobile blood cells such as leukocytes across the pulmonary capillaries into the alveolar lumen may also trigger a mitotic response. Other cells in the alveolar zone, such as capillary endothelial cells, interstitial cells, and alveolar macrophages, also proliferate. The result is a normal-looking organ, although excessive proliferation of fibroblasts may result in lung disease. In general, the lung appears to have a high capacity to repair itself and thus to deal with the many toxic insults presented by the environment.

CHRONIC RESPONSES OF THE LUNG TO INJURY

Emphysema

In emphysema, the lungs become larger and too compliant, caused by destruction of the walls without fibrosis. Destruction of the gas-exchanging surface area results in a distended, hyperinflated lung that no longer effectively exchanges oxygen and carbon dioxide as a result of both loss of tissue and air trapping (Figure 15–5). The major cause of human emphysema is, by far, cigarette smoke inhalation, although other toxicants also can

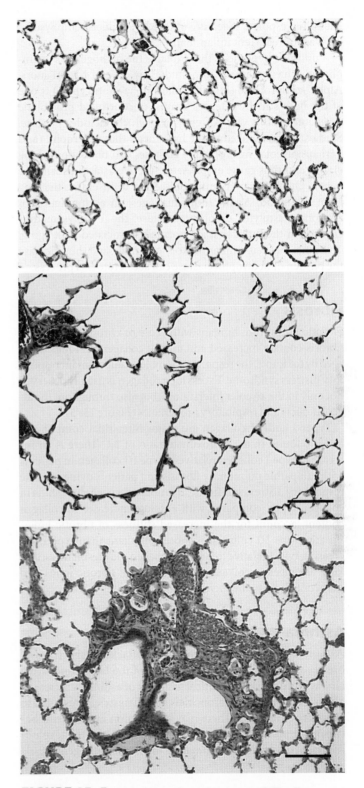

FIGURE 15–5 Rat models of emphysema and fibrosis. *Top panel.* Light micrograph of a normal rat lung. *Middle panel.* Lung of a spontaneously hypertensive (SH) rat 12 weeks after inhalation of tobacco smoke at a concentration of 90 mg/m³ of total suspended particulate material. Note extensive distension of alveoli (emphysema). *Bottom panel.* Lung of a rat 1 year after exposure (8 h/day, 5 days a week for 12 months) to chrysotile asbestos. Note accumulation of connective tissue around blood vessel and airways (fibrosis). Bar length: 100 μm. (Photograph courtesy of Dr. Kent E. Pinkerton, University of California, Davis.)

elicit this response. A feature of toxicant-induced emphysema is severe or recurrent inflammation.

A unifying hypothesis that explains the pathogenesis of emphysema has emerged from studies by several investigators. Alpha$_1$-antiprotease (initially called alpha$_1$-antitrypsin) is one of the body's main defenses against uncontrolled proteolytic digestion by this class of enzymes, which includes elastase. Studies in smokers led to the hypothesis that neutrophil (and perhaps alveolar macrophage) elastases can break down lung elastin and thus cause emphysema; these elastases usually are kept in check by alpha$_1$-antiprotease that diffuses into the lung from the blood. As the individual ages, an accumulation of random elastolytic events can cause the emphysematous changes in the lungs that are normally associated with aging. Toxicants that cause inflammatory cell influx and thus increase the burden of neutrophil elastase can accelerate this process.

Fibrosis

Fibrotic lungs from humans with acute or chronic pulmonary fibrosis contain increased amounts of collagen. In lungs damaged by toxicants, the response resembles adult or infant respiratory distress syndrome. Excess lung collagen is usually observed not only in the alveolar interstitium, but also throughout the alveolar ducts and respiratory bronchioles (Figure 15–5).

Types I and III collagen are major interstitial components and are found in an approximate ratio of 2:1. There is an increase in type I collagen relative to type III collagen in patients with idiopathic pulmonary fibrosis and patients dying of acute respiratory distress syndrome. It is not known whether shifts in collagen types, compared with absolute increases in collagen content, account for the increased stiffness of fibrotic lungs. Because type III collagen is more compliant than type I, increasing type I relative to type III collagen may result in a stiffer lung. Changes in collagen cross-linking in fibrotic lungs also may contribute to the increased stiffness.

Asthma

Asthma is characterized clinically by attacks of shortness of breath, which is caused by narrowing of the large conducting airways (bronchi). The clinical hallmark of asthma is increased airway reactivity of the bronchial smooth muscle in response to exposure to irritants. There may be common mechanisms between asthma and pulmonary fibrosis, with regard to the role of recurrent or chronic inflammation in disease pathogenesis.

Lung Cancer

Lung cancer is now the leading cause of death from cancer among men and women. Retrospective and prospective epidemiologic studies unequivocally show an association between tobacco smoking and lung cancer. Average smokers have a 10-fold and heavy smokers a 20-fold increased risk of developing lung cancer compared with nonsmokers. Many other agents also cause lung cancer (see Table 15–1).

Human lung cancers may have a latency period of 20 to 40 years, making the relationship to specific exposures difficult to establish. Many lung cancers in humans originate from the cells lining the airways, but during the last two decades a significant increase in peripheral adenocarcinomas has occurred. Compared with cancer in the lung, cancer in the upper respiratory tract is less common.

The potential mechanisms of lung carcinogenesis center on damage to DNA. An activated carcinogen or its metabolic product may interact with DNA. DNA damage caused by active oxygen species is another potentially important mechanism. Ionizing radiation leads to the formation of superoxide. Cigarette smoke contains high quantities of active oxygen species and other free radicals.

The Developing Lung

The developing lung is uniquely sensitive to many airborne and blood-borne toxicants. Children living in homes of active smokers have been found to suffer from middle ear infections and infections of the lower respiratory tract. Infants born to mothers who smoked had thickened and narrower airways compared with infants of nonsmoking mothers. Because development of the lung occurs during both the prenatal and postnatal periods, the stage of development during which toxicant exposure occurs may greatly influence the severity of the lesion.

AGENTS KNOWN TO PRODUCE LUNG INJURY IN HUMANS

During the past 20 years, a large body of knowledge of the cellular and molecular events that determine lung injury and repair has accumulated. Table 15–1 lists common toxicants that are known to produce acute and chronic lung injury in humans.

Airborne Agents that Produce Lung Injury in Humans

Lung Overload Caused by Particles—Investigators have observed a slowing of the rate of alveolar clearance when deposited lung burdens are high. Clearance mechanisms in the deep lung depending predominantly on phagocytosis and migration of pulmonary alveolar macrophages can be overwhelmed by quantities of respirable dusts far in excess of physiologic loads. Consequently, lung burdens of these dusts persist for months or years, and unphysiologic mechanisms of disease pathogenesis may come into play.

For example, exposure to asbestos fibers occurs frequently in mining and construction (specifically deconstruction) industries. Once the fibers are deposited in the lung, they are phagocytized by macrophages. Relatively long fibers are incompletely ingested and the macrophages cannot leave the alveoli. Release of lymphokines and growth factors stimulates collagen production and triggers an inflammatory sequence of events, leading to carcinogenesis.

TABLE 15–1 Industrial toxicants that produce lung disease.

Toxicant	Common Name of Disease	Occupational Source	Acute Effect	Chronic Effect
Asbestos	Asbestosis	Mining, construction, shipbuilding, manufacture of asbestos-containing material		Fibrosis, pleural calcification, lung cancer, pleural mesothelioma
Aluminum dust	Aluminosis	Manufacture of aluminum products, fireworks, ceramics, paints, electrical goods, abrasives	Cough, shortness of breath	Interstitial fibrosis
Aluminum abrasives	Shaver's disease, corundum smelter's lung, bauxite lung	Manufacture of abrasives, smelting	Alveolar edema	Interstitial fibrosis, emphysema
Ammonia		Ammonia production, manufacture of fertilizers, chemical production, explosives	Upper and lower respiratory tract irritation, edema	Chronic bronchitis
Arsenic		Manufacture of pesticides, pigments, glass, alloys	Bronchitis	Lung cancer, bronchitis, laryngitis
Beryllium	Berylliosis	Ore extraction, manufacture of alloys, ceramics	Severe pulmonary edema, pneumonia	Fibrosis, progressive dyspnea, interstitial granulomatosis, lung cancer, cor pulmonale
Cadmium oxide		Welding, manufacture of electrical equipment, alloys, pigments, smelting	Cough, pneumonia	Emphysema, cor pulmonale
Carbides of tungsten, titanium, tantalum	Hard metal disease	Manufacture of cutting edges on tools	Hyperplasia and metaplasia of bronchial epithelium	Peribronchial and perivascular fibrosis
Chlorine		Manufacture of pulp and paper, plastics, chlorinated chemicals	Cough, hemoptysis, dyspnea, tracheobronchitis, bronchopneumonia	
Chromium(VI)		Production of Cr compounds, paint pigments, reduction of chromite ore	Nasal irritation, bronchitis	Lung cancer, fibrosis
Coal dust	Pneumoconiosis	Coal mining		Fibrosis
Cotton dust	Byssinosis	Manufacture of textiles	Chest tightness, wheezing, dyspnea	Reduced pulmonary function, chronic bronchitis
Hydrogen fluoride		Manufacture of chemicals, photographic film, solvents, plastics	Respiratory irritation, hemorrhagic pulmonary edema	
Iron oxides	Siderotic lung disease; silver finisher's lung, hematite miner's lung, arc welder's lung	Welding, foundry work, steel manufacture, hematite mining, jewelry making	Cough	Silver finisher's lung: subpleural and perivascular aggregations of macrophages; hematite miner's lung: diffuse fibrosis-like pneumoconiosis; arc welder's lung: bronchitis
Isocyanates		Manufacture of plastics, chemical industry	Airway irritation, cough, dyspnea	Asthma, reduced pulmonary function
Kaolin	Kaolinosis	Pottery making		Fibrosis
Manganese	Manganese pneumonia	Chemical and metal industries	Acute pneumonia, often fatal	Recurrent pneumonia

(continued)

TABLE 15–1 Industrial toxicants that produce lung disease. (Continued)

Toxicant	Common Name of Disease	Occupational Source	Acute Effect	Chronic Effect
Nickel		Nickel ore extraction, smelting, electronic electroplating, fossil fuels	Pulmonary edema, delayed by 2 days (NiCO)	Squamous cell carcinoma of nasal cavity and lung
Oxides of nitrogen		Welding, silo filling, explosive manufacture	Pulmonary congestion and edema	Bronchiolitis obliterans
Ozone		Welding, bleaching flour, deodorizing	Pulmonary edema	Fibrosis
Phosgene		Production of plastics, pesticides, chemicals	Edema	Bronchitis, fibrosis
Perchloroethylene		Dry cleaning, metal degreasing, grain fumigating	Edema	Cancer, liver, and lung
Silica	Silicosis, pneumoconiosis	Mining, stone cutting, construction, farming, quarrying, sand blasting	Acute silicosis	Fibrosis, silicotuberculosis
Sulfur dioxide		Manufacture of chemicals, refrigeration, bleaching, fumigation	Bronchoconstriction, cough, chest tightness	Chronic bronchitis
Talc	Talcosis	Rubber industry, cosmetics		Fibrosis
Tin	Stanosis	Mining, processing of tin		Widespread mottling of x-ray without clinical signs
Vanadium		Steel manufacture	Airway irritation and mucus production	Chronic bronchitis

Oxygen—Oxygen toxicity is mediated through increased production of partially reduced oxygen products. In animals exposed to 95 to 100 percent oxygen, diffuse pulmonary damage develops and is usually fatal after 3 to 4 days. Type I epithelial cells and capillary endothelial cells develop necrotic changes. Capillary damage leads to leakage of proteinaceous fluid and formed blood elements into the alveolar space. Hyaline membranes formed by cellular debris and proteinaceous exudate are a characteristic sign of pulmonary oxygen toxicity. In animals returned to air after the development of acute oxygen toxicity, there is active cell proliferation.

Blood-borne Agents that Cause Pulmonary Toxicity in Humans

Paraquat—The bipyridylium herbicide paraquat (historically used for marijuana control) produces extensive lung injury when ingested by humans. In patients who survive the first few days of acute paraquat poisoning, progressive and eventually fatal lung lesions characterized by diffuse interstitial and intraalveolar fibrosis can develop. After initial widespread necrosis, extensive proliferation of fibroblasts in the alveolar interstitium follows. Paraquat accumulates in the cells of the lung. Once inside the cells, paraquat continuously cycles from its oxidized form to the

reduced form, with the concomitant formation of active oxygen species and eventual depletion of cellular NADPH.

Monocrotaline—Monocrotaline (MCT) is one of the many structurally related naturally occurring products that have been identified in grains, honey, and herbal teas. These compounds produce hepatocellular necrosis and veno-occlusive disease. MCT is metabolized in the liver by cytochrome P450 3A to a highly reactive pyrrole, a bifunctional alkylating agent, some of which is released from the liver and travels to other organs, such as the lung, where it initiates endothelial injury resulting in pulmonary hypertension and hypertrophy of the right side of the heart.

Bleomycin—Bleomycin is a widely used cancer chemotherapeutic agent that also produces pulmonary fibrosis. The sequence of damage includes necrosis of capillary endothelial and type I alveolar cells, edema formation and hemorrhage, delayed (after 1 to 2 weeks) proliferation of type II epithelial cells, and eventually thickening of the alveolar walls by fibrotic changes.

Cyclophosphamide and 1,3-Bis-(2-Chloroethyl)-1-Nitrosourea (BCNU)—Though widely used as an anticancer and immunosuppressive agent, cyclophosphamide produces hemorrhagic cystitis and pulmonary fibrosis. Cyclophosph-amide is metabolized by the cytochrome P450 system to two highly reactive metabolites: acrolein and phosphoramide mustard, which initiate lipid peroxidation. In humans, a dose-related pulmonary toxicity is often noticed first by a decrease in diffusion capacity, and subsequent pulmonary fibrosis can be fatal. Because BCNU inhibits pulmonary glutathione disulfide reductase, GSH/GSSG ratio may be disturbed, leaving lung cells unable to cope with oxidant stress.

Cationic Amphophilic Drugs—Several drugs with similar structural characteristics, such as the antiarrhythmic amiodarone and the anorexic chlorphentermine, elicit pulmonary lipidosis, presumably by inhibiting phospholipases A and B. Degradation of pulmonary surfactant is impaired, and the material accumulates in phagocytic cells.

EVALUATION OF TOXIC LUNG DAMAGE

Inhalation Exposure Systems

Monitoring and quantifying gaseous pollutants require either expensive detectors or very labor-intensive wet chemical analysis procedures after sampled gases from the chambers are bubbled through traps. Particle generation is difficult. Exposure chambers must allow for rapid attainment of the desired concentrations of toxicants, maintenance of desired levels homogeneously throughout the chamber, adequate capacity for experimental animals, and minimal accumulation of undesired products associated with animal occupancy (usually ammonia, dander, heat, and carbon dioxide). As a general rule, the total body volume of the animals should not exceed 5 percent of the chamber volume. Nose-only exposure chambers avoid some of these problems.

Pulmonary Function Studies

Commonly used tests include measurement of VC, TLC, functional RV, TV, airway resistance, and maximum flow (Figure 15–6). Additional tests evaluate the distribution of ventilation, lung and chest wall compliance, diffusion capacity, and the oxygen and carbon dioxide content of the arterial and venous blood.

The FEV_1 (forced expiratory volume during the first second of an active exhalation) is an easy test to administer to humans, does not require sophisticated equipment or a hospital setting, and is completely noninvasive. A reduction in FEV_1 is usually indicative of impaired ventilation such as that found in restrictive (increased lung stiffness) or obstructive (obstructed airflow) lung disease.

Analysis of breathing patterns has been widely used to assess the effects of irritants. This technique allows one to differentiate between sensory or upper airway irritants and "pulmonary" irritants. Highly water-soluble irritants such as ammonia, chlorine, and formaldehyde produce upper respiratory tract irritation, whereas less soluble gases such as nitrogen dioxide and

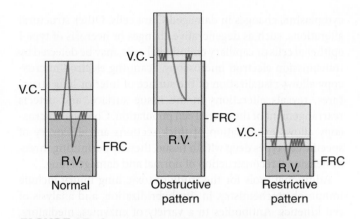

FIGURE 15–6 Typical lung volume measurements from individuals with normal lung function, obstructive airways disease, or restrictive lung disease. Note that there is (1) a slowing of forced expiration in addition to gas trapping (an increase in residual volume) in obstructive disease and (2) a general decrease in lung volumes in restrictive disease. Note that the measurements read from left to right. FRC = functional residual capacity.

ozone generate pulmonary irritation. The sensory irritant pattern has been described as slowing down respiratory frequency while increasing TV. Pulmonary irritants usually increase respiratory frequency and decrease minute volume. The result is rapid, shallow breathing.

To accomplish proper oxygenation of venous blood and elimination of CO_2, the gases have to diffuse across the air-blood barrier. Gas exchange can be evaluated by measuring the arterial partial pressure of both oxygen and CO_2. In general, blood gas analysis is a comparatively insensitive assay for disturbed ventilation because of the organism's buffering and reserve capacities. Although it is a useful tool in clinical medicine, only the most severe obstructive or restrictive pulmonary alterations cause signs of impaired gas exchange in animals. Measurement of diffusion capacity with CO, a gas that binds with 250 times higher affinity to hemoglobin than does oxygen, is more sensitive and is widely used in toxicology studies.

Morphologic Techniques

The pathology of acute and chronic injury may be described after examination of the respiratory tract by gross inspection and under the microscope. Morphologic evaluation should include the examination of nasal passages, the larynx, and major airways, as well as is the lung parenchyma. Careful consideration must be given to tissue fixation and preparation. The choice of fixative depends on how the lung will be further analyzed.

Ordinary paraffin sections of respiratory tract tissue are suitable for routine histopathologic analysis permitting detection of gross pathologic changes such as inflammation and the presence of cancerous tissue. Plastic or Epon sections about 1 μm thick are required for proper identification of different cell types lining the airways or alveoli and for recognition of cytoplasmic changes in damaged Clara cells. Other structural alterations, such as degenerative changes or necrosis of type I epithelial cells or capillary endothelial cells, may be detected by transmission electron microscopy. Scanning electron microscopy allows visualization of the surface of interior lung structures, reveals alterations in the tissue surface, and detects rearrangement of the overall cell population. Confocal microscopy allows examination of thick sections and discovery of specific cell types deep within tissue, thereby permitting three-dimensional reconstruction of normal and damaged lung.

Additional tools for the study of toxic lung injury include immunohistochemistry, in situ hybridization, and analysis of cell kinetics. Antibodies to a variety of enzymes, mediators, and other proteins are available. In situ hybridization allows one to visualize anatomical sites where a specific gene product is expressed, for example, collagen production in a fibrotic lung. Flow cytometry is valuable in the study of cell populations prepared from the lung. The technique requires dissociation of the lung parenchyma into its individual cell populations. Different lung cells then can be identified and isolated.

Pulmonary Lavage

The lungs of exposed and control animals are washed with multiple small volumes of isotonic saline. Current emphasis seems to be on the measurement of polymorphonuclear leukocytes, macrophages, and monocytes (and their phagocytotic capabilities) in the cellular fraction, and the measurement of several types of enzymes and total protein levels. Measurement of apparent changes in the permeability of the air–blood barrier by quantification of intravenously injected tracer in lung lavage fluid is another useful index of lung damage.

In Vitro Approaches

In vitro systems are particularly suited for the study of mechanisms that cause lung injury. The systems presented in the next sections are widely used.

Isolated Perfused Lung—The lung, in situ or excised, is perfused with blood or a blood substitute through the pulmonary arterial bed. At the same time, the lung is ventilated. Toxic agents can be introduced into the perfusate or the inspired air. Repeated sampling of the perfusate allows one to determine the rate of metabolism of drugs and the metabolic activity of the lung.

Lung Explants and Slices—Slices and explants from the conducting airways or the lung parenchyma allow one to examine biochemical and morphologic changes in the lung parenchyma without intervening complications from cells migrating into the tissue (e.g., leukocytes). If the lung is first inflated with agar, the alveolar spaces remain open in the explant. Slices prepared in this way can be kept viable for several weeks, and the mechanisms of development of chronic lesions can be studied.

Microdissection—Many inhalants act in circumscribed regions of the respiratory tract, such as the terminal bronchioles, a region especially rich in metabolically highly competent Clara cells. Microdissection of the airways consists of the stripping of small bronchi and terminal bronchioles from the surrounding parenchyma and maintenance of the isolated airways in culture. Specific biochemical reactions predominantly located in the cells of the small airways can then be studied with biochemical or morphologic techniques.

Organotypic Cell Culture Systems—Tissue culture systems permit epithelial cells to maintain their polarity, differentiation, and normal function similar to what is observed in vivo. Epithelial cell surfaces are exposed to air (or a gas phase containing an airborne toxic agent), while the basal portion is bathed by a tissue culture medium.

Isolated Lung Cell Populations—Many specific lung cell types have been isolated and maintained as primary cultures in vitro. Alveolar macrophages are easily obtained from human and animal lungs by lavage. Their function can be examined in vitro with or without exposure to appropriate toxic stimuli. Type II alveolar epithelial cells are isolated after digestion of the lung. Direct isolation of type I epithelial cells has also been successful. Systems for the isolation and culture of Clara cells and neuroepithelial cells are available. Lung fibroblasts are easily grown and have been studied in coculture with epithelial cells. Multiple primary cell cultures and cell lines have been established from lung tumors found in experimental animals and humans.

BIBLIOGRAPHY

Gardner DE (ed): *Toxicology of the Lung*, 4th ed. Boca Raton: CRC Press/Taylor & Francis, 2006.

Harding R, Pinkerton KE, Plopper CG (eds): *The Lung. Development, Aging and the Environment*. Holland: Elsevier, 2004.

Haschek WM, Rousseaux CG, Wallig MA (eds): *Handbook of Toxicologic Pathology*, 2nd ed., Vol. 2. Academic Press, San Diego, CA, 2002.

IARC (International Agency for Research on Cancer): *IARC Monographs on the Evaluation of the Carcinogenic Risk of Chemicals to Humans*. Volume 83 in *Tobacco Smoke and Involuntary Smoking*. Lyon, France: IARC, 2004.

Oberdorster G, Oberdorster E, Oberdorster J: Nanotoxicology: an emerging discipline evolving from studies of ultrafine particles. *Environ Health Perspect* 113:823–839, 2005.

QUESTIONS

1. Which of the following statements is FALSE regarding the role of mucus in the conducting airways?
   a. Pollutants trapped by mucus can be eliminated via expectoration or swallowing.
   b. Mucus is of a basic pH.
   c. The beating of cilia propels mucus out of the lungs.
   d. Mucus plays a role promoting oxidative stress.
   e. Free radical scavenging is believed to be a role of mucus.

2. Respiratory distress syndrome sometimes affects premature neonates due to lack of surfactant production by which of the following cell types?
   a. lung fibroblasts.
   b. type II pneumocytes.
   c. endothelial cells.
   d. alveolar macrophages.
   e. type I pneumocytes.

3. In a situation where there is an increased metabolic demand for oxygen, which of the following volume measurements will greatly increase?
   a. total lung capacity (TLC).
   b. residual volume (RV).
   c. functional residual capacity (FRC).
   d. tidal volume (TV).
   e. vital capacity (VC).

4. The free radicals that inflict oxidative damage on the lungs are generated by all of the following EXCEPT:
   a. tobacco smoke.
   b. neutrophils.
   c. ozone.
   d. monocytes.
   e. SO_2.

5. Which of the following gases would most likely pass all the way through the respiratory tract and diffuse into the pulmonary blood supply?
   a. O_3 (ozone).
   b. NO_2.
   c. H_2O.
   d. CO.
   e. SO_2.

6. All of the following statements regarding particle deposition and clearance are true EXCEPT:
   a. One of the main modes of particle clearance is via mucociliary escalation.
   b. Diffusion is important in the deposition of particles in the bronchial regions.
   c. Larger volumes of inspired air increase particle deposition in the airways.
   d. Sedimentation results in deposition in the bronchioles.
   e. Swallowing is an important mechanism of particle clearance.

7. Which of the following is not a common location to which particles are cleared?
   a. stomach.
   b. lymph nodes.
   c. pulmonary vasculature.
   d. liver.
   e. GI tract.

8. Pulmonary fibrosis is marked by which of the following?
   a. increased type I collagen.
   b. decreased type III collagen.
   c. increased compliance.
   d. elastase activation.
   e. decreased overall collagen levels.

9. Activation of what enzyme(s) is responsible for emphysema?
   a. antitrypsin.
   b. epoxide hydrolase.
   c. elastase.
   d. hyaluronidase.
   e. nonspecific proteases.

10. Which of the following measurements would NOT be expected from a patient with restrictive lung disease?
    a. decreased FRC.
    b. decreased RV.
    c. increased VC.
    d. decreased FEV_1.
    e. impaired ventilation.

Toxic Responses of the Nervous System

Virginia C. Moser, Michael Aschner,
Rudy J. Richardson, and Martin A. Philbert

- The central nervous system (CNS) is protected from the adverse effects of many potential toxicants by an anatomical blood–brain barrier.
- Neurons are highly dependent on aerobic metabolism because this energy is needed to maintain proper ion gradients.
- Individual neurotoxic compounds typically target the neuron, the axon, the myelinating cell, or the neurotransmitter system.

- Neuronopathy is the toxicant-induced irreversible loss of neurons, including its cytoplasmic extensions, dendrites and axons, and the myelin ensheathing the axon.
- Neurotoxicants that cause *axonopathies* cause axonal degeneration, and loss of the myelin surrounding that axon; however, the neuron cell body remains intact.
- Numerous naturally occurring toxins as well as synthetic chemicals may interrupt the transmission of impulses, block or accentuate transsynaptic communication, block reuptake of neurotransmitters, or interfere with second-messenger systems.

OVERVIEW OF THE NERVOUS SYSTEM

Several generalities that allow a basic understanding of the actions of neurotoxicants include (1) the privileged status of the nervous system (NS) with the maintenance of a biochemical barrier between the brain and the blood, (2) the importance of the high energy requirements of the brain, (3) the spatial extensions of the NS as long cellular processes and the requirements of cells with such a complex geometry, (4) the maintenance of an environment rich in lipids, (5) the transmission of information across extracellular space at the synapse, (6) the distances over which electrical impulses must be transmitted, coordinated, and integrated, and (7) development and regenerative patterns of the NS.

Blood–Brain Barrier

The central NS (CNS) is protected from the adverse effects of many potential toxicants by an anatomical barrier between the blood and the brain, or a "blood–brain barrier." To gain entry to the NS, molecules must pass into the cell membranes of endothelial cells of the brain rather than between endothelial cells, as they do in other tissues (Figure 16–1). The blood–brain barrier also contains xenobiotic transporters that transport some xenobiotics that have diffused through endothelial cells back into the blood. If not actively transported into the brain, the penetration of toxicants or their metabolites into the NS is largely related to their lipid solubility. However, spinal and

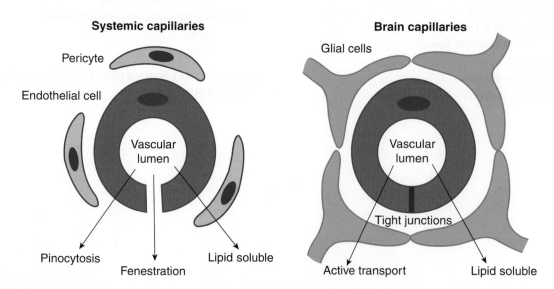

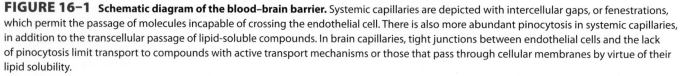

FIGURE 16–1 **Schematic diagram of the blood–brain barrier.** Systemic capillaries are depicted with intercellular gaps, or fenestrations, which permit the passage of molecules incapable of crossing the endothelial cell. There is also more abundant pinocytosis in systemic capillaries, in addition to the transcellular passage of lipid-soluble compounds. In brain capillaries, tight junctions between endothelial cells and the lack of pinocytosis limit transport to compounds with active transport mechanisms or those that pass through cellular membranes by virtue of their lipid solubility.

autonomic ganglia as well as a small number of other sites within the brain are not protected by blood–tissue barriers. The blood–brain barrier is incompletely developed at birth and even less so in premature infants. This predisposes the premature infant to brain injury by toxicants that later in life are excluded from the NS.

Energy Requirements

Neurons are highly dependent on aerobic metabolism because they must use this energy to maintain proper ion gradients. The brain is extremely sensitive to even brief interruptions in the supply of oxygen or glucose. Exposure to toxicants that inhibit aerobic respiration (e.g., cyanide) or to conditions that produce hypoxia (e.g., CO poisoning) leads to early signs of neuronal dysfunction.

Axonal Transport

Impulses are conducted over great distances at rapid speed, providing information about the environment to the organism in a coordinated manner that allows an organized response to be carried out at a specific site. However, the intricate organization of such a complex network places an unparalleled demand on the cells of the NS. Single cells, rather than being spherical and a few micrometers in diameter, are elongated and may extend over 1 m in length. Two immediate demands placed on the neuron are the maintenance of a much larger cellular volume requiring more protein synthesis and the transport of intracellular materials over great distances using various mechanisms. These demands require ATP.

Axonal transport moves protein products from the cell body to the appropriate site in the axon. *Fast axonal transport* carries a large number of proteins from their site of synthesis in the cell body into the axon. Many proteins associated with vesicles migrate through the axon at a rate of 400 mm/day (Figure 16–2). This process is dependent on microtubule-associated ATPase activity and the microtubule-associated

motor proteins, kinesin and dynein, that provide both the mechanochemical force in the form of a microtubule-associated ATPase and the interface between microtubules as the track and vesicles as the cargo. Vesicles are transported rapidly in an anterograde direction by kinesin, and they are transported in a retrograde direction by dynein. This mechanism of cytoplasmic transport is amplified within the NS, compared with other cells, by the distances encompassed by the axonal extensions of neurons.

The transport of some organelles, including mitochondria, constitutes an intermediate component of axonal transport, moving at 50 mm/day. The slowest component of axonal transport represents the movement of the cytoskeleton itself (Figure 16–2). The cytoskeleton is composed of microtubules formed by the association of tubulin subunits and neurofilaments formed by the association of three neurofilament protein subunits. Each of the elements of the cytoskeleton moves along the length of the axon at a specific rate. Overall, slow component A (SCa) represents retrograde axonal transport, whereas slow component B (SCb) is composed of the movement of the axonal cytoskeleton in an anterograde direction.

Neurofilaments and microtubules move at a rate of approximately 1 mm/day and make up the majority of SCa, the slowest moving component of axonal transport. Moving at only a slightly more rapid rate of 2 to 4 mm/day in an anterograde direction is SCb, which is composed of many proteins. Included in SCb are several structural proteins, such as the component of microfilaments (actin) and several microfilament-associated proteins (M2 protein and fodrin), as well as clathrin and many soluble proteins.

This continual transport of proteins from the cell body through the various components of forward-directed, or anterograde, axonal transport is the mechanism through which the neuron provides the distal axon with its complement of functional and structural proteins. Some vesicles are also moving in a retrograde direction and undoubtedly provide the cell body with information concerning the status of the distal axon.

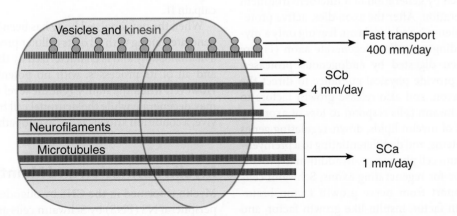

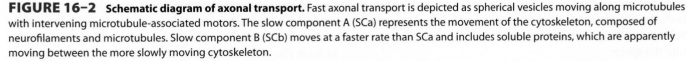

FIGURE 16–2 **Schematic diagram of axonal transport.** Fast axonal transport is depicted as spherical vesicles moving along microtubules with intervening microtubule-associated motors. The slow component A (SCa) represents the movement of the cytoskeleton, composed of neurofilaments and microtubules. Slow component B (SCb) moves at a faster rate than SCa and includes soluble proteins, which are apparently moving between the more slowly moving cytoskeleton.

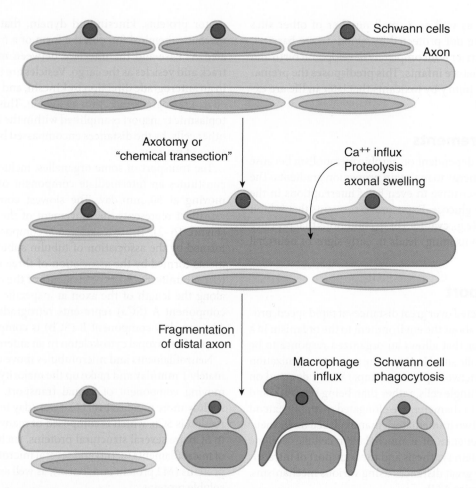

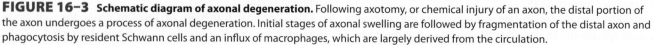

FIGURE 16–3 **Schematic diagram of axonal degeneration.** Following axotomy, or chemical injury of an axon, the distal portion of the axon undergoes a process of axonal degeneration. Initial stages of axonal swelling are followed by fragmentation of the distal axon and phagocytosis by resident Schwann cells and an influx of macrophages, which are largely derived from the circulation.

Axonal Degeneration

Following axotomy (cutting of an axon), there is degeneration of the distal nerve stump, referred to as *Wallerian degeneration,* which is followed by generation of a microenvironment supportive of regeneration. After the axon dies, active proteolysis digests the axolemma and axoplasm, leaving only a myelin sheath surrounding a swollen degenerate axon (Figure 16–3), which is then digested by endogenous proteases. Schwann cells then provide physical guidance to direct the regrowth of a new axon, and also release growth factors to stimulate growth. Schwann cells respond to loss of axons by decreasing synthesis of myelin lipids, down-regulating genes encoding myelin proteins, and dedifferentiating to a premyelinating mitotic Schwann cell phenotype. In addition to providing physical guidance for regenerating axons, Schwann cells provide trophic support from nerve growth factor, brain-derived nerve growth factor, insulin-like growth factor, and corresponding receptors produced by the associated Schwann cells. Resident and recruited macrophages and the denervated Schwann cells clear myelin debris so that a new axon can grow into the space.

Investigations have shown that degeneration of the distal axonal stump after transection is an active, synchronized process that can be delayed through decreasing temperature, preventing the entry of extracellular Ca^{2+} or inhibiting proteolysis by calpain II.

When the neuronal cell body has been lethally injured, it degenerates, along with all of its cellular processes. This process is a *neuronopathy* and is characterized by the loss of the cell body and all of its processes, with no potential for regeneration. However, when the injury is at the level of the axon, the axon may degenerate while the neuronal cell body continues to survive, a condition known as an "axonopathy" (Figure 16–4).

Myelin Formation and Maintenance

Myelin is formed in the CNS by oligodendrocytes and in the peripheral NS (PNS) by Schwann cells as concentric layers by the progressive wrapping of their cytoplasmic processes around the axon in successive loops (Figure 16–5). These cells exclude cytoplasm from the inner surface of their membranes to form the major dense line of myelin. In a similar process,

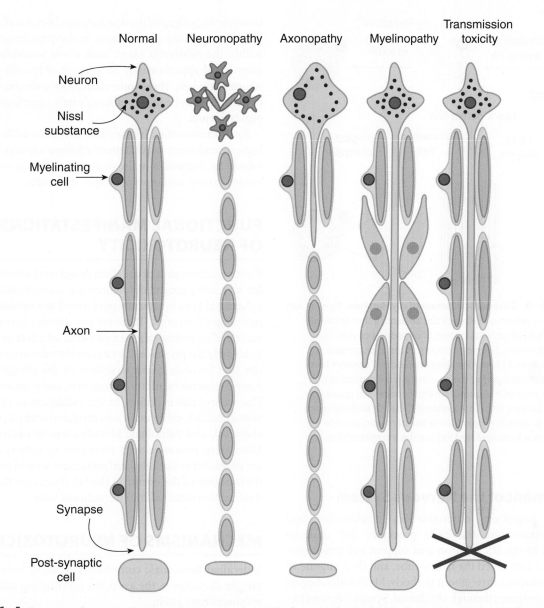

FIGURE 16–4 **Patterns of neurotoxic injury.** A neuronopathy results from the death of the entire neuron. Astrocytes often proliferate in response to the neuronal loss, creating both neuronal loss and gliosis. When the axon is the primary site of injury, the axon degenerates, while the surviving neuron shows only chromatolysis with margination of its Nissl substance and nucleus to the cell periphery. This condition is termed an axonopathy. Myelinopathies result from disruption of myelin or from selective injury to the myelinating cells. To prevent cross-talk between adjacent axons, myelinating cells divide and cover the denuded axon rapidly; however, the process of remyelination is much less effective in the CNS than in the PNS. Some compounds do not lead to cell death but exert their toxic effects by interrupting the process of neurotransmission, either through blocking excitation or by excessive stimulation.

the extracellular space is reduced on the extracellular surface of the bilayers, and the lipid membranes stack together.

The maintenance of myelin is dependent on a number of membrane-associated proteins and on metabolism of specific lipids present in myelin bilayers. Some toxic compounds interfere with this complex process of the maintenance of myelin and result in the toxic "myelinopathies" (Figure 16–4). In general, the loss of myelin, with the preservation of axons, is referred to as *demyelination*.

Neurotransmission

Intercellular communication is achieved in the NS through the synapse. Neurotransmitters released from one neuron act as the first messenger. Binding of the transmitter to the postsynaptic receptor is followed by modulation of an ion channel or activation of a second-messenger system, leading to changes in the responding cell. Various therapeutic drugs and toxic compounds impact the process of neurotransmission.

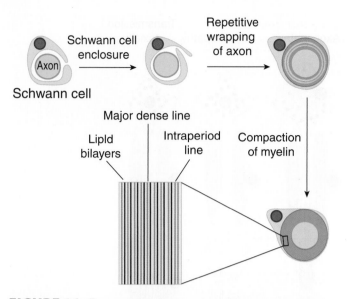

FIGURE 16–5 **Schematic diagram of myelination.** Myelination begins when a myelinating cell encircles an axon, either Schwann cells in the peripheral nervous system or oligodendrocytes in the central nervous system. Simple enclosure of the axon persists in unmyelinated axons. Myelin formation proceeds by a progressive wrapping of multiple layers of the myelinating cell around the axon, with extrusion of the cytoplasm and extracellular space to bring the lipid bilayers into close proximity. The intracellular space is compressed to form the major dense line of myelin, and the extracellular space is compressed to form the intraperiod line.

Development of the Nervous System

Replication, migration, differentiation, myelination, and synapse formation are the basic processes that underlie development of the NS. Neuron and support cell precursors replicate in an area called the neural tube, and then migrate to different destinations throughout the body. Myelination begins in utero and continues through childhood. Synaptic connectivity, the basis of neurologic function, is a dynamic process throughout life.

The immature NS is especially vulnerable to certain agents. The insufficient replacement of damaged neural cells, the slow formation of the blood–brain barrier, and the lack of key metabolic enzymes may influence NS sensitivity. Ethanol exposure during pregnancy can result in abnormalities in the fetus, including abnormal neuronal migration and diffuse abnormalities in the development of neuronal processes. The clinical result of fetal alcohol exposure is often mental retardation, with malformations of the brain and delayed myelination of white matter.

Environmental Factors Relevant to Neurodegenerative Diseases

It has been observed that individuals exposed to 1-methyl-4-phenyl-1,2,3,6-tetrahydropyridine (MPTP) at insufficient levels to result in immediate parkinsonism have developed however early signs of the disease years later. Small exposures to MPTP may cause a decrement in the population of neurons within the substantia nigra. Such a loss would most likely be silent until approximately 80 percent of the substantia nigra neurons are lost. These individuals with a diminished number of neurons may be more vulnerable to further loss of dopaminergic neurons.

An epidemic of dialysis-related dementia with some pathologic resemblance to Alzheimer's disease appears to have been related to aluminum in the dialysate, and its removal has prevented further instances of dialysis dementia.

FUNCTIONAL MANIFESTATIONS OF NEUROTOXICITY

Functional assessment uses functional test batteries as a means for screening potentially neurotoxic compounds. A group of behavioral tests is typically performed to evaluate a variety of neurologic functions. There are two distinct tiers of functional testing of neurotoxicants: a first tier in which tests may be used to identify the presence of a neurotoxic substance and a second tier that involves characterization of the effects of the compound on sensory, motor, autonomic, and cognitive functions. The second tier is critical to the validation of the behavioral tests as behavioral changes are correlated with physiologic, biochemical, and pathologic identification of neurotoxic injury. Ultimately, neurotoxicants identified by behavioral methods are evaluated at a cellular and molecular level to provide an understanding of the events in the NS that cause the neurologic dysfunction detected by observational tests.

MECHANISMS OF NEUROTOXICITY

Individual neurotoxic compounds typically have one of four targets: the neuron, the axon, the myelinating cell, or the neurotransmitter system.

Neuronopathies

Certain toxicants are specific for neurons, resulting in their injury or death. Neuron loss is irreversible and includes degeneration of all of its cytoplasmic extensions, dendrites and axons, and the myelin ensheathing the axon (Figure 16–4). Features of the neuron that place it at risk for the action of cellular toxicants include a high metabolic rate, a long cellular process that is supported by the cell body, and an excitable membrane that is rapidly depolarized and repolarized.

Although a large number of compounds are known to result in toxic neuronopathies (Table 16–1), all of these toxicants share certain features. Each toxic condition is the result of a cellular toxicant that has a predilection for neurons. The initial injury to neurons is followed by apoptosis or necrosis, leading to permanent loss of the neuron. These agents tend to be diffuse in their action, although they may show some selectivity in the degree of injury of different neuronal subpopulations.

TABLE 16-1 Compounds associated with neuronal injury (neuronopathies).

Neurotoxicant	Neurologic Findings	Cellular Basis of Neurotoxicity
Aluminum	Dementia, encephalopathy (humans), learning deficits	Spongiosis cortex, neurofibrillary aggregates, degenerative changes in cortex
6-Amino-nicotinamide	Not reported in humans; hind limb paralysis (experimental animals)	Spongy (vacuolar) degeneration in spinal cord, brainstem, cerebellum; axonal degeneration of the peripheral nervous system (PNS)
Arsenic	Encephalopathy (acute), peripheral neuropathy (chronic)	Brain swelling and hemorrhage (acute); axonal degeneration in PNS (chronic)
Azide	Insufficient data (humans); convulsions, ataxia (primates)	Neuronal loss in cerebellum and cortex
Bismuth	Emotional disturbances, encephalopathy, myoclonus	Neuronal loss, basal ganglia, and Purkinje cells of cerebellum
Carbon monoxide	Encephalopathy, delayed parkinsonism/dystonia	Neuronal loss in cortex, necrosis of globus pallidus, focal demyelination; blocks oxygen-binding site of hemoglobin and iron-binding sites of brain
Carbon tetrachloride	Encephalopathy (secondary to liver failure)	Enlarged astrocytes in striatum, globus pallidus
Chloramphenicol	Optic neuritis, peripheral neuropathy	Neuronal loss (retina), axonal degeneration (PNS)
Cyanide	Coma, convulsions, rapid death; delayed parkinsonism/dystonia	Neuronal degeneration, cerebellum, and globus pallidus; focal demyelination; blocks cytochrome oxidase/ATP production
Doxorubicin	Insufficient data (humans); progressive ataxia (experimental animals)	Degeneration of dorsal root ganglion cells, axonal degeneration (PNS)
Ethanol	Mental retardation, hearing deficits (prenatal exposure)	Microcephaly, cerebral malformations
Lead	Encephalopathy (acute), learning deficits (children), neuropathy with demyelination (rats)	Brain swelling, hemorrhages (acute), axonal loss in PNS (humans)
Manganese	Emotional disturbances, parkinsonism/dystonia	Degeneration of striatum, globus pallidus
Mercury, inorganic	Emotional disturbances, tremor, fatigue	Insufficient data in humans (may affect spinal tracts; cerebellum)
Methanol	Headache, visual loss or blindness, coma (severe)	Necrosis of putamen, degeneration of retinal ganglion cells
Methylazoxymethanol acetate (MAM)	Microcephaly, retarded development (rats)	Developmental abnormalities of fetal brain (rats)
Methyl bromide	Visual and speech impairment; peripheral neuropathy	Insufficient data
Methyl mercury (organic mercury)	Ataxia, constriction of visual fields, paresthesias (adult)	Neuronal degeneration, visual cortex, cerebellum, ganglia
	Psychomotor retardation (fetal exposure)	Spongy disruption, cortex, and cerebellum
1-Methyl-4-phenyl-1,2,3,6-tetrahydropyridine (MPTP)	Parkinsonism, dystonia (acute exposure)	Neuronal degeneration in substantia nigra
	Early onset parkinsonism (late effect of acute exposure)	Neuronal degeneration in substantia nigra
3-Nitropropionic acid	Seizures, delayed dystonia/grimacing	Necrosis in basal ganglia
Phenytoin (diphenyl-hydantoin)	Nystagmus, ataxia, dizziness	Degeneration of Purkinje cells (cerebellum)
Quinine	Constriction of visual fields	Vacuolization of retinal ganglion cells
Streptomycin (aminoglycosides)	Hearing loss	Degeneration of inner ear (organ of Corti)
Thallium	Emotional disturbances, ataxia, peripheral neuropathy	Brain swelling (acute), axonal degeneration in PNS
Trimethyltin	Tremors, hyperexcitability (experimental animals)	Loss of hippocampal neurons, amygdala pyriform cortex

The expression of these cellular events is often a diffuse encephalopathy, with global dysfunctions.

Doxorubicin—Doxorubicin (Adriamycin) injures neurons in the PNS, specifically those of the dorsal root ganglia and autonomic ganglia by intercalating with DNA and interfering with transcription. The vulnerability of sensory and autonomic neurons appears to reflect the lack of protection of these neurons by a blood–tissue barrier within ganglia.

Methyl Mercury—The neurons that are most sensitive to the toxic effects of methyl mercury are those that reside in the dorsal root ganglia, perhaps again reflecting the vulnerability of neurons not shielded by blood–tissue barriers. Methyl mercury exposure impairs glycolysis, nucleic acid biosynthesis, aerobic respiration, protein synthesis, and neurotransmitter release. In addition, there is evidence for enhanced oxidative injury and altered calcium homeostasis. Exposure to methyl mercury leads to widespread neuronal injury and subsequently to a diffuse encephalopathy.

Dopamine, 6-Hydroxydopamine, and Catecholamine Toxicity—The oxidation of catecholamines by monoamine oxidase (MAO) yields H_2O_2, a known cytotoxic metabolite. The metal ion-catalyzed autooxidation of catecholamines, especially dopamine, results in the production of catecholamine-derived quinones as well as superoxide anion.

6-Hydroxydopamine produces chemical sympathectomy in peripheral nerves after systemic administration. Oxidation of this catecholamine analog leads to production of reactive oxygen species with selective destruction of sympathetic innervation. The sympathetic fibers degenerate, resulting in an uncompensated parasympathetic tone, a slowing of the heart rate, and hypermotility of the gastrointestinal system.

Axonopathies

The neurotoxic disorders termed *axonopathies* are those in which the primary site of toxicity is the axon itself. The axon degenerates, and with it the myelin surrounding that axon; however, the neuron cell body remains intact (Figure 16–4). The toxicant results in a "chemical transection" of the axon at some point along its length, and the axon distal to the transection degenerates.

A critical difference exists in the significance of axonal degeneration in the CNS compared with that in the PNS: peripheral axons can regenerate, whereas central axons cannot. In the PNS, glial cells and macrophages support axonal regeneration. In the CNS, release of inhibitory factors from damaged myelin and astrocyte scarring actually interferes with regeneration. The clinical relevance of the disparity between the CNS and PNS is that partial to complete recovery can occur after axonal degeneration in the PNS, whereas the same event is irreversible in the CNS.

Axonopathies can be considered to result from a chemical transection of the axon. The number of axonal toxicants is large and increasing in number (Table 16–2). As the axons

degenerate, sensations and motor strength are first impaired in the most distal extent of the axonal processes, the hands and feet, resulting in a "glove-and-stocking" neuropathy. With time and continued injury, the deficit progresses to involve more proximal areas of the body and the long axons of the spinal cord.

Gamma-diketones—Humans develop a progressive sensorimotor distal axonopathy when exposed to high concentrations of a simple alkane, *n*-hexane, day after day in work settings or after repeated intentional inhalation of hexane-containing glues.

The ω-1 oxidation of *n*-hexane results ultimately in the γ-diketone, 2,5-hexanedione (HD), which reacts with amino groups in all tissues to form pyrroles that derivatize and cross-link neurofilaments, leading to development of neurofilament aggregates of the distal, subterminal axon. The neurofilament-filled axonal swellings distort nodal anatomy and impair axonal transport. The pathologic processes of neurofilament accumulation and degeneration of the axon are followed by the emergence of a clinical peripheral neuropathy.

Carbon Disulfide—Significant exposures of humans to CS_2 cause a distal axonopathy that is identical pathologically to that caused by hexane. Covalent cross-linking of neurofilaments occurs and CS_2 is itself the ultimate toxicant.

The clinical effects of exposure to CS_2 in the chronic setting are very similar to those of hexane exposure, with the development of sensory and motor symptoms occurring initially in a glove-and-stocking distribution. In addition to this chronic axonopathy, CS_2 can also lead to aberrations in mood and signs of diffuse encephalopathic disease.

IDPN—β,β′-Iminodipropionitrile (IDPN) causes a bizarre "waltzing syndrome" consisting of excitement, circling, head twitching, and over-alertness, which appears to result from degeneration of the vestibular sensory hair cells. In addition, administration of IDPN is followed by massive neurofilament-filled swellings of the proximal, instead of the distal, axon.

3,4-Dimethyl-2,5-hexanedione (DMHD) is an analog of HD that is 20 to 30 times more potent as a neurotoxicant and the neurofilament-filled swellings occur in the proximal axon, as in IDPN intoxication. DMHD intoxication leads to limb paralysis, whereas IDPN intoxication results in muscle atrophy but not paralysis.

Acrylamide—Acrylamide is a vinyl monomer used widely in water purification, paper manufacturing, mining, and waterproofing. It is also used extensively in biochemical laboratories, and is present in many foods prepared at high temperatures. Studies of acrylamide neuropathy revealed a distal axonopathy characterized by multiple axonal swellings. Repeated dosing results in a more proximal axonopathy, in a "dying back" process. These changes are caused by accumulations of neurofilaments at the nerve terminal. Recently it has been observed that nerve terminal degeneration occurs prior to development of axonopathy, suggesting that this degeneration is the primary lesion.

TABLE 16–2 Compounds associated with axonal injury (axonopathies).

Neurotoxicant	Neurologic Findings	Basis of Neurotoxicity
Acrylamide	Peripheral neuropathy (often sensory)	Axonal degeneration, axon terminal affected in earliest stages
p-Bromophenylacetyl urea	Peripheral neuropathy	Axonal degeneration in the peripheral nervous system (PNS) and central nervous system (CNS)
Carbon disulfide	Psychosis (acute), peripheral neuropathy (chronic)	Axonal degeneration, early stages include neurofilamentous swelling
Chlordecone (Kepone)	Tremors, in coordination (experimental animals)	Insufficient data (humans); axonal swelling and degeneration
Chloroquine	Peripheral neuropathy, weakness	Axonal degeneration, inclusions in dorsal root ganglion cells; also vacuolar myopathy
Clioquinol	Encephalopathy (acute), subacute myelooptic neuropathy (subacute)	Axonal degeneration, spinal cord, PNS, optic tracts
Colchicine	Peripheral neuropathy	Axonal degeneration, neuronal perikaryal filamentous aggregates; vacuolar myopathy
Dapsone	Peripheral neuropathy, predominantly motor	Axonal degeneration (both myelinated and unmyelinated axons)
Dichlorophenoxyacetate	Peripheral neuropathy (delayed)	Insufficient data
Dimethylaminopropionitrile	Peripheral neuropathy, urinary retention	Axonal degeneration (both myelinated and unmyelinated axons)
Ethylene oxide	Peripheral neuropathy	Axonal degeneration
Glutethimide	Peripheral neuropathy (predominantly sensory)	Insufficient data
Gold	Peripheral neuropathy (may have psychiatric problems)	Axonal degeneration, some segmental demyelination
n-Hexane	Peripheral neuropathy, severe cases have spasticity	Axonal degeneration, early neurofilamentous swelling, PNS, and spinal cord
Hydralazine	Peripheral neuropathy	Insufficient data
β,β'-Iminodipropionitrile	No data in humans; excitatory movement disorder (rats)	Proximal axonal swellings, degeneration of olfactory epithelial cells, vestibular hair cells
Isoniazid	Peripheral neuropathy (sensory), ataxia (high doses)	Axonal degeneration
Lithium	Lethargy, tremor, ataxia (reversible)	Insufficient data
Methyl n-butyl ketone	Peripheral neuropathy	Axonal degeneration, early neurofilamentous swelling, PNS, and spinal cord
Metronidazole	Sensory peripheral neuropathy, ataxia, seizures	Axonal degeneration, mostly affecting myelinated fibers; lesions of cerebellar nuclei
Misonidazole	Peripheral neuropathy	Axonal degeneration
Nitrofurantoin	Peripheral neuropathy	Axonal degeneration
Organophosphorus compounds (NTE inhibitors)	Abdominal pain (acute); peripheral neuropathy	Axonal degeneration
Paclitaxel (taxoids)	Delayed peripheral neuropathy (motor), spasticity	Axonal degeneration (delayed after single exposure), PNS, and spinal cord
Platinum (cisplatin)	Peripheral neuropathy	Axonal degeneration; microtubule accumulation in early stages
Pyridinethione (pyrithione)	Movement disorders (tremor, choreoathetosis)	Axonal degeneration (variable)
Vincristine (vinca alkaloids)	Cranial (most often trigeminal) neuropathy	Insufficient data
	Peripheral neuropathy, variable autonomic symptoms	Axonal degeneration (PNS), neurofibrillary changes (spinal cord, intrathecal route)

Organophosphorus Compounds—These compounds, which are used as pesticides and as additives in plastics and petroleum products, inhibit acetylcholinesterase and create a cholinergic excess. However, tri-*ortho*-cresyl phosphate (TOCP) causes a severe axonopathy without inducing cholinergic poisoning.

Some hydrophobic organophosphorus compounds readily enter the NS, where they alkylate or phosphorylate macromolecules and lead to delayed-onset neurotoxicity. Whereas "nontoxic" organophosphorus esters inhibit most of the esterase activity in the NS, there is another esterase activity, or *neuropathy target esterase* (NTE), that is inhibited by the neurotoxic organophosphorus esters. Furthermore, there is a good correlation between the potency of a given organophosphorus ester as an axonal toxicant and its potency as an inhibitor of NTE.

The degeneration of axons does not commence immediately after acute organophosphorus ester exposure but is delayed for 7 to 10 days between the acute high-dose exposure and the clinical signs of axonopathy. The axonal lesion in the PNS appears to be readily repaired, and the peripheral nerve becomes refractory to degeneration after repeated doses. By contrast, axonal degeneration in the long tracks of the spinal cord is progressive.

Pyridinethione—Zinc pyridinethione has antibacterial and antifungal properties and is a component of shampoos that are effective in the treatment of seborrhea and dandruff. Only the pyridinethione moiety is absorbed following ingestion, with the majority of zinc eliminated in the feces. Pyridinethione appears to interfere with the fast axonal transport systems, impairs the turnaround of rapidly transported vesicles, and slows the retrograde transport of vesicles. Aberration of the fast axonal transport systems most likely contributes to the accumulation of tubular and vesicular structures in the distal axon (Figure 16–6). As these materials accumulate in one region of

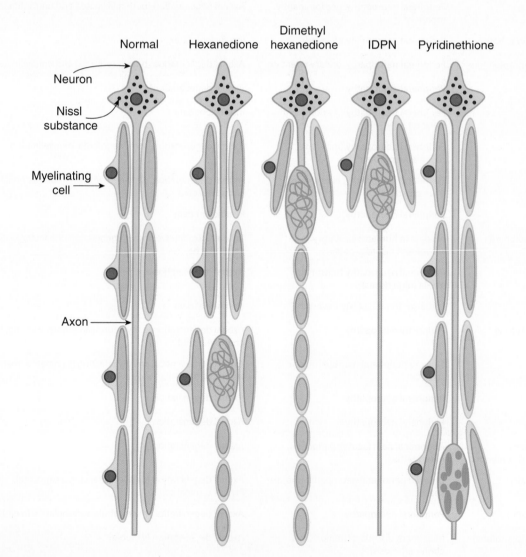

FIGURE 16–6   Diagram of axonopathies. Whereas 2,5-hexanedione results in the accumulation of neurofilaments in the distal regions of the axon, 3,4-dimethyl-2,5-hexanedione results in identical accumulation within the proximal segments. These proximal neurofilamentous swellings are quite similar to those that occur in the toxicity of β,β′-iminodipropionitrile (IDPN), although the distal axon does not degenerate in IDPN axonopathy but becomes atrophic. Pyridinethione results in axonal swellings that are distended with tubulovesicular material, followed by distal axonal degeneration.

TABLE 16–3 Compounds associated with injury of myelin (myelinopathies).

Neurotoxicant	Neurologic Findings	Basis of Neurotoxicity
Acetylethyltetramethyl tetralin (AETT)	Not reported in humans; hyperexcitability, tremors (rats)	Intramyelinic edema; pigment accumulation in neurons
Amiodarone	Peripheral neuropathy	Axonal degeneration and demyelination; lipid-laden lysosomes in Schwann cells
Cuprizone	Not reported in humans; encephalopathy (experimental animals)	Status spongiosis of white matter, intramyelinic edema (early stages); gliosis (late)
Disulfiram	Peripheral neuropathy, predominantly sensory	Axonal degeneration, swellings in distal axons
Ethidium bromide	Insufficient data (humans)	Intramyelinic edema, status spongiosis of white matter
Hexachlorophene	Irritability, confusion, seizures	Brain swelling, intramyelinic edema in CNS and PNS, late axonal degeneration
Lysolecithin	Effects only on direct injection into PNS or CNS (experimental animals)	Selective demyelination
Perhexilene	Peripheral neuropathy	Demyelinating neuropathy, membrane-bound inclusions in Schwann cells
Tellurium	Hydrocephalus, hind limb paralysis (experimental animals)	Demyelinating neuropathy, lipofuscinosis (experimental animals)
Triethyltin	Headache, photophobia, vomiting, paraplegia (irreversible)	Brain swelling (acute) with intramyelinic edema, spongiosis of white matter

the axon, the axon degenerates in its more distal regions beyond the accumulated structures. The earliest signs are diminished grip strength and changes of the axon terminal, leading to a peripheral neuropathy.

Microtubule-associated Neurotoxicity—The vinca alkaloids and colchicine, which bind to tubulin and inhibit the association of this protein subunit to form microtubules, produce peripheral neuropathies in patients. Although generally mild, they are often accompanied by a disabling myopathy that can lead to the inability to walk. Paclitaxel (Taxol), which stabilizes the assembled polymerized form of tubules, causes sensorimotor axonopathy and autonomic neuropathy in high doses.

The morphology of the axon is, of course, different in the two situations. In the case of colchicine, the axon appears to undergo atrophy and there are fewer microtubules within the axons. In contrast, following exposure to paclitaxel, microtubules are present in great numbers and are aggregated in arrays. Both situations probably interfere with the process of fast axonal transport, and both result in a peripheral neuropathy.

Myelinopathies

Myelin provides electrical insulation of neuronal processes, and its absence leads to a slowing of conduction and aberrant conduction of impulses between adjacent processes. Exposure to toxicants can result in either separation of the myelin lamellae, termed *intramyelinic edema*, or the selective loss of myelin, termed *demyelination*. Remyelination in the CNS occurs to

only a limited extent after demyelination. However, Schwann cells in the PNS are capable of remyelinating the axon.

All the compounds in Table 16–3 lead to a myelinopathy.

Hexachlorophene—Hexachlorophene, or methylene 2,2′-methylenebis(3,4,6-trichlorophenol), caused neurotoxicity when newborn infants were bathed with the compound to avoid staphylococcal skin infections. Following skin absorption of this hydrophobic compound, hexachlorophene enters the NS and results in intramyelinic edema, which leads to the formation of vacuoles creating a "spongiosis" of the brain. Hexachlorophene causes intramyelinic edema that leads to segmental demyelination. Swelling of the brain causes increased intracranial pressure, axonal degeneration, along with degeneration of photoreceptors in the retina. Humans exposed acutely to hexachlorophene may have generalized weakness, confusion, and seizures. Progression may occur, to include coma and death.

Tellurium—The neurotoxicity of tellurium in young rats alters the synthesis of myelin lipids in Schwann cells, because of various lipid abnormalities. As biochemical changes occur, lipids accumulate in Schwann cells, which eventually lose their ability to maintain myelin in the PNS.

Lead—Lead exposure in animals results in a peripheral neuropathy with prominent segmental demyelination. In young children, acute massive exposures to lead result in severe cerebral edema, perhaps from damage to endothelial cells. Children absorb lead more readily, and the very young do not have the protection of the blood–brain barrier. Chronic lead intoxication

TABLE 16–4 Compounds associated with neurotransmitter-associated toxicity.

Neurotoxicant	Neurologic Findings	Basis of Neurotoxicity
Amphetamine and methamphetamine	Tremor, restlessness (acute); cerebral infarction and hemorrhage; neuropsychiatric disturbances	Bilateral infarcts of globus pallidus, abnormalities in dopaminergic, serotonergic, cholinergic systems Acts at adrenergic receptors (PNS)
Atropine	Restlessness, irritability, hallucinations	Blocks cholinergic receptors (anticholinergic)
Cocaine	Increased risk of stroke and cerebral atrophy (chronic users); increased risk of sudden cardiac death; movement and psychiatric abnormalities, especially during withdrawal Decreased head circumference (fetal exposure)	Infarcts and hemorrhages; alteration in striatal dopamine neurotransmission Structural malformations in newborns
Domoic acid	Headache, memory loss, hemiparesis, disorientation, seizures	Neuronal loss, hippocampus and amygdala, layers 5 and 6 of neocortex Kainate-like pattern of excitotoxicity
Kainate	Insufficient data in humans; seizures in animals (selective lesioning compound in neuroscience)	Degeneration of neurons in hippocampus, olfactory cortex, amygdala, thalamus Binds AMPA/kainate receptors
β-N-Methylamino-L-alanine (BMAA)	Weakness, movement disorder (monkeys)	Degenerative changes in motor neurons (monkeys) Excitotoxic probably via NMDA receptors
Muscarine (mushrooms)	Nausea, vomiting, headache	Binds muscarinic receptors (cholinergic)
Nicotine	Nausea, vomiting, convulsions	Binds nicotinic receptors (cholinergic) low-dose stimulation; high-dose blocking
β-N-Oxalylamino-L-alanine (BOAA)	Seizures	Excitotoxic probably via AMPA class of glutamate receptors

in adults results in peripheral neuropathy, gastritis, colicky abdominal pain, anemia, and the prominent deposition of lead in particular anatomical sites, creating lead lines in the gums and in the epiphyses of long bones in children. Lead in the peripheral nerve of humans slows nerve conduction. The basis of lead encephalopathy is unclear, although an effect on the membrane structure of myelin and myelin membrane fluidity has been shown.

Astrocytes

Astrocytes perform and regulate a wide range of physiologic functions in the CNS. The astrocyte appears to be a primary means of defense in the CNS following exposure to neurotoxicants, as a spatial buffering system for osmotically active ions, and as a depot for the sequestration and metabolic processing of endogenous molecules and xenobiotics.

Ammonia—At high CNS concentrations, ammonia produces seizures, resulting from its depolarizing action on cell membranes, whereas at lower concentrations, ammonia produces stupor and coma, consistent with its hyperpolarizing effects. Ammonia intoxication is associated with astrocytic swelling and morphological changes. Increased intracellular ammonia concentrations have also been implicated in the inhibition of neuronal glutamate precursor synthesis, resulting in diminished glutamatergic neurotransmission, changes in

neurotransmitter uptake (glutamate), and changes in receptor-mediated metabolic responses of astrocytes to neuronal signals.

Nitrochemicals—Organic nitrates are used for peripheral vasodilatation and reduction of blood pressure (nitroglycerine) in treatment of cardiovascular disease. Other members of the class have neurotoxic properties: (1) 1,3-dinitrobenzene (DNB) produces gliovascular lesions that target astrocytes in the periaqueductal gray matter of the brainstem and deep cerebellar roof nuclei and (2) metronidazole is associated with peripheral neuropathy characterized by paresthesias and dysesthesias.

Neurotransmission-associated Neurotoxicity

Numerous naturally occurring toxins as well as synthetic chemicals interact with intercellular communication via the process of neurotransmission (Table 16–4). This group of compounds may interrupt the transmission of impulses, block or accentuate synaptic communication, block reuptake of neurotransmitters, or interfere with second-messenger systems. As the targets of these drugs are located throughout the body, the responses are not localized; however, the responses are stereotyped in that each member of a class tends to have similar biological effects.

In terms of toxicity, most of the side effects of these drugs may be viewed as short-term interactions that are easily reversible. However, long-term use is associated with irreversible tardive dyskinesias, or facial grimaces.

Nicotine—Nicotine exerts its effects by binding to a subset of nicotinic cholinergic receptors. Smoking and "pharmacologic" doses of nicotine accelerate heart rate, elevate blood pressure, and constrict blood vessels within the skin as a result of stimulation of the ganglionic sympathetic NS.

The rapid rise in circulating levels of nicotine after acute overdose leads to excessive stimulation of nicotinic receptors, a process that is followed rapidly by ganglionic paralysis. Initial nausea, rapid heart rate, and perspiration are followed shortly by marked slowing of heart rate with a fall in blood pressure. Somnolence and confusion may occur, followed by coma; if death results, it is often the result of paralysis of the muscles of respiration.

Exposure to lower levels for longer duration, in contrast, is very common. The complications of smoking include cardiovascular disease, cancers, and chronic pulmonary disease. Chronic exposure to nicotine has effects on the developing fetus. Along with decreased birth weights, attention-deficit disorders are more common in children whose mothers smoke cigarettes during pregnancy.

Cocaine and Amphetamines—The euphoric and addictive properties of cocaine derive from enhanced dopaminergic neurotransmission, by blocking the dopamine reuptake transporter (DAT). Acute toxicity due to excessive intake, or overdose, may result in unanticipated death.

Although cocaine increases maternal blood pressure during acute exposure in pregnant animals, the blood flow to the uterus actually diminishes. Depending on the level of the drug in the mother, the fetus may develop marked hypoxia. Women who used cocaine during pregnancy had more miscarriages and placental hemorrhages (abruptions) than drug-free women.

In addition to deleterious effects on fetal growth and development, cocaine abuse is associated with an increased risk of cerebrovascular disease, cerebral perfusion defects, and cerebral atrophy in adults, along with neurodegenerative changes.

Like cocaine, amphetamines exert their effects in the CNS, altering catecholamine neurotransmission by competing for uptake via plasma membrane transporters and by disrupting the vesicular storage of dopamine. Amphetamines have been associated with an increased risk of abnormal fetal growth and development, increased risk of cerebrovascular disease, and increased risk of psychiatric and neurologic problems in chronic abusers.

Excitatory Amino Acids—Glutamate and certain other acidic amino acids are excitatory neurotransmitters within the CNS. The toxicity of glutamate can be blocked by certain glutamate antagonists, and the concept has emerged that the toxicity of excitatory amino acids may be related to such conditions as hypoxia, epilepsy, and neurodegenerative diseases.

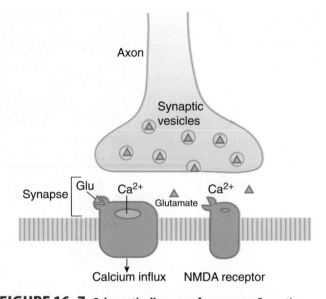

FIGURE 16–7 Schematic diagram of a synapse. Synaptic vesicles are transported to the axonal terminus, and released across the synaptic cleft to bind to the postsynaptic receptors. Glutamate, as an excitatory neurotransmitter, binds to its receptor and opens a calcium channel, leading to the excitation of the postsynaptic cell.

Glutamate is the main excitatory neurotransmitter of the brain and its effects are mediated by several subtypes of receptors (Figure 16–7) called *excitatory amino acid receptors* (EAARs). The two major subtypes of glutamate receptors are those that are ligand-gated directly to ion channels (ionotropic) and those that are coupled with G proteins (metabotropic). Ionotropic receptors may be further subdivided by their specificity for binding kainate, quisqualate, α-amino-3-hydroxy-5-methylisoxazole-4-propionic acid (AMPA), and N-methyl-D-aspartate (NMDA). The entry of glutamate into the CNS is regulated at the blood–brain barrier, and glutamate exerts its effects in the circumventricular organ of the brain in which the blood–brain barrier is least developed. Within this site of limited access, glutamate injures neurons, apparently by opening glutamate-dependent ion channels, ultimately leading to neuronal swelling and neuronal cell death. The only known related human condition is the "Chinese restaurant syndrome," in which consumption of large amounts of monosodium glutamate as a seasoning may lead to a burning sensation in the face, neck, and chest.

The cyclic glutamate analog kainate, isolated from a seaweed in Japan, is extremely potent as an excitotoxin, being a hundredfold more toxic than glutamate, and is selective at a molecular level for the kainate receptor. Like glutamate, kainate selectively injures dendrites and neurons and shows no substantial effect on glia or axons. Injected into a region of the brain, it can destroy the neurons of that area without disrupting all of the fibers that pass through the same region. Kainate has become a tool for neurobiologists to explore the anatomy and function of the NS. Kainate, through its selective action on neuronal cell bodies, has provided a greater understanding of

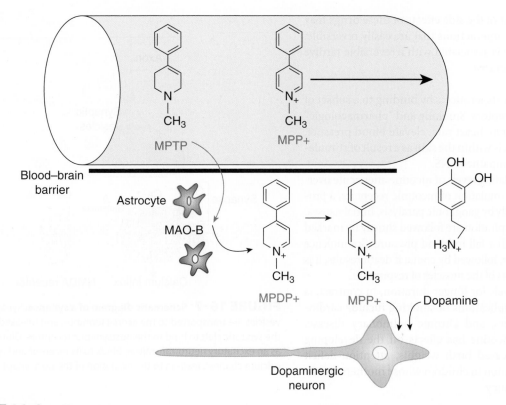

FIGURE 16–8 **MPTP toxicity.** MPP$^+$, either formed elsewhere in the body following exposure to MPTP or injected directly into the blood, is unable to cross the blood–brain barrier. In contrast, MPTP gains access and is oxidized in situ to MDDP$^+$ and MPP$^+$. The same transport system that carries dopamine into the dopaminergic neurons also transports the cytotoxic MPP$^+$.

the functions of cells within a specific region of the brain, whereas previous lesioning techniques addressed only regional functions. This void in understanding and the epidemiologic evidence that some neurodegenerative diseases may have environmental contributors inspire a heightened desire to appreciate more fully the effects of elements of our environment on the NS.

Development of permanent neurologic deficits occurred in individuals accidentally exposed to high doses of the EAAR agonist domoic acid, an analog of glutamate. The acute illness most commonly presented as gastrointestinal disturbance, severe headache, and short-term memory loss. A subset of the more severely afflicted patients had chronic memory deficits and motor neuropathy. Neuropathologic investigation of patients who died within 4 months of intoxication showed neurodegeneration that was most prominent in the hippocampus and amygdala.

Models of Neurodegenerative Disease

MPTP—A contaminant formed during meperidine synthesis, 1-methyl-4-phenyl-1,2,3,6-tetrahydropyridine (MPTP) (Figure 16–8), produces over hours to days the signs and symptoms of irreversible Parkinson's disease. Autopsy studies have dem-

onstrated marked degeneration of dopaminergic neurons in the substantia nigra, with degeneration continuing many years after exposure. It appears that MPTP is metabolized to a molecule that enters the dopaminergic neurons of the substantia nigra, resulting in their deaths.

Although not identical, MPTP neurotoxicity and Parkinson's disease are strikingly similar. The symptomatology of each reflects a disruption of the nigrostriatal pathway: masked facies, difficulties in initiating and terminating movements, resting "pill-rolling" tremors, rigidity, and bradykinesias are all features of both conditions.

Manganese—As an essential trace metal that is found in all tissues, manganese (Mn) is required for normal metabolism of amino acids, proteins, lipids, and carbohydrates, acting as a cofactor of synthesis enzymes. Excessive exposure to Mn produces neurotoxicity resulting in psychologic and neurologic disturbances, including delusions, hallucinations, depression, disturbed equilibrium, compulsive or violent behavior, weakness, and apathy, followed by extrapyramidal motor system defects such as tremors, muscle rigidity, ataxia, bradykinesia, and dystonia. Mn toxicity causes a loss of dopamine neurons in the substantia nigra, and as in Parkinson's disease, oxidative stress appears to play a significant role in the disorder.

CHEMICALS THAT INDUCE DEPRESSION OF NERVOUS SYSTEM FUNCTION

Generalized depression of CNS function is produced by a variety of volatile solvents that are small lipophilic molecules. Human exposures range from chronic low-level concentrations encountered in environmental or occupational setting to high-level concentrations intentionally generated through solvent abuse. Recent research has implicated interactions with ligand-gated ion channels as well as voltage-gated calcium channels as the mechanism of generalized depression.

BIBLIOGRAPHY

Bellinger D: *Human Developmental Neurotoxicity*. New York: Taylor and Francis, 2006.

Berent S, Albers JW: *Neurobehavioral Toxicology: Neuropsychological and Neurological Perspectives*. New York: Taylor and Francis, 2005.

Dobbs MR: *Clinical Neurotoxicology: Syndromes, Substances, Environments*. Philadelphia: Saunders Elsevier, 2009.

Massaro EJ (ed): *Handbook of Neurotoxicology*. Totowa, NJ: Humana Press, 2002.

Webster LR: *Neurotoxicity Syndromes*. New York: Nova Biomedical, 2007.

QUESTIONS

1. Which of the following statements regarding axons and/ or axonal transport is FALSE?
   a. Single nerve cells can be over 1 m in length.
   b. Fast axonal transport is responsible for movement of proteins from the cell body to the axon.
   c. Anterograde transport is accomplished by the protein kinesin.
   d. The motor proteins, kinesin and dynein, are associated with microtubules.
   e. A majority of the ATP in nerve cells is used for axonal transport.

2. Which of the following statements is not characteristic of Schwann cells in Wallerian degeneration?
   a. Schwann cells provide physical guidance needed for the regrowth of the axon.
   b. Schwann cells release trophic factors that stimulate growth.
   c. Schwann cells act to clear the myelin debris with the help of macrophages.
   d. Schwann cells increase synthesis of myelin lipids in response to axonal damage.
   e. Schwann cells are responsible for myelination of axons in the peripheral nervous system.

3. Prenatal exposure to ethanol can result in mental retardation and hearing deficits in the newborn. What is the cellular basis of the neurotoxicity?
   a. neuronal loss in cerebellum.
   b. acute cortical hemorrhage.
   c. microcephaly.
   d. loss of hippocampal neurons.
   e. degeneration of the basal ganglia.

4. Which of the following characteristics is LEAST likely to place a neuron at risk of toxic damage?
   a. high metabolic rate.
   b. ability to release neurotransmitters.
   c. long neuronal processes supported by the soma.
   d. excitable membranes.
   e. large surface area.

5. The use of meperidine contaminated with MPTP will result in a Parkinson's disease-like neurotoxicity. Where is the most likely site in the brain that MPTP exerts its toxic effects?
   a. cerebellum.
   b. cerebral cortex.
   c. brainstem.
   d. substantia nigra.
   e. hippocampus.

6. Which of the following statements regarding the PNS and the CNS is TRUE?
   a. Nerve impulse transduction is much faster in the CNS than in the PNS.
   b. PNS axons can regenerate, whereas CNS axons cannot.
   c. Remyelination does not occur in the CNS.
   d. Oligodendrocytes perform remyelination in the PNS.
   e. In the CNS, oligodendrocyte scarring interferes with axonal regeneration.

7. Platinum (cisplatin) results in which of the following neurologic problems?
   a. peripheral neuropathy.
   b. trigeminal neuralgia.
   c. spasticity.
   d. gait ataxia.
   e. tremor.

8. Which of the following is NOT characteristic of axonopathies?
   a. There is degeneration of the axon.
   b. The cell body of the neuron remains intact.
   c. Axonopathies result from chemical transaction of the axon.
   d. A majority of axonal toxicants cause motor deficits.
   e. Sensory and motor deficits are first noticed in the hands and feet following axonal degeneration.

9. All of the following statements regarding lead exposure are true EXCEPT:
   a. Lead exposure results in peripheral neuropathy.
   b. Lead slows peripheral nerve conduction in humans.
   c. Lead causes the transection of peripheral axons.
   d. Segmental demyelination is a common result of lead ingestion.
   e. Lead toxicity can result in anemia.

10. Regarding excitatory amino acids, which of the following statements is FALSE?
    a. Glutamate is the most common excitatory amino acid in the CNS.
    b. Excitotoxicity has been linked to conditions such as epilepsy.
    c. Overconsumption of monosodium glutamate (MSG) can result in a tingling or burning sensation in the face and neck.
    d. An ionotropic glutamate receptor is coupled to a G protein.
    e. Glutamate is toxic to neurons.

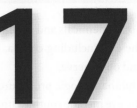
Toxic Responses of the Ocular and Visual System[1]

Donald A. Fox and William K. Boyes

---

[1]This chapter has been reviewed by the National Health and Environmental Effects Research Laboratory, U.S. EPA, and approved for publication.

INTRODUCTION TO OCULAR AND VISUAL SYSTEM TOXICOLOGY

Environmental and occupational exposure to toxic chemicals, gases, and vapors as well as side effects resulting from therapeutic drugs frequently results in structural and functional alterations in the eye and central visual system. The retina and central visual system are especially vulnerable to toxic insult.

EXPOSURE TO THE EYE AND VISUAL SYSTEM

Ocular Pharmacodynamics and Pharmacokinetics

Toxic chemicals and systemic drugs can affect all parts of the eye (Figure 17–1; Table 17–1). Factors determining whether a chemical can reach a particular ocular site of action include physiochemical properties of the chemical, concentration and duration of exposure, and movement across ocular compartments and barriers. The cornea, conjunctiva, and eyelids are often exposed directly to chemicals, gases, and particles. The first site of action is the tear film, a three-layered structure with both hydrophobic and hydrophilic properties. The outermost thin tear film layer is secreted by the meibomian (sebaceous) glands. This superficial lipid layer protects the underlying thicker aqueous layer that is produced by the lacrimal glands. The third layer is the very thin mucoid layer that is secreted by the goblet cells of the conjunctiva and acts as an interface between the hydrophilic layer of the tears and the hydrophobic layer of the corneal epithelial cells.

The avascular cornea is considered the external barrier to the internal ocular structures. Greater systemic absorption occurs through contact with the vascularized conjunctiva (Figure 17–2). The human cornea has several distinct layers through which a chemical must pass in order to reach the anterior chamber. The first is the corneal epithelium of stratified squamous, nonkeratinized cells with tight junctions. The permeability of the corneal epithelium is low and only lipid-soluble chemicals readily pass through this layer. Bowman's

membrane separates the epithelium from the stroma. The corneal stroma makes up 90 percent of the corneal thickness and is composed of water, collagen, and glycosaminoglycans, which permits hydrophilic chemicals to easily dissolve in this thick layer. The inner edge of the corneal stroma is bounded by a thin basement membrane, called Descemet's membrane, which is secreted by the corneal endothelium. The innermost layer of the cornea, the corneal endothelium, is composed of a single layer of cells that are surrounded by lipid membranes. The permeability of the corneal endothelial cells to ionized chemicals is relatively low.

The two separate vascular systems in the eye are: (1) the uveal blood vessels, which include the vascular beds of the iris, ciliary body, and choroid, and (2) the retinal vessels. In the anterior segment of the eye, there is a blood–aqueous barrier that has relatively tight junctions between the endothelial cells of the iris capillaries and nonpigmented cells of the ciliary epithelium. The major function of the ciliary epithelium is to produce aqueous humor from the plasma filtrate present in the ciliary processes.

In humans and several widely used experimental animals (e.g., monkeys, pigs, dogs, rats, and mice), the retina has a dual circulatory supply: choroidal and retinal. The retina consists of the outer plexiform layer (OPL), inner nuclear layer (INL), inner plexiform layer (IPL), and ganglion cell layer (GCL). The endothelial cells of capillaries of the retinal vessels have tight junctions forming the blood–retinal barrier. However, at the level of the optic disk, the blood–retinal barrier is lacking and thus hydrophilic molecules can enter the optic nerve (ON) head by diffusion from the extravascular space and cause selective damage at this site of action. The outer or distal retina, which consists of the retinal pigment epithelium (RPE), rod and cone photoreceptor outer segments (ROS and COS) and inner segments (RIS and CIS), and the photoreceptor outer nuclear layer (ONL) are avascular. These areas of the retina are supplied by the choriocapillaris: a dense, one-layered network of fenestrated vessels formed by the short posterior ciliary arteries and located next to the RPE. Consistent with their known structure and function, these capillaries have loose endothelial junctions and abundant fenestrae; they are highly permeable to large proteins.

for causing undue pain and distress to the tested animals. These criticisms have spawned development of alternative methods or strategies to evaluate compounds for their potential to cause ocular irritation.

Ophthalmologic Evaluations

There are many ophthalmologic procedures for evaluating the health of the eye. Procedures available range from fairly routine clinical screening evaluations to sophisticated techniques for very targeted purposes. Examination of the adnexa includes evaluating the eyelids, lacrimal apparatus, and palpebral (covering the eyelid) and bulbar (covering the eye) conjunctiva. The anterior structures or anterior segment include the cornea, iris, lens, and anterior chamber. The posterior structures, referred to as the *ocular fundus,* include the retina, retinal vasculature, choroid, ON, and sclera. The adnexa and surface of the cornea can be examined initially with the naked eye, a hand-held light, or a slit-lamp biomicroscope, using a mydriatic drug (which causes pupil dilation) if the lens is to be observed. The width of the reflection of a thin beam of light projected from the slit-lamp is an indication of the thickness of the cornea and may be used to evaluate corneal edema. Lesions of the cornea can be better visualized with the use of fluorescein dye, which is retained where there is an ulceration of the corneal epithelium. Examination of the fundus requires use of a mydriatic drug and a direct or an indirect ophthalmoscope.

An ophthalmologic examination of the eye may also involve an examination of the pupillary light reflex. The direct pupillary reflex involves shining a bright light into the eye and observing the reflexive pupil constriction in the same eye. The consensual pupillary reflex is observed in the eye not stimulated. Both the direct and consensual pupillary light reflexes are dependent on function of a reflex arc involving cells in the retina, which travel through the ON, optic chiasm, and optic tract (OT) to project to neurons in the pretectal area. The absence of a pupillary reflex is indicative of damage somewhere in the reflex pathway, and differential impairment of the direct or consensual reflexes can indicate the location of the lesion. The presence of a pupillary light reflex, however, is not synonymous with normal visual function. Pupillary reflexes can be maintained even with substantial retinal damage. In addition, lesions in visual areas outside of the reflex pathway, such as in the visual cortex, may also leave the reflex function intact.

Electrophysiologic Techniques

Most electrophysiologic or neurophysiologic procedures for testing visual function in a toxicologic context involve stimulating the eyes with visual stimuli and electrically recording potentials generated by visually responsive neurons. The most commonly used procedures are the flash-evoked electroretinogram (ERG), visual-evoked potentials (VEPs), and, less often, the electrooculogram (EOG).

ERGs are typically elicited with a brief flash of light and recorded from an electrode placed in contact with the cornea.

A typical ERG waveform includes an a-wave that reflects the activation of photoreceptors and a b-wave that reflects the activity of retinal bipolar cells (BC) and associated membrane potential changes in Müller cells (MC). A standard set of ERG procedures includes the recording of (1) a response reflective of only rod photoreceptor function in the dark-adapted eye, (2) the maximal response in the dark-adapted eye, (3) a response developed by cone photoreceptors, (4) oscillatory potentials, and (5) the response to rapidly flickered light.

Flash-elicited VEPs are recorded from electrodes overlying visual (striate) cortex, and they reflect the activity of the retinogeniculostriate pathway and the activity of cells in the visual cortex. Pattern-elicited VEPs (PEPs), which are widely used in human clinical evaluations, have diagnostic value.

The EOG is generated by a potential difference between the front and back of the eye, which originates primarily within the RPE. The magnitude of the EOG is a function of the level of illumination and health status of the RPE. Electrodes placed on the skin on a line lateral or vertical to the eye measure potential changes correlated with eye movements as the relative position of the ocular dipole changes. Thus, the EOG finds applications in assessing both RPE status and measuring eye movements. The EOG is also used in monitoring eye movements during the recording of other brain potentials, so that eye movement artifacts are not misinterpreted as brain-generated electrical activity.

Behavioral and Psychophysical Techniques

Behavioral testing procedures typically vary the parameters of the visual stimulus and then determine whether the subject can discriminate or perceive the stimulus. *Contrast sensitivity* refers to the ability to resolve small differences in luminance contrast, such as the difference between subtle shades of gray or a series of visual patterns that differ in pattern size, or the luminance changes across the pattern in a sinusoidal profile. Contrast sensitivity functions are dependent primarily on the neural as opposed to the optic properties of the visual system. The assessment of visual acuity and contrast sensitivity has been recommended for field studies of humans potentially exposed to neurotoxic substances.

Color vision deficits are either inherited or acquired. Most acquired color vision deficits, such as those caused by drug and chemical exposure, begin with a reduced ability to perform blue–yellow discriminations. With increased or prolonged low-level exposure, the color confusion can progress to the red–green axis as well. Because of the rarity of inherited tritanopia, it is generally assumed that blue–yellow deficits, when observed, are acquired deficits. Generally, disorders of the outer retina produce blue–yellow deficits, whereas disorders of the inner retina and ON produce red–green perceptual deficits. Bilateral lesions in the visual cortex can also lead to color blindness.

Assessment of color vision in human toxicologic evaluations includes the Farnsworth–Munson 100 Hue (FM-100) test and the simplified 15-chip tests using either the saturated hues of the Farnsworth D-15 or the desaturated hues of the

Lanthony Desaturated Panel D-15. The Farnsworth–Munson procedure involves arrangement of 85 chips in order of progressively changing color. The relative chromatic value of successive chips induces those with color perception deficits to abnormally arrange the chips. The pattern is indicative of the nature of the color perception anomaly. The FM-100 is considered more diagnostically reliable but takes considerably longer to administer than the similar but more efficient Farnsworth and Lanthony tests. The desaturated hues of the Lanthony D-15 are designed to better identify subtle acquired color vision deficits.

TARGET SITES AND MECHANISMS OF ACTION: CORNEA

The cornea provides three essential functions. First, it must provide a clear refractive surface and the curvature of the cornea must be correct for the visual image to be focused at the retina. Second, the cornea provides tensile strength to maintain the appropriate shape of the globe. Third, the cornea protects the eye from external factors, including potentially toxic chemicals.

The cornea is transparent to wavelengths of light ranging between 310 nm (UV) and 2500 nm (IR). Exposure to UV light below this range can damage the cornea. It is most sensitive to wavelengths of approximately 270 nm. Excessive UV exposure leads to photokeratitis and corneal pathology, the classic example being welder's-arc burns. Also, the cornea can be damaged by topical or systemic exposure to chemicals.

Direct chemical exposure to the eye requires emergency medical attention. Products at pH extremes ≤2.5 or ≥11.5 can cause severe ocular damage and permanent loss of vision. Damage that extends to the corneal endothelium is associated with poor repair and recovery. The most important therapy is immediate and adequate irrigation with large amounts of water or saline, whichever is most readily available. The extent of damage to the eye and the ability to achieve a full recovery are dependent on the nature of the chemical, the concentration and duration of exposure, and the speed and magnitude of the initial irrigation.

Acids

Among the most significant acidic chemicals in terms of the tendency to cause clinical ocular damage are hydrofluoric acid, sulfurous acid, sulfuric acid, and chromic acid, followed by hydrochloric and nitric acid and finally acetic acid. Injuries may be mild if contact is with weak acids or with dilute solutions of strong acids. Compounds with a pH between 2.5 and 7 produce pain or stinging, but with only a brief contact, they will cause no lasting damage. Following mild burns, the corneal epithelium may become turbid as the corneal stroma swells (chemosis). Mild burns are typically followed by rapid regeneration of the corneal epithelium and full recovery. In more severe burns, the epithelium of the cornea and conjunctiva become opaque and necrotic and may disintegrate over the course of a few days. In severe burns, there may be no sensation of pain because the corneal nerve endings are destroyed.

Acid chemical burns of the cornea occur through hydrogen ion-induced denaturing and coagulation of proteins. As epithelial cell proteins coagulate, glycosaminoglycans precipitate and stromal collagen fibers shrink. These events cause the cornea to become cloudy. The protein coagulation and shrinkage of the collagen is protective in that it forms a barrier and reduces further penetration of the acid. The collagen shrinkage, however, contracts the eye and can lead to a dangerous acute increase in intraocular pressure.

Bases or Alkalies

Compounds with a basic pH are potentially even more damaging to the eye than are strong acids. Among the compounds of clinical significance in terms of frequency and severity of injuries are ammonia or ammonium hydroxide, sodium hydroxide (lye), potassium hydroxide (caustic potash), calcium hydroxide (lime), and magnesium hydroxide. One reason that caustic agents are so dangerous is their ability to rapidly penetrate the ocular tissues. The toxicity of these substances is a function of their pH, being more toxic with increasing pH values. Rapid and extensive irrigation after exposure and removal of particles, if present, is the immediate therapy of choice.

Two phases of injury may be observed with caustic burns. There is an acute phase from time of exposure up to 1 week. Depending on the extent of injury, direct damage from exposure is observed in the cornea, adnexia, and possibly the iris, ciliary body, and lens. Strong alkali substances attack membrane lipids, causing necrosis, hydration of the collagen matrix, and corneal swelling. Intraocular pressure may increase. Conversely, if the alkali burn extends to involve the ciliary body, the intraocular pressure may decrease due to reduced formation of aqueous humor. The acute phase of damage is typically followed by initiation of corneal repair. The repair process may involve corneal neovascularization along with regeneration of the corneal epithelium. Approximately 2 to 3 weeks after alkali burns, however, damaging ulceration of the corneal stroma often occurs as a result of inflammatory infiltration of polymorphonuclear leukocytes and fibroblasts and the release of degratory proteolytic enzymes. Stromal ulceration usually stops when the corneal epithelium is restored.

Organic Solvents

When organic solvents are splashed into the eye, the result is typically a painful immediate reaction. Exposure of the eye to solvents should be treated rapidly with abundant water irrigation. Highly lipophilic solvents can damage the corneal epithelium and produce swelling of the corneal stroma. Most organic solvents cause minimal chemical burns to the cornea. In most cases, the corneal epithelium will be repaired over the course of a few days and there will be no residual damage. Exposure to solvent vapors may produce small transparent vacuoles in the corneal epithelium, which may be asymptomatic or associated with moderate irritation and tearing.

Surfactants

These compounds have water-soluble (hydrophilic) properties at one end of the molecule and lipophilic properties at the other end that help to dissolve fatty substances in water and also serve to reduce water surface tension. The widespread use of these agents in soaps, shampoos, detergents, cosmetics, and similar consumer products leads to abundant opportunities for exposure to ocular tissues. Many of these agents may be irritating or injurious to the eye. In general, cationic surfactants tend to be stronger irritants and more injurious than the other types, and anionic compounds more so than neutral ones. Because these compounds are soluble in both aqueous and lipid media, they readily penetrate the sandwiched aqueous and lipid barriers of the cornea.

TARGET SITES AND MECHANISMS OF ACTION: LENS

The lens of the eye plays a critical role in focusing the visual image on the retina. The lens is a biconvex transparent body, encased in an elastic capsule, and located between the pupil and the vitreous humor (Figure 17–1). The mature lens has a dense inner nuclear region surrounded by the lens cortex. The high transparency of the lens to visible wavelengths of light is a function of its chemical composition, approximately two-thirds water and one-third protein, and the special organizational structure of the lenticular proteins. Nutrients are provided from the aqueous and vitreous fluids and are transported into the lens substance through a system of intercellular gap-type junctions. The lens is a metabolically active tissue that maintains careful electrolyte and ionic balance. The lens continues to grow throughout life, with new cells added to the epithelial margin of the lens as the older cells condense into a central nuclear region. The dramatic growth of the lens is illustrated by its increasing weight, from approximately 150 mg at 20 years of age to approximately 250 mg at 80 years of age.

Cataracts are decreases in the optic transparency of the lens that ultimately can lead to functional visual disturbances. Cataracts can occur at any age; they can also be congenital. Risk factors for the development of cataracts include aging, diabetes, low antioxidant levels, and exposure to a variety of environmental factors, including exposure to UV radiation and visible light, trauma, smoking, and exposure to a large variety of topical and systemic drugs and chemicals. Several different mechanisms of action have been hypothesized to account for the development of cataracts. Formation of high-molecular-weight aggregates involves the oxidation of protein thiol groups, which leads to a reduction in lens transparency and also impairments in membrane transport and permeability.

Light and Phototoxicity

The most important oxidizing agents are visible light and UV radiation, particularly UV-A (320 to 400 nm) and UV-B (290 to 320 nm), and other forms of electromagnetic radiation. Light- and UV-induced photooxidation leads to generation of reactive oxygen species, and oxidative damage that can accumulate over time. Higher energy UV-C (100 to 290 nm) is even more damaging. At sea level, the atmosphere filters out virtually all UV-C and all but a small fraction of UV-B derived from solar radiance. The cornea absorbs about 45 percent of light with wavelengths below 280 nm, but only about 12 percent between 320 and 400 nm. The lens absorbs much of the light between 300 and 400 nm and transmits 400 nm and above to the retina. Absorption of light energy in the lens triggers a variety of photoreactions, including the generation of fluorophores and pigments that lead to the yellow-brown coloration of the lens. Sufficient exposure to infrared radiation, as occurs to glassblowers, or microwave radiation will also produce cataracts through direct heating of the ocular tissues.

Drugs and other chemicals can mediate photoinduced toxicity in the cornea, lens, or retina. This occurs when the chemical structure allows absorption of light energy and the subsequent generation of activated intermediates, free radicals, and reactive oxygen species. The propensity of chemicals to cause phototoxic reactions can be predicted using photophysical and in vitro procedures.

Corticosteroids

There are two proposed mechanisms by which systemic treatment with corticosteroids may cause cataracts. Corticosteroids alter lens epithelium electrolyte balance, which disrupts the normal lens epithelial cell structure causing gaps to appear between the lateral epithelial cell borders. Another theory is that corticosteroid molecules react with lens crystallin proteins, producing corticosteroid–crystallin adducts that would be light-scattering complexes.

Naphthalene

Accidental exposure to naphthalene results in cortical cataracts and retinal degeneration. The metabolite 1,2-dihydro-1,2-dihydroxynaphthalene (naphthalene dihydrodiol) is the cataract-inducing agent. Subsequent studies showed that aldose reductase in the rat lens is the enzyme responsible for the formation of naphthalene dihydrodiol, and that treatment with aldose reductase inhibitors prevents naphthalene-induced cataracts.

Phenothiazines

Schizophrenics receiving phenothiazine drugs develop pigmented deposits in their eyes and skin. The phenothiazines combine with melanin to form a photosensitive product that reacts with sunlight, causing formation of the deposits in lens and cornea. The amount of pigmentation is related to the dose of the drug, with the annual yearly dose being the most predictive dose metric. More recent epidemiologic evidence demonstrates a dose-related increase in the risk of cataracts from use of nonantipsychotic phenothiazines.

TARGET SITES AND MECHANISMS OF ACTION: RETINA

The adult mammalian retina contains 9 distinct layers plus the RPE, 10 major types of neurons, and 3 cells with glial functions (Figure 17–1). The nine layers of the neural retina are the nerve fiber layer (NFL), GCL, IPL, INL, OPL, ONL, RIS and CIS, and the ROS and COS. The RPE is a single layer of cuboidal epithelial cells that lies on Bruch's membrane adjacent to the vascular choroid. Between the RPE and photoreceptor outer segments lies the subretinal space, which is similar to the brain ventricles. The major types of neurons are the rod (R) and cone (C) photoreceptors, (depolarizing) ON-rod and ON-cone BC, (hyperpolarizing) OFF-cone BC, horizontal cells (HC), numerous subtypes of amacrine cells (AC), an interplexiform cell (IPC), and retinal ganglion cells. The three cells with glial functions are the MC, fibrous astrocytes, and microglia. The somas of the MCs are in the INL. The end feet of the MCs in the proximal or inner retina along with a basal lamina form the internal limiting membrane (ILM) of the retina, which is similar to the pial surface of the brain. In the distal retinal, the MC end feet join with the photoreceptors and zonula adherens to form the external limiting membrane (ELM), which is located between the ONL and RIS/CIS.

The mammalian retina is highly vulnerable to toxicant-induced structural and/or functional damage due to (1) the presence of a highly fenestrated choriocapillaris that supplies the distal or outer retina as well as a portion of the inner retina; (2) the very high rate of oxidative mitochondrial metabolism, especially that in the photoreceptors; (3) high daily turnover of rod and cone outer segments; (4) high susceptibility of the rod and cones to degenerate due to inherited retinal dystrophies as well as associated syndromes and metabolic disorders; (5) presence of specialized ribbon synapses and synaptic contact sites; (6) presence of numerous neurotransmitter and neuromodulatory systems, including extensive glutamatergic, GABAergic, and glycinergic systems; (7) presence of numerous and highly specialized gap junctions used in the information signaling process; (8) presence of melanin in the choroid and RPE and also in the iris and pupil; (9) a very high choroidal blood flow rate, as high as 10 times that of the gray matter of the brain; and (10) the additive or synergistic toxic action of certain chemicals with ultraviolet and visible light.

Each of the retinal layers can undergo specific as well as general toxic effects. These alterations and deficits include but are not limited to visual field deficits, scotopic vision deficits such as night blindness and increases in the threshold for dark adaptation, cone-mediated (photopic) deficits such as decreased color perception, decreased visual acuity, macular and general retina edema, retinal hemorrhages and vasoconstriction, and pigmentary changes.

Retinotoxicity of Systemically Administered Therapeutic Drugs

Cancer Chemotherapeutics—Ocular toxicity is a common side effect of cancer chemotherapy, resulting in blurred vision, diplopia, decreased color vision and visual acuity, optic/retrobular neuritis, transient cortical blindness, and demyelination of the ONs. If not detected at an early stage of toxicity, the ocular complications are often irreversible even after chemotherapy is discontinued.

Chloroquine and Hydroxychloroquine—Chloroquine and hydroxychloroquine can cause irreversible loss of retinal function. Chloroquine, its major metabolite desethylchloroquine, and hydroxychloroquine have high affinity for melanin, which results in these drugs accumulating in the choroid and RPE, ciliary body, and iris during and following drug administration. Prolonged exposure of the retina to these drugs, especially chloroquine, may lead to an irreversible retinopathy. Doses of hydroxychloroquine less than 400 mg per day appear to produce little or no retinopathy even after prolonged therapy.

The clinical findings accompanying chloroquine retinopathy can be divided into early and late stages. The early changes include (1) the pathognomonic "bull's-eye retina" visualized as a dark, central pigmented area involving the macula, surrounded by a pale ring of depigmentation, which, in turn, is surrounded by another ring of pigmentation; (2) a diminished EOG; (3) possible granular pigmentation in the peripheral retina; and (4) visual complaints such as blurred vision and problems discerning letters or words. Late-stage findings, which can occur during or even following cessation of drug exposure, include (1) a progressive scotoma, (2) constriction of the peripheral fields commencing in the upper temporal quadrant, (3) narrowing of the retinal artery, (4) color and night blindness, (5) absence of a typical retinal pigment pattern, and (6) very abnormal EOGs and ERGs. These late-stage symptoms are irreversible.

Digoxin and Digitoxin—The cardiac glycosides digoxin and digitoxin induce visual system abnormalities such as decreased vision, flickering scotomas, and altered color vision. The photoreceptors are a primary target site of these cardiac glycosides. The retina has the highest number of Na^+,K^+-ATPase sites of any ocular tissue, which are potently inhibited by digoxin and digitoxin.

Indomethacin—Chronic administration of 50 to 200 mg per day of indomethacin for 1 to 2 years has been reported to produce corneal opacities, discrete pigment scattering of the RPE perifoveally, paramacular depigmentation, decreases in visual acuity, altered visual fields, increases in the threshold for dark adaptation, blue–yellow color deficits, and decreases in ERG and EOG amplitudes. Decreases in the ERG a- and b-wave amplitudes, with larger changes observed under scotopic dark-adapted than light-adapted conditions, have been reported. On cessation of drug treatment, the ERG waveforms and color vision changes return to near normal, although the pigmentary changes are irreversible. The mechanism of retinotoxicity is unknown.

Tamoxifen—Chronic high-dose therapy (180 to 240 mg per day for ~2 years) produces widespread axonal degeneration in the macular and perimacular areas. Clinical symptoms include a permanent decrease in visual acuity and abnormal visual fields, as the axonal degeneration is irreversible. Chronic low-dose tamoxifen (20 mg per day) can result in a small increase in the incidence of keratopathy, with minimal alterations in visual function. Following cessation of low-dose tamoxifen therapy, most of the keratopathy and retinal alterations, except the corneal opacities and retinopathy, are reversible.

Retinotoxicity of Known Neurotoxicants

Inorganic Lead—Lead poisoning (mean blood lead [BPb] ≥80 µg/dL) in humans produces amblyopia, blindness, optic neuritis or atrophy, peripheral and central scotomas, paralysis of eye muscles, and decreased visual function. Moderate- to high-level lead exposure produces scotopic and temporal visual system deficits in occupationally exposed factory workers, and developmentally lead-exposed monkeys and rats. This lead exposure dosage produces irreversible retinal deficits in the experimental animals. Occupational lead exposure produces concentration- and time-dependent alterations in the retina such that higher levels of lead directly and adversely affect both the retina and ON, whereas lower levels of lead appear to primarily affect the rod photoreceptors and the rod pathway. Furthermore, these retinal and oculomotor alterations were, in most cases, correlated with the blood lead levels and occurred in the absence of observable ophthalmologic changes, CNS symptoms, and abnormal performance test scores. Thus, these measures of temporal visual function may be among the most sensitive for the early detection of the neurotoxic effects of inorganic lead.

Methanol—Formic acid is the toxic metabolite of methanol that mediates the metabolic acidosis as well as the retinal and ON toxicity observed in humans, monkeys, and rats with a decreased capacity for folate metabolism. Human and nonhuman primates are highly sensitive to methanol-induced neurotoxicity due to their limited capacity to oxidize formic acid. The toxicity occurs in several stages. It first occurs as a mild CNS depression, followed by an asymptomatic 12 to 24 h latent period, followed by a syndrome consisting of formic acidemia, uncompensated metabolic acidosis, ocular and visual toxicity, coma, and possibly death. Acute methanol poisoning results in profound and permanent structural alterations in the retina and ON, and visual impairments ranging from blurred vision to decreased visual acuity and light sensitivity to blindness. Formate is directly toxic to Müller glial cell function as well as rod and cone photoreceptors. The mechanism of formate toxicity appears to involve a disruption in oxidative phosphorylation in photoreceptors, Müller glial cells, and ON.

Organic Solvents—Organic solvents produce structural alterations in rods and cones as well as functional alterations such as color vision deficits, decreased contrast sensitivity, and altered visual-motor performance. Dose–response color vision loss and decreases in the contrast sensitivity function occur in workers exposed to organic solvents such as trichlorethylene, alcohols, xylene, toluene, n-hexane, styrene, mixtures of these, and others. Adverse effects usually occur only at concentrations above the occupational exposure limits.

Organophosphates—Various organophosphates produce retinotoxicity and chronic ocular damage. The evidence for organophosphate-induced retinal toxicity is strongest for fenthion (dimethyl 3-methyl-4-methylthiophenyl phosphorothionate).

TARGET SITES AND MECHANISMS OF ACTION: OPTIC NERVE AND TRACT

The ON consists primarily of RGC axons carrying visual information from the retina to several distinct anatomical destinations in the CNS. Disorders of the ON may be termed *optic neuritis, optic neuropathy,* or *ON atrophy,* referring to inflammation, damage, or degeneration, respectively, of the ON. *Retrobulbar neuritis* refers to inflammation or involvement of the orbital portion of the ON posterior to the globe. Among the symptoms of ON disease are reduced visual acuity, contrast sensitivity, and color vision. Toxic effects observed in the ON may originate from damage to the ON fibers themselves or to the RGC somas that provide axons to the ON. A number of toxic and nutritional disorders can adversely affect the ON. Deficiency of thiamine, vitamin B_{12}, or zinc results in degenerative changes in ON fibers. A condition referred to as *alcohol–tobacco amblyopia* or simply as *toxic amblyopia* is observed in habitually heavy users of these substances and is associated with nutritional deficiency.

Carbon Disulfide

Carbon disulfide (CS_2) damages the peripheral and CNSs. In the visual system, workers exposed to CS_2 experience loss of visual function accompanied by observable lesions in the retinal vasculature. Central scotoma, depressed visual sensitivity in the peripheral visual field, optic atrophy, pupillary disturbances, blurred vision, and disorders of color perception have all been reported. The retinal and ON pathology produced by CS_2 are likely a direct neuropathologic action and not the indirect result of vasculopathy.

Ethambutol

The dextro isomer of ethambutol produces dose-related alterations in the visual system, such as blue–yellow and red–green dyschromatopsias, decreased contrast sensitivity, reduced visual acuity, and visual field loss. The earliest visual symptoms appear to be a decrease in contrast sensitivity and color vision. Impaired red–green color vision is the most frequently observed and reported complaint. The symptoms are primarily associated with one of the two forms of retrobulbar neuritis (i.e., optic neuropathy). The most common form, seen in almost all cases, involves the central ON fibers and typically results in a central or paracentral scotoma in the visual field and is associated with impaired red–green color vision and decreased visual acuity, whereas the second form involves the peripheral ON fibers and typically results in a peripheral scotoma and visual field loss.

TARGET SITES AND MECHANISMS OF ACTION: THE CENTRAL VISUAL SYSTEM

Many areas of the cerebral cortex are involved in the perception of visual information. The primary visual cortex receives the primary projections of visual information from the thalamus (LGN) and also from the superior colliculus. Neurons from the thalamus project to the visual cortex maintaining a topographic representation of the receptive field origin in the retina.

Lead

In addition to the well-documented retinal effects of lead (see above), lead exposure during adulthood or perinatal development produces structural, biochemical, and functional deficits in the visual cortex of humans, nonhuman primates, and rats. Quantitative morphometric studies in monkeys exposed to high levels of lead from birth or infancy to 6 years of age revealed a decrease in visual cortex (areas V1 and V2), cell volume density, and a decrease in the number of initial arborizations among pyramidal neurons. These alterations could partially contribute to the alterations in the amplitude and latency measures of the flash-evoked and pattern-reversal-evoked potentials in lead-exposed children, workers, monkeys, and rats, and the alterations in tasks assessing visual function in lead-exposed children.

Methyl Mercury

Visual deficits are a prominent feature of methyl mercury intoxication in adult humans. Methyl mercury-poisoned individuals experience a striking and progressive constriction of the visual field (peripheral scotoma). The narrowing of the visual world gives impression of looking through a long tunnel, hence the term *tunnel vision*. The damage is most severe in the regions of primary visual cortex subserving the peripheral visual field, with relative sparing of the cortical areas representing the central vision. Methyl mercury-poisoned individuals also experience poor night vision that is also attributable to peripheral visual field losses.

BIBLIOGRAPHY

Bartlett JD, Jaanus SD: *Clinical Ocular Pharmacology*, 5th ed. Boston: Butterworth-Heinemann, 2008.

Fraunfelder FT, Fraunfelder FW, Chambers WA: *Clinical Ocular Toxicology: Drugs, Chemicals, and Herbs*. Philadelphia: Elsevier Saunders, 2008.

Smolin G, Foster CS, Azar DT, Dohlman CH: *Smolin and Thoft's The Cornea: Scientific Foundations and Clinical Practice*. Philadelphia: Lippincott Williams and Wilkins, 2005.

QUESTIONS

1. In which of the following locations would one NOT find melanin?
   a. iris.
   b. ciliary body.
   c. retinal pigment epithelium (RPE).
   d. uveal tract.
   e. sclera.

2. Systemic exposure to drugs and chemicals is most likely to target which of the following retinal sites?
   a. RPE and ganglion cell layer.
   b. optic nerve and inner plexiform layer.
   c. RPE and photoreceptors.
   d. photoreceptors and ganglion cell layer.
   e. inner plexiform layer and RPE.

3. Which of the following structures is NOT part of the ocular fundus?
   a. retina.
   b. lens.
   c. choriod.
   d. sclera.
   e. optic nerve.

4. Drugs and chemicals in systemic blood have better access to which of the following sites because of the presence of loose endothelial junctions at that location?
   a. retinal choroid.
   b. inner retina.
   c. optic nerve.
   d. iris.
   e. ciliary body.

5. All of the following statements regarding ocular irritancy and toxicity are true EXCEPT:
   a. The Draize test involves instillation of a potentially toxic liquid or solid into the eye.
   b. The effect of the irritant in the Draize test is scored on a weighted scale for the cornea, iris, and conjunctiva.
   c. The Draize test usually uses one eye for testing and the other as a control.
   d. The Draize test has strong predictive value in humans.
   e. The cornea is evaluated for opacity and area of involvement in the Draize test.

6. Which of the following statements regarding color vision deficits is FALSE?
   a. Inheritance of a blue–yellow color deficit is common.
   b. Bilateral deficits in the visual cortex can lead to color blindness.
   c. Disorders of the outer retina produce blue–yellow deficits.
   d. Drug and chemical exposure most commonly results in blue–yellow color deficits.
   e. Disorders of the optic nerve produce red–green deficits.

7. A substance with which of the following pH values would be most damaging to the cornea?
   a. 1.0.
   b. 3.0.
   c. 7.0.
   d. 10.0.
   e. 12.0.

8. Which of the following statements concerning the lens is FALSE?
   a. UV radiation exposure is a common environmental risk factor for developing cataracts.
   b. Cataracts are opacities of the lens that can occur at any age.
   c. The lens continues to grow throughout one's life.
   d. Naphthalene and organic solvents both can cause cataracts.
   e. Topical treatment with corticosteroids can cause cataracts.

9. Which of the following is NOT a reason why the retina is highly vulnerable to toxicant-induced damage?
   a. presence of numerous neurotransmitter systems.
   b. presence of melanin in the RPE.
   c. high choroidal blood flow rate.
   d. high rate of oxidative mitochondrial metabolism.
   e. lack of gap junctions.

10. A deficiency in which of the following vitamins can result in degeneration of optic nerve fibers?
    a. vitamin A.
    b. vitamin B_3.
    c. vitamin C.
    d. vitamin B_{12}.
    e. vitamin E.

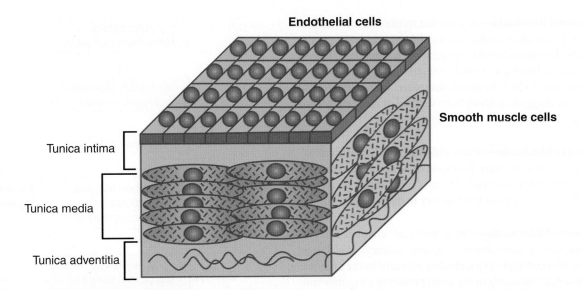

FIGURE 18–4 **Acute and chronic toxic exposure-induced heart failure and the transition from heart hypertrophy to heart failure.** Acute exposure to drugs or xenobiotics can cause cardiac arrhythmia, which is often observed. But if the toxic insult is too severe, then myocardial apoptosis and necrosis become predominant leading to dilated cardiomyopathy and heart failure. However, the heart often survives from toxic insults through adaptive mechanisms involving upregulation of hypertrophic genes and heart hypertrophy. Heart hypertrophy increases the risk for QT prolongation and sudden cardiac death, and also activates neurohormonal regulatory mechanisms including elevation of plasma concentration of sympathetic neural transmitters and angiotensins. These compensatory mechanisms in turn activate counter-regulatory mechanisms such as ANP, BNP, and TNF-α. A long-term action of the counter-regulatory mechanisms leads to myocardial remodeling and the transition from heart hypertrophy to heart failure.

produced by progressive cardiac hypertrophy, with impaired compliance of the ventricular walls and reduced diastolic ventricular filling.

Biomarkers for Cardiac Toxicity

In clinical practice and experimental approach, biomarkers are referred to as indexes of myocardial injury measured from blood samples. Molecules that are released from the myocardium under various injury conditions are readily detectable from blood samples. Table 18–1 lists current biomarkers of cardiac toxicity and the injuries/abnormalities they indicate.

GENERAL MECHANISMS OF CARDIOTOXICITY

Interference with Ion Homeostasis

Cardiac function is dependent on tight regulation of ion channel activity and ion homeostasis. Any xenobiotic that disrupts ion movement or homeostasis may induce a cardiotoxic reaction composed principally of disturbances in heart rhythm. Stress-induced Ca^{2+} overload in myocardial cells increases the likelihood of arrhythmia. Electrolyte imbalances exert a greater effect on compromised hearts.

Inhibition of Na^+,K^+-ATPase—Na^+,K^+-ATPase reduces intracellular Na^+ in exchange for extracellular K^+. Inhibition of cardiac Na^+,K^+-ATPase will increase resting intracellular Na^+

concentrations. This, in turn, will increase intracellular Ca^{2+} concentrations through Na^+/Ca^{2+} exchange, and the elevated intracellular Ca^{2+} and Ca^{2+} stores thus contribute to the inotropic actions of these agents.

TABLE 18–1 **Biomarkers for cardiac toxicity.**

Biomarker	Tissue Location	Proposed Cardiac Abnormality Indicated by Elevated Levels
Creatine kinase		
CK-MM	Skeletal muscle, myocardium	—
CK-BB	Brain, kidney	—
CK-MB	Myocardium	Acute myocardial infarction; peak values observed 18–24 h after infarction
Myoglobin	All muscle types, including myocardium	Acute myocardial infarction; peak values observed 1–4 h after infarction
B-type natriuretic peptide (BNP)	Ventricular myocardium	Volume pressure overload; ventricular wall tension; chronic heart failure
C-reactive protein (CRP)	Liver	Systemic and vascular inflammation
Cardiac troponins	Cardiomyocytes	Irreversible myocardial injury (i.e., myocardial infarction)

Na⁺ Channel Blockade—Agents that inhibit Na⁺ channels in cardiac cells will alter cardiac excitability by requiring greater membrane depolarization for opening of Na⁺ channels. Effects of Na⁺ channel blockade include reduction of conduction velocity, prolonged QRS duration, decreased automaticity, and inhibition of triggered activity from delayed or early afterdepolarizations.

K⁺ Channel Blockade—Many different K⁺ channels are expressed in the human heart. Blockade of K⁺ channels increases action potential duration and increases refractoriness (the cell undergoing repolarization is refractory to depolarization).

Ca²⁺ Channel Blockade—The L-type Ca²⁺ channel contributes to excitation–contraction coupling, whereas the T-type Ca²⁺ channels contribute to pacemaker potential in the SA node. Blockade of Ca²⁺ channels in the heart produces a negative inotropic effect due to reductions in Ca²⁺-induced Ca²⁺ release.

Altered Coronary Blood Flow

Catecholamines such as epinephrine normally enhance coronary blood flow indirectly through increased release of metabolic vasodilators and through a relative increase in diastolic duration at higher heart rates where epinephrine stimulation of beta-adrenergic receptors increases heart rate, contractility, and myocardial oxygen consumption. In contrast, the direct effect of sympathomimetics on the coronary vasculature includes coronary vasospasm through activation of alpha-adrenergic receptors. When beta-adrenergic receptors are blocked or during underlying pathophysiologic conditions of the heart, the direct actions of sympathomimetics may predominate, leading to coronary vasoconstriction.

With ischemic disease, relief of the offending cause of ischemia (e.g., thrombolytic therapy following acute myocardial infarction) provides reperfusion of the myocardium. However, depending on the duration of ischemia, a reversible contractile dysfunction remains for 1 to several days following reperfusion. And, reperfusion of the myocardium leads to subsequent tissue damage that may be reversible or permanent, a phenomenon known as ischemia–reperfusion (I/R) injury.

Intracellular acidosis, inhibition of oxidative phosphorylation, and ATP depletion are consequences of myocardial ischemia. Mechanisms proposed to account for the reperfusion injury include the generation of toxic oxygen radicals, Ca²⁺ overload, changes in cellular pH, uncoupling of mitochondrial oxidative phosphorylation, and physical damage to the sarcolemma.

Oxidative Stress

Reactive oxygen species are generated during myocardial ischemia and at the time of reperfusion. In atherosclerosis, oxidative alteration of low-density lipoprotein is thought to be involved in the formation of atherosclerotic plaques. Figure 18–5 summarizes the adverse effects of reactive oxygen radicals

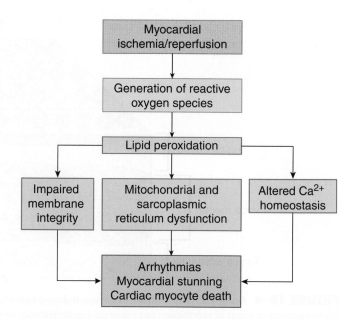

FIGURE 18–5 Deleterious effects of reactive oxygen species in myocardial ischemia and reperfusion.

generated during myocardial ischemia and reperfusion. Doxorubicin and ethanol may induce cardiotoxicity through generation of reactive oxygen species.

Organellar Dysfunction

Sarcolemmal Injury, SR Dysfunction, and Ca²⁺ Overload—All cells contain elaborate systems for the regulation of intracellular Ca²⁺. Because extracellular Ca²⁺ concentrations are typically several orders of magnitude higher than resting intracellular free Ca²⁺, the sarcolemmal membrane must prevent a rapid influx of Ca²⁺ and subsequent Ca²⁺ overload (sustained elevated intracellular free Ca²⁺ concentration). The principal Ca²⁺ regulatory organelle in cardiac myocytes is the sarcoplasmic reticulum (SR). Alterations of cardiac Ca²⁺ homeostasis by toxicants may perturb the regulation of cellular functions.

Mitochondrial Injury—ATP, the energy source required for work in most biological systems, is obtained mainly through the oxidative phosphorylation of adenine diphosphate (ADP) in the mitochondria. Oxidative phosphorylation can be affected at various sites along the respiratory chain by using different chemical inhibitors, such as rotenone, cyanide, or antimycin A. Conversely, uncouplers such as 2,4-dinitrophenol stimulate electron flow and respiration but prevent the formation of ATP by short-circuiting the normal flow of protons through ATP synthetase.

Apoptosis and Oncosis

In the early periods following myocardial infarction, ischemic injury, I/R injury, or toxicant-induced injury, cardiac myocyte death likely occurs through apoptotic pathways, whereas necrosis occurs at later time points following the insult. Several peptides and cytokines directly activate apoptotic signaling pathways and death of cardiac myocytes in vitro. Atrial natriuretic peptide (ANP), angiotensin II (also a hypertrophic growth stimulus), tumor necrosis factor alpha (TNF-α), and Fas ligand are elevated in the blood and myocardium during the progression of various cardiac diseases. Xenobiotics associated with induction of cardiac myocyte apoptosis in vitro include cocaine, daunorubicin, doxorubicin, isoproterenol, norepinephrine, and staurosporine.

CARDIOTOXICANTS

Pharmaceutical Agents

The cardiotoxicity of a cardiovascular drug often represents an overexpression of its principal pharmacologic effect on the heart. For example, digitalis, quinidine, and procainamide may induce cardiac arrhythmias as an exaggerated pharmacologic action of the drugs. In contrast, drugs may produce cardiotoxicity by actions that are not necessarily related to their intended therapeutic use and principal pharmacologic effects. Table 18–2 summarizes key pharmaceutical agents with their prominent cardiotoxic effects and proposed mechanisms of toxicity.

Alcohol and Alcoholic Cardiomyopathy—The acute toxicity of ethanol includes a reduced conductivity and a decreased threshold for ventricular fibrillation (rapid, repetitive excitation of the ventricles). Chronic consumption of ethanol by humans has been associated with myocardial abnormalities, arrhythmias, and a condition known as alcoholic cardiomyopathy that may present similar symptoms as congestive heart failure. Alcohol is believed to be the causal chemical in up to 40 percent of all patients with nonischemic, dilated cardiomyopathy. Metabolites from the metabolism of ethanol may lead to lipid peroxidation of cardiac myocytes or oxidation of cytosolic and membraneous protein thiols. For example, direct effects of acetaldehyde on the myocardium include inhibition of protein synthesis, inhibition of Ca^{2+} sequestration by the SR, alterations in mitochondrial respiration, and disturbances in the association of actin and myosin.

Cardiac Glycosides—Cardiac glycosides (digoxin and digitoxin) used for the treatment of congestive heart failure inhibit Na^+,K^+-ATPase, elevate intracellular Na^+, activate Na^+/Ca^{2+} exchange, and increase the availability of intracellular Ca^{2+} for contraction. Cardiotoxicity may result from Ca^{2+} overload, and arrhythmias may occur. Cardiac glycosides may also make the resting membrane potential less negative or induce delayed afterdepolarizations and premature ventricular contractions. Cardiac glycosides also exhibit parasympathomimetic activity through vagal stimulation; however, at higher doses, sympathomimetic effects may occur as sympathetic outflow is enhanced. The principal adverse cardiac effects of cardiac glycosides include slowed AV conduction with potential block, ectopic beats, and bradycardia. During overdose, ventricular tachycardia may develop and progress to ventricular fibrillation.

Sympathomimetics—Catecholamine-induced cardiotoxicity includes increased heart rate, enhanced myocardial oxygen demand, and an overall increase in systolic arterial blood pressure. These actions may cause myocardial hypoxia and, if severe enough, lead to the production of necrotic lesions in the heart. High concentrations of catecholamines also produce coronary insufficiency resulting from coronary vasospasm, decreased levels of high-energy phosphate stores caused by mitochondrial dysfunction, increased sarcolemmal permeability leading to electrolyte alterations, altered lipid metabolism resulting in the accumulation of fatty acids, intracellular Ca^{2+} overload, and apoptosis of cardiac myocytes.

Anthracyclines and Other Antineoplastic Agents—Doxorubicin and daunorubicin are antineoplastic agents whose clinical usefulness is limited because of cardiotoxicity. The acute effects mimic anaphylactic-type responses, such as tachycardia and various arrhythmias. These effects are usually manageable and most likely are due to the potent release of histamine from mast cells sometimes observed in acute dosing. Long-term exposure to anthracyclines often results in the development of cardiomyopathies and, in severe stages, congestive heart failure. Major hypotheses that have been suggested to account for the onset of anthracycline-induced cardiomyopathy are listed in Table 18–2.

Centrally Acting Drugs

Tricyclic Antidepressants—Standard tricyclic antidepressants have significant cardiotoxic actions, particularly in cases of overdose, that include EKG abnormalities and sudden cardiac death. As a result of peripheral alpha-adrenergic blockade, postural hypotension is a prevalent cardiovascular effect. Although many adverse effects are related to anticholinergic effects and adrenergic actions of these agents, the tricyclics also may have direct cardiotoxic actions on cardiac myocytes and Purkinje fibers, depressing inward Na^+ and Ca^{2+} and outward K^+ currents.

Antipsychotic Agents—Many antipsychotic agents exert profound cardiovascular effects, most commonly orthostatic hypotension. Antipsychotic drugs may alter cardiovascular function through indirect actions on the autonomic and central nervous systems and through direct actions on the myocardium. Direct effects on the myocardium include negative inotropic actions and quinidine-like effects.

General Anesthetics—The inhalational general anesthetics may reduce cardiac output by 20 to 50 percent, depress contractility, and produce arrhythmias. These anesthetics may sensitize the heart to the arrhythmogenic effects of endogenous epinephrine or to beta-receptor agonists. Halothane, as a prototype, may block Ca^{2+} channels, may disrupt Ca^{2+} homeostasis associated with the SR, and may modify the responsiveness of the contractile proteins to activation by Ca^{2+}.

Local Anesthetics—Local anesthetics interfere with the transmission of nerve impulses in other excitable organs, including the heart and circulatory system. The cardiotoxicity of

TABLE 18–2 Cardiotoxicity of key pharmaceutical agents.

Agents	Cardiotoxic Manifestations	Proposed Mechanisms of Cardiotoxicity
Ethanol	↓ Conductivity (acute) Cardiomyopathy (chronic)	Acetaldehyde (metabolite) Altered $[Ca^{2+}]_i$ homeostasis Oxidative stress Mitochondrial injury
Antiarrhythmic drugs		
Class I (disopyramide, encainide, flecainide, lidocaine, mexiletine, moricizine, phenytoin, procainamide, propafenone, quinidine, tocainide)	↓ Conduction velocity Proarrhythmogenic	Na^+ channel blockade
Class II (acebutolol, esmolol, propranolol, sotalol)	Bradycardia, heart block	β-Adrenergic receptor blockade
Class III (amiodarone, bretylium, dofetilide, ibutilide, quinidine, sotalol)	↑ Action potential duration QTc interval prolongation Proarrhythmogenic	K^+ channel blockade
Class IV (diltiazem, verapamil)	↓ AV conduction Negative inotropic effect Negative chronotropic effect Bradycardia	Ca^{2+} channel blockade
Inotropic drugs and related agents		
Cardiac glycosides (digoxin, digitoxin)	Action potential duration AV conduction Parasympathomimetic (low doses) Sympathomimetic (high doses)	Inhibition of Na^+,K^+-ATPase, $\uparrow[Ca^{2+}]_i$
Ca^{2+}-sensitizing agents (adibendan, levosimendan, pimobendan)	↓ Diastolic function? Proarrhythmogenic	↑ Ca^{2+} sensitivity Inhibition of phosphodiesterase
Other Ca^{2+}-sensitizing agents (allopurinol, oxypurinol)	?	Inhibition of xanthine oxidase
Catecholamines (dobutamine, epinephrine, isoproterenol, norepinephrine)	Tachycardia Cardiac myocyte death	$β_1$-Adrenergic receptor activation Coronary vasoconstriction Mitochondrial dysfunction ↑ $[Ca^{2+}]_i$ Oxidative stress Apoptosis
Bronchodilators (albuterol, bitolterol, fenoterol, formeterol, metaproterenol, pirbuterol, procaterol, salmeterol, terbutaline)	Tachycardia	Nonselective activation of $β_1$-adrenergic receptors
Nasal decongestants (ephedrine, ephedrine alkaloids, ma huang, phenylephrine, phenylpropanolamine, pseudoephedrine)	Tachycardia	Nonselective activation of $α_1$-adrenergic receptors
Appetite suppressants (amphetamines, fenfluramine, phentermine)	Tachycardia Pulmonary hypertension Valvular disease	↑ Serotonin? Na^+ channel blockade?
Antineoplastic drugs		
Anthracyclines (daunorubicin, doxorubicin, epirubicin)	Cardiomyopathy Heart failure	Altered $[Ca^{2+}]_i$ homeostasis Oxidative stress Mitochondrial injury Apoptosis
5-Fluorouracil Cyclophosphamide	Proarrhythmogenic Cardiac myocyte death	Coronary vasospasm? 4-Hydroxycyclophosphamide (metabolite) Altered ion homeostasis
Antibacterial drugs		
Aminoglycosides (amikacin, gentamicin, kanamycin, netilmicin, streptomycin, tobramycin)	Negative inotropic effect	↓ $[Ca^{2+}]_i$
Macrolides (azithromycin, clarithromycin, dirithromycin, erythromycin)	↑ Action potential duration QTc interval prolongation Proarrhythmogenic	K^+ channel blockade

(continued)

TABLE 18-2 Cardiotoxicity of key pharmaceutical agents. (Continued)

Agents	Cardiotoxic Manifestations	Proposed Mechanisms of Cardiotoxicity
Fluoroquinolones (grepafloxacin, moxifloxacin, sparfloxacin)	↑ Action potential duration QTc interval prolongation Proarrhythmogenic	K^+ channel blockade
Tetracycline	Negative inotropic effect	↓ $[Ca^{2+}]_i$
Chloramphenicol	Negative inotropic effect	↓ $[Ca^{2+}]_i$
Antifungal drugs		
Amphotericin B	Negative inotropic effect	Ca^{2+} channel blockade? Na^+ channel blockade? ↑ Membrane permeability?
Flucytosine	Proarrhythmogenic Cardiac arrest	5-fluorouracil metabolite Coronary vasospasm?
Antiviral drugs		
Nucleoside analog reverse transcriptase inhibitors (stavudine, zalcitabine, zidovudine)	Cardiomyopathy	Mitochondrial injury Inhibition of mitochondrial DNA polymerase Inhibition of mitochondrial DNA synthesis Inhibition of mitochondrial ATP synthesis
Centrally acting drugs		
Tricyclic antidepressants (amitriptyline, desipramine, doxepin, imipramine, protriptyline)	ST segment elevation QTc interval prolongation Proarrhythmogenic Cardiac arrest	Altered ion homeostasis Ca^{2+} channel blockade Na^+ channel blockade K^+ channel blockade
Selective serotonin reuptake inhibitors (fluoxetine)	Bradycardia Atrial fibrillation	Ca^{2+} channel blockade Na^+ channel blockade
Phenothiazine antipsychotic drugs (chlorpromazine, thioridazine)	Anticholinergic effects Negative inotropic effect QTc interval prolongation PR interval prolongation	Ca^{2+} channel blockade?
Other antipsychotic drugs (clozapine)	Blunting of T waves ST segment depression	
General inhalational anesthetics (enflurane, desflurane, halothane, isoflurane, methoxyflurane, sevoflurane)	Negative inotropic effect Decreased cardiac output Proarrhythmogenic	Ca^{2+} channel blockade Altered Ca^{2+} homeostasis β-Adrenergic receptor sensitization
Other general anesthetics (propofol)	Negative inotropic effect	Ca^{2+} channel blockade Altered Ca^{2+} homeostasis β-Adrenergic receptor sensitization
Local anesthetics		
Cocaine	Sympathomimetic effects Ischemia/myocardial Proarrhythmogenic Cardiac arrest Cardiac myocyte death	Na^+ channel blockade Coronary vasospasm, infarction Altered Ca^{2+} homeostasis Mitochondrial injury Oxidative stress Apoptosis
Other local anesthetics (bupivacaine, etidocaine, lidocaine, procainamide)	Decreased excitability ↓ Conduction velocity Proarrhythmogenic	Na^+ channel blockade
Antihistamines (astemizole, terfenadine)	↑ Action potential duration QTc interval prolongation Proarrhythmogenic	K^+ channel blockade
Immunosuppressants (rapamycin, tacrolimus)	Cardiomyopathy Heart failure	Altered Ca^{2+} homeostasis

(continued)

TABLE 18–2 Cardiotoxicity of key pharmaceutical agents. (Continued)

Agents	Cardiotoxic Manifestations	Proposed Mechanisms of Cardiotoxicity
Miscellaneous drugs		
Cisapride	↑ Action potential duration QTc interval prolongation Proarrhythmogenic	K+ channel blockade
Methylxanthines (theophylline)	↑ Cardiac output Tachycardia Proarrhythmogenic	Altered Ca^{2+} homeostasis Inhibition of phosphodiesterase
Sildenafil	?	Inhibition of phosphodiesterase
Radiocontrast agents (diatrizoate meglumine, iohexol)	Proarrhythmogenic Cardiac arrest	Apoptosis?

cocaine includes its ability to act as a local anesthetic and block nerve conduction by reversibly inhibiting Na+ channels. In the heart, cocaine decreases the rate of depolarization and the amplitude of the action potential, slows conduction speed, and increases the effective refractory period. Cocaine also inhibits norepinephrine and dopamine reuptake into sympathetic nerve terminals. The net effect of these two pharmacologic actions is to elicit and maintain ventricular fibrillation. In addition, cocaine causes cardiac myocyte death and myocardial infarction, but the mechanism of action remains to be elucidated.

Antihistamines—Second-generation antihistamines terfenadine and astemizole have been associated with life-threatening torsade de pointes arrhythmias. Electrophysiologic effects include altered repolarization, notched inverted T waves, prolonged QT interval, AV block, ventricular tachycardia, or fibrillation. These antihistamines produce cardiac arrhythmias by blocking the delayed rectifier K+ channel and prolonging action potential duration in cardiac myocytes.

Naturally Occurring Substances

Table 18–3 summarizes the cardiotoxicity of various naturally occurring substances, including cardiotoxic manifestations and proposed mechanisms of toxicity.

Steroids and Related Hormones—The myocardium expresses steroid receptors and the heart serves as a target organ for steroid effects. Also, cardiac tissue can synthesize steroid hormones, although the capacity for synthesis may be much lower than more classic steroid synthesizing tissue.

Estrogens—Estrogens alter cardiac fibroblast proliferation; they have been shown to both increase and decrease proliferation of these cells. Furthermore, antiapoptotic effects of estrogen in cardiac myocytes have been reported.

Progestins—Naturally occurring and synthetic progestins serve an opposing role to estrogens. The effects of progestins on lipid metabolism are similar to those of androgens. Unfortunately, estrogen treatment opposed with progestins may negate the cardiovascular benefits of estrogens on lipid metabolism. Very little is known about the direct effects of progestins on the heart.

Androgens—Anabolic steroids increase LDL and decrease HDL cholesterol. Increasing evidence suggests that the anabolic-androgenic steroids may exert direct cardiotoxic actions, including mitochondrial swelling, dissolution of sarcomeric contractile units, and rapid Ca^{2+} fluxes (both directions) in cardiac myocytes. In humans, high-dose anabolic-androgenic steroid use has been associated with cardiac hypertrophy and myocardial infarction.

Glucocorticoids—Chronic glucocorticoid therapy often results in elevated total, LDL, and HDL cholesterols. Furthermore, glucocorticoids are known to cause Na+ and water retention through mineralocorticoid receptor activation, which could produce hypertension during chronic therapy. Glucocorticoids appear to directly stimulate cardiac fibrosis by regulating cardiac collagen expression independently of hemodynamic alterations. Moreover, glucocorticoids may induce hypertrophic growth and alter expression of several ion transporters.

Thyroid Hormones—Triiodothyronine and thyroxine exert profound effects on the cardiovascular system. Hypothyroid states are associated with decreased heart rate, contractility, and cardiac output, whereas hyperthyroid states are associated with increased heart rate, contractility, cardiac output, ejection fraction, and heart mass. Peripheral vascular resistance is either unchanged or decreased regardless of thyroid status. Thyroid hormones promote hypertrophic growth of cardiac myocytes, alter expression of cardiac SR Ca^{2+} handling proteins, and may promote arrhythmias.

Cytokines—The cardiovascular effects of cytokines can be classified as proinflammatory, anti-inflammatory, or cardioprotective. Many of these cytokines are elevated during cardiovascular diseases such as I/R injury, myocardial infarction, and

TABLE 18–3 Cardiotoxicity of naturally occurring substances.

Agents	Cardiotoxic Manifestations	Proposed Mechanisms of Cardiotoxicity
Estrogens Natural estrogens (17β-estradiol, estrone, estriol) Synthetic estrogens (diethylstilbestrol, equilin, ethinyl estradiol, mestranol, quinestrol) Nonsteroidal estrogens (bisphenol A, diethylstilbestrol, DDT, genistein)	QTc interval prolongation? Cardioprotection?	Gender differences in K^+ channel expression? Antiapoptotic effects? Antioxidant activity? ↑ Na^+,K^+-ATPase activity? Ca^{2+} channel blockade? Other mechanisms?
Progestins (desogestrel, hydroxyprogesterone, medroxyprogesterone, norethindrone, norethynodrel, norgestimate, norgestrel, progesterone)	Enhanced toxicity of cocaine?	Mechanisms?
Androgens Natural androgens (androstenedione, dehydroepiandrosterone, dihydrotestosterone, testosterone) Synthetic androgens (boldenone, danazol, fluoxymesterone, methandrostenolone, methenolone, methyltestosterone, nandrolone, oxandrolone, oxymetholone, stanozolol)	Myocardial infarction Cardiac hypertrophy	Mitochondrial injury? Altered Ca^{2+} homeostasis? Other mechanisms?
Glucocorticoids Natural glucocorticoids (corticosterone, cortisone, hydrocortisone) Synthetic glucocorticoids (e.g., dexamethasone, methylprednisolone, prednisolone, prednisone)	Cardiac hypertrophy Cardiac fibrosis	Increased collagen expression Other mechanisms?
Mineralocorticoids (aldosterone)	Cardiac fibrosis Heart failure	Increased collagen expression Other mechanisms?
Thyroid hormones (thyroxine, triiodothyronine)	Tachycardia Positive inotropic effect Increased cardiac output Cardiac hypertrophy Proarrhythmogenic	Altered Ca^{2+} homeostasis
Cytokines Interleukin-1β Interleukin-2 Interleukin-6 Interferon-γ Tumor necrosis factor-α	Negative inotropic effect Cardiac myocyte death Negative inotropic effect Negative inotropic effect Cardomyopathy Proarrhythmogenic Negative inotropic effect Cardiac myocyte death	↑ Nitric oxide synthase expression Apoptosis ↑ Nitric oxide synthase expression ↑ Nitric oxide synthase expression ↑ Nitric oxide synthase expression Altered ion homeostasis ↑ Nitric oxide synthase expression ↑ Sphingosine production ↓ Ca^{2+} transients Apoptosis

congestive heart failure. In addition, cardiac myocytes may serve as the synthetic source of many of these cytokines.

Interleukin-1β—IL-1β is known to exert negative inotropic actions and induce apoptosis of cardiac myocytes. The effects of IL-1β on cardiac myocytes are likely mediated through induction of nitric oxide synthase and/or increased production of nitric oxide.

Tumor Necrosis Factor Alpha—TNF-α induces apoptotic death of target cells, including cardiac myocytes. It also exerts negative inotropic effects on cardiac myocytes.

Animal and Plant Toxins—Animal toxins in the venom of snakes, spiders, scorpions, and marine organisms have profound effects on the cardiovascular system. There are also a number of plants—such as foxglove, oleander, and monkshood—that contain toxic constituents and have adverse effects on the cardiovascular system.

Industrial Agents

Table 18–4 provides a summary of selected industrial agents with their prominent cardiotoxic effects and proposed mechanisms of cardiotoxicity.

TABLE 18–4 Cardiotoxicity of selected industrial agents.

Agents	Cardiotoxic Manifestations	Proposed Mechanisms of Cardiotoxicity
Solvents Toluene (paint products)	Proarrhythmogenic	↓ Parasympathetic activity ↑ Adrenergic sensitivity Altered ion homeostasis
Halogenated hydrocarbons (carbon tetrachloride, chloroform, chloropentafluoroethane, 1,2-dibromotetra-fluoromethane, dichlorodifluoromethane, *cis*-dichloroethylene, *trans*-dichloroethylene, dichlortetrafluorethane, difluoroethane, ethyl bromide, ethyl chloride, fluorocarbon 502, heptafluoro-1-iodo-propane, 1,2-hexafluoroethane, isopropyl chloride, methyl bromide, methyl chloride, methylene chloride, monochlorodifluoroethane, monochlorodifluoromethane, octafluorocyclobutane, propyl chloride, 1,1,1-trichloroethane, trichloroethane, trichloroethylene, trichlorofluoromethane, trichloromonofluoroethylene, trichlorotrifluoroethane, trifluoroiodomethane, trifluorobromomethane)	Proarrhythmogenic Negative inotropic effect Decreased cardiac output	↓ Parasympathetic activity ↑ Adrenergic sensitivity Altered ion homeostasis Altered coronary blood flow
Ketones (e.g., acetone, methyl ethyl ketone)	Proarrhythmogenic	↓ Parasympathetic activity ↑ Adrenergic sensitivity Altered ion homeostasis
Heavy metals (Cadmium, cobalt, lead) (Barium, lanthanum, manganese, nickel)	Negative inotropic effect Cardiac hypertrophy Proarrhythmogenic Proarrhythmogenic	Complex formation Altered Ca^{2+} homeostasis Ca^{2+} channel blockade

Solvents—Industrial solvents act on the nervous system, which in turn is responsible for regulating cardiac electrical activity. Because of their high lipid solubility, solvents may disperse into cell membranes and affect membrane fluidity, signal transduction, and oxidative phosphorylation. Their influence on cardiac function may also involve the release of circulating hormones such as catecholamines, vasopressin, and serotonin. From a more general perspective, industrial solvents typically produce a depressant effect on the CNS and an attenuation of myocardial contractility.

Halogenated Alkanes—Halogenated alkanes encompass a wide range of industrial and pharmaceutical agents. Their highly lipophilic nature allows them to cross the blood–brain barrier readily, where they produce CNS depression. Halogenated hydrocarbons depress heart rate, contractility, and conduction. Some of these agents sensitize the heart to the arrhythmogenic effects of β-adrenergic receptor agonists.

OVERVIEW OF VASCULAR PHYSIOLOGY

As a complex network of vessels of varying size and complexity, the vascular system delivers oxygen and nutrients to tissues throughout the body and removes the waste products of cellular metabolism. Oxygenated blood returning from the lungs to the heart is emptied into the aorta, which gradually branches off, giving rise to smaller vessels that reach individual organs (Figure 18–6). Blood returns to the heart for reoxygenation

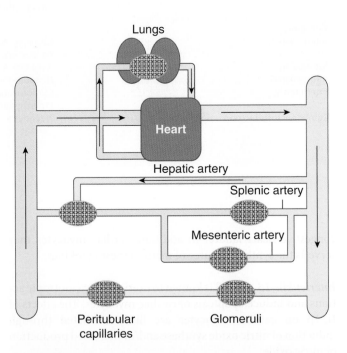

FIGURE 18–6 Schematic diagram of vascular supply to selected organs. The capillary beds represented by a meshwork connecting the arteries (*right*) with the veins (*left*); the distribution of the vasculature in several organs (liver, kidney, and lung) indicates the importance of the vascular system in toxicology.

glands) span the epidermis and are embedded in the dermis. In thickness, the dermis makes up approximately 90 percent of the skin and has largely a supportive function. Separating the dermis from underlying tissues is a layer of adipocytes, whose accumulation of fat has a cushioning action. The blood supply to the epidermis originates in the capillaries located in the rete ridges at the dermal–epidermal junction. Capillaries also supply the bulbs of the hair follicles and the secretory cells of the eccrine (sweat) glands. The ducts from these glands carry a dilute salt solution to the surface of the skin, where its evaporation provides cooling.

The interfollicular epidermis is a stratified squamous epithelium consisting primarily of keratinocytes, which are tightly attached to each other and to the basement membrane. Melanocytes are distributed sparsely in the dermis, with occasional concentrations beneath the basal lamina and in the papillae of hair follicles. In the epidermis, these cells are stimulated by ultraviolet light to produce melanin granules. The granules are extruded and taken up by the surrounding keratinocytes, which thereby become pigmented. Migrating through the epidermis are numerous Langerhans cells (LCs), which are important participants in the immune response of skin to foreign agents.

Keratinocytes of the basal layer make up the germinative compartment. When a basal cell divides, one of the progeny detaches from the basal lamina and migrates outward. As cells move toward the skin surface, they undergo a remarkable program of terminal differentiation. They gradually express new protein markers and accumulate keratin proteins. At the granular layer, the cells become flattened and increase in volume nearly 40-fold. Lipid granules fuse with the plasma membrane, replacing the aqueous environment in the intercellular space with their contents. Meanwhile, the plasma membranes of these cells become permeable and cell organelles are degraded, while a protein envelope is synthesized immediately beneath the plasma membrane. The membrane is altered characteristically by the loss of phospholipid and the addition of sphingolipid.

This program of terminal differentiation, beginning as keratinocytes leave the basal layer, produces the outermost layer of the skin, the stratum corneum. No longer viable, the mature cells (called *corneocytes*) are ~80 percent keratin in content. They are gradually shed from the surface and replaced from beneath. The process typically takes 2 weeks for basal cells to reach the stratum corneum and another 2 weeks to be shed from the surface. In instances in which the outer layer is deficient due to disease or physical or chemical trauma, the barrier to the environment that the skin provides is inferior to that provided by normal, healthy skin.

Percutaneous Absorption

The stratum corneum is the primary barrier to percutaneous absorption. Diseases (e.g., psoriasis) or other conditions (e.g., abrasion and wounding) that compromise this barrier can permit greatly increased uptake of poorly permeable substances.

The viable layer of epidermis provides a much less effective barrier, because hydrophilic agents readily diffuse into the intercellular water, whereas hydrophobic agents can partition into cell membranes, and each can diffuse readily to the blood supply in the rete ridges of the dermis.

The stratum corneum prevents water loss from underlying tissues by evaporation. Its hydrophobic character reflects the lipid content of the intercellular space. The lipids, a major component being sphingolipids, have a high content of long-chain ceramides, removal of which seriously compromises barrier function as measured by transepidermal water loss. The stratum corneum is ordinarily hydrated (typically 20 percent water), the moisture residing in corneocyte protein, but it can take up a great deal more water on prolonged immersion, thereby reducing the effectiveness of the barrier to agents with a hydrophilic character. Indeed, occlusion of the skin with plastic wrap, permitting the retention of perspiration underneath, is a commonly employed technique to enhance uptake of agents applied to the skin surface. Penetration from the air is generally too low to be of concern.

Uptake through the skin is now incorporated in pharmacokinetic modeling to estimate potential risks from exposures. The degree of uptake depends on the details of exposure conditions, being proportional to solute concentration (assuming it is dilute), time, and the amount of skin surface exposed. In addition, two intrinsic factors contribute to the absorption rate of a given compound: its hydrophobicity, which affects its ability to partition into epidermal lipid, and its rate of diffusion through this barrier. A measure of the first property is the commonly used octanol/water partitioning ratio (K_{ow}). This is particularly relevant for exposure to contaminated water, such as occurs during bathing or swimming. However, partitioning of an agent into the skin is greatly affected by its solubility in or adhesion to the medium in which it is applied (including soil). Similarly, very hydrophobic compounds, once in the stratum corneum, may diffuse only very slowly into less hydrophobic regions below. The second property is an inverse function of molecular weight (MW) or molecular volume. Thus, hydrophobic agents of low MW permeate the skin better than those of high MW or those that are hydrophilic. For small molecules, hydrophobicity is a dominant factor in penetration.

Diffusion through the epidermis is considerably faster at some anatomical sites than others. A list in order of decreasing permeability under steady-state conditions gives the following hierarchy: foot sole > palm > scrotum > forehead > abdomen. Absorption through the epidermal appendages is generally neglected, despite the ability of agents to bypass the stratum corneum by this route, because the combined appendageal surface area is a small fraction of the total available for uptake. However, penetration through the appendages can be appreciable.

Transdermal Drug Delivery—Specially designed patches are currently in use to deliver drugs such as clonidine, estradiol, testosterone, nitroglycerin, scopolamine, fentanyl, and nicotine for therapeutic purposes. Advantages of this approach over oral dosing include providing a steady infusion for extended periods (typically 1 to 7 days) thereby avoiding large variations in plasma concentration, preventing exposure to the acidic pH of the stomach, and avoiding biotransformation in the gastrointestinal tract or from first-pass removal by the liver.

Measurements of Penetration—Volunteers are dosed, plasma and/or urine concentrations are measured at suitable intervals, and amounts excreted from the body are estimated. For in vitro work, excised split-thickness skin can be employed in special diffusion chambers, though care is needed to preserve the viability of the living layer of epidermis. The agent is removed for measurement from the underside by a fluid into which it partitions, thereby permitting continued penetration. A simpler setup commonly employed uses cadaver skin with the lower dermis removed. This lacks biotransformation capability but retains the barrier function of the stratum corneum. To simplify determination of penetration kinetics, skin flaps may be employed and the capillary blood flow monitored to measure penetration. For this purpose, pig skin has particular utility. A promising variation minimizing species differences is to use skin grafts on experimental animals for these measurements. Human skin persists well on athymic mice and retains its normal barrier properties.

Biotransformation

The ability of the skin to metabolize agents that diffuse through it contributes to its barrier function. This influences the potential biological activity of xenobiotics and topically applied drugs, leading to their degradation or their activation as skin sensitizers or carcinogens. The epidermis and pilosebaceous units are the major sites of such activity in the skin. Enzymes participating in biotransformation that are expressed in skin include multiple forms of cytochrome P450, epoxide hydrolase, UDP-glucuronosyltransferase, quinone reductase, and glutathione transferases. Other metabolic enzyme activities detected in human epidermal cells include sulfatases, β-glucuronidase, N-acetyltransferases, esterases, and reductases. The intercellular region of the stratum corneum has catabolic activities (e.g., proteases, lipases, glycosidases, and phosphatase).

CONTACT DERMATITIS

Of all occupational skin diseases, contact dermatitis accounts for over 90 percent of reported causes. Contact dermatitis falls into the two major categories of irritant and allergic forms. Both involve inflammatory processes and can have indistinguishable clinical characteristics of erythema (redness), induration (thickening and firmness), scaling (flaking), and vesiculation (blistering) on areas directly contacting the chemical agent. Figure 19–2 shows examples of many types of contact dermatitis as a result of occupational skin toxicity.

Irritant Dermatitis

Irritant dermatitis is a nonimmune-related response caused by the direct action of an agent on the skin. Extrinsic variables such as concentration, pH, temperature, duration, repetitiveness of contact, and occlusion impact significantly on the appearance of the eruption. Strong acids, bases, solvents, and unstable or reactive chemicals rank high among the many possible human irritants.

Strongly noxious substances such as those with extreme pH can produce an immediate irreversible and potentially scarring dermatitis following a single exposure. This acute irritant phenomenon is akin to a chemical burn and has been described as an "etching" reaction. More commonly, single exposures to potentially irritating chemicals will not produce significant reactions; repeated exposures eventually result in either an eczematous dermatitis with clinical changes characteristic of allergic contact dermatitis or a fissured, thickened eruption without a substantial inflammatory component. Chemicals inducing the latter two reactions are termed *marginal irritants*.

Divergent etiologies make it difficult to assign a specific mechanism for the pathophysiology of irritant dermatitis. Direct corrosives, solvents, oxidizing and reducing agents, and dehydrating agents act as irritants by disrupting the keratin ultrastructure or directly injuring critical cellular macromolecules or organelles. Marginal irritants require multifactorial variables to create disease and may not be capable of producing reactions under all circumstances. The varying time courses necessary to produce dermatitis by known irritants result from the differing rates of percutaneous absorption that depend on the specific agent selected.

No single testing method has been successful in determining the irritancy potential of specific chemicals. Several tests exploit various contributory factors necessary to elicit irritant contact dermatitis. These tests involve either a single or repeated application of the same material to the skin. The use of animals in the testing of potentially irritant chemicals is based on a variety of epicutaneous (epidermal surface) methods and has continued for decades. Generally, both intact skin and abraded skin of albino rabbits are tested with various materials under occluded patches. The patches are removed in 24 h and the tested areas of the skin are evaluated at this time and again in 1 to 3 days.

The in vitro Corrositex assay tests the ability of a chemical to penetrate a hydrated collagen matrix barrier and produce a color change in the underlying aqueous chemical detection system. The relative corrosiveness of a chemical is determined by the time required to penetrate the collagen and enter the liquid buffer with pH indicator dyes.

In the repeat insult patch test, used primarily in humans for the evaluation of potential allergic sensitization, chemicals are placed on the skin under occlusion for 3 to 4 weeks. The test materials are replaced every 2 to 3 days to maintain an adequate reservoir in the patch site. The test is functionally similar to the cumulative irritancy test, where daily patches are applied under occlusion for 2 weeks in parallel with control substances.

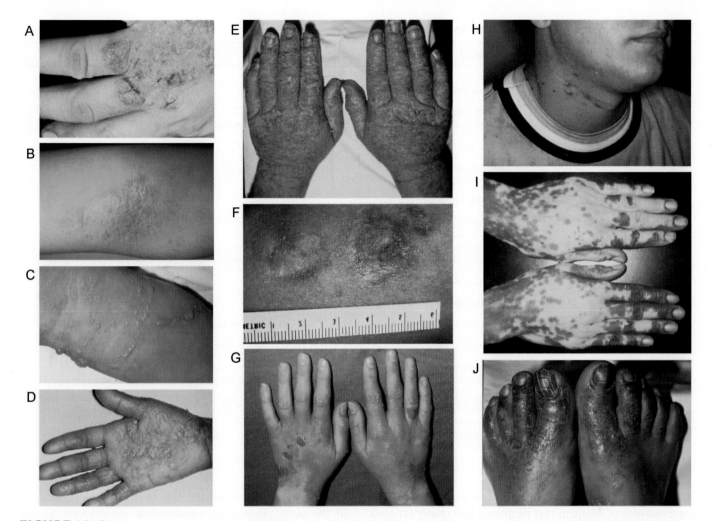

FIGURE 19–2 **Examples of occupational skin toxicity.** The panels, available at the NIOSH website (http://www.cdc.gov/niosh/topics/skin/occderm-slides/ocderm1.html), are a small selection from the 140-slide NIOSH program "Occupational Dermatoses—A Program for Physicians" prepared by Drs. E. Shmunes, M.M. Key, J.B. Lucas, and J.S. Taylor. (*A*. Eczema from cutting oil. *B*. Atopic irritant dermatitis. *C*. Burn from ethylene oxide. *D*. Burn from alkali exposure. *E*. Sensitization to dichromate. *F*. Beryllium granulomas. *G*. Phototoxicity from lime juice. *H*. Acne from cutting oil. *I*. Leukoderma from rubber antioxidants. *J*. Hyperpigmentation from mercaptobenzothiazole.)

The chamber scarification test modifies the aforementioned tests by abrading the skin to expose the upper dermis. All of these provocative tests rely on overt clinical changes such as erythema and induration (hardening) at the site of challenge with a potential irritant.

Chemical Burns

Extremely corrosive and reactive chemicals may produce immediate coagulative necrosis that results in substantial tissue damage, with ulceration and sloughing. Sometimes referred to as a third-degree chemical burn, the damage does not have a primary inflammatory component and thus may not be classified as an irritant reaction. In addition to the direct effects of the chemical, necrotic tissue can act as a chemical reservoir resulting in either continued cutaneous damage or percutaneous absorption and systemic injury after exposure.

Table 19–2 lists selected corrosive chemicals that are important clinically.

Allergic Contact Dermatitis

Allergic contact dermatitis represents a delayed (type IV) hypersensitivity reaction. Only minute quantities of material are necessary to elicit overt reactions. This is distinct from irritant contact dermatitis, where the intensity of the reaction is proportional to the dose applied. An estimated 20 percent of all contact dermatitis is allergic in nature.

For allergic contact dermatitis to occur, one must first be sensitized to the potential allergen. Subsequent contact elicits the classic clinical and pathologic findings. To mount an immune reaction to a sensitizer, one must be genetically prepared to become sensitized, have a sufficient contact with a sensitizing chemical, and then have repeated contact later.

TABLE 19–2 Selected chemicals causing skin burns.

Chemical	Comment
Ammonia	Potent skin corrosive Contact with compressed gas can cause frostbite
Calcium oxide (CaO)	Severe chemical burns Extremely exothermic reaction—dissolving in water can cause heat burns
Chlorine	Liquid and concentrated vapors cause cell death and ulceration
Ethylene oxide	Solutions and vapors may burn Compressed gas can cause frostbite
Hydrogen chloride (HCl)	Severe burning with scar formation
Hydrogen fluoride (HF)	Severe, painful, slowly healing burns from high concentration Lower concentration causes delayed cutaneous injury Systemic absorption can lead to electrolyte abnormalities and death Calcium-containing topical medications and quaternary ammonium compounds are used to limit damage
Hydrogen peroxide	High concentration causes severe burns and blistering
Methyl bromide	Liquid exposure produces blistering, deep burns
Nitrogen oxides	Moist skin facilitates the formation of nitric acid causing severe yellow-colored burns
Phosphorus	White phosphorus continues to burn on skin in the presence of air
Phenol	Extremely corrosive even in low concentrations Systemic absorption through burn sites may result in cardiac arrhythmias, renal disease, and death
Sodium hydroxide	High concentration causes deep burns, readily denatures keratin
Toluene diisocyanate	Severe burns with contact Skin contact rarely may result in respiratory sensitization

Contact dermatitis may occur on exposure to any number of the thousands of allergens that people are potentially exposed to daily. Table 19–3 lists frequent allergens based on common exposure patterns. Contact with esoteric allergens frequently occurs in the workplace.

There are several allergens—like nickel, chromium, cobalt, and some food flavorings—that are also ingested with great frequency. In cases where an individual has a contact sensitivity to an agent that is systemically administered (orally), a generalized skin eruption with associated symptoms such as headache, malaise, and arthralgia may occur. Less dramatic eruptions may include flaring of a previous contact dermatitis to the same substance, vesicular hand eruptions, and an eczematous eruption in flexural areas. Systemic contact dermatitis may produce a delayed-type hypersensitivity reaction and/or deposition of immunoglobulins and complement components in the skin. Such deposits are potent inducers of a secondary inflammatory response and are responsible for the initial pathophysiology of many blistering and connective tissue diseases of the skin.

Cross-reactions between chemicals may occur if they share similar functional groups critical to the formation of complete allergens (hapten plus carrier protein). These reactions may cause difficulties in controlling contact dermatitis, because avoidance of known allergens and potentially cross-reacting substances is necessary for improvement. Table 19–4 lists common cross-reacting substances. Proper diagnosis can be hampered by concomitant sensitization to two different chemicals in the same product or simultaneous sensitization to two chemicals in different products.

Diagnosis and Testing—In order to find the responsible chemical causing allergic contact dermatitis, patch testing is commonly employed. On the washed backs of patients, patches are placed containing a small amount of a potential allergen. Diagnostic patch testing utilizes standardized concentrations of material dissolved or suspended in petrolatum or water that are placed on stainless steel chambers adhering to acrylic tape. Chambers are left in place for 48 h, and an initial reading is performed at the time the patches are removed. A subsequent reading 24 to 96 h later is also made, because delayed reactions commonly occur. Reactions are graded as positive if erythema (redness) and induration (skin thickening) occur at the test site. Strict adherence to established protocols is necessary to draw conclusions about the clinical relevance of the reactions. Avoidance and substitution of the offending agent will lead to improvement in the majority of cases in a few weeks. Cross-reacting chemicals must be noted during interpretation (Table 19–4).

In animal testing, a chemical is applied to intact or abraded skin or through intradermal injection with or without adjuvant. The skin reaction to a subsequent challenge with the chemical is observed and graded, in an attempt to identify causative agents.

TABLE 19–3 Common contact allergens.

Source	Common Allergens	
Topical medications/hygiene products	**Antibiotics** Bacitracin Neomycin Polymyxin Aminoglycosides Sulfonamides	**Therapeutics** Benzocaine Fluorouracil Idoxuridine α-Tocopherol (vitamin E) Corticosteroids
	Preservatives Benzalkonium chloride Formaldehyde Formaldehyde releasers Quaternium-15 Imidazolidinyl urea Diazolidinyl urea DMDM hydantoin Methylchloroisothiazolone	**Others** Cinnamic aldehyde Ethylenediamine Lanolin p-Phenylenediamine Propylene glycol Benzophenones Fragrances Thioglycolates
Plants and trees	Abietic acid Balsam of Peru Rosin (colophony)	Pentadecylcatechols Sesquiterpene lactone Tuliposide A
Antiseptics	Chloramine Chlorhexidine Chloroxylenol Dichlorophene Dodecylaminoethyl glycine HCl	Glutaraldehyde Hexachlorophene Thimerosal (Merthiolate) Mercurials Triphenylmethane dyes
Rubber products	Diphenylguanidine Hydroquinone Mercaptobenzothiazole p-Phenylenediamine	Resorcinol monobenzoate Benzothiazolesulfenamides Dithiocarbamates Thiurams
Leather	Formaldehyde Glutaraldehyde	Potassium dichromate
Paper products	Abietic acid Formaldehyde Nigrosine	Rosin (colophony) Triphenyl phosphate Dyes
Glues and bonding agents	Bisphenol A Epichlorohydrin Formaldehyde Acrylic monomers Cyanoacrylates	Epoxy resins p-(t-Butyl)formaldehyde resin Toluene sulfonamide resins Urea formaldehyde resins
Metals	Chromium Cobalt	Mercury Nickel

PHOTOTOXICOLOGY

In the course of life, the skin is exposed to radiation that spans the electromagnetic spectrum, including ultraviolet, visible, and infrared radiation from the sun, artificial light sources, and heat sources. In general, the solar radiation reaching the earth that is most capable of inducing skin changes extends from 290 to 700 nm, the ultraviolet and visible spectra. For any form of electromagnetic radiation to produce a biological change, it must first be absorbed. The absorption of light in deeper, more vital structures of the skin is dependent on chromophores, epidermal thickness, and water content that differ from region to region on the body. The chromophores melanin and amino acids are capable of absorbing UV-B (290 to 320 nm) radiation.

Biologically, the most significant chromophore is DNA, because the resultant damage from radiation potentially will have lasting effects on the structure and function of the tissue.

Adverse Responses to Electromagnetic Radiation

After exposure, the most evident acute feature of UV radiation exposure is erythema (redness or sunburn). The minimal erythema dose (MED), the smallest dose of UV light needed to induce an erythematous response, varies greatly from person to person. Vasodilation responsible for the color change is accompanied by significant alterations in inflammatory mediators released from local inflammatory cells as well as from injured keratino-

TABLE 19–4 Common cross-reacting chemicals.

Chemical	Cross-reactor
Abietic acid	Pine resin (colophony)
Balsam of Peru	Pine resin, cinnamates, benzoates
Bisphenol A	Diethylstilbestrol, hydroquinone monobenzyl ether
Canaga oil	Benzyl salicylate
Chlorocresol	Chloroxylenol
Diazolidinyl urea	Imidazolidinyl urea, formaldehyde
Ethylenediamine di-HCl	Aminophylline, piperazine
Formaldehyde	Arylsulfonamide resin, chloroallyl-hexaminium chloride
Hydroquinone	Resorcinol
Methyl hydroxybenzoate	Parabens, hydroquinone monobenzyl ether
p-Aminobenzoic acid	p-Aminosalicylic acid, sulfonamide
Phenylenediamine	Parabens, p-aminobenzoic acid
Propyl hydroxybenzoate	Hydroquinone monobenzyl ether
Phenol	Resorcinol, cresols, hydroquinone
Tetramethylthiuram disulfide	Tetraethylthiuram mono- and disulfide

cytes, and may be responsible for several of the systemic symptoms associated with sunburn, such as fever, chills, and malaise. UV-B (290 to 320 nm) is the most effective solar band to cause erythema in human skin. Environmental conditions that affect UV-induced injury include duration of exposure, season, altitude, body site, skin pigmentation, and previous exposure. A substantially greater dosage of UV-A (320 to 400 nm) reaches the earth compared with UV-B (up to 100-fold); however, its efficiency in generating erythema in humans is about 1000-fold less than that of UV-B. Overt pigment darkening is another typical response to UV exposure. This may be accomplished by enhanced melanin production by melanocytes or by photooxidation of melanin. Tanning or increased pigmentation usually occurs within 3 days of UV light exposure, whereas photooxidation is evident immediately. The tanning response is most readily produced by exposure in the UV-B band. The tanning response serves to augment the protective effects of melanin in the skin. However, the immediate pigment-darkening characteristic of UV-A and visible light exposure does not confer improved photoprotection.

Commensurate with melanogenesis, UV radiation will provoke skin thickening primarily in the stratum corneum, and this response lends significant defense against subsequent UV insult. Chronic exposure to radiation induces a variety of characteristic skin changes that depend greatly on the baseline skin pigmentation of the individual as well as the duration and location of the exposure. Lighter skinned people tend to suffer from chronic skin changes with greater frequency than darker individuals, and locations such as the head, neck, hands, and upper chest are more readily involved due to their routine exposures. Pigmentary changes—such as freckling and hypomelanotic areas, wrinkling, telangiectasias (fine superficial blood vessels), actinic keratoses (precancerous lesions), and malignant skin lesions, for example, basal and squamous cell carcinomas and malignant melanomas—are all consequences of chronic exposure to UV light. One significant pathophysiologic response of chronic exposure to UV light is the pronounced decrease of epidermal LCs, which may result in lessened immune surveillance of neoantigens on malignant cells, thus allowing such transformation to proceed unabated. Exposures to ionizing radiation may produce a different spectrum of disease, depending on the dose delivered. Large acute exposures will result in local redness, blistering, swelling, ulceration, and pain. After a latent period or following subacute chronic exposures, characteristic changes such as epidermal thinning, freckling, telangiectasias (dilated capillaries), and nonhealing ulcerations may occur. Also, a variety of skin malignancies have been described years after the skin's exposure to radiation.

Aside from the toxic nature of electromagnetic radiation, natural and environmental exposures to certain bands of light are vital for survival. Ultraviolet radiation is critical for the conversion of 7-dehydrocholesterol to previtamin D_3, a required precursor for normal endogenous production of vitamin D. Blue light in the 420- to 490-nm range can photoisomerize bilirubin (a red blood cell breakdown product) in the skin, rendering urinary excretion of this neurotoxic metabolite by infants with elevated serum bilirubin. In addition, the toxic effects of UV light have been exploited for decades through artificial light sources for treatment of hyperproliferative skin disorders like psoriasis.

Photosensitivity

An abnormal sensitivity to UV and visible light, photosensitivity may result from endogenous or exogenous factors. Various genetic diseases, such as xeroderma pigmentosum, and the autoimmune disease lupus erythematosus impair the cell's ability to repair UV light-induced damage. In hereditary or chemically induced porphyrias, enzyme abnormalities disrupt the biosynthetic pathways producing heme, leading to accumulation of porphyrin precursors or derivatives throughout the body. These compounds in general fluoresce when exposed to light of 400 to 410 nm (Soret band), and in this excited state interact with cellular macromolecules or with molecular oxygen to generate toxic-free radicals. Chlorinated aromatic hydrocarbons induce this syndrome. A "constitutional" sensitivity to light (porphyria cutanea tarda) can be precipitated by alcohol, estrogens, or certain antibiotics in individuals with hereditary abnormalities in porphyrin synthesis, and an "acquired" sensitivity in general by hexachlorobenzene and mixtures of polyhalogenated aromatic hydrocarbons.

Phototoxicity—Phototoxic reactions from exogenous chemicals may be produced by systemic or topical administration or

Toxic Responses of the Reproductive System

Paul M. D. Foster and L. Earl Gray Jr.

INTRODUCTION

Chemicals can adversely affect reproduction in males and females. Recent trends in human fertility point to the potential for declines in normal human reproduction and suggest that exposure to environmental chemicals and drugs may contribute to these declines. The reproductive cycle is outlined in Figure 20–1.

THE REPRODUCTIVE CYCLE

Numerous complex processes are orchestrated in a precise and sequential order for optimal performance at different stages of the life cycle of animals and humans. Following fertilization of an egg by a sperm, the resulting zygote must be transported along the oviduct while maturing into an early embryo. This embryo must then implant in the uterus successfully, differentiate, produce a placenta, and undergo normal embryogenesis and fetal development.

Acquisition of sexual maturity involves the generation of gametes by the gonads. For parental animals, once their reproductive life span has finished, the process of reproductive senescence then occurs. These processes all involve complex interplay between tissues and cells, under hormonal control that provides the critical signals and precise timing of these events. All these processes can be targets for the action of specific agents that can disturb events leading to adverse effects on reproduction, such that the normal production of viable offspring cannot occur.

REPRODUCTIVE DEVELOPMENT AND SEXUAL DIFFERENTIATION

During the seventh week of human gestation, the male and female morphological characteristics begin to develop. Gonadal differentiation depends on signals from the Y chromosome, which contains the genes necessary to induce testicular morphogenesis. One of these signals is the *SRY* gene, which is the sex-determining region on the short arm of the Y chromosome and acts as a "switch" to initiate transcription of other genes that contribute to testicular organogenesis. In the absence of the SRY protein, the gonad remains indifferent for a short period of time before differentiating into an ovary.

Interstitial Leydig cells produce the male sex hormone testosterone, which induces masculine differentiation of the Wolffian duct and external genitalia. Figure 20–2 provides a diagrammatic representation of sexual differentiation in the human male. In rodent and human species, fetal testicular androgen production is necessary for proper testicular devel-

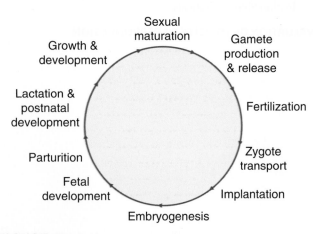

FIGURE 20–1 The reproductive cycle.

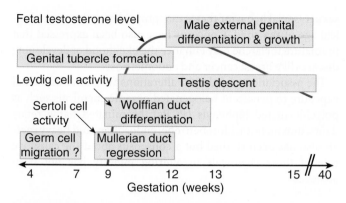

FIGURE 20–2 **Male sexual differentiation in humans during gestation.** (Reproduced with permission from Klonisch T, Fowler PA, Hombach-Klonisch S: Molecular and genetic regulation of testis descent and external genitalia development. *Dev Biol* 270:1–18, 2004. Elsevier Science.)

opment, normal male sexual differentiation, and differentiation of the Wolffian ducts into the epididymides, vasa deferentia, and seminal vesicles.

Androgens derived from the Leydig interstitial cells stimulate the mesonephric (or Wolffian) ducts to form the male genital ducts, while Sertoli cells produce Müllerian-inhibiting substance (or anti-Müllerian hormone), which suppresses development of the paramesonephric (Müllerian) ducts, or female genital ducts.

In the humans, the external genitalia are indistinguishable until the 9th week of gestation, and not fully differentiated until the 12th week of development. Development of the external genitalia coincides with gonadal differentiation. Fetal testicular androgens are responsible for the induction of masculinization of the androgynous external genitalia. Thus, male, but not female, reproductive tract development is totally hormonally dependent and inherently more susceptible to endocrine disruption.

GAMETOGENESIS

The mammalian oocyte (Figure 20–3) begins meiosis during fetal development but arrests partway through meiosis I and does not complete the first division until ovulation; the second division is completed only if the egg is fertilized. In the males, meiosis begins at puberty and is a continuous process, with spermatocytes progressing from prophase to the meiotic second division in little more than a week. This difference in strategy has implications for the action of toxicants and critical time periods when these cells may be vulnerable to attack.

NEONATAL DEVELOPMENT

Late in gestation and at birth, male rats display longer anogenital distances (AGD) than do female rats with neonatal male AGD being more than twice as long as females. There are homologous sex differences in humans. In many mammalian species, including humans and rats, males of the species engage in more aggressive play than do females. Both AGD and behavior can be altered by exposure to hormonal and antihormonal agents.

INFANTILE DEVELOPMENT

During the infantile period of development, emergence of the nipple buds and areolae in females as well as maturation of the hypothalamic–pituitary axis occurs. Emergence of the nipple buds is prevented in males by prenatal androgen-induced atrophy of the nipple anlagen. Prenatal androgen-treated females may display reproductive tract malformations (retained male tissues or vaginal agenesis).

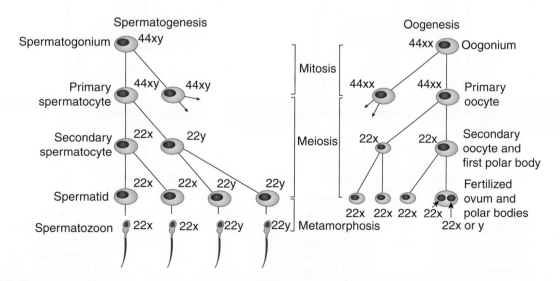

FIGURE 20–3 **Cellular replication (mitosis) and cellular reductive divisions (meiosis) involved in spermatogenesis, oogenesis, and fertilization.**

PUBERTAL DEVELOPMENT

Puberty is initiated by activation of the hypothalamic–pituitary–gonadal (HPG) and hypothalamic–pituitary–adrenal (HPA) axes (see Figure 20–4). At the onset, the HPG axis releases gonadotropin-releasing hormone (GnRH) pulses with increasing frequency and amplitude that induces complimentary pulsatile secretions of luteinizing hormone (LH) and follicle-stimulating hormone (FSH) from the anterior pituitary. In turn, LH and FSH stimulate the gonads inducing gonadarche characterized by the onset of gonadal hormone production. In the females, secretion of androgens from theca cells and estradiol from granulosa cells of maturing follicles prior to ovulation is followed by secretion of progesterone from the corpus luteum after ovulation. In the males, LH stimulates testicular synthesis and secretion of androgens and insulin-like peptide 3 hormone from the Leydig cells of males.

Premature thelarche and premature adrenarche are often referred to as pseudoprecocious puberty when the full spectrum of pubertal changes does not occur. Premature thelarche in girls and gynecomastia in boys result from direct exposure to estrogen-containing personal care and "natural" products. Untoward consequences of these conditions may occur with prolonged exposure, including shortened stature due to effects of estrogens on the growth plates of the long bones and sexual–social behavior that is inappropriate for the chronological age of the child. Concerns have also been expressed that premature thelarche may enhance the likelihood of developing diseases like breast cancer and endometriosis.

The association of pubertal alterations with environmental exposure to persistent halogenated organic chemicals such as polychlorinated biphenyls (PCBs), brominated flame retardants, dioxin, hexachlorobenzene, endosulfan, and heavy metals also has been studied but a consensus about the causative role of these chemicals in altering puberty has not been achieved.

Rodent Models of Puberty

Rodents are important animal models in the study of the effects of toxicants on puberty. In the laboratory rats, the standard landmarks of puberty are the age of preputial separation (PPS) in the males, and the ages of vaginal opening (VO) and first estrus in females.

Onset of pubertal landmarks in rats can be altered after acute in utero and/or lactational exposures to 2,3,7,8-tetrachlorodibenzo-p-dioxin (TCDD), busulfan, androgens, and endocrine-disrupting chemicals (EDCs). Also, onset of pubertal landmarks in rats is delayed after peripubertal exposures to antiandrogenic chemicals. Throughout puberty and into adulthood, the sex

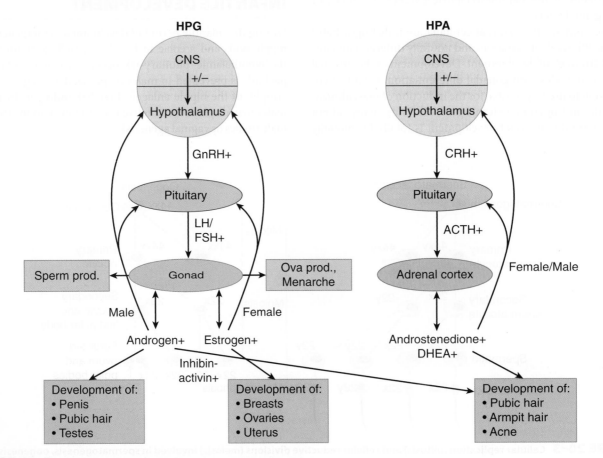

FIGURE 20–4 Endocrine control of puberty in males and females.

accessory glands and other androgen-dependent tissues (i.e., muscles and nervous system) continue to depend on testosterone and 5α-dihydrotestosterone for maturation and maintenance of function.

SEXUAL MATURITY

Hypothalamo-pituitary–Gonadal Axis

FSH and LH are glycoproteins synthesized and released from the pituitary gland. Hypothalamic neuroendocrine neurons secrete specific releasing or release-inhibiting factors into the hypophyseal portal system, which carries them to the adenohypophysis, where they act to stimulate or inhibit the release of anterior pituitary hormones. GnRH acts on gonadotropic cells, thereby stimulating the release of FSH and LH.

The neuroendocrine neurons have nerve terminals containing monoamines (norepinephrine, dopamine, and serotonin) that impinge on them. Reserpine, chlorpromazine, and monoamine oxidase (MAO) inhibitors modify the content or actions of brain monoamines that affect gonadotropin production.

In the females (Figure 20–5), LH acts on thecal cells of the ovary to induce steroidogenesis, particularly the production of progesterone and androgens that are transferred to the granulosa cells that can be stimulated by FSH to produce estradiol. These steroids provide feedback on the hypothalamus and pituitary to regulate gonadotropin production.

Similarly in the males (Figure 20–6), FSH acts primarily on the Sertoli cells, but it also appears to stimulate the mitotic activity of spermatogonia. LH stimulates steroidogenesis in the interstitial Leydig cells. A defect in the function of the testis (in

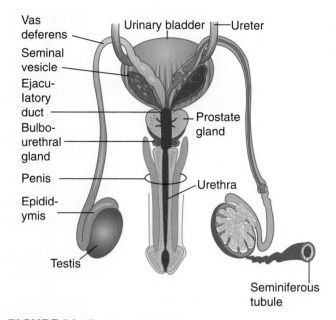

FIGURE 20–6 **Male reproductive system.**

the production of spermatozoa or testosterone) will tend to be reflected in increased levels of FSH and LH in serum because of the lack of the negative feedback effect of testicular hormones.

The HPG feedback system is a very delicately modulated hormonal process. Toxicants that alter the hepatic and/or renal biotransformation of endogenous sex steroid may be expected to interfere with the pituitary feedback system.

Ovarian Function

Oogenesis—About 400,000 follicles are present at birth in each human ovary. After birth, many undergo atresia, and those that survive are continuously reduced in number. Any chemical that damages the oocytes will accelerate the depletion of the pool and can lead to reduced fertility in females. About one-half of the numbers of oocytes present at birth remain at puberty; the number is reduced to about 25,000 by 30 years of age. About 400 primary follicles will yield mature ova during a woman's reproductive life span. During the approximately three decades of fecundity, follicles in various stages of growth can always be found. After menopause, follicles are no longer present in the ovary.

Although ovarian weight does not fluctuate during the estrous cycle, ovarian weight and histology can provide very useful information about the effects of toxicants on the female reproductive system. Ovarian weight can be reduced by either depletion of oocytes or disruption of the HPG axis. Toxicants induce various ovarian lesions, including polyovular follicles, oocyte depletion, interstitial cell hyperplasia, corpora albicans, and an absence of corpora lutea.

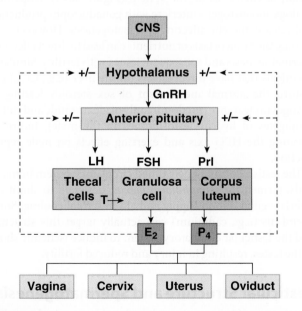

FIGURE 20–5 **Endocrine control of the female reproductive cycle.** CNS = central nervous system; GnRH = gonadotrophin-releasing hormone; LH = luteinizing hormone; FSH = follicle-stimulating hormone; Prl = prolactin; T = testosterone; E_2 = estradiol; P_4 = progesterone.

Case Study: Busulfan—Busulfan is an alkylating agent used to treat several diseases in humans, including chronic myelogenous leukemia, certain myeloproliferative disorders such as severe

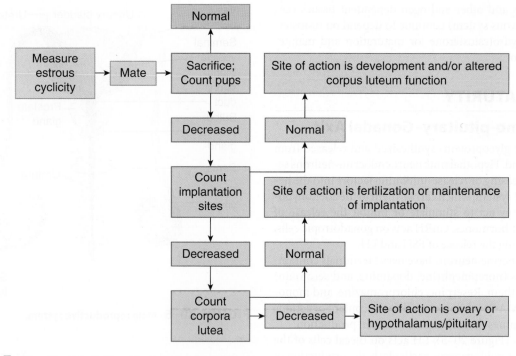

FIGURE 20–7 Sites of action for female reproductive toxicants.

thrombocytosis, and polycythemia vera. Busulfan causes ovarian failure and prevents or delays the onset of puberty in girls.

In rodents, administration of busulfan specifically inhibits germ cell development. Offspring display permanent reproductive and CNS alterations. The most severely affected females do not display estrous cycles or spontaneous sexual behavior as a consequence of this exposure. Even though the gonads of both sexes are affected at similar dosage levels, fertility and gonadal hormone production are much more easily disrupted in female than male offspring, because the steroid-producing cells in the ovary fail to differentiate in the absence of the oocyte. A diagrammatic representation of the sites of actions of female reproductive toxicants is presented in Figure 20–7.

Ovarian Cycle

The cyclic release of pituitary gonadotropins involving the secretion of ovarian progesterone and estrogen is depicted in Figure 20–8. These female sex steroids determine ovulation and prepare the female accessory sex organs to receive the male sperm. This axis can be disrupted, resulting in infertility at any level of the endocrine system. For example, chemicals that block the LH surge transiently can prevent or delay ovulation, resulting in infertility or lower fecundity due to delayed fertilization of ova.

TESTICULAR STRUCTURE AND FUNCTION

The blood–testis barrier between the lumen of an interstitial capillary and the lumen of a seminiferous tubule impedes or

prevents the free exchange of chemicals/drugs between the blood and the fluid inside the seminiferous tubules.

Targets for Toxicity

For an adult male, there are numerous potential targets for the action of chemicals on the system (Figure 20–9). Dopamine analogs and estrogens interfere with gonadotropin production and release, thereby affecting spermatogenesis. However, perturbing the homeostasis of nutrients can lead to direct effects on spermatogenesis and subsequent issues with fertility. Similarly, chemicals that have direct effects on the liver (e.g., CCl_4) can disturb the normal metabolism of sex steroids leading to changes in clearance (predominantly of glucuronide and sulfate conjugates of hydroxytestosterones in the male), indirectly affecting the HPG axis and exerting effects on male reproduction.

The testis also has a finely tuned circulatory system in mammals, termed the *pampiniform plexus*, designed to shunt the arterial venous blood supply and aid in scrotal cooling. Some chemicals (e.g., cadmium) can actually target this structure and the testicular circulatory system to induce ischemic shock to the testes, resulting in injury and reduced fertility.

Testicular Structure and Spermatogenesis

Spermatogenesis is an extremely ordered process in the rat. The spermatogonia have populations that act as the stem cells for the seminiferous tubules and a proportion of these cells then undergo a series of mitotic divisions to increase numbers and move into meiotic prophase, and are then committed to

Comparative endocrinology of menstrual and estrous cycles and early pregnancy

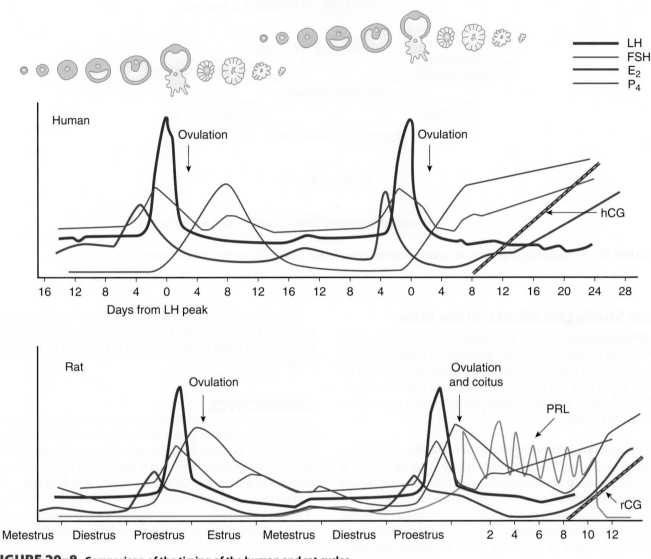

FIGURE 20-8 Comparison of the timing of the human and rat cycles.

becoming spermatozoa, which are released into the lumen of the seminiferous tubule.

Different biochemical events can go on during the different stages and indeed this can provide clues as to potential modes of action of chemicals that produce stage-specific lesions. Such occurrences do occur regularly with certain phthalate esters, glycol ethers, and antiandrogenic agents.

Once sperms are released into the seminiferous tubule lumen and proceed to the epididymis, they can also be the target of toxicant action. Chlorosugars and epichlorohydrin have both been shown to inhibit energy metabolism in sperm, preventing them from functioning normally. The number of environmental chemicals that produce adverse responses in human males is not large. All of these have been shown to induce effects in rodents and especially the rat, although there may be differences in sensitivity based on dose.

Posttesticular Processes

During the movement along the epididymal tubule, fluid is removed by active transport and this stage of the process is one that can be interfered with by toxicants, resulting in an inappropriate environment for normal sperm development.

Erection and Ejaculation

Little is known concerning the effects of chemicals on erection or ejaculation. Pesticides, particularly the organophosphates, are known to affect neuroendocrine processes involved in erection and ejaculation. Many drugs act on the autonomic nervous system and affect potency. Impotence, the failure to obtain or sustain an erection, is rarely of endocrine origin; more often, the cause is psychological.

Potential target sites

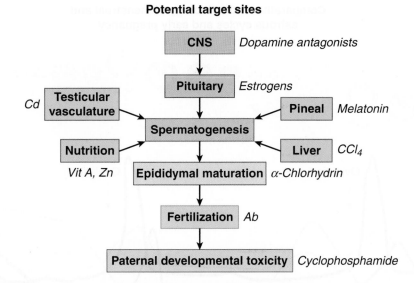

FIGURE 20–9 Potential target sites for male reproductive toxicants. Examples of agents shown in italics.

Case Studies for Effects on the Male

***m*-Dinitrobenzene**—*m*-Dinitrobenzene (*m*-DNB) has been extensively studied for its ability to produce a rapid deleterious effect on the rat testis. Testicular weight remained reduced for many weeks after the treatment period with significant dose-related effects on fertility (measured by pregnancy rate and implantation success).

Ethylene Glycol Monomethyl Ether (EGME)—EGME has been shown to produce testicular toxicity in a wide variety of species, including nonmammals. A number of studies have described Sertoli cell vacuoles, swollen germ cell mitochondria, and a breakdown of the membrane between the Sertoli cell and the pachytene spermatocyte. This is followed within hours by the death of (probably those) pachytene spermatocytes.

EGME is metabolized to active intermediates methoxyacetaldehyde and methoxyacetic acid (MAA). Treating animals with MAA produces identical testicular lesions as that of the parent compound. The lesion is not characteristic of a low-androgen testicular lesion, and reduced accessory sex organ weights are not a prominent feature associated with the early testicular pathology.

PREGNANCY

Because the transition from early to midpregnancy in the rat requires hormones from the feto-placental unit, if implantation or uterine decidualization is blocked by a chemical, then the female would resume her estrous cycles and the corpora lutea would regress. Chemicals that induce whole-litter loss at mid- to late pregnancy may cause abortions in some of the females, whereas others fail to deliver and appear pregnant for an unusually long period of time.

Many abortifacients induce pregnancy loss by reducing progesterone levels in the rat. Generally, reducing midpregnancy progesterone levels by half or more is sufficient to terminate pregnancy.

SENESCENCE

Perinatal exposure to toxicants with estrogenic activity can defeminize the HPG axis such that the female rats are acyclic and infertile, whereas less affected females display the "delayed anovulatory syndrome" and become anovulatory and acyclic at an early age.

In males, a decrease in androgen is noted in around 20 percent of fit 60-year-old men, but the value of androgen supplementation is not clear with regard to reproductive senescence.

ENDOCRINE DISRUPTION

Currently, the potential effects of EDCs on human health and the proven effects of EDCs on wildlife are a major focus among the scientific community. It has been suggested that in utero exposure to environmental estrogens, antiandrogens, or chemicals like phthalates or 2,3,7,8-TCDD could be responsible for the reported 50 percent decline in sperm counts in some areas and the apparent increase in cryptorchid testes, testicular cancer, and hypospadias.

Phthalate exposures have been associated with reduced AGD in boys and lower testosterone levels in men. In females, exposure to EDCs during development could contribute to earlier age of puberty and to increased incidences of endometriosis and breast cancer. Besides pesticides and other toxic substances in the environment, many compounds that are phytosterols, estrogens, antibiotics, beta-blockers, antiepileptics, and lipid-regulating agents have significant endocrine-disrupting activity and are capable of inducing reproductive toxicity.

In the area of wildlife toxicology and ecosystem health, it is apparent that clear-cut cause and effect relationships exist between exposure to EDCs and adverse effects in several vertebrate classes from fish to mammals.

Known Effects of EDCs in Humans and Animals

The list of chemicals that are known to affect humans, domestic animals, and/or wildlife via functional developmental toxicity or endocrine mechanisms includes 2,3,7,8-TCDD, PCBs and polychlorinated dibenzofurans (PCDFs), methylmercury, ethinylestradiol, alkylphenols, plant sterols, fungal estrogens, androgens, chlordecone, DBCP, dichlorodiphenyltrichloroethane (DDT), and other organochlorine compounds. In addition to these xenobiotics, over 30 different drugs taken during pregnancy have been found to alter human development as a consequence of endocrine disruption. These drugs are not limited to estrogens, like diethylstilbestrol (DES). EDCs are known to alter human development via several mechanisms besides the estrogen receptor (ER), including binding to retinoic acid (RAR and RXR) receptors, and inhibiting synthesis of steroidogenic enzymes or thyroid hormones. Findings on the effects of background levels of PCBs on the neurobehavioral development of the child have contributed to the concerns about the effects of EDCs on human health via alteration of hormone function.

Human Sexual Differentiation—Exposure to hormonally active chemicals during sex differentiation can produce pseudohermaphroditism. Androgenic drugs like danazol and methyltestosterone can masculinize human females (i.e., "female pseudohermaphroditism"). The drug aminoglutethimide, which alters steroid hormone synthesis in a manner identical to many fungicides, also masculinizes human females following in utero exposure.

Transplacental exposure of the developing fetus to DES causes clear cell adenocarcinoma of the vagina, as well as gross structural abnormalities of the cervix, uterus, and fallopian tube. These DES-exposed women are more likely to have an adverse pregnancy outcome, including spontaneous abortions, ectopic pregnancies, and premature delivery. Some of the pathological effects that develop in males following fetal DES exposure appear to result from an inhibition of androgen action or synthesis (underdevelopment or absence of the vas deferens, epididymis, and seminal vesicles) and anti-Müllerian duct factor (persistence of the Müllerian ducts).

Known Effects of Plant and Fungal Products in Animals and Humans—Although most naturally occurring environmental estrogens are relatively inactive, the phytoestrogen miroestrol is almost as potent as estradiol in vitro and even more potent than estradiol when administered orally. In addition, many plant estrogens occur in such high concentrations that they induce reproductive alterations in domestic animals. "Clover disease," which is characterized by dystocia, prolapse of the uterus, and infertility, is observed in sheep that graze on highly estrogenic clover pastures. Permanent infertility can be produced in ewes by much lower amounts of estrogen over a longer time period than are needed to produce "clover disease."

Known Effects of Organochlorine Compounds in Humans—Several pesticides and toxic substances have been shown to alter human reproductive function. An accidental high-dose in utero exposure to PCBs and PCDFs has been associated with reproductive alterations in boys, increased stillbirths, low birth weights, malformations, and IQ and behavioral deficits. In addition to the effects associated with this inadvertent exposure, subtle adverse effects were seen in infants and children exposed to relatively low levels of PCBs and PCDFs.

One metabolite of DDT (mitotane, o,p'-DDD) was found to alter adrenal function with sufficient potency to be used as a drug to treat adrenal steroid hypersecretion associated with adrenal tumors. In addition, lower doses of mitotane restored menstruation in women with spanomenorrhea associated with hypertrichosis.

Occupational Exposures—Occupational exposure to pesticides and other toxic substances (i.e., chlordecone and DBCP) in the workplace has been associated with reduced fertility, lowered sperm counts, and/or endocrine alterations in male workers. Workers exposed to high levels of chlordecone, an estrogenic and neurotoxic organochlorine pesticide, displayed intoxication, severe neurotoxicity, and abnormal testicular function. Male workers involved in the manufacture of 4,4′-diaminostilbene-2,2′-disulfonic acid (DAS), a key ingredient in the synthesis of dyes and fluorescent whitening agents, had lower serum testosterone levels and reduced libido as compared with control workers. Thus, it is surprising that occupational exposures to potential EDCs at effective concentrations have not been entirely eliminated from the workplace.

Environmental Androgens

Androgenic activity has been detected in several complex environmental mixtures. Pulp and paper mill effluents (PME) include a chemical mixture that binds androgen receptors (AR) and induces androgen-dependent gene expression in vitro. This mode of action is consistent with the masculinized female mosquitofish (*Gambusia holbrooki*) collected from contaminated sites. Male-biased sex ratios of fish embryos have been reported in broods of eelpout (*Zoarces viviparus*) in the vicinity of a large kraft pulp mill on the Swedish Baltic coast, suggesting that masculinizing compounds in the effluent were affecting gonadal differentiation and skewing sex ratios. Effluents from beef-cattle concentrated animal feeding operations have been shown to display androgenicity.

Environmental Antiandrogens

Fungicides—Vinclozolin and procymidone are two members of the dicarboximide fungicide class that act as AR antagonists. These pesticides, or their metabolites, competitively inhibit the binding of androgens to AR, leading to an inhibition of androgen-dependent gene expression.

Administration of vinclozolin during sexual differentiation demasculinizes and feminizes the male rat offspring such that treated males display female-like AGD at birth, retained nipples, hypospadias, suprainguinal ectopic testes, a blind vaginal pouch, and small to absent sex accessory glands.

Procymidone induces shortening of the AGD in male pups, and older males display retained nipples, hypospadias, cryptorchidism, cleft phallus, a vaginal pouch, and reduced sex accessory gland size. Fibrosis, cellular infiltration, and epithelial hyperplasia are noted in the dorsolateral and ventral prostatic and seminal vesicular tissues in adult offspring.

Linuron (Herbicide)—This herbicide binds rat and human AR and inhibits DHT–hAR-induced gene expression in vitro. In utero linuron exposure produces male rats displaying epididymal and testicular abnormalities. Also, fetal testosterone production is significantly reduced in linuron-treated fetal males.

Phthalates (Plasticizers)—In utero, some phthalate esters alter the development of the male rat reproductive tract at relatively low dosages. Prenatal exposures to DBP, benzylbutyl phthalate (BBP), di-isononyl phthalate (DINP), and diethylhexylphthalate (DEHP) cause a syndrome of effects, including underdevelopment and agenesis of the epididymis and other androgen-dependent tissues and testicular abnormalities. The phthalates are unique in their ability to induce agenesis of the gubernacular cords, a tissue whose development is dependent on the peptide hormone insulin-like peptide 3.

Environmental Estrogens

Methoxychlor is an estrogenic pesticide that produces estrogen-like effects. The active metabolites activate estrogen-dependent gene expression in vitro and in vivo in the female rats, thereby stimulating a uterotropic response, accelerating VO and inducing constant estrus, and reducing infertility. In the ovariectomized female rats, methoxychlor also induces estrogen-dependent reproductive and nonreproductive behaviors, including female sex behaviors, running wheel activity, and food consumption.

When given to the dam during pregnancy and lactation, both male and female offspring are affected. Females display irregular estrous cycles and reduced fecundity. Male fertility is unaffected at doses up to 200 mg/kg per day.

Ethinylestradiol is a synthetic derivative of estradiol that is in almost all modern formulations of combined oral contraceptive pills. This drug is found in many aquatic systems contaminated by sewage effluents, originating principally from human excretion. Thus, ethinylestradiol plays a major role in causing widespread endocrine disruption in wild populations of fish species and other lower vertebrate species.

EDC Screening Programs

The Endocrine Disruptor Screening and Testing Advisory Committee (EDSTAC) proposed a tiered screening (tier 1) and testing (tier 2) strategy for EDCs. The recommended screening battery was designed to detect alterations of HPG function; estrogen, androgen, and thyroid hormone synthesis; and AR- and ER-mediated effects in mammals and other taxa.

In Vivo Mammalian Assays—EDSTAC recommended the laboratory rat as the species of choice for the endocrine screening and testing assays. The EDSTAC proposed three short-term in vivo mammalian assays for the tier 1 screening battery: the uterotropic, Hershberger, and pubertal female rat assays.

*Uterotropic Assay—*Estrogen agonists and antagonists are detected in a 3-day uterotropic assay using subcutaneous administration of the test compound. The selected uterotropic assays for estrogens and antiestrogens use either the intact juvenile or the castrated ovariectomized adult/juvenile female rat.

*Hershberger Assay—*The second in vivo assay in tier 1, the Hershberger assay, detects antiandrogenic activity simply by weighing androgen-dependent tissues in the castrated male rat. In this assay, weights of the ventral prostate, Cowper's glands, seminal vesicle (with coagulating glands and fluids), glans penis, and levator ani/bulbocavernosus muscles are measured after 10 days of oral treatment with the test compound. This assay is very sensitive for detection of androgens and antiandrogens.

*Pubertal Female Rat Assay—*The third in vivo mammalian/rat assay in the screening battery is the pubertal female rat assay. Weanling female rats are dosed daily by gavage for 21 days while the age at VO (puberty) is monitored. The females are necropsied at about 42 days of age. This assay detects alterations in thyroid hormone status, HPG function, inhibition of steroidogenesis, estrogens, and antiestrogens, and has been found to be highly reproducible and very sensitive to certain endocrine activities including estrogenicity, inhibition of steroidogenesis, and antithyroid activity.

TESTING FOR REPRODUCTIVE TOXICITY
Screens and Multigeneration Studies

Significant attention has focused on the development of "screens" for reproductive toxicity. The screens currently employed have been developed to prioritize chemicals for more comprehensive testing.

The most comprehensive assessment of reproductive toxicity would be provided by a protocol that exposes the animal model throughout the reproductive cycle (see Figure 20–1) and assesses multiple endpoints at different life stages during this continuous exposure. The protocol and guideline coming closest to this ideal is the multigeneration reproduction study (Figure 20–10) used for the assessment of chemicals, pesticides, and some food additives. Multigeneration studies

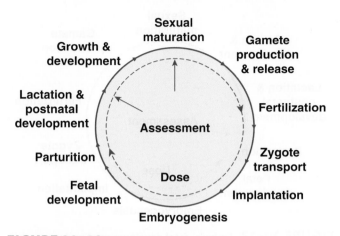

FIGURE 20–10 Multigeneration study.

normally encompass detailed measurements of reproductive performance (number of pregnant females from number of pairs mated, number of females producing a litter, litter size, and number of live pups with their birth weights and sex). Measurement of growth and analysis of the reproductive organs in the F_0 parental generation is conducted. Similar measurements to those undertaken for the F_0 are made on the F_1 parents, and the offspring are examined at birth (and sexually dimorphic endpoints may be collected such as AGD), at weaning, and at puberty (particularly the assessment of VO and time of first estrus in females and belanopreputial separation in males) in addition to the adult measurements of reproductive performance, organ weights, histology, etc.

Testing for Endocrine-disrupting Chemicals

In the tiered screening and testing approach, only chemicals that display positive reproducible responses in tier 1 screening (T1S) would continue evaluation in full-life cycle or multigenerational tests. In tier 2 testing (T2T), issues of dose–response, relevance of the route of exposure, sensitive life stages, and adversity are resolved.

Data should be summarized in a manner that clearly delineates the proportion of animals that are affected. In teratology studies, data are typically presented and analyzed in this manner, indicating the number of malformed/number observed on an individual and litter basis, whereas multigenerational studies are frequently presented and analyzed differently, even when clear teratogenic and other developmental responses are noted after birth. Multigenerational protocols are used in T2T because only these protocols expose the animals during all critical stages of development and examine reproductive function of offspring after they mature.

Although the EPA multigenerational test provides for a comprehensive evaluation of the F_0 or parental generation, too few F_1 animals (offspring with developmental exposure) are exam-

ined after maturity to detect anything but the most profound reproductive teratogens. F_0 animals within a dose group typically respond in a similar fashion to the chemical exposure; however, the response to toxicants in utero can vary greatly even within a litter with only a few animals displaying severe reproductive malformations in the lower dosage groups.

"Transgenerational" protocols typically use fewer litters (7 to 10 per dose group) but examine all of the animals in each litter. These protocols actually use fewer animals but provide enhanced statistical power to detect reproductive effects in the F_1 generation. The life-long exposure of both males and females in the F_1 generation, which allows one to detect effects induced in utero, during lactation, or from direct exposure after puberty, can confound the identification of when the effect was induced (i.e., during adulthood versus development) or of which sex was affected.

Some EDCs disrupt pregnancy by altering maternal ovarian hormone production in F_0 dams at dosage levels that appear to be without direct effect on the offspring. In such cases, the standard EPA multigenerational protocol with minor enhancements would be recommended, or a transgenerational protocol with exposure continued after weaning. The transgenerational or in utero lactational protocols fill a gap in the testing program for EDCs that should be used only on a case-by-case basis.

Testing Pharmaceuticals

In the case of pharmaceuticals, it is rare for multigeneration studies to be conducted, because it is not common for all the population to use a specific drug and exposure to the drug is over many different life stages, and not necessarily chronic. Typically three specific studies are undertaken:

1. **A study of fertility and early embryonic development** (see Figure 20–11). Parental adults are exposed to the test chemical for 2 weeks (females) or 4 weeks (males) prior to breeding and then during breeding. Females then continue their exposure through to implantation. Males can be

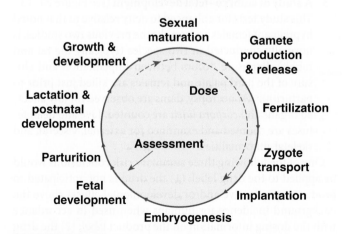

FIGURE 20–11 Fertility and early embryonic study.

Pre-and postnatal development study

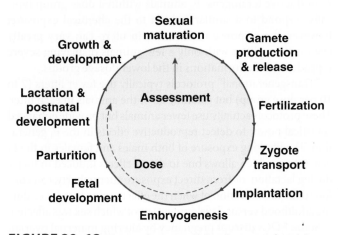

FIGURE 20–12 **Pre- and postnatal developmental toxicity study.** Dosing is from implantation until the litters are weaned.

Embryo–fetal development study

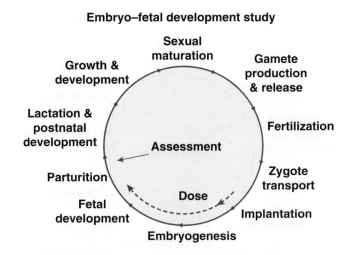

FIGURE 20–13 **Embryo–fetal developmental toxicity study as used by FDA guidelines.** Dosing starts at implantations and continues to closure of the hard palate with an assessment of fetuses just prior to parturition.

necropsied for the endpoints noted above for the multi-generation studies after pregnancy has been confirmed, and for the pregnant females, necropsy takes place any time after midgestation. Reproductive and target organs are weighed and examined histologically, sperm parameters are assessed in males, and the uterine implantation sites and ovarian *corpora lutea* are counted in females, as well as live and dead embryos.

2. **A study of effects on pre- and postnatal development including maternal function** (see Figure 20–12). In this study, pregnant females are exposed from implantation until weaning of their offspring (usually PND 21 in the rat). After cessation of exposure, selected offspring (one male and one female per litter) are raised to adulthood and then mated to assess reproductive competence. These animals are observed for maturation and growth (but are not exposed). Puberty indices, as employed in the multigeneration study, are measured. In addition, sensory function, reflexes, motor activity, learning, and memory are also evaluated.

3. **A study of embryo–fetal development** (see Figure 20–13). This study tests for enhanced toxicity relative to that noted in pregnant females and, unlike the previous two studies, is normally conducted in two species (typically the rat and rabbit). Exposure occurs between implantation and closure of the hard palate and females are killed just prior to parturition. At necropsy, dams are observed for any affected organs and *corpora lutea* are counted. Live and dead fetuses are counted and examined for external, visceral, and skeletal abnormalities.

One of the following three summary risk conclusions would be applied to the drug label: (1) the drug is not anticipated to produce reproductive and/or developmental effects above the background incidence for humans when used in accordance with the dosing information on the product label; (2) the drug may increase the incidence of adverse reproductive and/or de-velopmental events; or (3) the drug is expected to increase the incidence of adverse reproductive and/or developmental effects in humans when used according to the product label.

An examination of the reproductive cycle in a comparison of these three most likely options for FDA studies indicates an obvious gap in the exposure regime for the complete reproductive cycle, namely exposure of weanlings through puberty to adulthood. This exposure period has become of increasing interest to many companies developing drugs for specific administration to infants and juveniles, and "bridging-type" protocols have been developed to specifically address toxicity that may occur after exposure during this specific life stage.

EVALUATION OF TOXICITY TO REPRODUCTION

There are a number of general points that the investigator should note in any estimation of potential reproductive toxicity:

- Adequacy of experimental design and conduct. Was there sufficient statistical power in the evaluation(s)?
- Occurrence of common versus rare reproductive deficits. Biological versus statistical significance.
- Use of historical control data to place concurrent control data into perspective and to estimate population background incidence of various reproductive parameters and deficits.
- Known structure–activity relationships for inducing reproductive toxicity.
- Concordance of reproductive endpoints. Did a decrease in litter size relate to ovarian histology and changes in vaginal cytology?
- Did the reproductive deficits become more severe with increases in dose? Did histological changes at one dose level become decrements in litter size and then reductions in fertility at higher dose levels in any generation?

- Did the reproductive deficits increase in prevalence (more individuals and/or more litters) with dose level in any generation?
- Special care should be taken for decrements in reproductive parameters noted in the F_1 generation (and potentially later generations) that were not seen in the F_0 generation, which may suggest developmental, as well as reproductive, toxicity. Likewise, findings in an F_1 generation animal may (or may not) be reproduced in F_2 offspring. For example, effects in the F_1 generation on reproductive parameters may have resulted in the selection out of sensitive animals in the population, thus not producing F_2 offspring for subsequent evaluation.

BIBLIOGRAPHY

Kapp RW, Tyl RW (eds): *Reproductive Toxicology*. Boca Raton: CRC Press, 2009.

Norris DO, Carr JA (eds): *Endocrine Disruption: Biological Basis for Health Effects in Wildlife and Humans*. New York: Oxford University Press, 2006.

QUESTIONS

1. Which of the following cell types secretes anti-Müllerian hormone (AMH)?
   a. spermatogonium.
   b. Leydig cell.
   c. Sertoli cell.
   d. primary spermatocyte.
   e. spermatid.

2. Penile erections are dependent on:
   a. the CNS.
   b. sympathetic nerve stimulation.
   c. helicine (penile) artery constriction.
   d. corpora cavernosa smooth muscle relaxation.
   e. a spinal reflex arc.

3. The corpus luteum is responsible for the secretion of which of the following hormones during the first part of pregnancy?
   a. estradiol and hCG.
   b. progesterone and estradiol.
   c. progesterone and hCG.
   d. FSH and LH.
   e. FSH and progesterone.

4. All of the following statements regarding the hypothalamo-pituitary–gonadal axis are true EXCEPT:
   a. FSH increases testosterone production by the Leydig cells.
   b. FSH and LH are synthesized in the anterior pituitary.
   c. Estradiol provides negative feedback on the hypothalamus and the anterior pituitary.
   d. GnRH from the hypothalamus increases FSH and LH release from the anterior pituitary.
   e. The LH spike during the menstrual cycle is responsible for ovulation.

5. Which of the following statements is FALSE regarding gametal DNA repair?
   a. DNA repair in spermatogenic cells is dependent on the dose of chemical.
   b. Spermiogenic cells are less able to repair damage from alkylating agents.
   c. Female gametes have base excision repair capacity.
   d. Meiotic maturation of the oocyte decreases its ability to repair DNA damage.
   e. Mature oocytes and mature sperm no longer have the ability to repair DNA damage.

6. Reduction division takes place during the transition between which two cell types during spermatogenesis?
   a. spermatogonium and primary spermatocyte.
   b. primary spermatocyte and secondary spermatocyte.
   c. secondary spermatocyte and spermatid.
   d. spermatid and spermatozoon.
   e. spermatozoon and mature sperm.

7. Which of the following cell types is properly paired with the substance that it secretes?
   a. ovarian granulosa cells—progesterone.
   b. Leydig cells—ABP.
   c. ovarian thecal cells—estrogens.
   d. Sertoli cells—testosterone.
   e. gonadotroph—LH.

8. Which of the following statements regarding male reproductive capacity is FALSE?
   a. Klinefelter's syndrome males are sterile.
   b. FSH levels are often measured in order to determine male reproductive toxicity of a particular toxin.
   c. Divalent metal ions, such as An, Hg, and Cu, act as androgen receptor antagonists and affect male reproduction.
   d. The number of sperms produced per day is approximately the same in all males.
   e. ABP is an important biochemical marker for testicular injury.

9. Reduction of sperm production can be caused by all of the following diseases EXCEPT:
   a. hypothyroidism.
   b. measles.
   c. Crohn's disease.
   d. renal failure.
   e. mumps.

10. Of the following, which is LEAST likely to be affected by estrogen?
    a. nervous system.
    b. musculoskeletal system.
    c. digestive system.
    d. cardiovascular system.
    e. urinary system.

Toxic Responses of the Endocrine System

Charles C. Capen

INTRODUCTION

Endocrine glands are collections of specialized cells that synthesize, store, and release their secretions directly into the bloodstream. They are sensing and signaling devices located in the extracellular fluid compartment that are capable of responding to changes in the internal and external environments and coordinating multiple activities that maintain homeostasis.

PITUITARY GLAND

Normal Structure and Function

The pituitary gland (hypophysis) is divided into two major compartments: (1) the adenohypophysis (anterior lobe), composed of the pars distalis, pars tuberalis, and pars intermedia, and (2) the neurohypophyseal system, which includes the pars nervosa (posterior lobe), infundibular stalk, and hypothalamic nuclei (supraoptic and paraventricular) containing the neurosecretory neurons, which synthesize and package the neurohypophyseal hormones into secretory granules. The pars intermedia forms the thin cellular zone between the adenohypophysis and neurohypophysis. The arterial blood supply to the pituitary gland forms a capillary plexus that drains into the hypophyseal portal veins, which supply the adenohypophysis. The hypothalamic–hypophyseal portal system transports the hypothalamic-releasing and release-inhibiting hormones directly to the adenohypophysis, where they interact with their specific populations of trophic hormone-producing cells.

The pars distalis of the adenohypophysis is composed of multiple populations of endocrine cells that secrete the pituitary trophic hormones. The secretory cells are surrounded by abundant capillaries derived from the hypothalamic–hypophyseal portal system. The pars tuberalis functions primarily as a scaffold for the capillary network of the hypophyseal portal system during its course from the median eminence to the pars distalis.

Secretory cells in the adenohypophysis can be classified functionally into somatotrophs that secrete growth hormone (GH; somatotrophin), luteotrophs that secrete luteotropic hormone (LTH; prolactin), gonadotrophs, which secrete luteinizing hormone (LH) and follicle-stimulating hormone (FSH), thyrotrophs, which secrete thyroid-stimulating hormone (TSH), and chromophobes, which are involved with the synthesis of adrenocorticotropin hormone (ACTH) and melanocyte-stimulating hormone (MSH) in some species.

Each type of endocrine cell in the adenohypophysis is under the control of a specific releasing hormone from the hypothalamus (Figure 21–1). These releasing hormones are small peptides that are synthesized and secreted by neurons of the hypothalamus and are conveyed by the hypophyseal portal system to specific trophic hormone-secreting cells in the adenohypophysis. Each hormone stimulates the rapid release of preformed secretory granules containing a specific trophic hormone. Specific releasing hormones have been identified for TSH, FSH and LH, ACTH, and GH. Prolactin secretion is stimulated by a number of factors, the most important of which appears to be thyrotropin-releasing hormone (TRH). Dopamine serves as the major prolactin-inhibitory factor and suppresses prolactin secretion and ACTH production. Somatostatin (somatotrophin-release-inhibiting hormone, SRIH) inhibits the secretion of both GH and TSH. Control of pituitary trophic hormone secretion also is affected by negative feedback by the circulating concentration of target organ hormones.

The neurohypophyseal hormones (i.e., oxytocin and antidiuretic hormone) are synthesized in the cell body of hypothalamic neurons, packaged into secretory granules, transported by long axonal processes to the pars nervosa, and released into the bloodstream.

As the biosynthetic precursor molecules travel along the axons in secretion granules from the neurosecretory neurons, the precursors are cleaved into the active hormones and their respective neurophysins.

In addition to the specific trophic hormone-secreting cells, a population of supporting cells is also present in the adenohypophysis. These cells, referred to as stellate (follicular) cells, appear to provide a phagocytic or supportive function in addition to producing a colloid-like material that accumulates in follicles.

Mechanisms of Pituitary Toxicity

Pituitary tumors can be induced readily by sustained uncompensated hormonal derangements leading to increased synthesis and secretion of pituitary hormones. The absence of negative feedback inhibition of pituitary cells leads to unrestrained proliferation (hyperplasia initially, neoplasia later). For example, surgical removal or radiation-induced ablation of the thyroid or

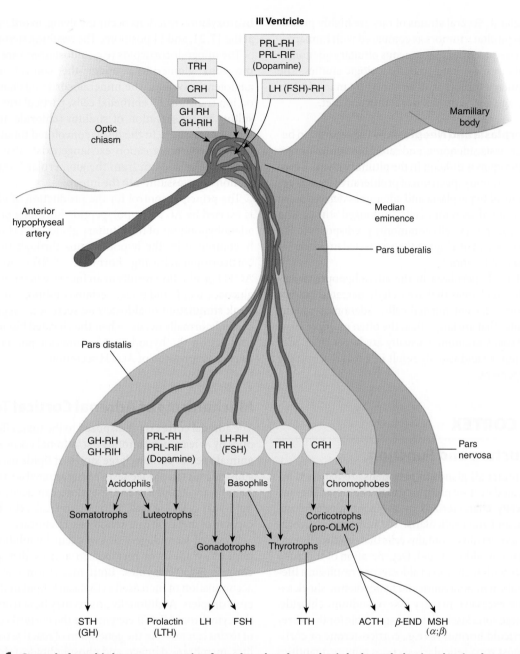

FIGURE 21–1 **Control of trophic hormone secretion from the adenohypophysis by hypothalamic-releasing hormones (RH) and release-inhibiting hormones (RIH).** The releasing and release-inhibiting hormones are synthesized by neurons in the hypothalamus, transported by axonal processes, and released into capillary plexus in the median eminence. They are transported to the adenohypophysis by the hypothalamic–hypophyseal portal system, where they interact with specific populations of trophic hormone-secreting cells to govern the rate of release of preformed hormones, such as growth hormone (GH), somatotropic hormone (STH), luteotropic hormone (LTH), luteinizing hormone (LH), follicle-stimulating hormone (FSH), thyrotropic hormone (TTH), adrenocorticotropic hormone (ACTH), and melanocyte-stimulating hormone (MSH). There are RIHs for those trophic hormones (e.g., prolactin and growth hormone) that do not directly influence the activity of target cells and result in production of a final endocrine product (hormone) that could exert negative feedback control.

interference with the production of thyroid hormones by the use of specific chemical inhibitors of thyroid hormone synthesis leads to a stimulation of TSH synthesis and secretion with elevated blood levels. The thyrotrophic cells in the adenohypophysis undergo prominent hypertrophy. Similarly, estrogens, caffeine, *N*-methylnitrosourea, and the neuroleptic agent sulpiride have been reported to cause the development of pituitary tumors.

Morphologic Alterations and Proliferative Lesions of Pituitary Cells

Calcitonin (CT) is produced in the posterior hypothalamus and median eminence where it normally exerts an effect on the hypothalamus–pituitary axis. CT receptors have been identified in the hypothalamus and lower numbers of receptors are found in the pituitary gland. Several strains of rats are highly predisposed to develop pituitary tumors as compared with humans.

There is a high frequency of spontaneous pituitary adenomas in laboratory rats in most long-term toxicologic studies. The incidence of pituitary tumors is determined by many factors including strain, age, sex, reproductive status, and diet.

Pituitary Hyperplasia and Neoplasia—The separation between focal hyperplasia, adenoma, and carcinoma utilizing histopathologic techniques is difficult in the pituitary gland. There appears to be a continuous spectrum of proliferative lesions between diffuse or focal hyperplasia and adenomas derived from a specific population of secretory cells. Prolonged stimulation of a population of secretory cells commonly predisposes to the subsequent development of a higher than expected incidence of focal hyperplasia and tumors.

Focal ("nodular") hyperplasia in the adenohypophysis appears as multiple small areas that are well demarcated but not encapsulated from adjacent normal cells. Adenomas usually are solitary nodules that are larger than the often multiple areas of focal hyperplasia. Carcinomas usually are larger than adenomas in the pituitary and usually result in a macroscopically detectable enlargement.

ADRENAL CORTEX

Normal Structure and Function

The adrenal (suprarenal) glands in mammals are flattened bilobed organs located in close proximity to the kidneys. The cortex is histologically characterized by the zona glomerulosa, zona fasciculata, and zona reticularis. The mineralocorticoid-producing zona glomerulosa contains cells that produce mineralocorticoids (namely, aldosterone). Degeneration of this zone or an interference with secretion of aldosterone results in a life-threatening retention of potassium and hypovolemic shock associated with the excessive urinary loss of sodium, chloride, and water. The large zona fasciculata is responsible for the secretion of glucocorticoid hormones (e.g., corticosterone or cortisol). The innermost zona reticularis secretes minute quantities of adrenal sex hormones.

The adrenal cortical cells contain large cytoplasmic lipid droplets consisting of cholesterol and other steroid hormone precursors. The lipid droplets are in close proximity to the smooth endoplasmic reticulum and large mitochondria, which contain the specific hydroxylase and dehydrogenase enzyme systems required to synthesize the different steroid hormones. There are no secretory granules in the cytoplasm, because there is direct secretion without significant storage of preformed steroid hormones.

The common biosynthetic pathway from cholesterol involves the formation of pregnenolone, the basic precursor for the three major classes of adrenal steroids. Pregnenolone is formed after two hydroxylation reactions at the carbon 20 and 22 positions of cholesterol and a subsequent cleavage between these two carbon atoms. In the zona fasciculata, pregnenolone is first converted to progesterone by two microsomal enzymes. Three subsequent hydroxylation reactions occur involving, in order, carbon atoms at the 17, 21, and 11 positions. The resulting steroid is cortisol.

The mineralocorticoids (e.g., aldosterone) are secreted from the zona glomerulosa under the control of the renin–angiotensin system. The mineralocorticoids have their effects on ion transport by epithelial cells, particularly renal cells, resulting in conservation of sodium (chloride and water) and loss of potassium. In the distal convoluted tubule of the mammalian nephron, a cation exchange exists that promotes the resorption of sodium from the glomerular filtrate and the secretion of potassium into the lumen.

The principal control for the production of glucocorticoids is exerted by ACTH, a polypeptide hormone produced in the adenohypophysis of the pituitary gland. ACTH release is largely controlled by the hypothalamus through the secretion of corticotropin-releasing hormone (CRH). An increase in ACTH production results in an increase in circulating levels of glucocorticoids and under certain conditions also can result in weak stimulation of aldosterone secretion. Negative feedback control normally occurs when the elevated blood levels of cortisol act on the hypothalamus, anterior pituitary, or both to cause a suppression of ACTH secretion.

Mechanisms of Adrenal Cortical Toxicity

The adrenal cortex is predisposed to the toxic effects of xenobiotics by at least two factors. *First,* adrenal cortical cells of most animal species contain large stores of lipids used primarily as substrate for steroidogenesis. Many adrenal cortical toxic compounds are lipophilic and therefore can accumulate in these lipid-rich cells. *Second,* adrenal cortical cells have enzymes capable of metabolizing xenobiotic chemicals.

Impaired steroidogenesis can occur by inhibition of cholesterol biosynthesis or metabolism and by disruption of cytochrome P-450 enzymes. Both mechanisms will lead to the accumulation of increased cytoplasmic lipid in the form of discrete droplets. Additionally, toxins may be activated by many of the cytochrome P-450 enzymes in the cortical cells. Activation of toxins can result in the generation of reactive oxygen metabolites, membrane damage, and phospholipidosis in the cells.

Classes of chemicals toxic for the adrenal cortex include short-chain (three- or four-carbon) aliphatic compounds, lipidosis inducers, and amphiphilic compounds. The most potent aliphatic compounds include acrylonitrile, 3-aminopropionitrile, 3-bromopropionitrile, 1-butanethiol, and 1,4-butanedithiol. By comparison, lipidosis inducers can cause the accumulations of neutral fats, which may cause a reduction or loss of organellar function and eventual cell destruction. Compounds causing lipidosis include aminoglutethimide, amphenone, and anilines. Biologically active cationic amphiphilic compounds, including chloroquine, triparanol, and chlorphentermine, produce a generalized phospholipidosis with microscopic phospholipid-rich inclusions that affect the functional integrity of lysosomes.

Many of the chemicals that cause morphologic changes in the adrenal glands also affect cortical function. Chemically induced changes in adrenal function may result either from blockage of the action of adrenocorticoids at peripheral sites or by inhibition of synthesis and/or secretion of hormone. In the first mechanism, many steroidal antagonists act by competing with or binding to steroid hormone–receptor sites, thereby either reducing the number of available receptor sites or altering their binding affinity. Cortexolone (11α-deoxycortisol), an antiglucocorticoid, and spironolactone, an antimineralocorticoid, are two examples of peripherally acting adrenal cortical hormone antagonists.

Xenobiotics may affect adrenal steroidogenesis. For example, chemicals causing increased lipid droplets often inhibit the utilization of steroid precursors, including the conversion of cholesterol to pregnenolone. Chemicals that affect the fine structure of mitochondria and smooth endoplasmic reticulum often impair the activity of 11α-, 17α-, and 21-hydroxylases, respectively, and are associated with lesions primarily in the zonae reticularis and fasciculata. Atrophy of the zona glomerulosa may reflect specific inhibition of aldosterone synthesis or secretion, either directly (e.g., inhibition of 18α-hydroxylation) or indirectly (e.g., suppression of the renin–angiotensin system) by chemicals such as spironolactone and captopril.

Pathological Alterations and Proliferative Lesions in Cortical Cells

Cortical hypertrophy due to impaired steroidogenesis or hyperplasia due to long-term stimulation often is present when the adrenal cortex is increased in size. Small adrenal glands often are indicative of degenerative changes or trophic atrophy of the adrenal cortex. Nodular lesions that distort and enlarge one or both adrenal glands suggest that a neoplasm is present.

Lesions of adrenal cortical cells associated with chemical injury may be classified as follows: endothelial damage with acrylonitrile, mitochondrial damage with DMNM, o,p′-DDD, amphenone, endoplasmic reticulum disruption with triparanol, lipid aggregation with aniline, lysosomal phospholipid aggregation with chlorophentermine, and secondary effects due to embolization by medullary cells with acrylonitrile. Damage to mitochondria and smooth endoplasmic reticulum occurs after exposure to chemical agents inhibiting steroidogenesis.

ADRENAL MEDULLA

Normal Structure and Function

The bulk of the medulla is composed of chromaffin cells, which synthesize and store catecholamines. Human adrenal medullary cells may contain both norepinephrine and epinephrine within a single chromaffin cell. The adrenal medulla also contains variable numbers of ganglion cells and the small granule-containing (SGC) cells or small intensely fluorescent (SIF) cells. SIF cells lie intermediate between chromaffin cells and ganglion cells and may function as interneurons. The adrenal medullary cells also contain serotonin and histamine as well as several neuropeptides including enkephalins, neurotensin, and neuropeptide Y.

Mechanisms of Adrenal Medullary Toxicity

Proliferative lesions of the medulla develop as a result of various mechanisms. For example, the long-term administration of GH is associated with an increased incidence of pheochromocytomas as well as tumors at other sites. Prolactin-secreting pituitary tumors also play a role in the development of proliferative medullary lesions. In addition, several neuroleptic compounds that increase prolactin secretion by inhibiting dopamine production have been associated with an increased incidence of proliferative lesions of medullary cells in rats. Drugs that increase the incidence of adrenal medullary proliferative lesions include nicotine, reserpine, zomepirac, isoretinoin, nafarelin (LHRH analog), atenolol, terazosin, ribavirin, and pamidronate (bisphosphonate).

Environmental and dietary factors may be more important than genetic factors as determinants of the incidence of adrenal medullary proliferative lesions in rats. Incidence can be reduced by lowering the carbohydrate content of the diet. Several agents, including sugar alcohols, that increase the incidence of adrenal medullary lesions increase absorption of calcium from the gut. Calcium ions, cyclic nucleotides, and prostaglandins may mediate both hormonal secretion and cellular proliferation. The fact that vitamin D is the most potent stimulus of medullary chromaffin cell proliferation supports the hypothesis that altered calcium homeostasis is involved in pheochromocytoma pathogenesis.

THYROID GLAND (FOLLICULAR CELLS)

Normal Structure and Function

The thyroid consists of follicles of varying size (20 to 250 μm) that contain colloid produced by the follicular cells (thyrocytes). Follicular cells have extensive profiles of rough endoplasmic reticulum and a large Golgi apparatus in their cytoplasm for synthesis and packaging substantial amounts of protein that are then transported into the follicular lumen.

Biosynthesis of Thyroid Hormones—Thyroglobulin is a high-molecular-weight glycoprotein synthesized in successive subunits on the ribosomes of the endoplasmic reticulum in follicular cells. Iodine is bound to the tyrosyl residues in thyroglobulin at the apical surface of follicular cells to form successively monoiodotyrosine (MIT) and diiodotyrosine (DIT). These biologically inactive iodothyronines subsequently are coupled together to form the biologically active triiodothyronine (T_3) and thyroxine (T_4) that are secreted by the thyroid gland. Thyroperoxidase oxidizes iodide ion (I^-) taken up by follicular cells into reactive iodine (I_2), which binds to the tyrosine residues in thyroglobulin. Thyroperoxidase also functions as a coupling enzyme to combine MIT and DIT to form T_3 or two DITs to form T_4. Transport of iodide has been shown to be associated with a sodium–iodide (Na^+–I^-) symporter (NIS) linked to the transport of Na^+.

Thyroid Hormone Secretion—Negative feedback control of thyroid hormone secretion is accomplished by coordinated response to circulating levels of thyroid hormones (especially T_3). A decrease in thyroid hormone concentration in plasma is sensed by groups of neurosecretory neurons in the hypothalamus that synthesize and secrete TRH into the hypophyseal portal circulation. TSH is conveyed to thyroid follicular cells where it activates adenyl cyclase, and increases the rate of biochemical reactions concerned with the synthesis and secretion of thyroid hormones.

Species Differences in Thyroid Hormone Economy

Long-term perturbations of the pituitary–thyroid axis by xenobiotics, iodine deficiency, partial thyroidectomy, and natural goitrogens in food are likely to predispose rats to a higher incidence of proliferative lesions in response to chronic TSH stimulation than in human thyroids. This greater sensitivity of the rodent thyroid is related to the shorter plasma half-life of thyroxine T_4 in rats than in humans.

Mechanisms of Thyroid Tumorigenesis

Chronic treatment of rodents with goitrogenic compounds results in the development of follicular cell adenomas. Thiouracil and its derivatives, brassica seeds, erythrosine, sulfonamides, and other compounds directly interfere with thyroid hormone synthesis or secretion in the thyroid gland, increase thyroid hormone catabolism and subsequent excretion into the bile, or disrupt the peripheral conversion of T_4 to T_3. The ensuing decrease in circulating thyroid hormone levels results in a compensatory increased secretion of pituitary TSH. TSH stimulation of the thyroid gland leads to proliferative changes of follicular cells that include hypertrophy, hyperplasia, and ultimately, neoplasia in rodents.

Xenobiotics that Directly Inhibit Thyroid Hormone Synthesis

Blockage of Iodine Uptake—Thyroid hormone biosynthesis occurs extracellularly within the follicular lumen. Essential raw materials, such as iodide, are transported rapidly against a concentration gradient into the lumen, and oxidized by a thyroid peroxidase to reactive iodine (I_2) (Figure 21–2). This transport of iodide ion is linked to the transport of Na^+. The iodine transport system in the thyroid gland can be selectively inhibited by competitive anion inhibitors, thereby blocking the

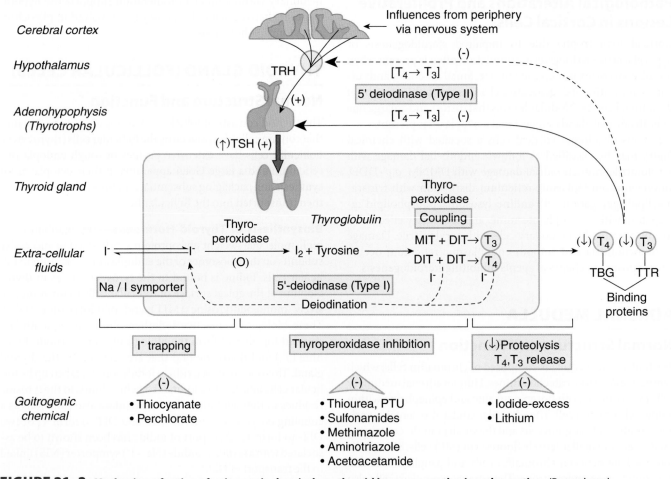

FIGURE 21–2 **Mechanism of action of goitrogenic chemicals on thyroid hormone synthesis and secretion.** (Reproduced with permission from Dunlop RH, Malbert C, Capen CC, O'Brien TD: Pathophysiology of Endocrine Homeostasis: Examples IN *Veterinary Pathophysiology*, Blackwell Publishing, 2004.)

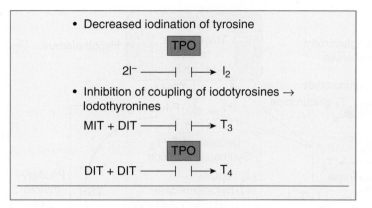

FIGURE 21–3 Mechanisms by which xenobiotic chemicals decrease thyroid hormone synthesis by inhibiting thyroperoxidase (TPO) in follicular cells.

ability of the gland to iodinate tyrosine residues in thyroglobulin and synthesize thyroid hormones.

Inhibition of Thyroid Peroxidase Resulting in an Organification Defect—The stepwise binding of iodide to the tyrosyl residues in thyroglobulin requires oxidation of inorganic iodide to molecular iodine (I_2) by thyroid peroxidase (Figure 21–2). Classes of chemicals that inhibit the organification of thyroglobulin include (1) the thionamides (such as thiourea, thiouracil, propylthiouracil [PTU], methimazole, carbimazole, and goitrin); (2) aniline derivatives (e.g., sulfonamides, *para*-aminobenzoic acid, *para*-aminosalicylic acid, and amphenone); (3) substituted phenols (such as resorcinol, phloroglucinol, and 2,4-dihydroxybenzoic acid); and (4) miscellaneous inhibitors (e.g., aminotriazole, antipyrine, and iodopyrine). Many of these chemicals inhibit thyroid peroxidase, which disrupts both the iodination of tyrosyl residues in thyroglobulin and the coupling reaction of MIT and DIT to form T_3 and T_4 (Figure 21–3). Inhibition of gap-junction intercellular communication by PTU or a low-iodine diet may increase thyroid follicular cell proliferation by disrupting the passage of regulatory substance(s) through these channels.

Blockage of Thyroid Hormone Release by Excess Iodide and Lithium

Relatively few chemicals selectively inhibit the secretion of thyroid hormone from the thyroid gland (Figure 21–2). An excess of iodine inhibits secretion of thyroid hormone and occasionally can result in goiter and subnormal function (hypothyroidism) in animals and human patients. Lithium carbonate inhibits the release of thyroid hormones and occasionally results in the development of goiter.

Hepatic Microsomal Enzyme Induction

Glucuronidation is the rate-limiting step in the biliary excretion of T_4 and sulfation for the excretion of T_3. Chemicals that induce these enzyme pathways may result in chronic stimulation of the thyroid by disrupting the hypothalamic–pituitary–thyroid axis (Figure 21–4). Microsomal enzyme inducers are more effective in reducing serum T_4 than serum T_3. Xenobiotics that induce liver microsomal enzymes and disrupt thyroid function in rats include CNS-acting drugs (e.g., phenobarbital and benzodiazepines), calcium channel blockers (e.g., nicardipine and bepridil), spironolactone, retinoids, chlorinated hydrocarbons (e.g., chlordane, DDT, and TCDD), and polyhalogenated biphenyls (PCB and PBB), among others. Most hepatic microsomal enzyme inducers have no apparent intrinsic carcinogenicity or mutagenicity. Their promoting effect on thyroid tumors usually is greater in rats than in mice, with males often developing a higher incidence of tumors than females.

There is no convincing evidence that humans treated with drugs or exposed to chemicals that induce hepatic microsomal enzymes are at increased risk for the development of thyroid or liver cancer. In fact, relatively high microsomal enzyme-inducing doses of phenobarbital have been used chronically as an anticonvulsant, sometimes for lifetime exposures, to control seizure activity in human beings without the onset of thyroid cancer.

Secondary Mechanisms of Thyroid Tumorigenesis and Risk Assessment

Many chemicals disrupt one or more steps in the synthesis and secretion of thyroid hormones, resulting in subnormal levels of T_4 and T_3 and an associated increased secretion of TSH (Figure 21–4). In the secondary mechanism of thyroid oncogenesis in rodents, the specific xenobiotic or physiologic perturbation evokes the chronic hypersecretion of TSH that promotes the development of proliferative lesions derived from follicular cells.

In contrast to rats and mice, humans are relatively resistant to the development of thyroid cancer, with an incidence of approximately 1 percent of the population. A few human patients with congenital defects in thyroid hormone synthesis

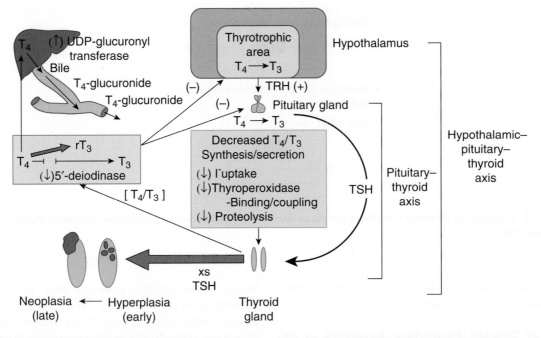

FIGURE 21–4 Multiple sites of disruption of the hypothalamic–pituitary–thyroid axis by xenobiotic chemicals. Chemicals can exert direct effects by disrupting thyroid hormone synthesis or secretion and indirectly influence the thyroid through an inhibition of 5'-deiodinase or by inducing hepatic microsomal enzymes (e.g., T_4–UDP-glucuronyltransferase). All of these mechanisms can lower circulating levels of thyroid hormones (T_4 and/or T_3), resulting in a release from negative feedback inhibition and increased secretion of thyroid-stimulating hormone (TSH) by the pituitary gland. The chronic hypersecretion of TSH predisposes the sensitive rodent thyroid gland to develop an increased incidence of focal hyperplastic and neoplastic lesions (adenomas) by a secondary (epigenetic) mechanism.

and elevated circulating TSH levels as well as thyrotoxic patients with Graves' disease appear to be at a greater risk of developing thyroid tumors. The literature suggests that prolonged stimulation of the human thyroid by TSH will induce neoplasia only in exceptional circumstances, possibly by acting together with some other metabolic or immunologic abnormality.

THYROID C CELLS

Normal Structure and Function

CT is secreted by C cells (parafollicular or light cells) in the mammalian thyroid gland. C cells contain numerous small membrane-limited secretory granules in the cytoplasm in which the CT activity is localized.

CT is a polypeptide hormone that is secreted continuously under conditions of normocalcemia. The rate of secretion of CT is increased greatly in response to elevations in blood calcium. C cells store substantial amounts of CT in their secretory granules. In response to hypercalcemia, there is a rapid discharge of stored hormone from C cells into interfollicular capillaries. The hypercalcemic stimulus, if sustained, is followed by hypertrophy of C cells. Hyperplasia of C cells occurs in response to long-term hypercalcemia.

CT exerts its function by interacting with target cells, primarily in bone and kidney. CT antagonizes the action of parathyroid hormone on mobilizing calcium from bone but synergistically decreases the renal tubular reabsorption of phosphorus. CT and parathyroid hormone, acting in concert, provide a dual negative feedback control mechanism to maintain the life-sustaining concentration of calcium ion in extracellular fluids within narrow limits.

Morphologic Alterations and Proliferative Lesions of Thyroid C Cells

There are two types of C-cell hyperplasia: diffuse and focal (nodular) (Figure 21–5). In diffuse hyperplasia, the numbers of C cells are increased throughout the thyroid lobe to a point where they may be more numerous than follicular cells. In focal C-cell hyperplasia, the accumulations of proliferating C cells are of a lesser diameter than five average colloid-containing thyroid follicles, with minimal evidence of compression of adjacent follicles. C-cell adenomas are discrete, expansive masses of C cells larger than five average colloid-containing thyroid follicles. C cells composing an adenoma may be subdivided by fine connective tissue septae and capillaries into small neuroendocrine packets. Occasional

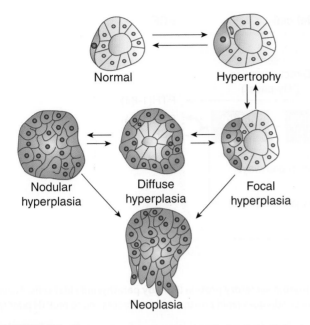

FIGURE 21–5 **Focal and nodular hyperplasia of C cells in the thyroid often precedes the development of C-cell neoplasms.**

amyloid deposits may be found both in nodular hyperplasia and in adenomas.

C-cell carcinomas often result in enlargement of one or both thyroid lobes due to the extensive proliferation of C cells. Immunoperoxidase reactions for CT generally are more intense in diffuse or nodular hyperplasia, whereas in adenomas and carcinomas CT immunoreactivity varies between tumors and different regions of a tumor. Hyperplastic C cells adjacent to adenomas and carcinomas usually are intensely positive for CT.

PARATHYROID GLAND

To maintain a constant concentration of calcium despite marked variations in intake and excretion, endocrine control consists of the interactions of three major hormones—parathyroid hormone (PTH), CT, and cholecalciferol (vitamin D) (Figure 21–6). Disruption of the regulation of calcium balance in animals results in hyper- or hypocalcemia and can lead to metabolic disease and death.

PTH is the principal hormone involved in the minute-to-minute, fine regulation of blood calcium in mammals. In general, the most important biologic effects of PTH are to: (1) elevate the blood concentration of calcium, (2) decrease the blood concentration of phosphorus, (3) increase the urinary excretion of phosphorus by a decreased rate of tubular reabsorption, (4) increase the renal tubular reabsorption of calcium, (5) increase the rate of skeletal remodeling and the net rate of bone resorption, (6) increase the numbers of osteoclasts on bone surfaces and the rate of osteolysis, (7) increase the urinary excretion of hydroxyproline, (8) activate adenylate cyclase in target cells, and (9) accelerate the formation of the principal active vitamin D metabolite.

Normal Structure and Function of Chief Cells

Biosynthesis of Parathyroid Hormone—Parathyroid chief cells in humans and many animal species store relatively

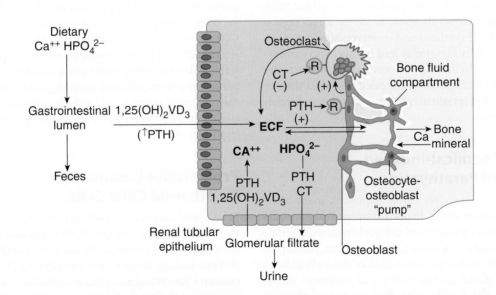

FIGURE 21–6 **Interrelationship of parathyroid hormone (PTH), calcitonin (CT), and 1,25-dihydroxycholecalciferol (1,25(OH)$_2$VD$_3$) in the regulation of calcium (Ca) and phosphorus in extracellular fluids.** Receptors for PTH are on osteoblasts and for CT on osteoclasts in bone. PTH and CT are antagonistic in their action on bone but synergistic in stimulating the renal excretion of phosphorous. Vitamin D exerts its action primarily on the intestine to enhance the absorption of both calcium and phosphorus.

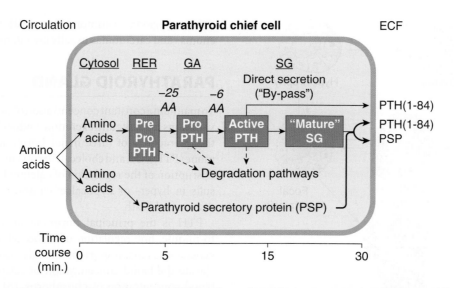

Circulation   **Parathyroid chief cell**   ECF

FIGURE 21–7 **Biosynthesis of parathyroid hormone (PTH) and parathyroid secretory protein (PSP) by parathyroid chief cells.** Active PTH is synthesized as a larger biosynthetic precursor molecule (preproPTH) that undergoes rapid posttranslational processing to proPTH prior to secretion from chief cells as active PTH (amino acids 1 to 84).

small amounts of preformed hormone, but they respond quickly to variations in the need for hormone by changing the rate of hormone synthesis (Figure 21–7). Under certain conditions of increased demand (e.g., a low calcium ion concentration in the extracellular fluid compartment), PTH may be released directly from chief cells without being packaged into secretion granules.

Control of Parathyroid Hormone Secretion—The parathyroid glands have a unique feedback controlled by the concentration of calcium (and to a lesser extent magnesium) ion in serum. Serum Ca^{2+} binds to a Ca receptor on the chief cell, which permits the serum Ca^{2+} to regulate chief cell function. The concentration of blood phosphorus has no direct regulatory influence on PTH synthesis and secretion; however, an elevated blood phosphorus level may lead indirectly to parathyroid stimulation by decreasing the production of the active form of vitamin D ($1,25$-$(OH)_2$-cholecalciferol), and thereby diminishing the rate of intestinal calcium absorption and thusly serum calcium levels.

Xenobiotic Chemical-induced Toxic Injury of Parathyroids

Ozone—One to 5 days after ozone exposure, many chief cells undergo compensatory hypertrophy and hyperplasia with areas of capillary endothelial cell proliferation, interstitial edema, degeneration of vascular endothelium, formation of platelet thrombi, leukocyte infiltration of the walls of larger vessels in the gland, and disruption of basement membranes. Inactive chief cells with few secretory granules predominate in the parathyroids in the later stages of exposure to ozone.

Aluminum—Patients with chronic renal failure treated by hemodialysis with aluminum-containing fluids or orally administered drugs containing aluminum often had normal or minimal elevations of immunoreactive parathyroid hormone (iPTH), little histologic evidence of osteitis fibrosa in bone, and a depressed response by the parathyroid gland to acute hypocalcemia. Aluminum appears to decrease diglyceride synthesis, which is reflected in a corresponding decrease in synthesis of phosphatidylcholine and triglyceride.

L-Asparaginase—Parathyroid chief cells appear to be selectively destroyed by L-asparaginase. Chief cells were predominately inactive and degranulated, with large autophagic vacuoles present in the cytoplasm of degenerating cells. Cytoplasmic organelles concerned with synthesis and packaging of secretory products were poorly developed in chief cells. Rabbits developed hyperphosphatemia, hypomagnesemia, hyperkalemia, azotemia, and acute hypocalcemia. The development of hypocalcemia and tetany is common in the rabbit, but some human patients receiving the drug also have developed hypocalcemia.

Proliferative Lesions of Parathyroid Chief Cells

Parathyroid adenomas are solitary nodules that are sharply demarcated from adjacent parathyroid parenchyma. Adenomas are usually endocrinologically inactive in adult-aged rats from chronic toxicity studies. The parathyroid glands that do not contain a functional adenoma also undergo trophic atrophy in response to the hypercalcemia.

Few chemicals or experimental manipulations increase the incidence of parathyroid tumors. Parathyroid adenomas have been noted infrequently following the administration of the pesticide rotenone in 2-year bioassay studies in Fischer rats. Irradiation significantly increases the incidence of parathyroid adenomas in inbred Wistar albino rats.

TESTIS

Structure and Endocrinologic Regulation of Leydig (Interstitial) Cells

Leydig (interstitial) cell tumors are among the most frequently occurring endocrine tumors in rodents in chronic carcinogenicity studies. In contrast, the incidence of Leydig cell tumors in human patients is extremely rare, on the order of 1 in 5 million, with age peaks at approximately 30 and 60 years. The most common and clinically important testicular neoplasms in men are of germ cell origin (e.g., seminona). By comparison, germ cell tumors are rare in rodents either as a spontaneous lesion or following exposure to large doses of xenobiotic chemicals.

Endocrinologic regulation of Leydig cells involves the coordinated activity of the hypothalamus and anterior pituitary with negative feedback control exerted by the blood concentration of gonadal steroids (Figure 21–8). Hypothalamic gonadotropin-releasing hormone (GnRH) stimulates the pulsatile release of both LH and FSH from the adenohypophysis. LH is the major trophic factor controlling the activity of Leydig cells and the synthesis of testosterone. The blood levels of testosterone exert negative feedback on the hypothalamus and, to a lesser extent, on the adenohypophysis. FSH binds to receptors on Sertoli cells in the seminiferous tubules and, along with the local concentration of testosterone, is critical in

spermatogenesis. Testosterone, by controlling GnRH release, is one important regulator of FSH secretion by the pituitary gland. The seminiferous tubules also produce a glycopeptide, designated as inhibin, which exerts negative feedback on the release of FSH.

Pathology of Leydig (Interstitial) Cell Tumors

To standardize the classification of focal proliferative lesions of Leydig cells between studies with different xenobiotic chemicals and different testing laboratories, the following diagnostic criteria were established: (1) hyperplasia was defined as a focal collection of Leydig cells with little atypia and a diameter of less than one seminiferous tubule; (2) an adenoma was defined as a mass of Leydig cells larger in diameter than one seminiferous tubule with some cellular atypia and compression of adjacent tubules.

Mechanisms of Leydig (Interstitial) Cell Tumor Development

Pathogenic mechanisms important in the development of proliferative lesions of Leydig cells include irradiation, the species and strain differences mentioned previously, cryptorchidism, a compromised blood supply to the testis, or heterotransplantation into the spleen. Hormonal imbalances include increased estrogenic steroids in mice and hamsters, and elevated pituitary gonadotrophins resulting from the chronic administration of androgen receptor antagonists, 5α-reductase inhibitors, GnRH agonists, and aromatase inhibitors. Loss of negative feedback

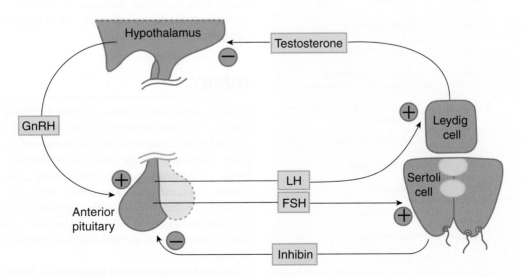

FIGURE 21–8 Hypothalamus–anterior pituitary gland–gonadal axis in the endocrine control of Leydig and Sertoli cells by luteinizing hormone (LH) and follicle-stimulating hormone (FSH).

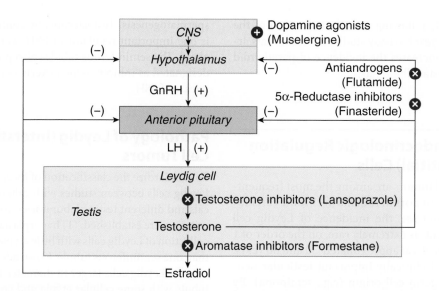

FIGURE 21–9 **Regulation of the hypothalamic–pituitary–testis (HPT) axis and control points for potential disruption by xenobiotic chemicals. Symbols: (+) feedback stimulation; (–) feedback inhibition; (⊕) receptor stimulation; (⊗) enzyme or receptor inhibition.** (Modified with permission from Cook JC, et al: Rodent Leydig cell tumorigenesis: a review of the physiology, pathology, mechanisms, and relevance to humans, *Crit Rev Toxicol* 29(2):169–261, 1999.)

control and the resulting overproduction of LH cause the proliferative changes in Leydig cells (Figure 21–9). Xenobiotics that increase the incidence of proliferative lesions of Leydig

TABLE 21–1 Selected examples of drugs that increase the incidence of proliferative lesions of Leydig cells in chronic exposure studies in rats or mice.

Name	Species	Clinical Indication
Indomethacin	Rat	Anti-inflammatory
Lactitol	Rat	Laxative
Metronidazole	Rat	Antibacterial
Muselergine	Rat	Parkinson's disease
Buserelin	Rat	Prostatic and breast carcinoma, endometriosis
Cimetidine	Rat	Reduction of gastric acid secretion
Flutamide	Rat	Prostatic carcinoma
Gemfibrozil	Rat	Hypolipidemia
Spironolactone	Rat	Diuretic
Nararelin	Rat	LHRH analog
Tamoxifen	Mouse	Antiestrogen
Vidarabine	Rat	Antiviral
Clofibrate	Rat	Hypolipidemia
Finasteride	Mouse	Prostatic hyperplasia

cells in chronic carcinogenicity studies in rats are listed in Table 21–1.

Although several hormonal imbalances result in an increased incidence of Leydig cell tumors in rodents, several disease conditions associated with chronic elevations in serum LH (including Klinefelter's syndrome and gonadotroph adenomas of the pituitary gland) in human patients have not been associated with an increased development of this type of rare testicular tumor. Likewise, compounds similar to those in Table 21–1 have not resulted in an increased incidence of Leydig cell neoplasia in humans. In summary, Leydig cell tumors are a frequently occurring tumor in rats, often associated mechanistically with hormonal imbalances; however, they are not an appropriate model for assessing risk to human males of developing this testicular tumor.

OVARY

Ovarian tumors in rodents can be subdivided into: epithelial tumors, sex cord–stromal tumors, germ cell tumors, tumors derived from nonspecialized soft tissues of the ovary, and tumors metastatic to the ovary from distant sites. Epithelial tumors of the ovary include cystadenomas and cystadenocarcinomas, tubulostromal adenomas, and mesothelioma. The tubular (or tubulostromal) adenomas are the most important of the ovarian tumors in mice, and they are uncommon in rats, rare in other animal species, and not recognized in the ovaries of women.

Ovarian tumors derived from the sex cords and/or ovarian stroma include the granulosal cell tumors, luteoma, thecoma, Sertoli cell tumor, tubular adenoma (with contributions from ovarian stroma), and undifferentiated sex cord–stromal tumors. The granulosal cell tumor is the most common of this group, which accounts for 27 percent of naturally occurring ovarian tumors in mice. Granulosal cell tumors may develop within certain tubular or tubulostromal adenomas following a long-term perturbation of endocrine function associated with genic deletion, irradiation, oocytotoxic chemicals, and neonatal thymectomy.

Ovarian Tumors Associated with Xenobiotic Chemicals

Nitrofurantoin—When fed at high doses to mice for 2 years, nitrofurantoin increased the incidence of the tubular or tubulostromal type of ovarian tumors. Nitrofurantoin caused sterility due to destruction of ovarian follicles and subsequent hormonal imbalances. Mice administered nitrofurantoin had a consistent change in the ovarian cortex, termed *ovarian atrophy,* which was characterized by an absence of Graafian follicles, developing ova, and corpora lutea; by focal or diffuse hyperplasia; and by varying numbers of polygonal, often vacuolated, sex cord-derived stromal cells between the tubular profiles. The ovaries were small with irregular surfaces, and had scattered eosinophilic stromal cells between tubular profiles.

Selective Estrogen Receptor Modulators—Selective estrogen receptor modulators (SERMs) have estrogen agonist effects on some tissues and estrogen antagonist actions on other tissues. The SERM tamoxifen has estrogen antagonist effects on the breast and an estrogen agonist effect on bone and also may stimulate the uterine endometrium. The SERM raloxifene has estrogen agonist effects on bone and serum lipids but estrogen antagonist actions on the uterus and breast. Tamoxifen, toremifene, and raloxifene have been reported to increase the incidence of ovarian tumors when administered chronically to mice.

Summary: Ovarian Tumorigenesis in Rodents

Examination of the literature supports the hypothesis that the unique intense hyperplasia of ovarian surface epithelium and stromal cells, leading eventually to tubular adenomas and occasionally granulosa cell tumors, develops secondarily to chronic pituitary gonadotropic hormone stimulation (Figure 21–10). Factors that destroy or greatly diminish the numbers of ovarian follicles—such as senescence, genetic deletion of follicles, x-irradiation, drugs, nitrofurantoin, and early thymectomy with the development of autoantibodies to oocytes—diminish sex steroid hormone secretion by the ovary. This results in elevated circulating levels of gonadotropins, especially LH, due to decreased negative feedback on the hypothalamic–pituitary axis by estrogens and possibly other humoral factors produced by the Graafian follicles. The long-term stimulation of stromal (interstitial) cells, which have receptors for LH, and, indirectly, the ovarian surface epithelium appears to place the mouse ovary at increased risk for developing the unique tubular or tubulostromal adenomas.

Studies using sterile mutant mice support the concept of a secondary (hormonally mediated) mechanism of ovarian carcinogenesis. Multiple pathogenetic factors that either destroy or diminish the numbers of Graafian follicles in the ovary result in decreased sex hormone secretion (especially estradiol-17β), leading to a compensatory overproduction of pituitary gonadotrophins (particularly LH) (Figure 21–10), which places

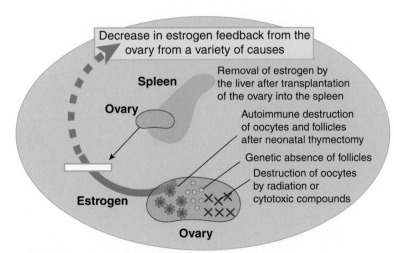

FIGURE 21–10 Multiple pathogenic mechanisms in ovarian tumorigenesis of mice resulting in decreased negative feedback by diminished levels of gonadal steroids, particularly estrogen.

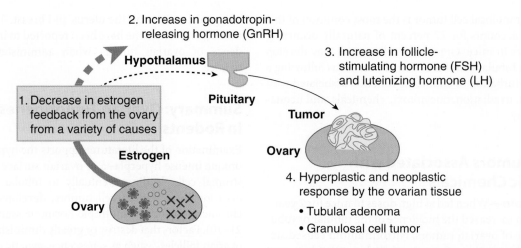

FIGURE 21-11 Decreased circulating estrogens release the hypothalamus–pituitary gland from negative feedback inhibition. The increased gonadotropin levels (LH and FSH) result in the mouse ovary being at a greater risk of developing tubular adenomas in chronic studies.

the mouse ovary at an increased risk for developing tumors (Figure 21–11). The intense proliferation of ovarian surface epithelium and stromal (interstitial) cells with the development of unique tubular adenomas in response to sterility does not appear to have a counterpart in the ovaries of human adult females.

BIBLIOGRAPHY

Eldridge JC, Stevens JT: *Endocrine Toxicology*, 3rd ed. London: Informa Healthcare, 2009.

Gardner DG, Shoback DM, Greenspan FS: *Greenspan's Basic and Clinical Endocrinology*. New York: McGraw-Hill, 2007.

Harvey PW, Everett DJ, Springall CJ (eds): *Adrenal Toxicology*. New York: Humana Healthcare, 2009.

QUESTIONS

1. The inability to release hormones from the anterior pituitary would NOT affect the release of which of the following?
   a. LH.
   b. PRL.
   c. ADH.
   d. TSH.
   e. ACTH.

2. Which of the following statements regarding pituitary hormones is TRUE?
   a. The hypothalamic–hypophyseal portal system transports releasing hormones to the neurohypophysis.
   b. Dopamine enhances prolactin secretion from the anterior pituitary.
   c. Somatostatin inhibits the release of GH.
   d. The function of chromophobes in the anterior pituitary is unknown.
   e. Oxytocin and ADH are synthesized by hypothalamic nuclei.

3. 21-Hydroxylase deficiency causes masculinization of female genitals at birth by increasing androgen secretion from which region of the adrenal gland?
   a. zona glomerulosa.
   b. zona reticularis.
   c. adrenal medulla.
   d. zona fasciculata.
   e. chromaffin cells.

4. Which of the following statements regarding adrenal toxicity is TRUE?
   a. The adrenal cortex and adrenal medulla are equally susceptible to fat-soluble toxins.
   b. Adrenal cortical cells lack the enzymes necessary to metabolize xenobiotic chemicals.
   c. Pheochromocytomas of the adrenal medulla can cause high blood pressure and clammy skin due to increased epinephrine release.
   d. Xenobiotics primarily affect the hydroxylase enzymes in the zona reticularis.
   e. Vitamin D is an important stimulus for adrenal cortex steroid secretion.

5. Chemical blockage of iodine transport in the thyroid gland:
   a. affects export of T_3 and T_4.
   b. prevents reduction to I_2 by thyroid peroxidase.
   c. decreases TRH release from the hypothalamus.
   d. interrupts intracellular thyroid biosynthesis.
   e. mimics goiter.

6. Chromaffin cells of the adrenal gland are responsible for secretion of which of the following?
   a. aldosterone.
   b. epinephrine.
   c. corticosterone.
   d. testosterone.
   e. estradiol.

7. The parafollicular cells of the thyroid gland are responsible for secreting a hormone that:
   a. increases blood glucose levels.
   b. decreases plasma sodium levels.
   c. increases calcium storage.
   d. decreases metabolic rate.
   e. increases bone resorption.

8. Parathyroid adenomas resulting in increased PTH levels would be expected to cause which of the following?
   a. hypocalcemia.
   b. hyperphosphatemia.
   c. increased bone formation.
   d. osteoporosis.
   e. rickets.

9. Which of the following vitamins increases calcium and phosphorus absorption in the gut?
   a. vitamin D.
   b. niacin.
   c. vitamin A.
   d. vitamin B_{12}.
   e. thiamine.

10. All of the following statements regarding ovarian tumor formation are true EXCEPT:
    a. Many ovarian tumors develop secondary to chronic GnRH stimulation.
    b. Increased sex steroid hormone secretion by the ovary is a risk factor for ovarian cancer.
    c. Tamoxifen has been shown to increase the incidence of ovarian tumors in mice.
    d. A decreased number of Graafian follicles results in decreased estrogen and progesterone secretion.
    e. The germinal epithelium surrounding the ovary is a common site of ovarian tumors.

C H A P T E R

22

Toxic Effects of Pesticides

Lucio G. Costa

INTRODUCTION

Pesticides can be defined as any substance or mixture of substances deliberately added to the environment and intended for preventing, destroying, repelling, or mitigating pests. Pesticides may be more specifically identified as insecticides (insects), herbicides (weeds), fungicides (fungi and molds), rodenticides (rodents), acaricides (mites), molluscides (snails and other mollusks), miticides (mites), larvicides (larvae), and pediculocides (lice). In addition, for regulatory purposes, plant growth regulators, repellants, and attractants (pheromones) often also fall in this broad classification of chemicals.

ECONOMICS AND PUBLIC HEALTH

Consideration of the use of pesticides must balance the benefits versus the possible risks of injury to human health or degradation of environmental quality. Pesticides play a major role in the control of vector-borne diseases, which represent a major threat to the health of large human populations. When introduced in 1942, DDT appeared to hold immense promise of benefit to agriculture and public health by controlling vector-borne diseases. However, because of its bioaccumulation in the environment and its effects on bird reproduction, DDT was eventually banned in most countries by the mid-1970s. When DDT was banned in 1996 in South Africa, less than 10,000 cases of malaria were registered in that country. By 2000, the number of malaria cases had increased to 62,000, but with the reintroduction of DDT at the end of that year, cases were down to 12,500.

Excessive loss of food crops to insects or other pests contributes to economic loss and possible starvation. In developed countries, pesticides allow production of abundant, inexpensive, and attractive fruits and vegetables, as well as grains. Along with insecticides, herbicides and fungicides play a major role in this endeavor.

Use of Pesticides

In the past 20 years, use of pesticides (as amount of active ingredient) has plateaued. Pesticides are often, if not always, used as multiagent formulations, in which the active ingredient is present together with other ingredients to allow mixing, dilution, application, and stability. These other ingredients are lumped under the term "inert" or "other." Though they do not have pesticidal action, such inert ingredients may not always be devoid of toxicity; thus, an ongoing task of manufacturers and regulatory agencies is to assure that inert ingredients do not pose any unreasonable risk of adverse health effects.

Exposure

Exposure to pesticides can occur via the oral or dermal routes or by inhalation. High oral doses, leading to severe poisoning and death, are achieved as a result of pesticide ingestion for suicidal intent, or of accidental ingestion, commonly due to storage of pesticides in improper containers. Chronic low doses, on the other hand, are consumed by the general population as pesticide residues in food or as contaminants in drinking water. Regulations exist to ensure that pesticide residues are maintained at levels below those that would cause any adverse effects. Workers involved in the production, transport, mixing and loading, and application of pesticides, as well as in harvesting of pesticide-sprayed crops, are at the highest risk for pesticide exposure. Dermal exposure during normal handling or application of pesticides, or in case of accidental spillings, occurs in body areas not covered by protective clothing, such as the face or the hands, or by inhalation. Furthermore, pesticides deposited on clothing may penetrate the skin and/or potentially expose others, if clothes are not changed and washed on termination of exposure.

Human Poisoning

Pesticides are not always selective for their intended target species, and adverse health effects can occur in nontarget species, including humans. In the general population and in occupationally exposed workers, concerns range from acute human poisoning to a possible association between pesticide exposure and increased risk of cancer. With several million poisonings causing hospital admission and a couple hundred thousand deaths,

TABLE 22-1 WHO-recommended classification of pesticides by hazard.

| | | LD$_{50}$ in Rat (mg/kg Body Weight) | | | |
| | | Oral | | Dermal | |
Class		Solids	Liquids	Solids	Liquids
Ia	Extremely hazardous	5 or less	20 or less	10 or less	40 or less
Ib	Highly hazardous	5–50	20–200	10–100	40–400
II	Moderately hazardous	50–500	200–2000	100–1000	400–4000
III	Slightly hazardous	Over 500	Over 2000	Over 1000	Over 4000
IV+	Unlikely to present hazard in normal use	Over 2000	Over 3000	Over 4000	Over 6000

the World Health Organization (WHO) has recommended a classification of pesticides by hazard, where acute oral or dermal toxicities in rats were considered (Table 22–1).

Regulatory Mandate

In the United States, the Environmental Protection Agency (EPA) regulates pesticide use under the Federal Insecticide,

TABLE 22-2 Basic toxicology testing requirements for pesticide registration.

Test	Animal Species[1]
Acute lethality (oral, dermal, inhalation)	Rat, mouse, guinea pig, rabbit
Dermal irritation	Rabbit, rat, guinea pig
Dermal sensitization	Guinea pig
Eye irritation	Rabbit
Acute delayed neurotoxicity	Hen
Genotoxicity studies (in vitro, in vivo)	Bacteria, mammalian cells, mouse, rat, *Drosophila*
Teratogenicity	Rabbit, rodent (mouse, rat, hamster)
2- to 4-week toxicity study (oral, dermal, inhalation)	Rat, mouse
90-Day toxicity study (oral)	Rat
Chronic toxicity study (oral; 6 months to 2 years)	Rat, dog
Oncogenicity study	Rat, mouse
Reproductive/fertility study	Rat
Developmental neurotoxicity study	Rat

[1]Substantial efforts are being devoted to develop alternative nonanimal test systems. As of 2006, only one in vitro test (for primary irritation) has been validated and accepted by EU regulatory bodies (OECD).

Fungicide and Rodenticide Act (FIFRA) and the Federal Food, Drug and Cosmetic Act (FFDCA). Under FIFRA, EPA registers pesticides for use, whereas under FFDCA, EPA establishes maximum allowable levels of pesticide residues (tolerances) in foods and animal feeds, which are enforced by other federal agencies.

The Food Quality & Protection Act gives EPA the mandate to assess risks of pesticides to infants and children, which are based on dietary consumption patterns of children, possible susceptibility of infants and children to pesticides, and cumulative effects of compounds that share the same mechanism of toxicity. Additional regulations concerning pesticides are present in other laws, such as the Safe Drinking Water Act or the Clean Air Act.

Under FIFRA, all pesticides sold or distributed in the United States must be registered by the EPA. To register a pesticide or a formulated product, a large number of studies (over 140) are required, a process that takes several years and costs between $50 and $100 million. The database includes information on product and residue chemistry, environmental fate, toxicology, biotransformation/degradation, occupational exposure and reentry protection, spray drift, environmental impact on no-target species (birds, mammals, aquatic organisms, plants, and soil), environmental persistence and bioaccumulation, as well as product performance and efficacy. Table 22–2 lists basic toxicology data needed for new pesticide registration.

Other nations, such as Canada, Japan, and most European countries, have legislated similar procedures for pesticide registration. The European Union (EU) has created a harmonized Union-wide framework for pesticide regulation. The WHO provides guidance, particularly with the setting of acceptable daily intake (ADI) values for pesticides.

INSECTICIDES

Insecticides play a most relevant role in the control of insect pests, particularly in developing countries. All of the chemical insecticides in use today are neurotoxicants, and act by poisoning the nervous systems of the target organisms (Table 22–3). The central nervous system of insects is highly developed and

TABLE 22–3 Molecular targets of the major classes of insecticides.

Target	Insecticide	Effect
Acetylcholinesterase	Organophosphates	Inhibition
	Carbamates	Inhibition
Sodium channels	Pyrethroids (types I and II)	Activation
	DDT	Activation
	Dihydropyrazoles	Inhibition
Nicotinic acetylcholine receptors	Nicotine	Activation
	Neonicotinoids	Activation
GABA receptors-gated chloride channels	Cyclodienes	Inhibition
	Phenylpyrazoles	Inhibition
	Pyrethroids (type II)	Inhibition
Glutamate-gated chloride channels[1]	Avermectins	Activation
Octopamine receptors[2]	Formamidines	Activation
Mitochondrial complex I	Rotenoids	Inhibition

[1]Found only in insects. In mammals, avermectins activate $GABA_A$ receptors.
[2]In mammals, formamidines activate alpha$_2$-adrenoceptors.

not unlike that of mammals. As a class, insecticides have high acute toxicity toward nontarget species compared with other pesticides. Some of them, most notably the organophosphates, are involved in a great number of human poisonings and deaths each year.

Organophosphorus Compounds

The general structure of OP insecticides can be represented by:

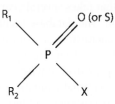

where X is the so-called leaving group that is displaced when the OP phosphorylates acetylcholinesterase (AChE), and is the most sensitive to hydrolysis; R_1 and R_2 are most commonly alkoxy groups (i.e., OCH_3 or OC_2H_5), though other chemical substitutes are also possible; either an oxygen or a sulfur (in this case the compound should be defined as a phosphorothioate) is also attached to the phosphorus with a double bond. Based on chemical differences, OPs can be divided into several subclasses, which include phosphates, phosphorothioates, phosphoramidates, phosphonates, and others. Figure 22–1 shows the chemical structures of some commonly used OPs.

Biotransformation—For all compounds that contain a sulfur bound to the phosphorus, a metabolic bioactivation is necessary for their biological activity to be manifest, as only

compounds with a P=O moiety are effective inhibitors of AChE. Oxidative desulfuration (leads to the formation of an "oxon," or oxygen analog of the parent insecticide) and thioether oxidation (formation of a sulfoxide, S=O, followed by the formation of a sulfone, O=S=O) are catalyzed by cytochrome P450s. Catalytic hydrolysis by phosphotriesterases, known as A-exterases (which are not inhibited by OPs), plays an important role in the detoxication of certain OPs. Noncatalytic hydrolysis of OPs also occurs when these compounds phosphorylate serine esterases classified as B-esterases.

Signs and Symptoms of Toxicity and Mechanism of Action—OP insecticides have high acute toxicity, with oral LD_{50} values in rat often below 50 mg/kg. For several OPs, acute dermal toxicity is also high. Inhibition of AChE by OPs causes accumulation of acetylcholine at cholinergic synapses, with overstimulation of muscarinic and nicotinic cholinergic receptors. As these receptors are localized in most organs of the body, a "cholinergic syndrome" ensues, which includes increased sweating and salivation, profound bronchial secretion, bronchoconstriction, miosis, increased gastrointestinal motility, diarrhea, tremors, muscular twitching, and various central nervous system effects (Table 22–4). Whereas respiratory failure is a hallmark of severe OP poisoning, mild poisoning and/or early stages of an otherwise severe poisoning may display no clear-cut signs and symptoms.

OPs with a P=O moiety phosphorylate a hydroxyl group on serine in the active (esteratic) site of the enzyme, impeding its action on the physiological substrate. Phosphorylated AChE is hydrolyzed by water slowly, and the rate of "spontaneous reactivation" depends on the chemical nature of the R substituents. Reactivation of phosphorylated AChE does not occur once the enzyme-inhibitor complex has "aged," which occurs when there is loss (by nonenzymatic hydrolysis) of one of the two alkyl (R) groups. When phosphorylated AChE has aged, the enzyme is considered to be irreversibly inhibited, and synthesis of new enzyme is required to restore activity, a process that may take days.

Treatment of Poisoning—Procedures aimed at decontamination and/or at minimizing absorption depend on the route of exposure. In case of dermal exposure, contaminated clothing should be removed, and the skin washed with alkaline soap. In case of ingestion, procedures to reduce absorption from the gastrointestinal tract do not appear to be very effective. Atropine, a muscarinic receptor antagonist, prevents the action of accumulating acetylcholine on these receptors. Atropine is preferably given intravenously to prevent the signs of excess cholinergic stimulation. The administration of pralidoxime (2-PAM) early after OP exposure can help prevent AChE aging, but its effectiveness is controversial. Diazepam may be used to relieve anxiety in mild cases, and to reduce muscle fasciculations and control convulsions in the more severe cases.

The Intermediate Syndrome—A second distinct manifestation of exposure to OPs is the so-called intermediate

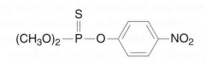

Methylparathion

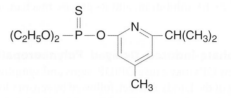

Azinphosmethyl (Guthion)

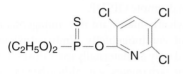

Chlorpyrifos

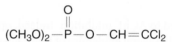

Diazinon

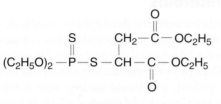

Malathion

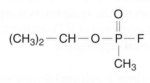

Dichlorvos

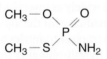

Metamidophos

Sarin

FIGURE 22–1 **Structures of some organophosphorus insecticides and of the nerve agent sarin.** Note that most commonly used compounds are organophosphorothioates (i.e., have a P=S bond), but some, including sarin, have a P=O bond and do not require metabolic activation.

TABLE 22–4 Signs and symptoms of acute poisoning with anticholinesterase compounds.

Site and Receptor Affected	Manifestations
Exocrine glands (M)	Increased salivation, lacrimation, perspiration
Eyes (M)	Miosis, blurred vision
Gastrointestinal tract (M)	Abdominal cramps, vomiting, diarrhea
Respiratory tract (M)	Increased bronchial secretion, bronchoconstriction
Bladder (M)	Urinary frequency, incontinence
Cardiovascular system (M)	Bradycardia, hypotension
Cardiovascular system (N)	Tachycardia, transient hypertension
Skeletal muscles (N)	Muscle fasciculations, twitching, cramps, generalized weakness, flaccid paralysis
Central nervous system (M, N)	Dizziness, lethargy, fatigue, headache, mental confusion, depression of respiratory centers, convulsions, coma

M = muscarinic receptors; N = nicotinic receptors.

syndrome, which is seen in 20 to 50 percent of acute OP poisoning cases. The syndrome develops 1 to several days after the poisoning, during recovery from cholinergic manifestations, or in some cases, when patients have completely recovered from the initial cholinergic crisis. Prominent features include a marked weakness of respiratory, neck, and proximal limb muscles. Mortality due to respiratory paralysis and complications ranges from 15 to 40 percent, and recovery in surviving patients takes up to 15 days. The intermediate syndrome is not an effect of AChE inhibition, and its precise mechanisms are unknown.

Organophosphate-induced Delayed Polyneuropathy (OPIDP)—A few OPs may cause OPIDP. Signs and symptoms include tingling of the hands and feet, followed by sensory loss, progressive muscle weakness and flaccidity of the distal skeletal muscles of the lower and upper extremities, and ataxia. These may occur 2 to 3 weeks after a single exposure, when signs of both the acute cholinergic and the intermediate syndromes have subsided. OPIDP can be classified as a distal sensorimotor axonopathy.

OPIDP is not related to AChE inhibition. Indeed, one of the compounds involved in several epidemics of this neuropathy is tri-*ortho*-cresyl phosphate (TOCP), a very poor AChE inhibitor. The target for OPIDP is an esterase, present in nerve tissues as well as other tissues (e.g., lymphocytes), named neuropathy target esterase (NTE). Several OPs, certain carbamates, and sulfonyl fluorides can inhibit NTE. Other compounds that inhibit NTE but cannot undergo the aging reaction are not neuropathic, indicating that inhibition of NTE catalytic activity is not the mechanism of axonal degeneration.

Long-term Toxicity—There is still controversy on possible long-term effects of OPs. The possibility exists that low exposure to OPs, at doses that produce no cholinergic signs, may lead to long-term adverse health effects, particularly in the central and peripheral nervous systems. Chronic exposure of animals to OPs, at doses that significantly inhibit AChE but may not be associated with clinical signs, results in the development of tolerance to their cholinergic effects (which is mediated, at least in part, by down-regulation of cholinergic receptors), and has been associated with neurobehavioral abnormalities, particularly at the cognitive level.

Carbamates

Carbamate insecticides are derived from carbamic acid, and most are *N*-methylcarbamates. Acute oral toxicity ranges from moderate to low toxicity, such as carbaryl, to extremely high toxicity, such as aldicarb. Dermal skin penetration by carbamates is increased by organic solvents and emulsifiers present in most formulations. Carbamates are susceptible to a variety of enzyme-catalyzed biotransformation reactions, and the principal pathways involve oxidation and hydrolysis. The mechanism of toxicity of carbamates is by inhibition of AChE, which is rapidly reversible.

The signs and symptoms of carbamate poisoning include miosis, urination, diarrhea, salivation, muscle fasciculation, and CNS effects (Table 22–4). Acute intoxication by carbamates is generally resolved within a few hours. The treatment of carbamate intoxication relies on the use of atropine. Carbamates can inhibit NTE, but because carbamylated NTE cannot age, they are thought to be unable to initiate OPIDP. Additionally, when given before a neuropathic organophosphate, carbamates offer protection against OPIDP, but when given after, they can promote OPIDP.

Methylcarbamates are not mutagenic, and there is no evidence of carcinogenicity. Embryotoxicity or fetotoxicity is observed only at maternally toxic doses. Limited evidence suggests that carbamates (e.g., aldicarb) may be more acutely toxic to young animals than to adults, possibly because of lower detoxication.

Pyrethroids

Pyrethrins were first developed as insecticides from extracts of the flower heads of *Chrysanthemum cinerariaefolium*, whose insecticidal potential was appreciated in ancient China and Persia. Because pyrethrins decompose rapidly on exposure to light, the synthetic pyrethroid analogs were developed. Because of their high insecticidal potency, relatively low mammalian toxicity, lack of environmental persistence, and low tendency to induce insect resistance, pyrethroids now account for more than 25 percent of the global insecticide market. The pyrethroids are used widely as insecticides both in the house and in agriculture, in medicine for the topical treatment of scabies and head lice, and in tropical countries in soaked bed nets to prevent mosquito bites. Pyrethroids alter the normal function of insect nerves by modifying the kinetics of voltage-sensitive sodium channels, which mediate the transient increase in the sodium permeability of the nerve membrane that underlies the nerve action potential.

On absorption, pyrethroids are very rapidly metabolized through two major biotransformation routes: hydrolysis of the ester linkage, which is catalyzed by hepatic and plasma carboxylesterases, and oxidation of the alcohol moiety by cytochrome P450s. These initial reactions are followed by further oxidations, hydrolysis, and conjugation with sulfate or glucuronide.

Signs and Symptoms of Toxicity and Mechanism of Action—Based on toxic signs in rats, pyrethroids have been divided into two types (Table 22–5). The pyrethroids disrupt voltage-gated sodium channels in mammals and insects. Pyrethroids bind to the α subunit of the sodium channel and slow the activation (opening), as well as the rate of inactivation (closing), of the sodium channel, leading to a stable hyperexcitable state. The higher sensitivity of insects to pyrethroid toxicity, compared with mammals, is believed to result from a combination of higher sensitivity of insect sodium channels, lower body temperature (as pyrethroids show a negative temperature coefficient of action), and slower biotransformation. Type II pyrethroids bind to and inhibit GABA$_A$-gated chloride channels at higher concen-

TABLE 22–5 Classification of pyrethroid insecticides based on toxic signs in rats.

Syndrome	Signs and Symptoms	Examples
Type I (T syndrome)	Aggressive sparring Increased sensitivity to external stimuli Whole-body tremors Prostration	Allethrin Bioallethrin Resmethrin Phenothrin
Type II (CS syndrome)	Pawing and burrowing Profuse salivation Coarse tremor Choreoathetosis Clonic seizures	Deltamethrin Fenvalerate Cypermethrin Cyhalothrin

trations than those sufficient to affect sodium channels (10^{-7} M versus 10^{-10} M). This effect is believed to contribute to the seizures that accompany severe type II pyrethroid poisoning.

Young animals are more sensitive to the acute toxicity of the pyrethroids deltamethrin and cypermethrin probably because of a lesser capacity for metabolic detoxification.

On occupational exposure, the primary adverse effect resulting from dermal contact with pyrethroids is paresthesia. Symptoms include continuous tingling or pricking or, when more severe, burning. The condition reverses in about 24 h, and topical application of vitamin E has been shown to be an effective treatment. Paresthesia is presumably due to pyrethroid-induced abnormal repetitive activity in skin nerve terminals. Chronic studies with pyrethroids indicate that at high dose levels they cause slight liver enlargement often accompanied by some histopathologic changes. There is little evidence of teratogenicity and mutagenicity. An increased rate of lymphoma incidence in rodents has been reported for deltamethrin, but the effect was not dose-dependent.

Organochlorine Compounds

The organochlorine insecticides include the chlorinated ethane derivatives, such as DDT and its analogs; the cyclodienes, such as chlordane, aldrin, dieldrin, heptachlor, endrin, and toxaphene; the hexachlorocyclohexanes, such as lindane; and the caged structures mirex and chlordecone. Their acute toxicity is moderate (less than that of organophosphates), but chronic exposure may be associated with adverse health effects particularly in the liver and endocrine disruption of the reproductive system.

DDT and Its Analogs—DDT is effective against a wide variety of agricultural pests, as well as against insects that transmit some of the world's most serious diseases, such as typhus, malaria, and yellow fever. DDT has a moderate oral acute toxicity and its dermal absorption is very limited. In humans, oral doses of 10 to 20 mg/kg produce illness, but doses as high as 285 mg/kg have been ingested accidentally without fatal results. Toxicity from dermal exposure in humans is also low, as evidenced by the lack of significant adverse health effects when thousands of

people were liberally dusted with this compound. On absorption, DDT distributes in all tissues, and the highest concentrations are found in adipose tissue.

Acute exposure to high doses of DDT causes motor unrest, increased frequency of spontaneous movements, abnormal susceptibility to fear, and hypersusceptibility to external stimuli (light, touch, and sound). This is followed by the development of fine tremors, progressing to coarse tremors, and eventually tonic–clonic convulsions. In humans, the earliest symptom of poisoning by DDT is hyperesthesia of the mouth and lower part of the face, followed by paresthesia of the same area and of the tongue. Dizziness, tremor of the extremities, confusion, and vomiting follow; convulsions occur only in severe poisoning. Both in insects and in mammals, DDT interferes with the sodium channels in the axonal membrane by a mechanism similar to that of type I pyrethroids.

An important target for chronic DDT exposure is the liver. DDT and its breakdown product DDE increase liver weight and cause hepatic cell hypertrophy and necrosis, and they are potent inducers of cytochrome P450s, particularly CYP2B and CYP3A. Both DDE and DDD, another breakdown product, are carcinogenic in rodents, causing primarily an increase in hepatic tumors.

Hexachlorocyclohexanes and Cyclodienes—These two families of organochlorine insecticides comprise a large number of compounds that share a similar mechanism of neurotoxic action. Lindane is the γ isomer of benzene hexachloride (BHC; 1,2,3,4,5,6-hexachlorocyclohexane). Cyclodiene compounds include chlordane, dieldrin, aldrin (which is rapidly metabolized to dieldrin), heptachlor, and endrin. Toxaphene is a complex mixture of over 200 chlorinated bornanes and camphenes.

Lindane and cyclodienes have moderate to high acute oral toxicity (Figure 22–2). However, in contrast to DDT, these compounds are readily absorbed through the skin. The primary target for their toxicity is the central nervous system. Unlike DDT, tremor is essentially absent, but convulsions are a prominent aspect of poisoning. Lindane and cyclodienes bind to the picrotoxin-binding site on the chloride channel, thereby blocking its opening and antagonizing the inhibitory action of GABA.

Other Old and New Insecticides

Rotenoids—The roots of *Derris elliptica* and those of *Lonchocarpus utilis* and *Lonchocarpus urucu* in South America contain at least six rotenoid esters. The most abundant is rotenone, which is used as an agricultural insecticide/acaricide particularly in organic farming. Toxicity of rotenone in target and nontarget species is due to its ability to inhibit, at nanomolar concentrations, the mitochondrial respiratory chain, by blocking electron transport at NADH–ubiquinone reductase, the energy-conserving enzyme complex commonly known as complex I. Poisoning symptoms include initial increased respiratory and cardiac rates, clonic and tonic spasms, and muscular depression, followed by respiratory depression. Rotenone may play a role in the etiology of Parkinson's disease.

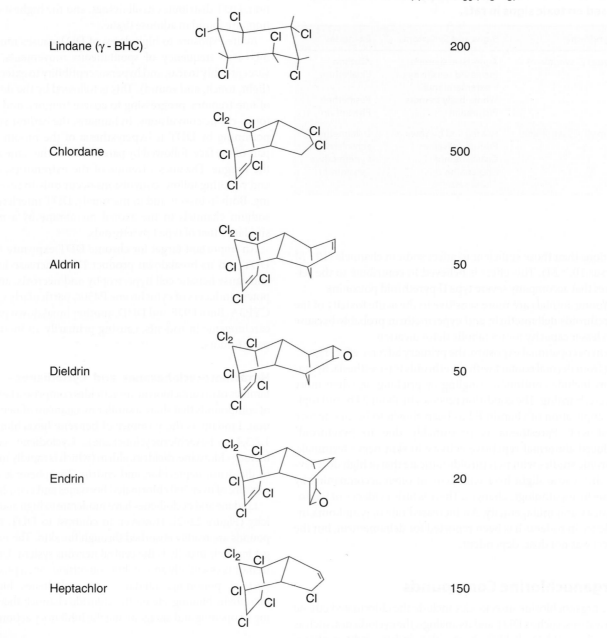

FIGURE 22-2 Structure and acute toxicity (oral LD$_{50}$ in rat) of selected organochlorine insecticides of different chemical classes.

Nicotine—Nicotine is an alkaloid extracted from the leaves of tobacco plants (*Nicotiana tabacum* and *Nicotiana rustica*), and is used as a free base or as the sulfate salt. Nicotine is a minor insecticide, and the signs and symptoms of poisoning include nausea, vomiting, muscle weakness, respiratory effects, headache, lethargy, and tachycardia. Most cases of poisoning with nicotine occur after exposure to tobacco products, or gum or patches. Workers who cultivate, harvest, or handle tobacco may experience green tobacco sickness, caused by dermal absorption of nicotine.

Avermectins—The avermectins are macrocyclic lactones that are isolated from the fermentation broth of *Streptomyces*

avermitilis. This fungus synthesizes eight individual avermectins that have antiparasitic activity. The semisynthetic derivatives of avermectin B$_{1a}$, emamectin benzoate, and ivermectin are used as insecticides, and for parasite control in human and veterinary medicine, respectively. Abamectin is used primarily to control mites, whereas emamectin benzoate is effective at controlling lepidopterian species in various crops and emerald ash borer in trees. Ivermectin is used as an antihelmintic and antiparasitic drug in veterinary medicine, and in humans it has proven to be an effective treatment for infection of intestinal threadworms, onchocerciasis (river blindness), and lymphatic filariasis. Signs and symptoms of intoxication include hyperexcitability, tremors, and incoordination, followed by ataxia and coma-like sedation.

INSECT REPELLENTS

DEET (*N*,*N*-diethyl-*m*-toluamide or *N*,*N*-diethyl-3-methylbenzamide) is very effective at repelling insects, flies, fleas, and ticks, and protection time increases with increasing concentrations. Subchronic toxicity studies in various species did not reveal major toxic effects and no significant effects of DEET were seen in mutagenicity, reproductive toxicity, and carcinogenicity studies. Acute and chronic neurotoxicity studies also provided negative results.

HERBICIDES

Herbicides are chemicals that are capable of either killing or severely injuring plants. Some of the various mechanisms by which herbicides exert their biological effects are shown in Table 22–6, together with examples for each class. Another method of classification pertains to how and when herbicides are applied. Thus, *preplanting* herbicides are applied to the soil before a crop is seeded, *preemergent* herbicides are applied to the soil before the time of appearance of unwanted vegetation, and *postemergent* herbicides are applied to the soil or foliage after the germination of the crop and/or weeds. Herbicides are also divided according to the manner they are applied to plants. *Contact* herbicides are those that affect the plant that was treated, whereas *translocated* herbicides are applied to the soil or to above-ground parts of the plant, and are absorbed and circulated to distant tissues. Nonselective herbicides will kill all vegetation, whereas selective compounds are those used to kill weeds without harming the crops.

A number of herbicides can cause dermal irritation and contact dermatitis, particularly in individuals prone to allergic reactions. Other compounds have generated much debate for their suspected carcinogenicity or neurotoxicity. The principal classes of herbicides associated with reported adverse health effects in humans are discussed below.

Chlorophenoxy Compounds

Chlorophenoxy herbicides are chemical analogs of auxin, a plant growth hormone, and produce uncontrolled and lethal growth in target plants. Because the auxin hormone is critical to the growth of many broad-leaved plants, but is not used by grasses, chlorophenoxy compounds can suppress the growth of weeds (e.g., dandelions) without affecting the grass. The most commonly used compound of this class is 2,4-dichlorophenoxyacetic acid (2,4-D).

Ingestion of 2,4-D has caused acute poisoning in humans, resulting in vomiting, burning of the mouth, abdominal pain, hypotension, myotonia, and CNS involvement including coma. Dermal exposure is the major route of unintentional exposure to 2,4-D in humans.

There are several case reports suggesting an association between exposure to 2,4-D and neurologic effects like peripheral neuropathy, demyelination and ganglion degeneration in the CNS, reduced nerve conduction velocity, myotonia, and behavioral alterations. The chlorophenoxy herbicides have attracted much attention because of an association between exposure and non-Hodgkin's lymphoma or soft-tissue sarcoma, found in a few epidemiological studies.

Bipyridil Compounds

Paraquat is a fast-acting, nonselective contact herbicide, used to control broad-leaved weeds and grasses in plantations and fruit orchards, and for general weed control. Paraquat has one of the highest acute toxicities among herbicides. On absorption, independent of the route of exposure, paraquat accumulates in the lung and the kidney. Paraquat is very poorly metabolized, and is excreted almost unchanged in the urine. It has minimal to no genotoxic activity, is not carcinogenic in rodents, has no effect on fertility, is not teratogenic, and only produces fetotoxicity at maternally toxic doses. The major toxicologic concerns for paraquat are related to its acute systemic effects, particularly in the lung, and secondarily, the kidney.

Once paraquat enters a cell, it undergoes alternate reduction followed by reoxidation, a process known as redox cycling. Intracellular redox cycling of paraquat would also result in the oxidation of NADPH, leading to its cellular depletion, which is augmented by the detoxification of hydrogen peroxide formed in the glutathione peroxidase/reductase enzyme system to regenerate GSH (Figure 22–3).

Damage to alveolar epithelial cells occurs within 24 h after acute exposure to lethal doses of paraquat. Damage progresses

TABLE 22–6 Some mechanisms of action of herbicides.

Mechanism	Chemical Classes (Example)
Inhibition of photosynthesis	Triazines (atrazine), substituted ureas (diuron), uracils (bromacil)
Inhibition of respiration	Dinitrophenols
Auxin growth regulators	Phenoxy acids (2,4-D), benzoic acids (dicamba), pyridine acids (picloram)
Inhibition of protein synthesis	Dinitroanilines
Inhibition of lipid synthesis	Aryloxyphenoxypropionates (diclofop)
Inhibition of specific enzymes • Glutamine synthetase • Enolpyruvylshikimate-3-phosphate synthetase • Acetalase synthase	 Glufosinate Glyphosate Sulfonylureas
Cell membrane disruptors	Bipyridyl derivatives (paraquat)

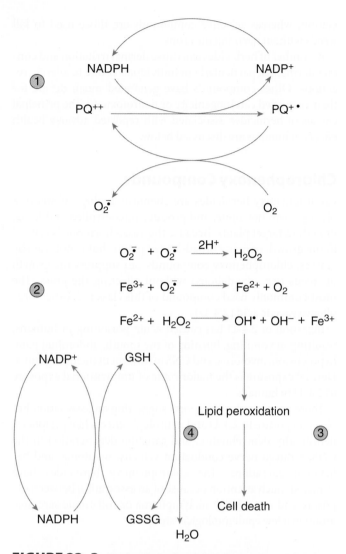

$$O_2^{\bar{\cdot}} + O_2^{\bar{\cdot}} \xrightarrow{2H^+} H_2O_2$$

$$Fe^{3+} + O_2^{\bar{\cdot}} \longrightarrow Fe^{2+} + O_2$$

$$Fe^{2+} + H_2O_2 \longrightarrow OH^\bullet + OH^- + Fe^{3+}$$

FIGURE 22–3 Mechanism of toxicity of paraquat. (1) Redox cycling of paraquat utilizing NADPH; (2) formation of hydroxy radicals leading to lipid peroxidation (3); (4) detoxication of H_2O_2 via glutathione reductase/peroxidase couple, utilizing NADPH. (Modified from Smith LL: Mechanism of paraquat toxicity in the lung and its relevance to treatment. *Hum Toxicol* 6:31–36, 1987, with permission from Palgrave Macmillan.)

in the following 2 to 4 days with loss of the alveolar epithelium, alveolar edema, extensive infiltration of inflammatory cells into the alveolar interstitium, and finally death due to severe anoxia. Survivors of this destructive first phase show extensive proliferation of fibroblasts in the lung. The second phase is characterized by attempts by the alveolar epithelium to regenerate and restore normal architecture, and presents as an intensive fibrosis. Individuals who survive the first phase may still die from the progressive loss of lung function several weeks after exposure.

The herbicide diquat presents a different toxicologic profile. Acute toxicity is somewhat lower. In contrast to paraquat, diquat does not accumulate in the lung, and no lung toxicity is seen on acute or chronic exposure. On chronic exposure, target organs for toxicity are the gastrointestinal tract, the kidney, and particularly the eye. Like paraquat, diquat can be reduced to form a free radical and then reoxidized in the presence of oxygen, with the concomitant production of superoxide anion. This process of redox cycling occurs in the eye and is believed to be the likely mechanism of cataract formation. Human clinical symptoms include nausea, vomiting, diarrhea, ulceration of mouth and esophagus, decline of renal functions, and neurologic effects, but no pulmonary fibrosis.

Chloroacetanilides

Representative compounds of this class of herbicides are alachlor, acetochlor, and metolachlor, which are used to control herbal grasses and broad-leaved weeds in a number of crops (corn, soybeans, and peanuts). Alachlor, acetochlor, and butachlor are probable human carcinogens (Group B2). The discovery of alachlor in well water led to cancellation of its registration in some countries, and to its restriction in others. Both are believed to be threshold-sensitive phenomena.

Triazines

The family of triazine herbicides comprises several compounds (atrazine, simazine, and propazine) that are extensively used for the preemergent control of broad-leaved weeds. Triazines have low acute oral and dermal toxicity, and chronic toxicity studies indicate primarily decreased body weight gain. There is no evidence that triazines are teratogenic, genotoxic, or developmental or reproductive toxicants. However, a more recent study has suggested a possible clastogenic effect. Though exposure to atrazine through residues in food commodities is very low, contamination of ground water and drinking water is common. Nevertheless, the known hormonal effects of triazines call for careful evaluation of the endocrine-disrupting effects of these herbicides.

Phosphonomethyl Amino Acids

The two compounds of this class are glyphosate (*N*-phosphonomethyl glycine) and glufosinate (*N*-phosphonomethyl homoalanine). Both are broad-spectrum nonselective systemic herbicides used for postemergent control of annual and perennial plants. Though both compounds contain a P=O moiety, they are organophosphonates and do not inhibit AChE.

Glyphosate—Glyphosate exerts its herbicidal action by inhibiting the enzyme 5-enolpyruvylshikimate-3-phosphate synthase, responsible for the synthesis of an intermediate in the biosynthesis of various amino acids. Although important in plant growth, this metabolic pathway is not present in mammals. It has no teratogenic, developmental, or reproductive effects. Genotoxicity and carcinogenicity studies in animals were negative.

Glyphosate is one of the most widely used herbicides, and the development of transgenic crops that can tolerate glyphosate treatment has expanded its utilization. Given its widespread use, including the home and garden market, accidental or intentional exposure to glyphosate is inevitable. The most widely used glyphosate product is Roundup® which is formulated as a concentrate containing water, 41 percent glyphosate (as isopropylamine salt), and 15 percent polyoxyethyleneamine (POEA). Mild intoxication results mainly in transient gastrointestinal symptoms. Moderate or severe poisoning presents with gastrointestinal bleeding, hypotension, pulmonary dysfunction, and renal damage.

Glufosinate—Glufosinate is a nonselective contact herbicide that acts by irreversibly inhibiting glutamine synthetase. Plants die as a consequence of the increased levels of ammonia. Mammals have other metabolizing systems that can cope with the effects on glutamine synthetase activity to a certain limit. There is no evidence of genotoxicity or carcinogenicity, or direct effects on reproductive performance and fertility. Developmental toxic effects were found in rabbits (premature deliveries, abortions, and dead fetuses). Symptoms include gastrointestinal effects, impaired respiration, neurologic disturbance, and cardiovascular effects.

FUNGICIDES

Fungal diseases are virtually impossible to control without chemical application. Fungicidal chemicals are derived from a variety of structures, ranging from simple inorganic compounds, such as copper sulfate, to complex organic compounds. Most fungicides are surface or plant protectants, and are applied prior to potential infection by fungal spores, either to plants or to postharvest crops. Other fungicides can be used therapeutically, to cure plants when an infestation has already begun. Still others are used as systemic fungicides that are absorbed and distributed throughout the plant.

With a few exceptions, fungicides have low acute toxicity in mammals. Some fungicides have been associated with severe epidemics of poisoning, and have thus been banned.

Captan and Folpet

Captan and folpet are broad-spectrum protectant fungicides; together with captafol, they are called chloroalkylthio fungicides, due to the presence of side chains containing chlorine, carbon, and sulfur. They are potent eye irritants, but only mild skin irritants. Dermal absorption is low. Captan and folpet, as well as thiophosgene, are mutagenic in in vitro tests; however, in vivo mutagenicity tests are mostly negative, possibly because of the rapid degradation of these compounds. Both fungicides induce the development of duodenal tumors in mice, and on this basis, they are classified by the USEPA as probable human carcinogens. Because of their structural similarity to the potent teratogen thalidomide, chloroalkylthio fungicides have been extensively tested in reproductive/developmental studies in multiple species, but no evidence of teratogenicity has been found.

Dithiocarbamates

The nomenclature of many of these compounds arises from the metal cations with which they are associated; thus, there are, for

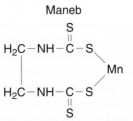

Maneb

Manganese ethylenebisdithiocarbamate

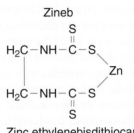

Zineb

Zinc ethylenebisdithiocarbamate

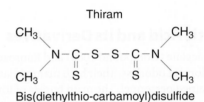

Thiram

Bis(diethylthio-carbamoyl)disulfide

FIGURE 22–4 **Structures of three dithiocarbamate fungicides.**

example, Maneb (Mn), Ziram and Zineb (Zn), and Mancozeb (Mn and Zn) (Figure 22–4). Thiram is an example of dithiocarbamate without a metal moiety (Figure 22–4). The dithiocarbamates have low acute toxicity by the oral, dermal, and respiratory routes. However, chronic exposure is associated with adverse effects that may be due to the dithiocarbamate acid or the metal moiety. These compounds are metabolized to a common metabolite, ethylenethiourea (ETU), which is responsible for the effects of dithiocarbamates on the thyroid, which include hypertrophy and hyperplasia of thyroid follicular cells that progress to adenomas and carcinomas. Similarly, dithiocarbamates alter thyroid hormone levels, and cause thyroid hypertrophy. Also, the structure of dithiocarbamate fungicides resembles that of disulfiram, which inhibits aldehyde dehydrogenase and may, after ingestion of ethanol, lead to elevated acetaldehyde levels.

Inorganic and Organometal Fungicides

Copper sulfate has overall low toxicity and remains one of the most widely used fungicides. Triphenyltin acetate is used as a fungicide, whereas tributyltin is utilized as an antifouling agent. Triphenyltin has moderate to high acute toxicity, but may cause reproductive toxicity and endocrine disruption. Organic mercury compounds, such as methylmercury, were used extensively as fungicides in the past for the prevention of seed-borne diseases in grains and cereals.

RODENTICIDES

Rats and mice can cause health and economic damages to humans. Rodents are vectors for several human diseases, including plague, endemic rickettsiosis, spirochetosis, and several others; they can occasionally bite people; they can consume large quantities of postharvest stored foods, and can contaminate foods with urine, feces, and hair. Rodenticides play an important role in rodent control. To be effective, yet safe, rodenticides must satisfy several criteria: (1) the poison must be very effective in the target species once incorporated into bait in small quantity; (2) baits containing the poison must not excite bait shyness, so that the animal will continue to eat it; (3) the manner of death must be such that survivors do not become suspicious of its cause; and (4) it should be species-specific, with considerably lower toxicity to other animals. Toxicologic problems can arise from acute accidental ingestions or from suicidal and homicidal attempts. Every year, thousands of accidental ingestions of rodenticide baits by children occur, most of which resolve without serious consequences.

Fluoroacetic Acid and Its Derivatives

Sodium fluoroacetate (Compound 1080) and fluoroacetamide are white in color and odorless. Their high mammalian toxicity limits use to trained personnel. The main targets of toxicity are the central nervous system and the heart. Initial gastrointestinal symptoms are followed by severe cardiovascular effects (ventricular tachycardia, fibrillation, and hypotension), as well as CNS effects (agitation, convulsions, and coma). Use of Compound 1080 in the United States is severely restricted primarily because of toxicity to nontarget animals, such as dogs.

Anticoagulants

In addition to their use as rodenticides, coumarin derivatives, including warfarin itself, are used as anticoagulant drugs and have become a mainstay for prevention of thromboembolic disease. Coumarins antagonize the action of vitamin K in the synthesis of clotting factors (factors II, VII, IX, and X). Their specific mechanism involves inhibition of vitamin K epoxide reductase, which regenerates the reduced vitamin K necessary for sustained carboxylation and synthesis of relevant clotting factors. Human poisonings by these rodenticides are rare because they are dispersed in grain-based baits. However, there are a significant number of suicide or homicide attempts or of accidental consumption of warfarin.

FUMIGANTS

These agents are active toward insects, mites, nematodes, weed seeds, fungi, or rodents, and have in common the property of being in the gaseous form at the time they exert their pesticidal action. They can be liquids that readily vaporize (e.g., ethylene dibromide), solids that can release a toxic gas on reaction with water (e.g., phosphine released by aluminum phosphide), or gases (e.g., methyl bromide). For soil fumigation, the compound is injected directly into the soil, which is then covered with plastic sheeting, which is sealed. Compounds used as fumigants are usually nonselective, highly reactive, and cytotoxic. They provide a potential hazard from the standpoint of inhalation exposure, and to a minor degree for dermal exposure or ingestion, in case of solids or liquids.

Methyl Bromide

Methyl bromide is a broad-spectrum pesticide, used for soil fumigation, commodity treatment, and structural fumigation. Acute exposure results in respiratory, gastrointestinal, and neurologic symptoms; the latter include lethargy, headache, seizures, paresthesias, peripheral neuropathy, and ataxia, and are considered to be more relevant than other toxic effects for human risk assessment. Acute and chronic neurotoxicity studies in rats have demonstrated behavioral effects and morphological lesions, which were concentration- and time-dependent. Methyl bromide is an odorless and colorless gas, but chloropicrin, with a pungent odor and eye irritation, is often used in conjunction with methyl bromide and other fumigant mixtures, to warn against potentially harmful exposures.

1,3-Dichloropropene

1,3-Dichloropropene is a soil fumigant, extensively utilized for its ability to control soil nematodes. It is an irritant, and can cause redness and necrosis of the skin. It is extensively metabolized, with the mercapturic acid conjugate being the major urinary metabolite. Data on genotoxicity are contradictory, and carcinogenicity studies in rodents have found an increase in benign liver tumors in rats but not in mice, after oral administration.

Sulfur

Elemental sulfur is an effective fumigant for the control of many plant diseases, particularly fungal diseases, and represents the most heavily used crop protection chemical in the United States. Sulfur finds its major uses in grapes and tomatoes, and can be used in organic farming. The primary health effect in humans associated with the agricultural use of elemental sulfur is dermatitis. In ruminants, excessive sulfur ingestion can cause cerebrocortical necrosis (polioencephalomalacia), possibly due to its conversion by microorganisms in the rumen to hydrogen sulfide.

BIBLIOGRAPHY

Marrs TT, Ballantyne B: *Pesticide Toxicology and International Regulation.* Hoboken NJ: John Wiley & Sons, 2004.
Yu SJ: *The Toxicology and Biochemistry of Insecticides.* Boca Raton: CRC Press/Taylor & Francis, 2008.

QUESTIONS

1. Which of the following does NOT contribute to the environmental presence of organochlorine insecticides?
   a. high water solubility.
   b. low volatility.
   c. chemical stability.
   d. low cost.
   e. slow rate of degradation.

2. All of the following are characteristic of DDT poisoning EXCEPT:
   a. paresthesia.
   b. hypertrophy of hepatocytes.
   c. increased potassium transport across the membrane.
   d. slow closing of sodium ion channels.
   e. dizziness.

3. Anticholinesterase agents:
   a. enhance the activity of AChE.
   b. increase ACh concentration in the synaptic cleft.
   c. only target the neuromuscular junction.
   d. antagonize ACh receptors.
   e. cause decreased autonomic nervous system stimulation.

4. All of the following symptoms would be expected following anticholinesterase insecticide poisoning EXCEPT:
   a. bronchodilation.
   b. tachycardia.
   c. diarrhea.
   d. increased blood pressure.
   e. dyspnea.

5. Which of the following insecticides blocks the electron transport chain at NADH–ubiquinone reductase?
   a. nicotine.
   b. carbamate esters.
   c. nitromethylenes.
   d. pyrethroid esters.
   e. rotenoids.

6. What is the main mechanism of pyrethroid ester toxicity?
   a. blockage of neurotransmitter release.
   b. inhibition of neurotransmitter reuptake.
   c. acting as a receptor agonist.
   d. causing hyperexcitability of the membrane by interfering with sodium transport.
   e. interfering with Cl⁻ transport across the axonal membrane.

7. Which of the following herbicides is NOT correctly paired with its mechanism of action?
   a. glufosinate—inhibition of glutamine synthetase.
   b. paraquat—interference with protein synthesis.
   c. glyphosate—inhibition of amino acid synthesis.
   d. chlorophenoxy compounds—growth stimulants.
   e. diquat—production of superoxide anion through redox cycling.

8. Captan:
   a. is an herbicide that inhibits root growth.
   b. is an insecticide that targets the reproductive organs.
   c. is a fungicide that could cause duodenal tumors.
   d. is an herbicide that stimulates growth.
   e. is a fungicide that is a known teratogen.

9. What is a mechanism of action of nicotine?
   a. Nicotine antagonizes ACh at the neuromuscular junction.
   b. Nicotine decreases the rate of repolarization of the axonal membrane.
   c. Nicotine interferes with sodium permeability.
   d. Nicotine acts as an ACh agonist in the synapse.
   e. Nicotine inhibits the release of neurotransmitter.

10. Which of the following is the most characteristic of warfarin poisoning?
    a. diarrhea.
    b. cyanosis.
    c. decreased glucose metabolism.
    d. hematomas.
    e. seizures.

Chronic Pulmonary Disease—Cadmium inhalation is toxic to the respiratory system in a fashion related to the dose and duration of exposure. Cadmium-induced obstructive lung disease in humans can be slow in onset, and results from chronic bronchitis, progressive fibrosis of the lower airways, and accompanying alveolar damage leading to emphysema. Pulmonary function is reduced with dyspnea, reduced vital capacity, and increased residual volume.

Other Toxicities—Cadmium toxicity affects calcium metabolism, and associated skeletal changes probably related to calcium loss include bone pain, osteomalacia, and/or osteoporosis. Epidemiologic studies suggest that cadmium may be an etiologic agent for essential hypertension. Heart mitochondria may be the site of the cadmium-induced reduction in myocardial contractility. Epidemiologic studies in humans have suggested a relationship between abnormal behavior and/or decreased intelligence in children and adults exposed to cadmium.

Lead

Lead is a ubiquitous toxic metal and is detectable in practically all phases of the inert environment and in all biological systems. The phasing out of leaded gasoline and the removal of lead from paint, solder, and water supply pipes have significantly lowered blood lead levels in the general population. Lead exposure in children still remains a major health concern.

Exposure—Lead-containing paint is a primary source of lead exposure in children. Major environmental sources of lead for infants and toddlers up to 4 years of age are hand-to-mouth transfer of lead-containing paint chips and dust from floors of older housing. Lead in household dust can also come from outside of the home (i.e., soil). A major route of exposure for the general population is from food and water. Dietary intake of lead has decreased dramatically in recent years. Other potential sources of lead exposure are recreational shooting, hand-loading ammunition, soldering, jewelry making, pottery making, gun smithing, glass polishing, painting, and stained glass crafting.

Toxicity—The toxic effects of lead and the minimum blood level at which an effect is likely to be observed are shown in Table 23–1 Lead can induce a wide range of adverse effects in humans depending on the dose and duration of exposure. The toxic effects range from inhibition of enzymes to the production of severe pathology or death. Children are most sensitive to effects in the central nervous system, whereas peripheral neuropathy, chronic nephropathy, and hypertension are concerns in adults. Other target tissues include the gastrointestinal, immune, skeletal, and reproductive systems. Effects on the heme biosynthesis provide a sensitive biochemical indicator even in the absence of other detectable effects.

Neurologic, Neurobehavioral, and Developmental Effects in Children—Symptoms of lead encephalopathy begin with leth-

TABLE 23–1 Summary of lowest observed effect levels for lead-related health effects.

Effect	Blood Lead Levels, µg/dL	
	Adult	Children
Neurologic		
Encephalopathy (overt)	80–100	100–120
Hearing deficits	20	—
IQ deficits	10–15	—
In utero effects	10–15	—
Nerve conduction velocity ↓	40	40
Hematologic		
Anemia	80–100	80–100
U-ALA ↑	40	40
B-EP ↑	15	15
ALA-D inhibition	10	10
Renal		
Nephropathy	40	40–60
Vitamin D metabolism	<30?	—

argy, vomiting, irritability, loss of appetite, and dizziness, progressing to obvious ataxia, and a reduced level of consciousness, which may progress to coma and death. Recovery is often accompanied by sequelae including epilepsy, mental retardation, and, in some cases, optic neuropathy and blindness.

The most sensitive indicators of adverse neurologic outcomes are psychomotor tests or mental development indices, and broad measures of IQ. Lead may act as a surrogate for calcium and/or disrupt calcium homeostasis. The stimulation of protein kinase C may result in alteration of the blood–brain barrier. Lead affects virtually every neurotransmitter system in the brain, including glutamatergic, dopaminergic, and cholinergic systems. All these systems play a critical role in synaptic plasticity and cellular mechanisms for cognitive function, learning, and memory.

Neurotoxic Effects in Adults—Adults with occupational exposure may demonstrate abnormalities in a number of measures in neurobehavior. Peripheral neuropathy is a classic manifestation of lead toxicity in adults. Footdrop and wristdrop may be observed in workers with excessive occupational exposure to lead. Peripheral neuropathy is characterized by segmental demyelination and possibly axonal degeneration.

Hematologic Effects—Lead has multiple hematologic effects, ranging from increased urinary porphyrins, coproporphyrins, δ-aminolevulinic acid (ALA), and zinc-protoporphyrin to anemia. The heme biosynthesis pathway and the sites of lead interference are shown in Figure 23–2. The most sensitive effects of

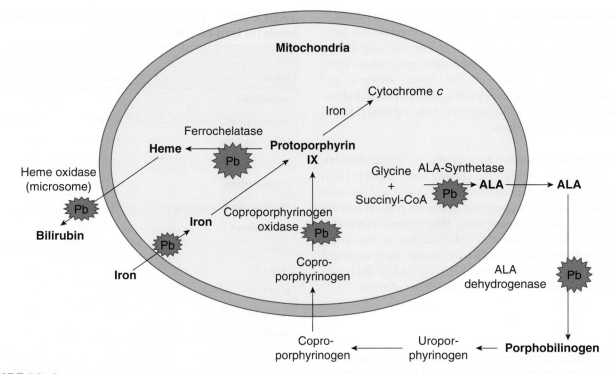

FIGURE 23–2 Lead interruption of heme biosynthesis. ALA, δ-aminolevulinate; Pb, sites for lead effects. The major lead inhibition sites are ALA dehydrogenase and ferrochelatase.

lead are the inhibition of δ-aminolevulinic acid dehydratase (ALAD) and ferrochelatase. ALAD catalyzes the condensation of two units of ALA to form phorphobilinogen (PBG). Inhibition of ALAD results in accumulation of ALA. Ferrochelatase catalyzes the insertion of iron into the protoporphyrin ring to form heme. Inhibition of ferrochelatase results in accumulation of protoporphyrin IX, which takes the place of heme in the hemoglobin molecule and, as the erythrocytes containing protoporphyrin IX circulate, zinc is chelated at the site usually occupied by iron. Anemia only occurs in very marked cases of lead toxicity.

Renal Toxicity—Acute lead nephrotoxicity consists of proximal tubular dysfunction and can be reversed by treatment with chelating agents. Chronic lead nephrotoxicity consists of interstitial fibrosis and progressive nephron loss, azotemia, and renal failure. Lead nephrotoxicity impairs the renal synthesis of heme-containing enzymes in the kidney, such as heme-containing hydroxylase involved in vitamin D metabolism causing bone effects. Hyperuricemia with gout occurs more frequently in the presence of lead nephropathy.

Effects on Cardiovascular System—The pathogenesis of lead-induced hypertension is multifactorial including: (1) inactivation of endogenous nitric oxide and cGMP, possibly through lead-induced reactive oxygen species; (2) changes in the renin–angiotensin–aldosterone system, and increases in sympathetic activity, important humoral components of hypertension; (3) alterations in calcium-activated functions of vascular

smooth muscle cells including contractility by decreasing Na^+/K^+-ATPase activity and stimulation of the Na^+/Ca^{2+} exchange pump; and (4) a possible rise in endothelin and thromboxane.

Other Toxic Effects—Lead may affect blood pressure via changes in plasma renin and in urinary kallikrein, alterations in calcium-activated functions of vascular smooth muscle cells, and changes in responsiveness to catecholamines. As an immunosuppressive agent, lead decreases immunoglobulins, peripheral B lymphocytes, and other components of the immunologic system. Retention and mobilization of lead in bone occur by the same mechanisms involved in regulating calcium influx and efflux. Lead also competes with calcium for gastrointestinal absorption. Lead is known to affect osteoblasts, osteoclasts, and chrondrocytes and has been associated with osteoporosis and delays in fracture repair. Lead toxicity has long been associated with sterility and neonatal deaths in humans. Lead, a 2B carcinogen, induces tumors of the respiratory and digestive systems. Epidemiologic studies suggest a relationship between occupational lead exposure and cancer of the lung, brain, and bladder among workers exposed to lead.

Mercury

Also called quicksilver, metallic mercury is in liquid state at room temperature. Mercury vapor (Hg^0) is much more hazardous than the liquid form. Mercury binds to other elements (such as chlorine, sulfur, or oxygen) to form inorganic mercurous (Hg^+) or mercuric (Hg^{2+}) salts.

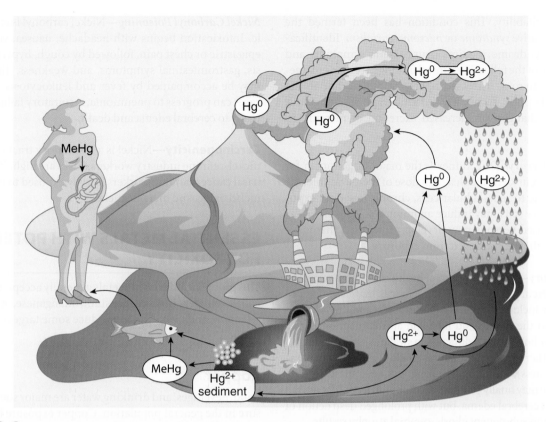

FIGURE 23–3 The movement of mercury in the environment. In nature, mercury vapor (Hg^0), a stable gas, evaporates from the earth's surface (both soil and water) and is emitted by volcanoes. Anthropogenic sources include emissions from coal-burning power stations and municipal incinerators. After ~1 year, mercury vapor is converted to soluble form (Hg^{2+}) and returned to the earth by rainwater. It may be converted back to the vapor by microorganisms and reemitted into the atmosphere. Thus, mercury may recirculate for long periods. Mercury attached to aquatic sediments is subjected to microbial conversion to methylmercury, starting with plankton, then herbivorous fish, and finally ascending to carnivorous fish and sea mammals. This biomethylation and biomagnification result in human exposure to methylmercury through consumption of fish, and pose the health risk to humans, especially the developing fetus.

Global Cycling and Ecotoxicology—Mercury exemplifies movement of metals in the environment (Figure 23–3). Atmospheric mercury, in the form of mercury vapor (Hg^0), is derived from natural degassing of the earth's crust and through volcanic eruptions as well as from evaporation from oceans and soils. Anthropogenic sources have become a significant contributor to atmospheric mercury. These include emissions from metal mining and smelting (mercury, gold, copper, and zinc), coal combustion, municipal incinerators, and chloralkali industries. Methylmercury enters the aquatic food chain starting with plankton, then herbivorous fish, and finally ascending to carnivorous fish and sea mammals. On the top of the food chain, tissue mercury can rise to levels 1800 to 80,000 times higher than levels in the surrounding water. This biomethylation and bioconcentration result in human exposure to methylmercury through consumption of fish.

Exposure

Dietary Exposure—Consumption of fish is the major route of exposure to methylmercury. Inorganic mercury compounds are also found in food. The source of inorganic mercurial is unknown but the amounts ingested are far below known toxic levels. Mercury in the atmosphere and in drinking water is generally so low that it does not constitute an important source of exposure to the general population.

Occupational Exposure—Inhalation of mercury vapor may occur from working in the chloralkali industry. Occupational exposure may occur during manufacture of a variety of scientific instruments and electrical control devices, in dentistry where mercury amalgams are used in tooth restoration, and in the extraction of gold.

Accidental Exposure—Elemental mercury exposure can occur from broken elemental mercury containers, medicinal devices, barometers, and melting tooth amalgam fillings to recover silver. Inhalation of large amounts of mercury vapor can be deadly.

Toxicity

Mercury Vapor—Inhalation of mercury vapor at extremely high concentrations may produce an acute, corrosive bronchitis and interstitial pneumonitis and, if not fatal, may be associated with central nervous system effects such as tremor or increased excitability. This condition has been termed the *asthenic-vegetative syndrome* or *micromercurialism*. Identification of the syndrome requires neurasthenic symptoms and three or more of the following clinical findings: tremor, enlargement of the thyroid, increased uptake of radioiodine in the thyroid, labile pulse, tachycardia, dermographism, gingivitis, hematologic changes, or increased excretion of mercury in urine.

Inorganic Mercury—The kidney is the major target organ for inorganic mercury. Although a high dose of mercuric chloride is directly toxic to renal tubular cells, chronic low-dose exposure to mercury salts may induce an immunologic glomerular disease. Exposed persons may develop proteinuria that is reversible after they are removed from exposure.

Methylmercury—The major human health effect from exposure to methylmercury is neurotoxicity. Clinical manifestations of neurotoxicity include paresthesia (a numbness and tingling sensation around the mouth and lips) and ataxia, manifested as a clumsy, stumbling gait, and difficulty in swallowing and articulating words. Other signs include neurasthenia (a generalized sensation of weakness), vision and hearing loss, and spasticity and tremor. These may finally progress to coma and death. The overall acute effect is cerebral edema, but with prolonged destruction of gray matter and subsequent gliosis, cerebral atrophy results.

Mechanism of Toxicity—High-affinity binding of divalent mercury to sulfhydryl groups of proteins in the cells is an important mechanism for producing nonspecific cell injury or even cell death. Other general mechanisms, such as the interruption of microtubule formation, inhibition of enzymes, oxidative stress, interruption of protein and DNA synthesis, and autoimmune responses, have also been proposed. Mercury causes overexpression of metallothionein and glutathione system-related genes in rat tissues.

Nickel

Metallic nickel is produced from sulfide and silicate-oxide ores. Nickel is used in various metal alloys, including stainless steels, and in electroplating. Occupational exposure to nickel occurs by inhalation of nickel-containing aerosols, dusts, or fumes, or dermal contact in workers engaged in nickel production (mining, milling, refinery, etc.) and nickel-using operations (melting, electroplating, welding, nickel–cadmium batteries, etc.). Nickel is ubiquitous in nature, and the general population is exposed to low levels of nickel in air, cigarette smoke, water, and food.

Toxicity
Contact Dermatitis—Nickel-induced contact dermatitis is the most common adverse health effect from nickel exposure and is found in 10 to 20 percent of the general population. It can result from exposure to airborne nickel, liquid nickel solutions, or prolonged skin contact with metal items containing nickel, such as coins and jewelry.

Nickel Carbonyl Poisoning—Nickel carbonyl is extremely toxic. Intoxication begins with headache, nausea, vomiting, and epigastric or chest pain, followed by cough, hyperpnea, cyanosis, gastrointestinal symptoms, and weakness. The symptoms may be accompanied by fever and leukocytosis. More severe cases can progress to pneumonia, respiratory failure, and eventually to cerebral edema and death.

Carcinogenicity—Nickel is a respiratory tract carcinogen in nickel-refining industry workers. Risks are highest for lung and nasal cancers among workers heavily exposed to nickel sulfide, nickel oxide, and metallic nickel.

ESSENTIAL METALS WITH POTENTIAL FOR TOXICITY

This group includes eight metals generally accepted as essential: cobalt, copper, iron, magnesium, manganese, molybdenum, selenium, and zinc. All can produce some target organ toxicity (Table 23–2).

Copper

Food, beverages, and drinking water are major sources of exposure in the general population. Copper exposure in industry is primarily from inhaled particulates in mining or metal fumes in smelting operations, welding, or related activities.

Toxicity—The most commonly reported adverse health effects of excess oral copper intake are gastrointestinal distress. Nausea, vomiting, and abdominal pain have been reported shortly after drinking solutions of copper sulfate or beverages stored in containers that readily release copper. Ingestion of drinking water with >3 mg Cu/L will produce gastrointestinal symptoms. Ingestion of large amounts of copper salts, most frequently copper sulfate, may produce hepatic necrosis and death.

Hereditary Disease of Copper Metabolism
Wilson's Disease—This is an autosomal recessive genetic disorder of copper metabolism characterized by the excessive accumulation of copper in liver, brain, kidneys, and cornea. Serum ceruloplasmin is low and serum copper not bound to ceruloplasmin is elevated. Urinary excretion of copper is high. Clinical abnormalities of the nervous system, liver, kidneys, and cornea are related to copper accumulation. Patients with Wilson's disease have impaired biliary excretion of copper, which is believed to be the fundamental cause of the copper overload. Reversal of abnormal copper metabolism is achieved by liver transplantation, confirming that the basic defect is in the liver. Clinical improvement can be achieved with chelation therapy.

Iron

Iron is an essential metal for erythropoiesis and a key component of hemoglobin, myoglobin, heme enzymes, metalloflavoprotein enzymes, and mitochondrial enzymes. In

TABLE 23–2 **Toxicity of several metals.**

Metal	CNS	GI Tract	Lung	Kidney	Liver	Heart	Blood	Skin
Aluminum	*		*					
Arsenic	*	*	*	*	*		*	
Beryllium			*					*
Bismuth				*	*			*
Cadmium	*	*	*	*	*	*		
Chromium	*		*	*	*			*
Cobalt	*	*	*			*		*
Copper		*					*	
Iron	*	*	*		*		*	
Lead	*			*			*	*
Manganese	*		*					
Mercury	*	*		*				
Nickel	*		*					*
Selenium		*		*				*
Zinc		*					*	

biological systems, iron mainly exists as the ferrous (+2) and ferric (+3) forms. Toxicologic considerations are important in terms of iron deficiency, accidental acute exposures, and chronic iron overload due to idiopathic hemochromatosis or as a consequence of excess dietary iron or frequent blood transfusions.

Toxicity—Acute iron poisoning from accidental ingestion of iron-containing dietary supplements is the most common cause of acute toxicity. Severe toxicity occurs after the ingestion of more than 0.5 g of iron or 2.5 g of ferrous sulfate. Toxicity occurs about 1 to 6 h after ingestion. Symptoms include abdominal pain, diarrhea, and vomiting. Of particular concern are pallor or cyanosis, metabolic acidosis, and cardiac collapse. Death may occur in severely poisoned children within 24 h.

Chronic iron toxicity from iron overload in adults is a relatively common problem. There are three basic ways in which excessive amounts of iron can accumulate in the body: (1) hereditary hemochromatosis due to abnormal absorption of iron from the intestinal tract, (2) excess intake via the diet or from oral iron preparations, and (3) repeated blood transfusions for some form of refractory anemia (*transfusional siderosis*). Increased body iron may play a role in the development of cardiovascular disease. It is suspected that iron may act as a catalyst to produce free radical damage resulting in artherosclerosis and ischemic heart disease. Some neurodegenerative disorders associated with aberrant iron metabolism in the brain include neuroferritinopathy, aceruloplasminemia, and manganism.

Zinc

An essential metal, zinc deficiency results in severe health consequences. However, zinc toxicity is relatively uncommon and occurs only at very high exposure levels. Zinc is present in most foodstuffs, water, and air. Occupational exposure to dusts and fumes of metallic zinc occurs in zinc mining and smelting. The zinc content of substances in contact with galvanized copper or plastic pipes may be high.

Essentiality and Deficiency—More than 300 catalytically active zinc metalloenzymes and 2000 zinc-dependent transcription factors exist. Zinc participates in a wide variety of metabolic processes, supports a healthy immune system, and is essential for normal growth and development during pregnancy, childhood, and adolescence. Zinc deficiency is related to poor dietary zinc intake, dietary phytate intake, chronic illness, or oversupplementation with iron or copper. Symptoms of zinc deficiency include growth retardation, appetite loss, alopecia, diarrhea, impaired immune function, cognitive impairments, dermatitis, delayed healing of wounds, taste abnormalities, and impaired sexual function. Therapeutic uses of zinc include the treatment of acute diarrhea in infants with severe zinc deficiency, the treatment of common cold by its antiviral and immunomodulatory effects, therapy for Wilson's disease to help reduce copper burden and to induce metallothionein, and the prevention of blindness in age-related macular degeneration.

Toxicity—Gastrointestinal distress and diarrhea have been reported following ingestion of beverages standing in galvanized cans. Following inhalation of zinc oxide, and to a lesser extent other zinc compounds, the most common effect is "metal-fume fever" characterized by fever, chest pain, chills, cough, dyspnea, nausea, muscle soreness, fatigue, and leukocytosis. Acute inhalation of high levels of zinc chloride as in the military use of "smoke bombs" results in more pronounced damage to the mucous membrane including interstitial edema, fibrosis, pneumonitis, bronchial mucosal edema, and ulceration. Following long-term exposure to lower doses of zinc, symptoms generally result from a decreased dietary copper absorption, leading to early symptoms of copper deficiency, such as decreased erythrocyte number or decreased hematocrit.

Neuronal Toxicity—Excess zinc released by oxidants can act as a potent neurotoxin, contributing to excitotoxic brain injury. The release of excess, toxic free zinc could be a factor that sets the stage for the later development of Alzheimer's disease.

METALS RELATED TO MEDICAL THERAPY

Metals that are used to treat a number of human illnesses, including aluminum, bismuth, gold, lithium, and platinum, exert some toxicity (Table 23–2).

Aluminum

Chemical compounds of aluminum occur typically in the trivalent valence state (Al^{3+}). As a hard trivalent ion, aluminum binds strongly to oxygen-donor ligands such as citrate and phosphate. Human exposure to aluminum comes primarily from food and secondarily from drinking water. Occupational exposures to aluminum occur during mining and processing, as well as in aluminum welding.

Toxicity—Most cases of aluminum toxicity in humans are observed in patients with chronic renal failure, or in persons exposed to aluminum in the workplace, with the lung, bone, and central nervous system as major target organs. Aluminum can produce developmental effects.

Lung and Bone Toxicity—Occupational exposure to aluminum dust can produce lung fibrosis in humans. Osteomalacia has been associated with excessive intake of aluminum-containing antacids in otherwise healthy individuals. This is assumed to be due to interference with intestinal phosphate absorption. Osteomalacia also can occur in uremic patients exposed to aluminum in the dialysis fluid. In these patients, osteomalacia may be a direct effect of aluminum on bone mineralization as bone levels are high.

Neurotoxicity—Aluminum is neurotoxic to experimental animals, with wide species and age variations. In susceptible animals, such as rabbits and cats, the most prominent early pathologic change is the accumulation of neurofibrillary tangles (NFTs) in large neurons, proximal axons, and dendrites of neurons of many brain regions. This is associated with loss of synapses and atrophy of the dendritic tree. In other species, impairment of cognitive and motor function and behavioral abnormalities are often observed.

Dialysis Dementia—A progressive, neurologic syndrome has been reported in patients on long-term intermittent hemodialysis for chronic renal failure. The first symptom in these patients is a speech disorder followed by dementia, convulsions, and myoclonus. The disorder, which typically arises after 3 to 7 years of dialysis treatment, may be due to aluminum intoxication. The aluminum content of brain, muscle, and bone increases in these patients. Sources of the excess aluminum may be from oral aluminum hydroxide commonly given to these patients or from aluminum in dialysis fluid derived from the tap water used to prepare the dialysate fluid. The high serum aluminum concentrations may be related to increased parathyroid hormone levels that are due to low blood calcium and osteodystrophy common in patients with chronic renal disease. The syndrome may be prevented by avoiding the use of aluminum-containing oral phosphate binders and by monitoring of aluminum in the dialysate.

Alzheimer's Disease—A possible relationship between aluminum and Alzheimer's disease has been a matter of speculation for decades. Elevated aluminum levels in Alzheimer's brains may be a consequence and not a cause of the disease. The reduced effectiveness of the blood–brain barrier in Alzheimer's might allow more aluminum into the brain. Also, recent studies have raised the possibility that the staining methods in earlier studies may have led to aluminum contamination. There are conflicting conclusions from studies examining the role of aluminum in Alzheimer's disease. However, there is increasing evidence suggesting a link between aluminum in the brain and other neurodegenerative diseases.

Lithium

Lithium is used in batteries, alloys, catalysts, photographic materials, and the space industry. Lithium hydride produces hydrogen on contact with water and is used in manufacturing electronic tubes, in ceramics, and in chemical analysis. Groundwater contamination with lithium from man-made waste disposal could be a risk factor for the aquatic environment. Lithium carbonate and lithium citrate are widely used for mania and bipolar disorders.

Toxicokinetics—Lithium is readily absorbed from the gastrointestinal tract. It is distributed to total body water with higher levels in kidney, thyroid, and bone as compared with other tissues. Excretion is chiefly through the kidneys with 80 percent of the filtered lithium reabsorbed. Lithium can substitute for sodium or potassium on several transport proteins.

Toxicity—Except for lithium hydride, no other salts are considered hazardous, nor is the metal very toxic itself. Lithium hydride is intensely corrosive and may produce burns on the skin because of the formation of hydroxides. The toxic responses to lithium include neuromuscular changes (tremor, muscle hyperirritability, and ataxia), central nervous system disorders (blackout spells, epileptic seizures, slurred speech, coma, psychosomatic retardation, and increased thirst), cardiovascular disturbances (cardiac arrhythmia, hypertension, and circulatory collapse), gastrointestinal symptoms (anorexia, nausea, and vomiting), and renal damage (albuminuria and glycosuria).

Chronic lithium nephrotoxicity and interstitial nephritis may occur with long-term exposure even when lithium levels remain within the therapeutic range. Chronic lithium-induced neurotoxicity, nephritis, and thyroid dysfunction may occur, especially in susceptible patients with nephrogenic diabetes insipidus, older age, abnormal thyroid function, and impaired renal function.

Platinum

Platinum compounds are used as automobile catalysts, in jewelry, in electronics, and in dental alloys.

Toxicity—Platinum can produce profound hypersensitivity reactions in susceptible individuals. The signs of hypersensitivity include urticaria, contact dermatitis of skin, and respiratory distress, ranging from irritation to an asthmatic syndrome, following exposure to platinum dust. The skin and respiratory changes, *platinosis,* are mainly confined to persons with a history of industrial exposure to soluble compounds such as sodium chloroplatinate.

Antitumor Effects of Platinum Complexes—The platinum-coordinated complexes are important antitumor agents, including cisplatin, carboplatin, and oxaliplatin. They are routinely administered, often in combination with other anticancer drugs, in the treatment of a wide spectrum of malignancies, especially advanced testicular cancer and also cancers of head and neck, bladder, esophagus, lung, and ovary.

Carcinogenic Effects of Platinum Complexes—Although cisplatin has antitumor activity in humans, it is considered to be a probable carcinogen in humans and is clearly carcinogenic in rodents. In fact, in mice deficient in metallothionein, cisplatin can induce tumors at clinically relevant doses.

Toxicities of Platinum Antitumor Complexes—Cisplatin produces proximal and distal tubular cell injury, mainly in the corticomedullary region, where the concentration of platinum is highest. Hearing loss can occur and can be unilateral or bilateral but tends to be more frequent and severe with repeated doses. Marked nausea and vomiting occur in most patients receiving the platinum complexes but can be controlled with ondansetron or high dose of corticosteroids.

BIBLIOGRAPHY

Hirner AV, Emons H (eds): *Organic Metal and Metalloid Species in the Environment: Analysis, Distribution, Processes and Toxicological Evaluation.* New York: Springer, 2004.

Nordberg GF, Fowler BA, Nordberg M, Friberg LT (eds): *Handbook on the Toxicology of Metals,* 3rd ed. Boston: Academic Press, 2007.

QUESTIONS

1. Which of the following is NOT a major excretory pathway of metals?
   a. sweat.
   b. urine.
   c. respiration.
   d. feces.
   e. hair.

2. Metallothioneins:
   a. are responsible for metal transport in the bloodstream.
   b. are involved in the biotransformation of metals.
   c. invoke hypersensitivity reactions.
   d. provide high-affinity binding of copper and mercury.
   e. are involved in extracellular transport of metals.

3. Which of the following metal-binding proteins is NOT correctly paired with the metal it binds?
   a. transferrin—iron.
   b. ceruloplasmin—copper.
   c. metallothioneins—zinc.
   d. ferritin—lead.
   e. albumin—nonspecific metal binding.

4. Which of the following groups is LEAST likely to chelate metals?
   a. —COOH.
   b. —Cl.
   c. —NH.
   d. —OH.
   e. —SH.

5. What is the mechanism of toxicity of arsenic (As)?
   a. inhibition of mitochondrial respiration.
   b. impairment of calcium uptake by membrane transporters.
   c. accumulation in renal corpuscle.
   d. abolition of sodium–potassium gradient.
   e. destruction of surfactant in the lungs.

6. Lead's toxicity is largely due to its ability to mimic and interfere with normal functioning of which of the following ions?
   a. Na^+.
   b. K^+.
   c. Cl^-.
   d. Fe^{2+}.
   e. Ca^{2+}.

7. Which of the following statements regarding mercury (Hg) toxicity is FALSE?
   a. A major source of environmental mercury is rainwater.
   b. Mercury vapor is much more dangerous than liquid mercury.
   c. Mercury vapor inhalation is characterized by fatigue and bradycardia.
   d. Microorganisms in bodies of water can convert mercury vapor to methylmercury.
   e. Methylmercury is the most important source of human mercury toxicity.

8. Which of the following is a common symptom of nickel exposure?
   a. renal failure.
   b. diarrhea.
   c. hepatic cirrhosis.
   d. contact dermatitis.
   e. tachycardia.

9. Which of the following statements regarding Wilson's disease is FALSE?
   a. Serum ceruloplasmin is high.
   b. Urinary excretion of copper is high.
   c. There is impaired biliary excretion of copper.
   d. The disease can be treated with liver transplantation.
   e. This is an autosomal recessive disorder.

10. Which of the following statements regarding metals and medical therapy is FALSE?
    a. There are elevated levels of aluminum in the brains of Alzheimer's patients.
    b. Lithium is used to treat depression.
    c. Chronic nephrotoxicity is a common result of excess aluminum exposure.
    d. Platinum is used as cancer treatment.
    e. Platinum salts can cause an allergic dermatitis.

24

Toxic Effects of Solvents and Vapors

James V. Bruckner, S. Satheesh Anand, and D. Alan Warren

INTRODUCTION

The term *solvent* refers to a class of liquid organic chemicals of variable lipophilicity and volatility, small molecular size, and lack of charge. Solvents undergo ready absorption across the lung, skin, and gastrointestinal (GI) tract. In general, the lipophilicity of solvents increases with increasing molecular weight, while volatility decreases. Solvents are frequently used to dissolve, dilute, or disperse materials that are insoluble in water. Most solvents are refined from petroleum. Many, such as naphthas and gasoline, are complex mixtures consisting of hundreds of compounds.

Solvents are classified largely according to molecular structure or functional group. Classes of solvents include aliphatic hydrocarbons, many of which are chlorinated (i.e., halocarbons), aromatic hydrocarbons, alcohols, ethers, esters/acetates, amides/amines, aldehydes, ketones, and complex mixtures that defy classification. The main determinants of a solvent's inherent toxicity are: (1) its number of carbon atoms; (2) whether it is saturated or has double or triple bonds between adjacent carbon atoms; (3) its configuration (i.e., straight chain, branched chain, or cyclic); and (4) the presence of functional groups. Subtle differences in chemical structure can translate into dramatic differences in solvent toxicity.

Nearly everyone is exposed to solvents during normal daily activities. Environmental exposures to solvents in air and groundwater use multiple exposure pathways (Figure 24–1). Though not reflected in Figure 24–1, household use of solvent-

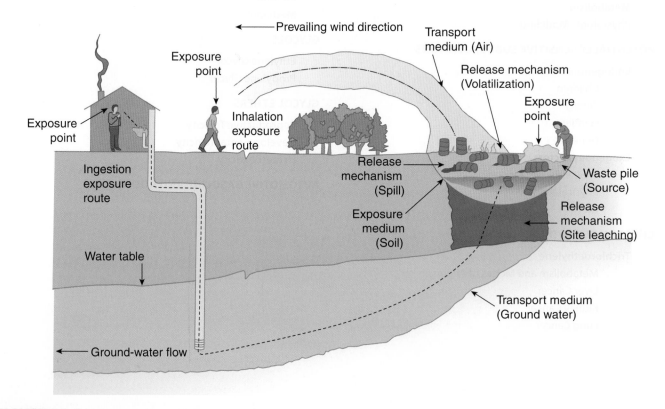

FIGURE 24–1 **Solvent exposure pathways and media.** (From EPA: *Risk Assessment Guidance for Superfund. Human Health Evaluation Manual Part A, Interim Final.* Washington, DC: Office of Emergency and Remedial Response, 1989.)

contaminated water may result in solvent intake from inhalation, and dermal and oral absorption. In many cases, environmental risk assessment requires that risks be determined for physiologically diverse individuals who are exposed to several solvents by multiple exposure pathways.

The Occupational Safety and Health Administration (OSHA) has established legally enforceable Permissible Exposure Limits (PELs) for over 100 solvents. The majority of existing PELs were adopted from the list of Threshold Limit Values (TLVs) published by the American Conference of Governmental Industrial Hygienists (ACGIH). Whereas the ACGIH's TLVs for an 8-h work day, 40-h work week are designed to be protective for a working lifetime, its Short-term Exposure Limits (STELs) and ceiling values are designed to protect against the acute effects of high-level, short-term solvent exposures. If warranted, the ACGIH will assign a skin notation to a solvent, indicating that significant dermal exposure is possible.

Most solvent exposures involve a mixture of chemicals, rather than a single compound. Whereas the assumption is frequently made that the toxic effects of multiple solvents are additive, solvents may also interact synergistically or antagonistically.

Although some solvents are less hazardous than others, all solvents can cause toxic effects. Most have the potential to induce narcosis and cause respiratory and mucous membrane irritation. Numerous solvents are animal carcinogens, but only a few are classified as known human carcinogens.

IS THERE A SOLVENT-INDUCED CHRONIC ENCEPHALOPATHY?

Considerable debate has examined whether chronic, low-level exposure to virtually any solvent or solvent mixture can produce a pattern of neurologic dysfunction referred to as *painter's syndrome, organic solvent syndrome, psychoorganic syndrome,* and *chronic solvent encephalopathy* (CSE). CSE is characterized by nonspecific symptoms (e.g., headache, fatigue, and sleep disorders) with or without changes in neuropsychological function. A reversible form of CSE, the *neuroasthenic syndrome,* consists of symptoms only. The "mild" and "severe" forms are accompanied by objective signs of neuropsychological dysfunction that may or may not be fully reversible. Well-designed and controlled clinical epidemiologic studies are needed to resolve this controversy of CSE.

SOLVENT ABUSE

Many solvents are intentionally inhaled in order to achieve a state of intoxication, with euphoria, delusions, and sedation as well as visual and auditory hallucinations. Solvent abuse is a unique exposure situation, in that participants repeatedly subject themselves to vapor concentrations high enough to produce effects as extreme as unconsciousness. These can be breathed in through the nose or the mouth by "sniffing" or "snorting" vapors from containers, spraying aerosols directly into the nose or mouth, "bagging" by inhaling vapors from

substances inside plastic or paper bags, or "huffing" from a solvent-soaked rag stuffed into the mouth. Solvents can be addicting and are often abused in combination with other drugs. Solvents present in relatively inexpensive household and commercial products are readily available to children and adolescents.

ENVIRONMENTAL CONTAMINATION

Most solvents enter the environment through evaporation (Figure 24–1). The majority of the more volatile organic compounds (VOCs) volatilize when products containing them (e.g., aerosol propellants, paint thinners, cleaners, and soil fumigants) are used as intended. Solvent loss into the atmosphere also occurs during production, processing, storage, and transport activities. Winds dilute and disperse solvent vapors across the world. Atmospheric concentrations of most VOCs are usually extremely low, though higher concentrations have been measured in urban areas, around petrochemical plants, and in the immediate vicinity of hazardous waste sites.

Solvent contamination of drinking water supplies is a major health concern. Solvents spilled onto the ground may permeate the soil and migrate until reaching groundwater or impermeable material. All solvents are soluble in water to some extent. Concentrations diminish rapidly after VOCs enter bodies of water, due primarily to dilution and evaporation. VOCs in surface waters rise to the surface or sink to the bottom, according to their density. VOCs on the surface will largely evaporate. VOCs on the bottom depend on solubilization in the water or on mixing by current or wave action to reach the surface. VOCs in groundwater tend to remain trapped until the water reaches the surface.

TOXICOKINETICS

Toxicokinetic (TK) studies delineate the uptake and disposition of chemicals in the body. Toxicity is a dynamic process, in which the degree and duration of injury of a target tissue depend on the net effect of toxicodynamic (TD) and TK processes, interaction with cellular components, and tissue repair.

Volatility and lipophilicity are two important properties of solvents that govern their absorption and deposition in the body. Lipophilicity also can vary from quite water soluble (e.g., glycols and alcohols) to quite lipid soluble (e.g., halocarbons and aromatic hydrocarbons). Many solvents have a relatively low molecular weight and are uncharged, enabling passive diffusion through membranes from areas of high to low concentration.

Absorption

Most systemic absorption of inhaled VOCs occurs in the alveoli, with some absorption occurring in the upper respiratory tract. Gases in the alveoli equilibrate almost instantaneously with blood in the pulmonary capillaries. Blood:air partition coefficients (PCs) of VOCs may be defined as the ratio of concentration of VOC achieved between two different media at equilibrium. More hydrophilic solvents have relatively high blood:air PCs, which favor extensive uptake. Because VOCs diffuse from areas of high to low concentration, increases in respiration (to maintain a high alveolar concentration) and in cardiac output/pulmonary blood flow (to maintain a large concentration gradient by removing capillary blood containing the VOC) enhance pulmonary absorption.

Solvents are well absorbed from the GI tract. Peak blood levels are observed within minutes of dosing, although the presence of food in the GI tract can delay absorption. It is usually assumed that 100 percent of an oral dose of most solvents is absorbed systemically. The vehicle or diluent in which a solvent is ingested can affect the absorption and TK of the compound.

Absorption of solvents through the skin can result in both local and systemic effects. Solvents penetrate the stratum corneum by passive diffusion. Determinants of the rate of dermal absorption of solvents include the chemical concentration, surface area exposed, exposure duration, integrity and thickness of the stratum corneum, and lipophilicity and molecular weight of the solvent.

Transport and Distribution

Solvents absorbed into portal venous blood from the GI tract are subject to uptake/elimination by the liver and exhalation by the lungs during their first pass along this absorption pathway. Those solvents that are well metabolized and quite volatile are most efficiently eliminated before they enter the arterial blood. Hepatic first-pass elimination depends on the chemical and the rate at which it arrives in the liver. Pulmonary first-pass elimination, in contrast, is believed to be a first-order process irrespective of the chemical concentration in the blood.

Solvents transported by the arterial blood are taken up according to rate of tissue blood flow and the tissue:blood PC of the solvent. Relatively hydrophilic solvents solubilize to different extents in plasma. Lipophilic solvents do not bind to plasma proteins or hemoglobin, but partition into hydrophobic sites in the molecules. They partition into phospholipids, lipoproteins, and cholesterol that are present in the blood.

Blood levels of solvents drop rapidly during the initial elimination phase. This redistribution phase is characterized by rapid diffusion of solvent from the blood into most tissues. Equilibration of adipose tissue is prolonged due to the small fraction of cardiac output (~3 percent) supplying fat depots. Body fat increases the volume of distribution and total body burden of lipophilic solvents.

Metabolism

Biotransformation can modulate the toxicities of solvents. Many solvents are poorly soluble in water and must be converted to relatively water-soluble derivatives, which may be more readily eliminated in the largely aqueous urine and/or bile.

Some solvents can undergo bioactivation to produce reactive metabolites that are cytotoxic and/or mutagenic.

Physiologic Modeling

Physiologically based toxicokinetic (PBTK) models are used to relate the administered dose to the tissue dose of a bioactive moiety or moieties. With knowledge of the physiology of the test animal and tissue, physiologically based toxicodynamic (PBTD) models can be developed. PBTK/TD models are well suited for species-to-species extrapolations, because human physiologic and metabolic parameter values can be entered and simulations of target tissue doses and effects in humans generated. Thus, solvent exposures necessary to produce the same target organ dose in humans as that found experimentally to cause an unacceptable cancer or noncancer incidence in test animals can be determined in some cases with reasonable certainty. In the limited number of cases where there may be species differences in tissue sensitivity, PBTD models can be used to forecast toxicologically effective target organ doses.

POTENTIALLY SENSITIVE SUBPOPULATIONS

Endogenous Factors

Children—Limited information is available on the toxic potential of solvents in children. Most age-dependent differences are less than an order of magnitude, usually varying no more than two- to threefold. The younger and more immature the subject, the more different is his or her response from that of adults.

GI absorption of solvents varies little with age, because most solvents are absorbed by passive diffusion. Systemic absorption of inhaled VOCs may be greater in infants and children than in adults owing to the relatively high cardiac output and respiratory rates despite their lower alveolar surface area. Extracellular water, expressed as percentage of body weight, is highest in newborns and gradually diminishes through childhood. Body fat content is high from ~1/2 to 3 years of age, and then steadily decreases until adolescence, when it increases again in females. Lipophilic solvents accumulate in adipose tissue, so more body fat would result in greater body burdens and slower clearance of the chemicals.

Changes in xenobiotic metabolism during maturation may impact susceptibility to solvent toxicity. P450 isoforms develop asynchronously. Increased rates of metabolism, urinary excretion, and exhalation by children should hasten elimination and reduce body burdens of solvents. However, the net effect of immaturity on solvent disposition and toxicity is difficult to predict.

Elderly—Age influences the distribution of xenobiotics in the body as well as their metabolism and elimination. With aging, body fat usually increases substantially at the expense of lean mass and body water. Thus, relatively polar solvents tend to reach higher blood levels during exposures. Relatively lipid-soluble solvents accumulate in adipose tissue and are released slowly. Cardiac output and renal and hepatic blood flows are diminished in the elderly.

The elderly, like infants and children, may be more or less sensitive to the toxicity of solvents than young adults. Greater organ system toxicity could be due to increased inflammatory damage or to age-related dysregulation of cytokines. Other major sources of variability and complexity in geriatric populations include inadequate nutrition, the prevalence of disease states, and the concurrent use of multiple medications.

Gender—Physiologic and biochemical differences between men and women have the potential to alter tissue dosimetry and health effects of certain solvents. Whereas most predictive models suggest effects of toxicants are independent of sex, physical differences, such as the tendency of men to have more lean body mass and a larger body size, could potentially cause physiologic differences.

Genetics—Genetic polymorphisms for biotransformation occur at different frequencies in different ethnic groups. Polymorphisms for xenobiotic-metabolizing enzymes may affect the quantity and quality of enzymes and the outcomes of exposures to solvents in different racial groups. Disentangling the influences of genetic traits from those of socioeconomic status, lifestyles, and geographic setting is difficult.

Exogenous Factors

P450 Inducers and Inhibitors—Preexposure to chemicals that induce or inhibit biotransformation enzymes can potentiate or reduce the toxicity of high doses of solvents that undergo metabolism. Inhibitors would generally be anticipated to enhance the toxicity of solvents that are metabolically inactivated and protect from solvents that undergo metabolic activation.

Physical Activity—Exercise increases alveolar ventilation and cardiac output/pulmonary blood flow. Polar solvents with relatively high blood:air PCs (e.g., acetone, ethanol, and ethylene glycol [EG]) are very rapidly absorbed into the pulmonary circulation. Alveolar ventilation is rate-limiting for these chemicals. In contrast, pulmonary blood flow and metabolism are rate-limiting for uptake of more lipophilic solvents. Heavy exercise can increase pulmonary uptake of relatively polar solvents as much as fivefold in human subjects. Light exercise doubles uptake of relatively lipid-soluble solvents, but no further increase occurs at higher workloads. Blood flow to the liver and kidneys diminishes with exercise, which may diminish biotransformation of metabolized solvents and urinary elimination.

Diet—The mere bulk of food in the stomach and intestines can inhibit systemic absorption of ingested chemicals by preventing contact of the chemical with the GI epithelium. VOCs in the GI tract partition into dietary lipids, largely remaining there until the lipids are emulsified and digested. Food intake results in increased splanchnic blood flow, which favors GI absorption, hepatic blood flow, and biotransformation. Foods may contain certain natural constituents, pesticides, and other chemicals that may enhance or reduce solvent metabolism.

CHLORINATED HYDROCARBONS

Trichloroethylene

1,1,2-Trichloroethylene (TCE) is a widely used solvent for metal degreasing. Although present data support weak associations between TCE exposure and multiple myeloma, Hodgkin's disease, and cancers of the prostate, skin, cervix, and kidney, this is a topic of much debate.

Metabolism and Modes of Action—Toxicities associated with TCE are predominantly mediated by metabolites rather than by the parent compound. Even the CNS-depressant effects of TCE are due in part to the sedative properties of the metabolites trichloroethanol (TCOH) and chloroform. After either oral or inhalational absorption, most of the TCE undergoes oxidation via cytochrome P450s, with a small proportion being conjugated with glutathione. Both of the following metabolic pathways are implicated in the carcinogenicity of TCE: reactive metabolite(s) of the GSH pathway in kidney tumors in rats and oxidative metabolites in liver and lung tumors in mice.

Liver Cancer—TCE induces liver cancer in B6C3F1 mice but not in rats. This differential susceptibility is due to the greater capacity of mice to metabolize TCE to an oxidative metabolite that stimulates peroxisome proliferation. Propagation results in an increased potential for oxidative DNA damage and decreased gap-junctional intercellular communication, both of which have been implicated in neoplastic transformation.

Kidney Cancer—TCE exposure by inhalation or the oral route results in kidney tumors in male but not female rats. The susceptibility of the male rat can be explained by its greater capacity for TCE metabolism via the GSH pathway. TCE-induced kidney tumors are believed to result from reactive metabolite(s) of this pathway alkylating cellular nucleophiles, including DNA. The resulting DNA mutations lead to alterations in gene expression, which in turn lead to neoplastic transformation and tumorigenesis via a genotoxic pathway.

Alternatively, proximal tubular cell cytotoxicity and subsequent tumor formation via a nongenotoxic mode of action could be induced by reactive metabolites that cause oxidative stress, alkylation of cytosolic and mitochondrial proteins, marked ATP depletion, and perturbations in Ca^{2+} homeostasis. Tubular necrosis ensues, with subsequent reparative proliferation that can alter gene expression and, in turn, alter the regulation of cell growth and differentiation. In fact, somatic mutations in the von Hippel-Lindau (VHL) tumor suppressor gene might be a specific and susceptible target of TCE.

Chronic tubular damage may be a prerequisite to TCE-induced renal cell cancer. Reactive metabolite(s) of the GSH pathway may have a genotoxic effect on the proximal tubule of the human kidney, but full development of a malignant tumor requires a promotional effect such as cell proliferation in response to tubular damage.

Lung Cancer—Inhaled TCE is carcinogenic to the mouse lung but not to that of the rat. Oral TCE is not carcinogenic to the lung, probably due to hepatic metabolism that limits the amount of TCE reaching the organ. The primary target of TCE within the mouse lung is the nonciliated Clara cell. Cytotoxicity to these cells is characterized by vacuolization and increases in cell replication in the bronchiolar epithelium. Clara cells of the mouse efficiently metabolize TCE to toxic metabolites. In mouse lung, Clara cells are more numerous and have a much higher concentration of metabolizing enzymes than rat lung.

Tetrachloroethylene

Tetrachloroethylene (perchloroethylene, PERC) is commonly used as a dry cleaner, fabric finisher, degreaser, rug and upholstery cleaner, paint and stain remover, solvent, and chemical intermediate. The highest exposures usually occur in occupational settings via inhalation. PERC is the third most frequently found chemical contaminant in groundwater at hazardous waste sites in the United States.

The systemic disposition and metabolism of PERC and TCE are quite similar. Both chemicals are well absorbed from the lungs and GI tract, distributed to tissues according to their lipid content, partially exhaled unchanged, and metabolized by P450s. PERC is oxidized by hepatic P450s to a much lesser degree than TCE, though trichloroacetic acid is a common major metabolite. GSH conjugation is a minor metabolic pathway, quantitatively, for TCE and PERC.

PERC's potential for causing cancer in humans is controversial. The many epidemiologic studies of cancer incidence and mortality in groups of persons occupationally exposed to PERC are equivocal and do not support a cause-and-effect relationship between either PERC or TCE and cancer. Cigarette smoking and alcohol consumption are important confounders for esophageal cancer. Kidney cancer incidences did not appear to be elevated.

Methylene Chloride

Methylene chloride (dichloromethane, MC) enjoys widespread use as a solvent in industrial processes, food preparation, degreasing agents, aerosol propellants, and agriculture. The primary route of exposure to this very volatile solvent is inhalation.

MC has limited systemic toxicity potential. High, repeated inhalation exposures produce slight, reversible changes in the livers of rodents. Persons subjected to high vapor levels manifest kidney injury occasionally. Carbon monoxide that is formed from MC binds to hemoglobin to produce dose-dependent increases in carboxyhemoglobin. Residual neurologic dysfunction in MC-exposed workers has been reported.

Occupational and environmental MC exposures are of concern primarily because of MC's carcinogenicity in rodents and its potential as a human carcinogen. Epidemiologic studies of employees exposed to MC have revealed that cancer risks from occupational exposure to MC, if any, are quite small.

Carbon Tetrachloride

Carbon tetrachloride (CCl_4) is a classic hepatotoxin, but kidney injury is often more severe in humans. There does not appear to be a good animal model for kidney toxicity.

Early signs of hepatocellular injury in rats include dissociation of polysomes and ribosomes from rough endoplasmic reticulum, disarray of smooth endoplasmic reticulum, inhibition of protein synthesis, and triglyceride accumulation. CCl_4 undergoes metabolic activation, producing lipid peroxidation, covalent binding, and inhibition of microsomal ATPase activity. Single cell necrosis, evident 5 to 6 h postdosing, progresses to maximal centrilobular necrosis within 24 to 48 h. Cellular regeneration is maximal 36 to 48 h postdosing. The rate and extent of tissue repair are important determinants of the ultimate outcome of liver injury.

Perturbation of intracellular calcium (Ca^{2+}) homeostasis appears to be part of CCl_4 cytotoxicity. Increased cytosolic Ca^{2+} levels may result from influx of extracellular Ca^{2+} due to plasma membrane damage and from decreased intracellular Ca^{2+} sequestration. Elevation of intracellular Ca^{2+} in hepatocytes can activate phospholipase A_2 and exacerbate membrane damage. Elevated Ca^{2+} may also be involved in alterations in calmodulin and phosphorylase activity as well as changes in nuclear protein kinase C activity. High intracellular Ca^{2+} levels activate a number of catabolic enzymes including proteases, endonucleases, and phospholipases, which kill cells via apoptosis or necrosis. Increased Ca^{2+} may stimulate the release of cytokines and eicosanoids from Kupffer cells, inducing neutrophil infiltration and hepatocellular injury. CCl_4 hepatotoxicity is obviously a complex, multifactorial process.

Chloroform

Chloroform ($CHCl_3$, trichloromethane) is used primarily in the production of the refrigerant chlorodifluoromethane (Freon 22). Measurable concentrations of $CHCl_3$ are found in municipal drinking water supplies. $CHCl_3$ is hepatotoxic and nephrotoxic. It can invoke CNS symptoms at subanesthetic concentrations similar to those of alcohol intoxication. Extremely high $CHCl_3$ exposures can sensitize the myocardium to catecholamines.

The metabolite phosgene covalently binds hepatic and renal proteins and lipids, which damages membranes and other intracellular structures, leading to necrosis and subsequent reparative cellular proliferation that promotes tumor formation in rodents by irreversibly "fixing" spontaneously altered DNA and clonally expanding initiated cells. The expression of certain genes, including *myc* and *fos,* is altered during regenerative cell proliferation in response to $CHCl_3$-induced cytotoxicity.

Although a rodent carcinogen, ingestion of CHCl₃ in small increments, similar to drinking water patterns of humans, fails to produce sufficient cytotoxic metabolite(s) per unit time to overwhelm detoxification mechanisms. Currently, CHCl₃ is classified as a probable human carcinogen (group B2).

AROMATIC HYDROCARBONS

Benzene

Benzene is derived primarily from petroleum and is used in the synthesis of other chemicals and as an antiknock agent in unleaded gasoline. Inhalation is the primary route of exposure in industrial and in everyday settings. Cigarette smoke is the major source of benzene in the home. Smokers have benzene body burdens which are 6 to 10 times greater than those of nonsmokers. Passive smoke can be a significant source of benzene exposure to nonsmokers. Gasoline vapor emissions and auto exhaust are the other key contributors to exposures of the general populace.

The hematopoietic toxicity of chronic exposure to benzene may manifest initially as anemia, leukopenia, thrombocytopenia, or a combination of these. Bone marrow depression appears to be dose-dependent in both laboratory animals and humans. Continued exposure may result in marrow aplasia and pancytopenia, an often fatal outcome. Survivors of aplastic anemia frequently exhibit a preneoplastic state, termed *myelodysplasia*, which may progress to myelogenous leukemia.

There is strong evidence from epidemiologic studies that high-level benzene exposures result in an increased risk of acute myelogenous leukemia (AML) in humans. Evidence of increased risks of other cancers in such populations is less compelling.

Various potential mechanisms require the complementary actions of benzene and several of its metabolites for toxicity. (1) A number of benzene metabolites bind covalently to GSH, proteins, DNA, and RNA. This can result in disruption of the functional hematopoietic microenvironment by inhibition of enzymes, destruction of certain cell populations, and alteration of the growth of other cell types. Covalent binding of hydroquinones to spindle-fiber proteins will inhibit cell replication. (2) Oxidative stress contributes to benzene toxicity. As the bone marrow is rich in peroxidase activity, phenolic metabolites of benzene can be activated there to reactive quinone derivatives, which can cause DNA damage, leading to cell mutation or apoptosis. Modulation of apoptosis may lead to aberrant hematopoiesis and neoplastic progression.

Toluene

Toluene is present in paints, lacquers, thinners, cleaning agents, glues, and many other products. It is also used in the production of other chemicals. Gasoline, which contains 5 to 7 percent toluene (w/w), is the largest source of atmospheric emissions and exposure of the general populace. Inhalation is the primary route of exposure, though skin contact occurs frequently. Toluene is a favorite of solvent abusers, who intentionally inhale high concentrations of the VOC.

Toluene is well absorbed from the lungs and GI tract. It rapidly accumulates in the brain, and subsequently, is deposited in other tissues according to their lipid content, with adipose tissue attaining the highest levels. Toluene is well metabolized, but a portion is exhaled unchanged.

The CNS is the primary target organ of toluene and other alkylbenzenes. Manifestations of exposure range from slight dizziness and headache to unconsciousness, respiratory depression, and death. Occupational inhalation exposure guidelines are established to prevent significant decrements in psychomotor functions. Acute encephalopathic effects are rapidly reversible on cessation of exposure. Subtle neurologic effects have been reported in some groups of occupationally exposed individuals. Severe neurotoxicity is sometimes diagnosed in persons who have abused toluene for a prolonged period. Clinical signs include abnormal electroencephalographic (EEG) activity, tremors, nystagmus, and cerebral atrophy as well as impaired hearing, vision, and speech. Magnetic resonance imaging has revealed permanent changes in brain structure, which correspond to the degree of brain dysfunction. These changes include ventricular enlargement, cerebral atrophy, and white matter hyperintensity, a characteristic profile termed *toluene leukoencephalopathy*.

Xylenes and Ethylbenzene

Large numbers of people are exposed to xylenes and ethylbenzene occupationally and environmentally. Xylenes and ethylbenzene, like benzene and toluene, are major components of gasoline and fuel oil. The primary uses of xylenes industrially are as solvents and synthetic intermediates. Most of the aromatics released into the environment evaporate into the atmosphere.

Similar to toluene, xylenes and other aromatic solvents are well absorbed from the lungs and GI tract, distributed to tissues according to tissue blood flow and lipid content, exhaled to some extent, well metabolized by hepatic P450s, and largely excreted as urinary metabolites. Acute lethality of hydrocarbons (i.e., CNS depression) varies directly with lipophilicity. There is limited evidence that chronic occupational exposure to xylenes is associated with residual neurologic effects.

Xylenes and ethylbenzene have limited capacity to adversely affect organs other than the CNS. Mild, transient liver and/or kidney toxicity have been reported occasionally in humans exposed to high vapor concentrations of xylenes. The majority of alkylbenzenes do not appear to be genotoxic or carcinogenic. Ethylbenzene and styrene are known animal carcinogens, but there are limited human data.

ALCOHOLS

Ethanol

Many humans experience greater exposure to ethanol (ethyl alcohol and alcohol) than to any other solvent. Ethyl alcohol is used as an additive in gasoline, as a solvent in industry, in many household products and pharmaceuticals, and in intoxicating beverages. Frank toxic effects are less important occupationally than injuries resulting from psychomotor impairment. Driving under the influence of alcohol is the major cause of fatal auto accidents. Blood alcohol level and the time necessary to achieve it are controlled largely by the rapidity and extent of ethanol consumption. Ethanol is distributed in body water and to some degree in adipose tissue. The alcohol is eliminated by urinary excretion, exhalation, and metabolism. The blood level in an average adult decreases by ~15 to 20 mg/dL per hour. Thus, a person with a blood alcohol level of 120 mg/dL would require 6 to 8 h to reach negligible levels.

Ethanol is metabolized to acetaldehyde by three enzymes: (1) alcohol dehydrogenase (ADH) catalyzes oxidation of most of the ethanol to acetaldehyde, which is rapidly oxidized by acetaldehyde dehydrogenase (ALDH) to acetate; (2) catalase, utilizing H_2O_2 supplied by the actions of NADPH oxidase and xanthine oxidase, will normally account for more than 10 percent of ethanol metabolism; (3) CYP2E1 of the hepatic microsomal ethanol oxidizing system (MEOS) will metabolize only a few percent.

ALDH activity is usually sufficiently high to metabolize large amounts of acetaldehyde to acetate. Caucasians, blacks, and Asians have varying percentages of different ALDH isozymes, which impact the efficiency of acetaldehyde metabolism. Some 50 percent of Asians have inactive ALDH, and these persons may experience flushing, headache, nausea, vomiting, tachycardia, and hyperventilation on ingestion of ethanol. Whereas this syndrome offers protection against developing alcoholism, it increases the risk of acetaldehyde-related cancers of the esophagus, stomach, colon, lung, head, and neck.

Gender differences in responses to ethanol are well recognized. Females exhibit slightly higher blood ethanol levels than men following ingestion of equivalent doses. This phenomenon is due in part to more extensive ADH-catalyzed metabolism of ethanol by the gastric mucosa of males and to the smaller volume of distribution in women for relatively polar solvents such as alcohols. Also, women are more susceptible to alcohol-induced hepatitis and cirrhosis.

Fetal alcohol syndrome (FAS) is the most common preventable cause of mental retardation. Diagnostic criteria for FAS include (1) heavy maternal alcohol consumption during gestation; (2) pre- and postnatal growth retardation; (3) craniofacial malformations including microcephaly; and (4) mental retardation. Less complete manifestations of gestational ethanol exposure are referred to as fetal alcohol effects or alcohol-related neurodevelopmental disorder. Overconsumption during all three trimesters of pregnancy can result in particular manifestations depending on the period of gestation during which insult occurs.

Human CYP2E1 is effective in production of reactive oxygen intermediates from ethanol that cause lipid peroxidation. Also, ethanol induces the release of endotoxin from gram-negative bacteria in the gut. The endotoxin is taken up by Kupffer cells, causing the release of inflammatory mediators, which are cytotoxic to hepatocytes.

Alcohol-induced tissue damage results from both nutritional disturbances and direct toxic effects. Malabsorption of thiamine, diminished enterohepatic circulation of folate, degradation of pyridoxal phosphate, and disturbances in the metabolism of vitamins A and D can occur. Prostaglandins released from endotoxin-activated Kupffer cells may be responsible for a hypermetabolic state in the liver. With the increase in oxygen demand, the viability of centrilobular hepatocytes would be most compromised due to their relatively poor oxygen supply. Metabolism of ethanol via ADH and ALDH results in a shift in the redox state of the cell. The resulting hyperlacticacidemia, hyperlipidemia, hyperuricemia, and hyperglycemia lead to increased steatosis and collagen synthesis.

Alcoholism can result in damage of extrahepatic tissues. Alcoholic cardiomyopathy is a complex process that may result from decreased synthesis of cardiac contractile proteins, attack of oxygen radicals, increases in endoplasmic reticulum Ca^{2+}-ATPase, and antibody response to acetaldehyde–protein adducts. Heavy drinking appears to deplete antioxidants and increases the risk of both hemorrhagic and ischemic strokes. The brain and pancreas may be adversely affected in alcoholics.

The associations between alcohol and cancers came primarily from epidemiologic case–control and cohort studies. Ethanol and smoking act synergistically to cause oral, pharyngeal, and laryngeal cancers. It is generally believed that alcohol induces liver cancer by causing cirrhosis or other liver damage and/or by enhancing the bioactivation of carcinogens.

Chronic ethanol consumption may promote carcinogenesis by: (1) production of acetaldehyde, a weak mutagen and carcinogen; (2) induction of CYP2E1 with conversion of procarcinogens to carcinogens; (3) depletion of SAM and, consequently, global DNA hypomethylation; (4) increased production of inhibitory guanine nucleotide regulatory proteins and components of extracellular signal-regulated kinase-mitogen-activated protein kinase signaling; (5) accumulation of iron and associated oxidative stress; (6) inactivation of the tumor suppressor gene *BRCA1* and increased estrogen responsiveness (primarily in the breast); and (7) impairment of retinoic acid metabolism.

Methanol

Methanol (methyl alcohol and wood alcohol) is found in a host of consumer products including windshield washer fluid, and is used in the manufacture of formaldehyde and methyl *tert*-butyl ether. Methanol can produce reversible sensory irritation and narcosis at airborne concentrations below those producing organ system pathology. Serious methanol toxicity is most commonly associated with ingestion. Acute methanol poisoning in humans is characterized by an asymptomatic period of 12 to 24 h followed by formic acidemia, ocular toxicity, coma, and in extreme cases death. Visual disturbances develop between 18 and 48 h after ingestion and range from mild photophobia and blurred vision to markedly reduced visual acuity and complete blindness.

The target of methanol within the eye is the retina, specifically the optic disk and optic nerve. Müller cells and rod and cone cells are altered functionally and structurally, because cytochrome *c* oxidase activity in mitochondria is inhibited, resulting in a reduction in ATP.

Though metabolized in liver, intraretinal conversion of methanol to formaldehyde and formate is critical. Metabolism of formate to CO_2 then occurs via a two-step, tetrahydrofolate (THF)-dependent pathway. Susceptibility to methanol toxicity is dependent on the relative rate of formate clearance. Conversion of formate to CO_2 is slower in primates than in rodents. In fact, formate acts as a direct ocular toxin and the acidotic state potentiates formate toxicity because the inhibition of cytochrome oxidase increases as pH decreases.

GLYCOLS

Ethylene Glycol

EG is a major constituent of antifreeze, deicers, hydraulic fluids, drying agents, and inks, and is used to make plastics and polyester fibers. The most important routes of exposure are dermal and accidental or intentional ingestion. EG is rapidly degraded in environmental media.

Acutely toxic to humans, EG is believed to cause over 100 deaths annually in the United States. Three clinical stages of acute poisoning entail: (1) a period of inebriation, the duration and degree depending on dose; (2) the cardiopulmonary stage 12 to 24 h after exposure, characterized by tachycardia and tachypnea, which may progress to cardiac failure and pulmonary edema; and (3) the renal toxicity stage 24 to 72 h postexposure. Metabolic acidosis can progress in severity during stages 2 and 3.

Absorption from the GI tract of rodents is very rapid and virtually complete. Dermal absorption in humans appears to be less extensive. EG is distributed throughout the body extracellular fluid. As illustrated in Figure 24–2, EG is metabolized by NAD^+-dependent ADH to glycolaldehyde and on to glycolic acid. Glycolic acid is oxidized to glyoxylic acid by glycolic acid oxidase and lactic dehydrogenase. Glyoxylic acid may be converted to formate and CO_2, or oxidized by glyoxylic acid oxidase to oxalic acid. Metabolic acidosis in humans appears to be due to accumulation of glycolic acid. Hypocalcemia can result from calcium chelation by oxalic acid to form calcium oxalate crystals. Deposition of these crystals in tubules of the kidney and small blood vessels in the brain is associated with damage of these organs. Additionally, hippuric acid crystals and direct cytotoxicity by other metabolites may act as damaging agents to the kidney in EG exposure. EG appears to have limited

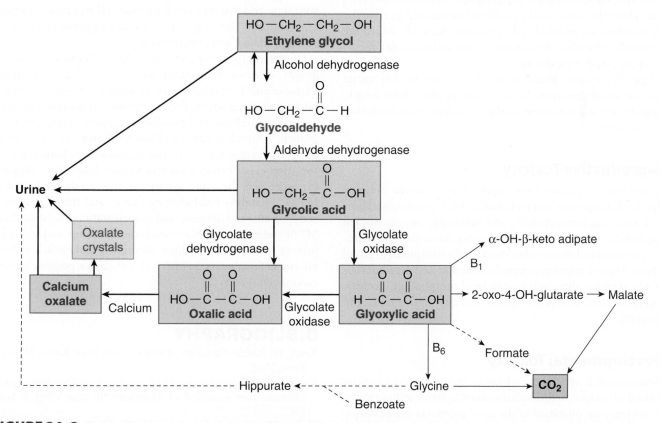

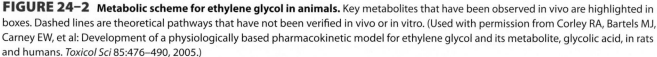

FIGURE 24–2 **Metabolic scheme for ethylene glycol in animals.** Key metabolites that have been observed in vivo are highlighted in boxes. Dashed lines are theoretical pathways that have not been verified in vivo or in vitro. (Used with permission from Corley RA, Bartels MJ, Carney EW, et al: Development of a physiologically based pharmacokinetic model for ethylene glycol and its metabolite, glycolic acid, in rats and humans. *Toxicol Sci* 85:476–490, 2005.)

chronic toxicity potential, exhibits no evidence of carcinogenicity, and does not appear to be a reproductive toxicant.

Propylene Glycol

Propylene glycol (PG) is used as an intermediate in the synthesis of polyester fibers and resins, as a component of automotive antifreeze/coolants, and as a deicing fluid for aircraft. As PG is "generally recognized as safe" by the FDA, it is a constituent of many cosmetics and processed foods. Furthermore, it serves as a solvent/diluent for a substantial number of oral, dermal, and intravenous drug preparations. The most important routes of exposure are ingesting and dermal contact. PG is readily metabolized by ADH to lactaldehyde, which is then oxidized by aldehyde dehydrogenase to lactate. Excessive lactate is primarily responsible for the acidosis. PG has a very low order of acute and chronic toxicity.

GLYCOL ETHERS

The glycol ethers include EG monomethyl ether, also called 2-methoxyethanol (2-ME; $CH_3—O—CH_2—CH_2—OH$), EG dimethyl ether ($CH_3—O—CH_2—CH_2—O—CH_3$), 2-butoxyethanol (2-BE; $CH_3—CH_2—CH_2—CH_2—O—CH_2—CH_2—OH$), and 2-ME acetate ($CH_3—CO—O—CH_2—CH_2—O—CH_3$). These solvents undergo rapid ester hydrolysis in vivo, and exhibit the same toxicity profile as unesterified glycols. The glycol ethers are metabolized to alkoxyacetic acids, which are regarded as the ultimate toxicants. Their acetaldehyde precursors have also been implicated.

Like glycol ether metabolism, glycol ether toxicity varies with chemical structure. With increasing alkyl chain length, reproductive and developmental toxicity decrease, whereas hematotoxicity increases.

Reproductive Toxicity

Epidemiologic studies have reported associations between glycol ether exposure and increased risk for spontaneous abortion, menstrual disturbances, and subfertility among women employed in the semiconductor industry. Reversible spermatotoxicity in males has been described for those exposed to glycol ethers. Typical responses include testicular and seminiferous tubule atrophy, abnormal sperm head morphology, necrotic spermatocytes, decreased sperm motility and count, and infertility.

Developmental Toxicity

Developmental toxicity in rodents includes a variety of minor skeletal variations, hydrocephalus, exencephaly, cardiovascular malformations, dilatation of the renal pelvis, craniofacial malformations, and digit malformations. There are significant associations for glycol ether exposure inducing cleft lip and neural tube defects such as spina bifida.

Hematotoxicity

Some glycol ethers are hemolytic to red blood cells. Typically, the osmotic balance of the cells is disrupted, they imbibe water and swell, their ATP concentration decreases, and hemolysis occurs. Humans are less susceptible than rodents to glycol ether-induced erythrocyte deformity and hemolysis.

AUTOMOTIVE GASOLINE AND ADDITIVES

Gasoline is a mixture of hundreds of hydrocarbons predominantly in the range of C_4 to C_{12}. Because its composition varies with the crude oil from which it is refined, the refining process, and the use of specific additives, generalizations regarding the toxicity of gasoline must be made carefully. Experiments conducted with fully vaporized gasoline may not be predictive of actual risk, because humans are exposed primarily to the more volatile components in the range of C_4 to C_5, which are generally less toxic than higher molecular-weight fractions.

The most extreme exposures occur to those intentionally sniffing gasoline for its euphoric effects. This dangerous habit can cause acute and chronic encephalopathies that are expressed as both motor and cognitive impairment. Ingestion of gasoline during siphoning events is typically followed by a burning sensation in the mouth and pharynx, as well as nausea, vomiting, and diarrhea resulting from GI irritation. Gasoline aspirated into the lungs may produce pulmonary epithelial damage, edema, and pneumonitis.

Oxygenated gasoline contains additives that boost its octane quality, enhance combustion, and reduce exhaust emissions. Benzene and 1,3-butadiene are classified as known or probable human carcinogens. The co-exposure of ethanol and gasoline shows additive and possibly synergistic toxic effects on growth, neurochemistry, and histopathology of the adrenal gland and respiratory tract. No significant epidemiologic association exists between methyl *tertiary*-butyl ether (MTBE) exposure and the acute symptoms commonly attributed to MTBE, including headache; eye, nose, and throat irritation; cough; nausea; dizziness; and disorientation. Because three MTBE animal cancer bioassays indicate kidney and testicular tumors in male rats and liver adenomas, leukemia, and lymphoma in female rats, MTBE is classified as a possible human carcinogen (group C).

BIBLIOGRAPHY

Karch SB: *Karch's Pathology of Drug Abuse*. Boca Raton, FL: CRC Press, 2002.

Patnaik P: *A Comprehensive Guide to the Hazardous Properties of Chemical Substances*, 3rd ed. Hoboken, NJ: John Wiley & Sons, 2007.

Philip RB: *Ecosystems and Human Health: Toxicology and Environmental Hazards*, 2nd ed. Boca Raton, FL: Lewis, 2001.

QUESTIONS

1. Which of the following statements regarding solvents is FALSE?
   a. Solvents can be absorbed from the GI tract and through the skin.
   b. Equilibration of absorbed solvents/vapors occurs most quickly in the lungs.
   c. Solvents are small molecules that lack charge.
   d. Volatility of solvents increases with molecular weight.
   e. Most solvents are refined from petroleum.

2. What is the route is in which most solvents enter the environment?
   a. chemical spills.
   b. contamination of drinking water.
   c. evaporation.
   d. improper waste disposal.
   e. wind.

3. All of the following statements are true EXCEPT:
   a. Most solvents can pass freely through membranes by diffusion.
   b. A solvent's lipophilicity is important in determining its rate of dermal absorption.
   c. Hydrophilic solvents have a relatively low blood:air partition coefficient.
   d. Biotransformation of a lipophilic solvent can result in the production of a mutagenic compound.
   e. Hepatic first-pass metabolism determines the amount of solvent absorbed in the GI tract.

4. Which of the following statements regarding age solvent toxicity is TRUE?
   a. GI absorption is greater in adults than it is in children.
   b. Polar solvents reach higher blood levels in the elderly than they do in children.
   c. Children are always more susceptible to solvent toxicity than are adults.
   d. Increased alveolar ventilation increases uptake of lipid-soluble solvents to a greater extent than water-soluble solvents.
   e. Increased body fat percentage increases clearance of solvent chemicals.

5. Huffing gasoline can result in which of the following serious health problems?
   a. renal failure.
   b. pneumothorax.
   c. Hodgkin's disease.
   d. encephalopathy.
   e. thrombocytopenia.

6. Which of the following statements regarding benzene is FALSE?
   a. High-level exposure to benzene could result in acute myelogenous leukemia (AML).
   b. Gasoline vapor emissions and auto exhaust are the two main contributors to benzene inhalation.
   c. Benzene is used as an ingredient in unleaded gasoline.
   d. Benzene metabolites covalently bind DNA, RNA, and proteins and interfere with their normal functioning within the cell.
   e. Reactive oxygen species can be derived from benzene.

7. Which of the following is NOT a criterion for fetal alcohol syndrome diagnosis?
   a. maternal alcohol consumption during gestation.
   b. pre- and postnatal growth retardation.
   c. microcephaly.
   d. ocular toxicity.
   e. mental retardation.

8. Which of the following is NOT an important enzyme in ethanol metabolism?
   a. alcohol dehydrogenase.
   b. formaldehyde dehydrogenase.
   c. CYP2E1.
   d. catalase.
   e. acetaldehyde dehydrogenase.

9. Which of the following is NOT associated with glycol ether toxicity?
   a. irreversible spermatotoxicity.
   b. craniofacial malformations.
   c. hematotoxicity.
   d. seminiferous tubule atrophy.
   e. cleft lip.

10. Which of the following statements regarding chlorinated hydrocarbons is FALSE?
    a. Toxicities of trichloroethylene (TCE) are mediated mostly by reactive metabolites, not the parent compound.
    b. Glutathione conjugation is an important metabolic step of both trichloroethylene (TCE) and perchloroethylene (PERC).
    c. Many chlorinated hydrocarbons are used as degreasing agents.
    d. Chloroform interferes with intracellular calcium homeostasis.
    e. Carbon tetrachloride causes hepatocellular and kidney toxicity.

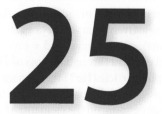

Toxic Effects of Radiation and Radioactive Materials

Naomi H. Harley

BASIC RADIATION CONCEPTS

   Alpha Particles

   Beta Particles, Positrons, and Electron Capture

   Gamma-ray (Photon) Emission

   Internal Conversion

INTERACTION OF RADIATION WITH MATTER

   Alpha Particles

   Beta Particles

   Gamma Rays

      The Photoelectric Effect

      The Compton Effect

      Pair Production

   Gamma-ray Energy Loss

MECHANISMS OF DNA DAMAGE AND MUTAGENESIS

   Energy Deposition in the Cell Nucleus

   Direct and Indirect Ionization

   DNA Damage

HUMAN STUDIES OF RADIATION TOXICITY

ENVIRONMENTAL AND DOMESTIC EPIDEMIOLOGY

   The Environmental Studies

   Meta-analysis of Environmental Epidemiology

   The Domestic Studies

   Meta-analysis of Domestic Epidemiology

   What Is Known about Radon Exposure

NATURAL RADIOACTIVITY AND RADIATION BACKGROUND

   Local Environmental Releases

KEY POINTS

- The four main types of radiation are due to alpha particles, electrons (negatively charged beta particles or positively charged positrons), gamma rays, and x-rays.
- Alpha particles are helium nuclei (consisting of two protons and two neutrons), with a charge of +2, that are ejected from the nucleus of an atom.
- Beta particle decay occurs when a neutron in the nucleus of an element is effectively transformed into a proton and an electron, which is ejected.
- Gamma-ray emission occurs in combination with alpha, beta, or positron emission or electron capture. Whenever the ejected particle does not utilize all the available energy for decay, the excess energy is released by the nucleus as photon or gamma-ray emission coincident with the ejection of the particle.
- Ionizing radiation loses energy when passing through matter by producing ion pairs (an electron and a positively charged atom residue).
- Radiation may deposit energy directly in DNA (direct effect) or may ionize other molecules closely associated with DNA, hydrogen, or oxygen, to form free radicals that can damage DNA (indirect effect).

347

BASIC RADIATION CONCEPTS

The four main types of radiation are due to alpha particles, electrons (negatively charged beta particles or positively charged positrons), gamma rays, and x-rays. An atom can decay to a product element through the loss of a heavy (mass = 4) charged (+2) alpha particle (He^{2+}) that consists of two protons and two neutrons. The alpha particle is ejected from the nucleus with energy depending on the element. After it loses its energy, it is a stable helium atom. An atom can decay by loss of a negatively or positively charged electron (e^-, a beta particle, or e^+, a positron). Gamma radiation results when the nucleus releases excess energy, usually after an alpha, beta, or positron transition. X-rays occur whenever an inner-shell orbital electron is removed and rearrangement of the atomic electrons results, with the release of the element's characteristic x-ray energy.

Alpha Particles

Alpha particles are helium nuclei (consisting of two protons and two neutrons), with a charge of +2, that are ejected from the nucleus of an atom. When an alpha particle loses energy, slows to the velocity of a gas atom, and acquires two electrons from the vast sea of free electrons present in most media, it becomes part of the normal background helium in the environment. The formula for alpha decay is:

$$_{Z}^{A}X \rightarrow {_{Z-2}^{A-4}}Y + He^{2+} + \text{gamma} + Q_\alpha$$

where Z is the atomic number and A the atomic weight.

The energy available in this decay is Q_α and is equal to the mass difference of the parent and the two products. The energy is shared among the particles and the gamma ray if one is present.

An example of alpha decay is given by the natural radionuclide radium (^{226}Ra):

$$_{86}^{226}\text{Ra} \rightarrow {_{84}^{222}}\text{Rn} + \text{alpha (5.2 MeV)}$$

The energy of alpha particles for most emitters lies in the range of 4 to 8 MeV. More energetic alpha particles exist but are seen only in very short-lived emitters such as those formed by reactions occurring in particle accelerators.

Beta Particles, Positrons, and Electron Capture

Beta particle decay occurs when a neutron in the nucleus of an element is effectively transformed into a proton and an electron. Subsequent ejection of the electron occurs, and the maximum energy of the beta particle equals the mass difference between the parent and the product nuclei. A gamma ray may also be present to share the energy, Q_β:

$$_{Z}^{A}X \rightarrow {_{Z+1}^{A}}Y + \text{beta} + Q_\beta$$

An example of beta decay is given by the natural radionuclide lead (^{210}Pb):

$$_{82}^{210}\text{Pb} \rightarrow {_{83}^{210}}\text{Bi} + \text{beta (0.015 MeV)} + \text{gamma (0.046 MeV)}$$

Unlike monoenergetic alpha particles in alpha decay, beta particles are emitted with a continuous spectrum of energy from zero to the maximum energy available for the transition. The reason for this is that the total available energy is shared in each decay or transition by two particles: the beta particle and an antineutrino. The total energy released in each transition is constant, but the observed beta particles then appear as a spectrum. The residual energy is carried away by the antineutrino, which is a particle with essentially zero mass and charge that cannot be observed without extraordinarily complex instrumentation. The beta particle, by contrast, is readily observed with conventional nuclear counting equipment.

Positron emission is similar to beta particle emission but results from the effective nucleon transformation of a proton to a neutron plus a positively charged electron. The atomic number decreases rather than increases, as it does in beta decay.

An example of positron decay is given by the natural radionuclide copper (^{64}Cu), which decays by beta emission 41 percent of the time, positron emission 19 percent of the time, and electron capture 40 percent of the time:

$$_{29}^{64}\text{Cu} \rightarrow {_{28}^{64}}\text{Ni} + \text{positron (0.66 MeV): 19\%}$$

$$_{29}^{64}\text{Cu} \rightarrow {_{30}^{64}}\text{Zn} + \text{beta (0.57 MeV): 41\%}$$

$$_{29}^{64}\text{Cu} \rightarrow {_{28}^{64}}\text{Ni electron capture: 40\%}$$

The energy of the positron appears as a continuous spectrum, similar to that in beta decay, where the total energy available for decay is shared between the positron and a neutrino. In the case of positron emission, the maximum energy of the emitted particle is the mass difference of the parent and product nuclide minus the energy needed to create two electron masses (1.02 MeV), whereas the maximum energy of the beta particle is the mass difference itself. This happens because in beta decay, the increase in the number of orbital electrons resulting from the increase in atomic number of the product nucleus cancels the mass of the electron lost in emitting the beta particle. This does not happen in positron decay, and there is an orbital electron lost as a result of the decrease in atomic number of the product and the loss of the electron mass in positron emission.

Electron capture competes with positron decay, and the resulting product nucleus is the same nuclide. In electron capture, an orbiting electron is acquired by the nucleus, and the transformation of a proton plus the electron to form a neutron takes place. In some cases, the energy available is released as a gamma-ray photon, but this is not necessary, and a monoenergetic neutrino may be emitted. If the 1.02 MeV required for positron decay is not available, positron decay is not kinetically possible and electron capture is the only mode observed.

Gamma-ray (Photon) Emission

Gamma-ray emission is not a primary process except in rare instances, but it occurs in combination with alpha, beta, or positron emission or electron capture. Whenever the ejected particle does not utilize all the available energy for decay, the excess energy is released by the nucleus as photon or gamma-ray emission coincident with the ejection of the particle.

One of the rare instances of pure gamma-ray emission is technetium 99m (^{99m}Tc), which has a 6.0-h half-life and is widely used in diagnostic medicine for various organ scans. Its decay product, ^{99}Tc, has a very long half-life (2.13×10^5 years), and as all ^{99}Tc is ultimately released to the environment, a background of this nuclide is emerging:

$$^{99m}_{43}\text{Tc} \rightarrow ^{99}_{43}\text{Tc} + \text{gamma (0.14 Mev)}$$

Internal Conversion

In many cases, the photon will not actually be emitted by the nucleus but the excess excitation energy will be transferred to an orbital electron. This electron is then ejected as a monoenergetic particle with energy equal to that of the photon minus the binding energy of the orbital electron. This process is known as internal conversion.

INTERACTION OF RADIATION WITH MATTER

Ionizing radiation, by definition, loses energy when passing through matter by producing ion pairs (an electron and a positively charged atom residue). A fraction of the energy loss raises atomic electrons to an excited state. The average energy needed to produce an ion pair, W, is numerically equal to 33.85 eV in air. This energy is roughly two times the ionization potential of most gases or other elements because it includes the energy lost in the excitation process. It is not clear what role the excitation plays, for example, in damage to targets in the cellular DNA. Ionization, by contrast, can break bonds in DNA, causing even double-strand breaks.

All particles and rays interact through their charge or field with atomic or free electrons in the medium through which they are passing. There is no interaction with the atomic nucleus except at energies above about 8 MeV, which is required for interactions that break apart the nucleus (spallation). Very high-energy cosmic-ray particles, for example, produce ^{3}H, ^{7}Be, ^{14}C, and ^{22}Na in the upper atmosphere by spallation of atmospheric oxygen and nitrogen.

Alpha Particles

The alpha particle is a heavy charged particle with a mass that is 7300 times that of the electrons with which it interacts. A massive particle interacting with a small particle has the interesting property that it can give a maximum velocity during energy transfer to the small particle of only two times the initial velocity of the heavy particle. The maximum energy that can be transferred per interaction is:

$$E_{\text{(maximum electron)}} = \frac{4}{7300} E_{\text{(alpha particle)}} \qquad (1)$$

Although alpha particles can lose perhaps 10 to 20 percent of their energy in traveling 10 mm in tissue (1 cm in air), each interaction can impart only the small energy in equation (1). Thus, alpha particles are characterized by a high energy loss per unit path length and a high ionization density along the track length. This is called a *high linear energy transfer* (LET) particle.

The energy loss in matter, dE/dx or stopping power, for alpha energies between 0.2 and 10 MeV, is given by:

$$\frac{dE}{dx} = 3.8 \times 10^{-25} \, C \frac{NZ}{E} \ln\left\{548\frac{E}{I}\right\} \text{ MeV/}\mu\text{m} \qquad (2)$$

where N is number of atoms per cubic centimeter in medium, Z the atomic number of medium, I the ionization potential of medium, E the energy of alpha particle, and C the charge correction for alpha particles with energy below 1.6 MeV.

A simple rule of thumb may be used to estimate the ionization potential of a compound or element:

$$I = 10(Z) \qquad (3)$$

When alpha particles are near the end of their range, the charge is not constant at +2 but can be +1 or even zero as the particle acquires or loses electrons. A correction factor, C, is needed for energies between 0.2 and 1.5 MeV to account for this effect. These factors vary from 0.24 at 0.2 MeV, 0.75 at 0.6 MeV, 0.875 at 1.0 MeV to 1.0 at 1.6 MeV.

For the case of tissue, equation (2) reduces to:

$$\frac{dE}{dx_{\text{tissue}}} = \left[0.126\frac{C}{E}\right] \ln\{7.99E\} \text{ MeV/}\mu\text{m} \qquad (4)$$

Example 1. Find the energy loss (stopping power) of a 0.6- and a 5-MeV alpha particle in tissue.

For a 0.6-MeV alpha particle:

$$\frac{dE}{dx} = \left[\frac{0.126(0.75)}{0.6}\right] \ln\{7.99 \times 0.6\} = 0.25 \text{ MeV/}\mu\text{m}$$

For a 5.0-MeV alpha particle:

$$\frac{dE}{dx} = \left[\frac{0.126(1.0)}{5.0}\right] \ln\{7.99 \times 5.0\} = 0.093 \text{ MeV/}\mu\text{m}$$

The slower moving (lower energy) alpha particle has more chance to interact with matter and the energy loss per unit distance is greater. The significance of this energy loss is seen in that it requires 33.85 eV to produce an ion pair; therefore, a 5-MeV alpha particle can produce (0.25 × 10^6 eV/μm)/(33.86 eV/ion pair) = 7400 ion pairs in 1 μm, or enough damage to cause a double-strand break.

Beta Particles

The equations for beta particle energy loss in matter cannot be simplified, as in the case of alpha particles, because of three factors:

1. Even at low energies of a few tenths of an MeV, beta particles are traveling near the speed of light and relativistic effects (mass increase) must be considered.
2. Electrons are interacting with particles of the same mass in the medium (free or orbital electrons), so large energy losses per collision are possible.
3. Radiative or bremsstrahlung energy loss occurs when electrons or positrons are slowing down in matter. Such a loss also occurs with alpha particles, but the magnitude of this energy loss is negligible.

Including the effects of these three factors, the energy loss for electrons and positrons has been well quantitated. Tabulations of energy loss in various media have been prepared with the ionization energy loss and the radiative loss detailed.

Gamma Rays

Photons do not have a mass or charge. The interaction between a photon and matter therefore is controlled by interaction of the electric and magnetic fields of the photon with the electron in the medium. There are three modes of interaction with the medium.

The Photoelectric Effect—The photon interaction with an orbital electron in the medium is complete, and the full energy of the photon is given to the electron.

The Compton Effect—Part of the photon energy is transferred to an electron, and the photon scatters (usually at a small angle from its original path) with reduced energy. The governing expressions are:

$$E' = E\frac{0.511}{1 + (1/a) - \cos\theta} \quad (5)$$

$$T = E\frac{a(1 - \cos\theta)}{1 + a(1 - \cos\theta)}$$

where E and E' are the initial and scattered photon energy (MeV), T the kinetic energy of electron (MeV), $a = E/0.511$, and θ the angle of photon scatter from its original path.

Pair Production—Pair production occurs whenever the photon energy is greater than the rest mass of two electrons, $2(0.511 \text{ MeV}) = 1.02 \text{ MeV}$. The electromagnetic energy of the photon can be converted directly to an electron–positron pair, with excess energy above 1.02 MeV appearing as kinetic energy given to these particles.

Gamma-ray Energy Loss

The loss of photons and energy loss from a photon beam as it passes through matter are described by two coefficients. The attenuation coefficient determines the fractional loss of pho-

tons per unit distance (usually in normalized units of g/cm², which is the linear distance times the density of the medium). The mass energy absorption coefficient determines the fractional energy deposition per unit distance traveled. The loss of photons from the beam is given by:

$$\frac{I}{I_0} = \exp\left(\frac{-\mu}{\rho d}\right) \quad (6)$$

where I is the intensity of photon beam (numbers of photons), I_0 the beam intensity, μ/ρ the attenuation coefficient in medium for energy considered (m²/kg), and d the thickness of medium in superficial density units kg/m² (thickness in m times density in kg/m³).

Superficial density is convenient in that it normalizes energy absorption in different media. For example, air and tissue have approximately the same energy absorption per kg/m², whereas in linear dimension, the energy absorption, say, per meter, is vastly different. The energy actually deposited in the medium per unit distance is calculated using the mass energy absorption

TABLE 25–1 Mass energy absorption coefficients for air and water.

Photon Energy, (MeV)	Air, μ_{en}/ρ (m²/kg)	Muscle, Striate (ICRU), μ_{en}/ρ (m²/kg)
0.01	0.46	0.49
0.015	0.13	0.14
0.02	0.052	0.055
0.03	0.015	0.016
0.04	0.0067	0.0070
0.05	0.0040	0.0043
0.06	0.0030	0.0032
0.08	0.0024	0.0026
0.10	0.0023	0.0025
0.15	0.0025	0.0027
0.20	0.0027	0.0029
0.30	0.0029	0.0032
0.40	0.0029	0.0032
0.50	0.0030	0.0033
0.60	0.0030	0.0033
0.80	0.0029	0.0032
1.00	0.0028	0.0031
1.50	0.0025	0.0028
2.00	0.0023	0.0026
3.00	0.0021	0.0023

coefficient as opposed to the overall attenuation coefficient and the energy loss is given by:

$$\Delta E = \left(\frac{\mu_{en}}{\rho}\right) E_0 \qquad (7)$$

where ΔE is the energy loss in medium per unit distance (MeV m²/kg), μ_{en}/ρ the mass energy absorption coefficient (m²/kg²), and E_0 the initial photon energy.

The values for μ_{en}/ρ as a function of gamma-ray energy are shown in Table 25–1 for air and muscle. Energy loss can be expressed per unit linear distance by multiplying by the density of the medium (kg/m³).

MECHANISMS OF DNA DAMAGE AND MUTAGENESIS

Energy Deposition in the Cell Nucleus

Ionizing radiation loses energy and slows down by forming ion pairs (a positively charged atom and an electron). Different ionization densities result from gamma rays, beta particles, and alpha particles. Their track structure is broadly characterized as from sparsely ionizing (or low-LET) to densely ionizing (high-LET) radiation. Each track of low-LET radiation, resulting from x-rays or gamma rays, consists of a few ionizations across an average-sized cell nucleus (e.g., an electron set in motion by a gamma ray crossing an 8-mm-diameter nucleus gives an average of about 70 ionizations, equivalent to about 5 mGy [500 mrad] absorbed dose). Individual tracks vary widely about this value because of the stochastic nature of energy deposition, that is, variability of ion pars per micrometer and path length through the nucleus. A high-LET alpha particle produces many thousands of ionizations and gives a relatively high dose to the cell. For example, a 4-MeV alpha-particle track yields, on average, about 30,000 ionizations (3 Gy, 300 rad) in an average-sized cell nucleus. However, within the nucleus, even low-LET gamma radiation will give some microregions of relatively dense ionization over the dimensions of DNA structures due to the low-energy electrons set in motion.

Direct and Indirect Ionization

Radiation tracks may deposit energy directly in DNA (direct effect) or may ionize other molecules closely associated with DNA, hydrogen or oxygen, to form free radicals that can damage DNA (indirect effect). Within a cell, the indirect effect occurs over very short distances, of the order of a few nanometers. The diffusion distance of radicals is limited by their reactivity. Although it is difficult to measure accurately the different contributions made by the direct and indirect effects to DNA damage caused by low-LET radiation, evidence from radical scavengers introduced into cells suggests that about 35 percent is exclusively direct and 65 percent has an indirect (scavengeable) component.

Both direct and indirect effects cause similar early damage to DNA; this is because the ion radicals produced by direct ionization of DNA may react further to produce DNA radicals similar to those produced by water-radical attack on DNA.

DNA Damage

Ionization frequently disrupts chemical bonding in cellular molecules. If the majority of ionizations occur as single isolated events (low-LET radiation), the disruptions are readily repaired by cellular enzymes. The average density of ionization by high-LET radiations is such that several ionizations may occur as the particle traverses a DNA double helix. Therefore, much of the damage from high-LET radiations, as well as a minority of the DNA damage from low-LET radiations, will derive from localized clusters of ionizations that can severely disrupt DNA structure. Although the extent of local clustering of ionizations in DNA from single tracks of low- and high-LET radiations will overlap, high-LET radiation tracks are more efficient at inducing larger clusters and hence more complex damage. Also, high-LET radiations will induce some very large clusters of ionizations that do not occur with low-LET radiations; the resulting damage may be irreparable and have unique cellular consequences. When a cell is damaged by high-LET radiation, each track will give large numbers of ionizations, so that the cell will receive a relatively high dose, and there will be a greater probability of correlated damage within a single DNA molecule. As a consequence, the irradiation of a population of cells or a tissue with a "low dose" of high-LET radiation results in a few cells being hit with a relatively high dose (one track) rather than in each cell receiving a small dose. In contrast, low-LET radiation is more uniformly distributed over the cell population. At doses of low-LET radiation in excess of about 1 mGy (for an average-sized cell nucleus of 8 mm in diameter), each cell nucleus is likely to be traversed by more than one sparsely ionizing track.

The interaction of ionizing radiation with DNA produces numerous types of damage. Table 25–2 lists some damage products that can be measured following low-LET irradiation of DNA, with a rough estimate of their abundance. Interactions can be classified according to the probability they will cause a single-strand DNA alteration, a double-strand break, or more complex DNA damage (e.g., a double-strand break with adjacent damage). Good agreement has been obtained between

TABLE 25–2 Estimated yields of DNA damage in mammalian cells caused by low-LET radiation exposures.

Type of Damage	Yield (Number of Defects per Cell), Gy⁻¹
Single-strand breaks	1000
Base damage[1]	500
Double-strand breaks	40
DNA protein cross-links	150

[1]Base excision enzyme-sensitive sites or antibody detection of thymine glycol.

TABLE 25–3 Lifetime cancer mortality per gray from five major epidemiologic studies (in parentheses, risk per Sievert for alpha emitters, wr = 20).[1]

Study	All Sites	Leukemia	Lung	Female Breast	Bone	Thyroid	Skin
Atom bomb whole-body, gamma	0.05	0.005	0.0085	0.002	0.0005	0.0008	0.0002
Uranium miner bronchial epithelium, alpha			(0.04) 0.0020				
Ankylosing spondylitis, spinal x-ray		0.0011	0.0008 0.0028	0.0015			
Tinea capitis, head x-ray						0.0010[2]	0.0030[3]
Radium ingestion, bone,[1] alpha (^{226}Ra)					0.004 (0.0002)		
Radium ingestion, bone,[4] alpha (^{224}Ra)					0.02 (0.0010)		

[1]The lifetime risk is calculated for an average skeletal dose of 10 Gy, assuming that the risk persists for 50 years. The risk is nonlinear and is about 0.01 Gy^{-1} at 100 Gy, for example.
[2]Thyroid mortality for males and females is estimated as 10 percent of incidence.
[3]The mortality for skin cancer is estimated as 1 percent of the incidence.
[4]The lifetime risk is calculated for an average skeletal dose of 10 Gy. The risk is nonlinear and is about 0.01 Gy^{-1} for a skeletal dose of 1 Gy.

these predictions and direct measurements of single-strand breaks. Although complex forms of damage are difficult to quantify with current experimental techniques, the use of enzymes that cut DNA at sites of base damage suggests that irradiation of DNA in solution gives complex damage sites consisting mainly of closely spaced base damage (measured as oxidized bases of abasic sites); double-strand breaks were associated with only 20 percent of the complex damage sites. It is expected that the occurrence of more complex types of damage will increase with increasing LET, and that this category of damage will be less repairable than the simpler forms of damage.

Some of the DNA damage caused by ionizing radiation is chemically similar to naturally occurring damage that "spontaneously" arises from the thermal instability of DNA as well as endogenous oxidative and enzymatic processes. Several metabolic pathways produce oxidative radicals within the cell, and these radicals can attack DNA to give both DNA base damage and breakage. The more complex types of damage caused by radiation may not occur spontaneously, because localized concentrations of endogenous radicals are less likely to be generated in the immediate vicinity of DNA.

HUMAN STUDIES OF RADIATION TOXICITY

There have been five major studies of the health detriment resulting from exposure of humans to ionizing radiation. Other studies of large worker populations exposed to very low levels of radiation and environmental populations exposed to radon are ongoing, but they are not expected to provide new data on the risk estimates from ionizing radiation. These worker or environmental populations are studied to ensure that there is no

inconsistency in the radiation risk data in extrapolating from the higher exposures. The basic studies on which the quantitative risk calculations are founded include radium exposures, A-bomb survivors, underground miners exposed to radon, patients irradiated with x-rays for ankylosing spondylitis, and children irradiated with x-rays for tinea capitis (ringworm).

The data from the five major studies are summarized in Table 25–3. This table shows the lifetime cancer risks that are significant. The risks are given in units of per gray (or per Sievert where appropriate for alpha emitters). Within the table, leukemia and cancers of the lung and female breast are the most critical. Osteogenic sarcoma is seen in the radium exposures. There is no clear linear dose–response for ^{224,226}Ra. The cancer risk to individual organs from different study groups is in general agreement regardless of radiation type or whole- or partial-body exposure.

ENVIRONMENTAL AND DOMESTIC EPIDEMOLOGY

The Environmental Studies

There are at least 24 published studies that attempt to define or detect the effect of radon exposure in the environment. The pattern emerging from the domestic studies indicates that the lung cancer risk from ^{222}Rn exposure is difficult to determine with accuracy or precision. This is mostly due to the high background lung cancer mortality caused by smoking.

Among the 24 published domestic studies, 13 are ecologic and 11 are case–control. Ecologic studies depend on relating the disease response of a population to some measure of a suspected causative agent. There usually are not enough data on all the variables involved in the disease to infer any reliable associations. Ecologic studies are the weakest type of epidemiologic exploration. Unless a biological marker for radon-induced lung cancer is found, it is unlikely that environmental epidemiology will be effective in assessing risk. The effects of radon in the environment are subtle compared with the overwhelming lung cancer mortality that results from smoking.

Meta-analysis of Environmental Epidemiology

A meta-analysis combined the published information from the largest domestic studies into one study without actually having the raw data available. The results in Figure 25–1 reveal that essentially no study found statistically significant cancer deaths due to radon, but the authors state that the combined trend in the relative risk with increasing exposure was statistically significant, with an estimated RR of 1.14 (95 percent CI = 1.0 to 1.3) at an exposure of 150 Bq/m³ (4 pCi/l).

The Domestic Studies

A large body of published information on residential exposure to radon has established the lung cancer risk from radon exposure. The results of the studies (odds ratio or relative risk) shown in

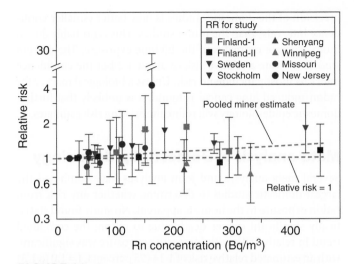

FIGURE 25–1 **Meta-analysis of eight domestic radon case-control studies.** Dashed line equals the extrapolation from miners, whereas the dotted line depicts a relative risk of 1. (From Lubin JH & Boice JD: Lung cancer risk from residential radon: Meta-analysis of eight epidemiologic studies, J Natl Cancer Instit 89(1):49-57, 1997, with permission from Oxford University Press.)

Figure 25–2 indicate that lung cancer risk from ²²²Rn exposure is evident at exposures of 100 Bq/m³. It is interesting that the

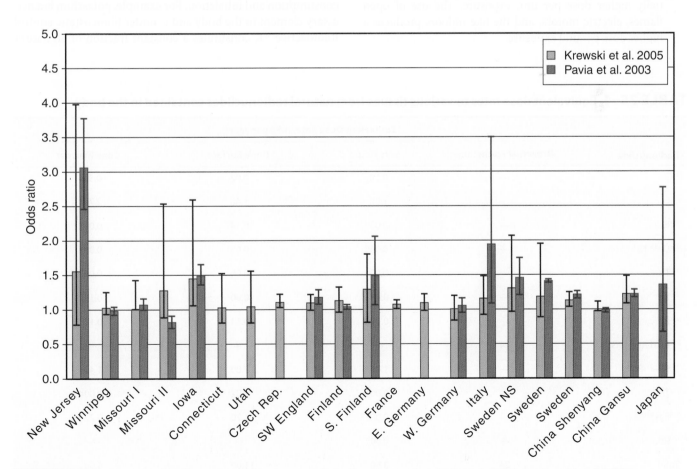

FIGURE 25–2 **Summary data for 21 domestic case–control studies.** Data are from Pavia et al. (2003) and Krewski et al. (2005).

precision of the domestic studies is now better (smaller confidence intervals) than the miner studies. This is probably due to more accurate estimates of the lifetime exposure. The present studies indicate a relative risk of about 1.2 but the confidence intervals mostly include no risk. Unless a biological marker for radon-induced lung cancer is found, it is unlikely that further domestic epidemiology will refine the existing risk estimates.

Meta-analysis of Domestic Epidemiology

Several meta-analyses and joint analyses have combined the largest domestic studies to determine whether any risk from radon exposure in the home is apparent. No study found statistically significant cancer deaths due to radon; the combined trend in relative risk with increasing exposure was significant, with an estimated relative risk of 1.14 (95 percent CI = 1.0 to 1.3) at an exposure of 150 Bq/m^3.

What Is Known about Radon Exposure

Four concepts have emerged from current radon research:

1. The mining epidemiology indicates that short exposure to high levels of radon and daughters produces a clear excess of lung cancer.
2. Particle size can change the actual dose delivered by radon to bronchial tissue, with small particles giving a substantially higher dose per unit exposure. The use of open flames, electric motors, and the like indoors produces a higher dose per unit exposure.
3. Smokers are at a higher risk from radon per unit exposure than are nonsmokers.
4. Urban areas almost universally have low radon, and apartment dwellers removed from the ground source have particularly low radon exposure at home.

The miners' data show clearly that there is a risk of lung cancer from exposure to high concentrations of radon delivered over short periods and temporal models can be derived from the data.

NATURAL RADIOACTIVITY AND RADIATION BACKGROUND

Occupational, accidental, and wartime experiences have provided the bases for all the current radiation risk estimates. For many years, the radioisotopes deposited internally were compared with ^{226}Ra to evaluate the maximum permissible body burden for a particular emitter. The present limits for external and internal radiation are based on dose estimates that, in turn, can be related to cancer risks. One standard of comparison has always been the exposure from natural background.

A substantial dose is received annually from cosmic radiation and from external terrestrial radiation present from uranium, thorium, and potassium in the earth's crust. Internal emitters are present in the body as a consequence of dietary consumption and inhalation. For example, potassium is a necessary element in the body and is under homeostatic control. Radioactive ^{40}K constitutes a constant fraction of all natural

TABLE 25–4 Equivalent dose rates to various tissues from natural radionuclides contained in the body.

Radionuclide	Equivalent Dose Rate, mSv per year			
	Bronchial Epithelium	Soft Tissue	Bone Surfaces	Bone Marrow
^{14}C	—	0.10	0.08	0.30
^{40}K	—	1.80	1.40	2.70
^{87}Rb	—	0.03	0.14	0.07
^{238}U–^{234}Th	—	0.046	0.03	0.004
^{230}Th	—	0.001	0.06	0.001
^{226}Ra	—	0.03	0.90	0.15
^{222}Rn	—	0.07	0.14	0.14
^{222}Rn daughters	24	—	—	—
^{210}Pb–^{210}Po	—	1.40	7.00	1.40
^{232}Th	—	0.001	0.02	0.004
^{228}Ra–^{224}Ra	—	0.0015	1.20	0.22
^{220}Rn	—	0.001	—	—
Total	24	3.50	11.00	5.00

TABLE 25-5 Estimated total effective dose rate for a member of the population in the United States and Canada from various sources of background radiation.

Source	Total Effective Dose Rate, mSv per year					
	Lung	Gonads	Bone Surface	Bone Marrow	Other Tissues	Total
Tissue weighting factor	0.12	0.25	0.03	0.12	0.48	1.0
Cosmic	0.03	0.07	0.008	0.03	0.13	0.27
Cosmogenic	0.001	0.002	—	0.004	0.003	0.01
Terrestrial	0.03	0.07	0.008	0.03	0.14	0.28
Inhaled	2.0	—	—	—	—	2.0
In body	0.04	0.09	0.03	0.06	0.17	0.40
Total	2.1	0.23	0.05	0.12	0.44	3.0

TABLE 25-6 Estimates of radionuclide released and collective effective dose from human-made environmental sources of radiation.

Source	Release (PBq)						Collective Effective Dose,[1] Person Sv	
	^{3}H	^{14}C	Noble Gases	^{90}Sr	^{131}I	^{137}Cs	Local and Regional	Global
Atmospheric nuclear testing	240,000	220		604	650,000	910		2,230,000
Local								
Semipalatinsk							4,600	
Nevada							500[2]	
Australia							700	
Pacific test site							160[2]	
Underground nuclear testing			50		15		200	
Nuclear weapons fabrication								
Early practice							8,000[3]	
Hanford							15,000[4]	
Chelyabinsk							1,000	10,000
Later practice							30,000	
Nuclear power production								
Milling and mining							2,700	
Reactor operation	140	1.1	3,200		0.04		3,700	
Fuel reprocessing	57	0.3	1,200	6.9	0.004	40	4,600	
Fuel cycle							300,000	100,000
Radioisotope production and use	2.6	1.0	52		6.0		2,000	

(continued)

TABLE 25–6 **Estimates of radionuclide released and collective effective dose from human-made environmental sources of radiation. (Continued)**

Source	^{3}H	^{14}C	Noble Gases	^{90}Sr	^{131}I	^{137}Cs	Local and Regional	Global
			Release (PBq)				Collective Effective Dose,[1] Person Sv	
Accidents								
Three Mile Island			370		0.0006		40	
Chernobyl					630	70		600,000
Kyshtym				5.4		0.04	2,500	
Windscale		1.2			0.7	0.02	2,000	
Palomares							3	
Thule							0	
SNAP 9A								2,100
Cosmos 954				0.003	0.2	0.003		20
Ciudad Juarez							150	
Mohammedia							80	
Goiania						0.05	60	
Total							380,000	23,100,000
Total collective effective dose (Person Sv)								23,500,000

[1]Truncated at 10,000 years
[2]External dose only
[3]From release of ^{131}I to the atmosphere
[4]From releases of radionuclides into the Techa River

potassium. Potassium delivers the largest internal dose from the diet of 0.15 mSv per year. However, the data are scanty on the dietary intake of other radionuclides in the U.S. population. Given the usual distribution of intakes across a large population, it is probable that other emitters, notably ^{210}Pb and its decay product ^{210}Po, could deliver a significant dose to a fraction of the population. For example, ^{210}Pb is found in all tobacco products and delivers a significant lung dose.

The largest dose received by the population is from the inhaled short-lived daughters of radon. These are present in all atmospheres because radon is released rather efficiently from the ^{226}Ra in rock and soil. The short-lived daughters, ^{218}Po, ^{214}Pb, and ^{214}Bi–^{214}Po, have an effective half-life of 30 min, but the 3.8-day parent radon supports their presence in the atmosphere.

Average outdoor concentrations in every state in the United States have been measured and summarized as 15 Bq/m^3, and indoors as 40 Bq/m^3. A structure such as a house prevents the rapid upward distribution of radon into the atmosphere, and substantial levels can build up indoors. The source of radon is the ground; therefore, levels in living areas above the ground are generally one third to one fifth the concentrations measured in basements. An effective barrier across the soil–building interface also inhibits the entry of radon to buildings. Ventilation with outdoor air reduces indoor radon. For this reason, industrial buildings with more substantial foundations and higher ventilation rates tend to have lower radon concentrations than do single-family (or detached) houses. Apartments above ground level have radon concentrations about half the average of those in single-family dwellings.

An average radon concentration indoors of 40 Bq/m^3 results in an equivalent dose to bronchial epithelium of 24 mSv per year or an effective dose of 2 mSv per year. The equivalent doses for other major natural internal emitters are shown in Table 25–4. The actual dose accumulated by an individual depends on dietary habits, location (Denver, e.g., at an altitude of 1.6 km, has double the average cosmic-ray exposure), and the dwelling. Table 25–5 provides estimated dose rates from various sources of background radiation.

Local Environmental Releases

Large- and small-scale accidents continue to release radioactivity into the environment. The accident at the Windscale nuclear power reactor in 1957 was a local incident in Great Britain.

The nearby population has been studied for over 30 years without the appearance of significant health effects. The nuclear power accident at Three Mile Island caused enormous financial damage, but the containment vessel was not breached and virtually no radioactivity escaped. In the accident at the Chernobyl nuclear power plant, containment failed and radioactivity was widespread over Europe. The United Nations Scientific Committee on the Effects of Atomic Radiation has summarized the committed dose from measurements made in the affected countries from various releases, and these are shown in Table 25–6. Local exposures and doses from accidents can only be anticipated to increase, as the use of radioactive materials industrially, for research, and for medical diagnosis increases.

BIBLIOGRAPHY

Bushong SC: *Radiologic Science for Technologists: Physics, Biology and Protection*, 9th ed. St. Louis: Mosby, 2008.

Forshier S: *Essentials of Radiation Biology and Protection*, 2nd ed. Albany, NY: Delmar, 2008.

Krewski D, Lubin JH, Zielinski JM, Alavanja M, Catalan VS, Field RW, Klotz JB, Létourneau EG, Lynch CF, Lyon JI, Sandler DP, Schoenberg JB, Steck DJ, Stolwijk JA, Weinberg C, Wilcox HB. Residential radon and risk of lung cancer: a combined analysis of 7 North American case-control studies. *Epidemiology* 16: 137-45, 2005.

Pavia M, Bianco A, Pileggi C, Angelillo IF. Meta-analysis of residential exposure to radon gas and lung cancer. *Bull World Health Organ.* 81:732-8, 2003.

QUESTIONS

1. Which of the following is NOT a main type of radiation?
   a. alpha particles.
   b. microwaves.
   c. beta particles.
   d. gamma rays.
   e. x-rays.

2. Which of the following statements regarding alpha particles is FALSE?
   a. Alpha particles are ejected from the nucleus of an atom.
   b. The atomic number decreases by two after emission of an alpha particle.
   c. The atomic weight decreases by two after emission of an alpha particle.
   d. Energies of most alpha particles range between 4 and 8 MeV.
   e. Alpha particles are helium nuclei.

3. Which of the following types of radiation is likely the MOST energetic?
   a. alpha particles.
   b. beta particles.
   c. positron emission.
   d. electron capture.
   e. photon emission.

4. Pair production and the Compton effect characterize which type of radiation's interaction with matter?
   a. alpha particles.
   b. beta particles.
   c. positron emission.
   d. electron capture.
   e. photon emission.

5. Which of the following statements regarding radiation DNA damage is FALSE?
   a. Ionizing radiation slows down by forming ion pairs.
   b. A main form of radiation DNA damage occurs by the production of free radicals.
   c. High-LET radiation causes more ionizations than does low-LET radiation.
   d. Most DNA damage caused by radiation happens directly.
   e. Direct and indirect ionization cause similar damage to DNA.

6. Low-LET radiation:
   a. causes large-scale ionizations throughout the cell.
   b. results from alpha particle emission.
   c. causes damage that is readily repaired by cellular enzymes.
   d. is also known as densely ionizing radiation.
   e. usually causes irreparable cell damage.

7. What is the most common type of DNA damage caused by low-LET radiation exposure?
   a. base damage.
   b. DNA protein cross-links.
   c. single-strand breaks.
   d. double-strand breaks.
   e. thymine-dimer formation.

8. Which of the following statements regarding radon exposure is FALSE?
   a. Miners are exposed to increased environmental radon levels.
   b. Radon exposure has been linked to the development of lung cancer.
   c. Smokers are at a higher risk from radon exposure.
   d. Radon levels are relatively higher in urban areas than in rural areas.
   e. The use of open flames indoors increases radon exposure.

9. The largest dose of radiation is received from which of the following sources?
   a. inhalation.
   b. in body.
   c. cosmic.
   d. cosmogenic.
   e. terrestrial.

10. The largest contributor to the effective dose of radiation in the U.S. population is which of the following?
    a. nuclear medicine.
    b. medical x-rays.
    c. terrestrial.
    d. internal.
    e. radon.

Toxic Effects of Terrestrial Animal Venoms and Poisons

John B. Watkins III

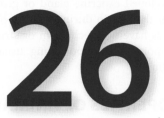

PROPERTIES OF ANIMAL TOXINS

ARTHROPODS

ARACHNIDA

Scorpions

Spiders

Agelenopsis Species (American Funnel Web Spiders)

Latrodectus Species (Widow Spiders)

Loxosceles Species (Brown or Violin Spiders)

Steatoda Species

Cheiracanthium Species (Running Spiders)

Theraphosidae Species (Tarantulas)

Ticks

CHILOPODA (CENTIPEDES)

DIPLOPODA (MILLIPEDES)

INSECTA

Heteroptera (True Bugs)

Hymenoptera (Ants, Bees, Wasps, and Hornets)

Formicidae (Ants)

Apidae (Bees)

Vespidae (Wasps)

Lepidoptera (Caterpillars, Moths, and Butterflies)

MULLOSCA (CONE SNAILS)

REPTILES

Lizards

Snakes

Snake Venoms

Enzymes

Polypeptides

Toxicology

Snakebite Treatment

Snake Venom Evolution

ANTIVENOM

KEY POINTS

- Venomous animals produce poison in a highly developed secretory gland or group of cells and can deliver their toxin during a biting or stinging act.
- Poisonous animals are those whose tissues, either in part or in their entirety, are toxic. Poisoning usually takes place through ingestion.
- The bioavailability of a venom is determined by its composition, molecular size, amount or concentration gradient, solubility, degree of ionization, and the rate of blood flow into that tissue as well as the properties of the engulfing surface itself.

- The distribution of most venom fractions is rather unequal, being affected by protein binding, variations in pH, and membrane permeability, among other factors.
- A venom may also be metabolized in several or many different tissues.
- Because of their protein composition, many toxins produce an antibody response; this response is essential in producing antisera.

Venomous animals are capable of producing a poison in a highly developed exocrine gland or group of cells and they can deliver their toxin during a biting or stinging act. Poisonous animals have no mechanism or structure for the delivery of their poisons, and poisoning usually takes place through ingestion.

PROPERTIES OF ANIMAL TOXINS

Venoms are very complex, containing polypeptides, high- and low-molecular-weight proteins, amines, lipids, steroids, glucosides, aminopolysaccharides, quinones, and free amino acids, as well as serotonin, histamine, and other substances. The complexity of snake venoms is illustrated in Figure 26–1.

Novel instrument developments have permitted researchers to tease out the complexity of natural venoms, thereby identifying the peptide and protein components of venom. Unfortunately, studying the chemistry, pharmacology, and toxicology of venoms requires isolating and dismantling the venoms and losing the synergy among multiple components. Nevertheless, advanced technology will permit peptide sequencing and the characterization of post-translational modifications, such as glycosylation, and the discovery of new pharmacophores.

Venom bioavailability is determined by its composition, molecular size, amount or concentration gradient, solubility, degree of ionization, and the rate of blood flow into that tissue as well as the properties of the engulfing surface itself. The venom can be absorbed by active or passive transport, facilitated

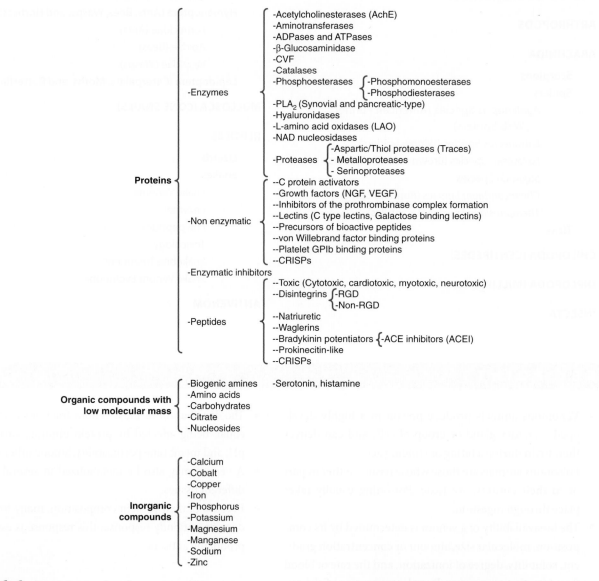

FIGURE 26–1 **Components of snake venoms.** ACE = angiotensin-converting enzyme; CRISP = cysteine-rich secretory protein; CVF = cobra venom factor-like proteins; LAO = L-amino acid oxidase; PLA$_2$ = phospholipase A$_2$; RGD = arginine–glycine–aspartate. (Reprinted with permission from Ramos OHP, Selistre-de-Araujo HS: Snake venom metalloproteases—structure and function of catalytic and disintegrin domains. *Comp Biochem Physiol, Part C* 142:328–346, 2006. Copyright © Elsevier.)

diffusion, or even pinocytosis. It is then transmitted into the vascular bed, sometimes directly or sometimes through lymphatic channels. The lymph circulation not only carries surplus interstitial fluid produced by the venom, but also transports the larger molecular components and other particulates back to the bloodstream.

The site of action of venom is dependent on its diffusion and partitioning along the gradient between the plasma and the tissues where the components are deposited. Once the toxin reaches a particular site, its entry to that site is dependent on the rate of blood flow into that tissue, the mass of the structure, and the partition characteristics of the toxin between the blood and the particular tissue. Receptor sites appear to have highly variable degrees of sensitivity. With complex venoms, there may be several to many receptor sites. There is also considerable variability in the sensitivity of those sites for the different components of a venom.

A venom may be metabolized in several or many different tissues. Some venom components are metabolized distant to the receptor site(s) and may never reach the primary receptor in a quantity sufficient to affect that site. The amount of toxin that tissues can metabolize without endangering the organisms may also vary. Organs or tissues may contain enzymes that catalyze a host of reactions, including deleterious ones. Once a venom component is metabolized or in some way altered, the end substance is excreted, principally through the kidneys. The intestines play a minor role. Excretion may be complicated by venom action on the kidneys.

ARTHROPODS

The more than a million species of arthropods are generally divided into 25 orders. Medically, only about 10 orders are of significant importance. These include the arachnids (scorpions, spiders, whip scorpions, solpugids, mites, and ticks), the myriapods (centipedes and millipedes), the insects (water bugs, assassin bugs, and wheel bugs), beetles (blister beetles), Lepidoptera (butterflies, moths, and caterpillars), and Hymenoptera (ants, bees, and wasps). Most arthropods do not have fangs or stings long or strong enough to penetrate human skin.

The number of deaths from arthropod stings and bites is not known. However, deaths from scorpion stings exceed several thousand a year, whereas spider bites probably do not account for more than 200 deaths a year worldwide. A common problem faced by physicians in suspected spider bites relates to the differential diagnosis. The arthropods most frequently involved in misdiagnoses were ticks (including their embedded mouthparts), mites, bedbugs, fleas (infected flea bites), Lepidoptera insects, flies, vesicating beetles, water bugs, and various stinging Hymenoptera. Among the disease states that were confused with spider or arthropod bites or stings were erythema chronicum migrans, erythema nodosum, periarteritis nodosum, pyroderma gangrenosum, kerion cell-mediated response to a fungus, Stevens–Johnson syndrome, toxic epidermal necrolysis, herpes simplex, and purpura fulminans.

Any other arthropod may bite or sting and not eject venom. Some arthropod envenomations give rise to the symptoms and signs of an existing undiagnosed subclinical disease. In some cases, stings or bites may induce stress reactions that bring the unrecognized disease to the surface.

ARACHNIDA

Scorpions

Of the more than 1000 species of scorpions, the stings of more than 75 can be considered of sufficient toxicity to warrant medical attention. Some of the more important scorpion species are noted in Table 26–1. The dangerous bark scorpion, *Centruroides exilicauda,* is often found hiding under the loose bark of trees or in dead trees or logs, and may frequent human dwellings. Straw to yellowish-brown or reddish-brown in color, it is often easily distinguishable from other scorpions in the same habitat by its long, thin telson, or tail, and its thin pedipalps, or pincer-like claws.

Many scorpion venoms contain low-molecular-weight proteins, peptides, amino acids, nucleotides, and salts, among other components. The neurotoxic fractions are generally classified on the basis of their molecular size, the short-chain toxins being composed of 20 to 40 amino acid residues with three or four disulfide bonds and appear to affect potassium or chloride channels; the long-chain toxins have 58 to 76 amino acids with four disulfide bonds and affect mainly the sodium channels. Toxins can selectively bind to a specific channel of excitable cells, thus impairing the initial depolarization of the action potential in the affected nerve and muscle.

The symptoms and signs of scorpion envenomation differ considerably depending on the species. The sting of members of the family Vejovidae gives rise to localized pain, swelling, tenderness, and mild parasthesia. Systemic reactions are rare, although weakness, fever, and muscle fasciculations have been reported. Envenomations by some members of the genus *Centruroides* may or may not produce initial pain in children.

TABLE 26–1 Location of some medically important scorpions.

Genus	Distribution
Androctonus species	North Africa, Middle East, Turkey
Buthus species	France and Spain to Middle East and North Africa, Mongolia, China
Buthotus species	Africa, Middle East, Central Asia
Centruroides species	North, Central, South America
Heterometrus species	Central and Southeast Asia
Leiurus species	North Africa, Middle East, Turkey
Mesobuthus species	Turkey, India
Parabuthus species	Southern Africa
Tityus species	Central and South America

However, the area becomes sensitive to touch, and merely pressing lightly over the injury will elicit an immediate retraction. The poisoned child becomes tense and restless and shows abnormal and random head and neck movements. Often the child will display roving eye movements. Tachycardia is usually evident within 45 min as well as some hypertension. Respiratory and heart rates are increased, and by 90 min the child may appear quite ill. Fasciculations may be seen over the face or large muscle masses, and the child may complain of generalized weakness and display some ataxia or motor weakness. Opisthotonos is not uncommon. The respiratory distress may proceed to respiratory paralysis. Excessive salivation may further impair respiratory function. Slurring of speech may be present, and convulsions may occur. If death does not occur, the child usually becomes asymptomatic within 36 to 48 h.

In adults the clinical picture is somewhat similar, but there are some differences. Almost all adults complain of immediate pain after the sting, regardless of the *Centruroides* species involved. Adults are tense and anxious, developing tachycardia, hypertension, and increased respirations. They may complain of difficulties in focusing and swallowing. In some cases, there is some general weakness and pain on moving the injured extremity. Ataxia and muscle incoordination may occur. Most adults are asymptomatic within 12 h but may complain of generalized weakness for 24 h or more.

Spiders

Of the 30,000 or so species, at least 200 have been implicated in significant bites on humans. Table 26–2 provides a short list of spiders, their toxins, and the targets of their toxins.

TABLE 26–2 Some significant spiders, their toxins, and the targets of the toxins.

Spider	Peptide	Target*
Acanthoscurria gomesiana	Gomesin	PLM
Agelenopsis aperta	ω-Afal-IVA	Ca²⁺
	μ-Afatoxin 1–6	Na⁺
Grammostola spatula	HaTx1,2	K⁺
	GsMTx2,4	MS
	GSTxSIA	Ca²⁺
Hadronyche versuta	ω-ACTX-Hv1a	Ca²⁺
	ω-ACTX-Hv2a	Ca²⁺
	δ-ACTX-Hv1a	Na⁺
Heteroscodra maculate	HmTx1,2	K⁺
Ornithoctonus huwena	Huwentoxin I	Ca²⁺
	Huwentoxin IV	Na⁺
Psalmopoeus cambridgei	PcTx1	ASIC
Phrixotrichus auratus	PaTx1,2	K⁺
Thrixopelma pruriens	ProTxI, II	Na⁺

*PLM = phospholipid membranes; Ca²⁺, K⁺, and Na⁺ = calcium, potassium, and sodium ion channels; MS = mechanosensitive ion channels; ASIC = acid-sensing ion channels.

Spider venoms are complex mixtures of low-molecular-weight components, including inorganic ions and salts, free acids, glucose-free amino acids, biogenic amines and neurotransmitters, and polypeptide toxins. Table 26–3 lists local and systemic effect for known cases of major spider groups in Australia.

***Agelenopsis* Species (American Funnel Web Spiders)—** These spiders contain three classes of agatoxins that target ion channels: (1) α-agatoxins appear to be use-dependent, noncompetitive antagonists of the glutamate receptor channels; (2) μ-agatoxins cause increased spontaneous release of neurotransmitter from presynaptic terminals and repetitive action potentials in motor neurons, and are specific for insect sodium channels; and (3) the four ω-agatoxins can be distinguished by sequence similarity and their spectrum of action against insect and vertebrate calcium channels.

***Latrodectus* Species (Widow Spiders)—**Found throughout the world in all continents with temperate or tropical climates, these spiders are commonly known as the black widow, brown widow, or red-legged, hourglass, poison lady, deadly spider, red-bottom spider, T-spider, gray lady spider, and shoebutton spider. Although both male and female widow spiders are venomous, only the female has fangs large and strong enough to penetrate the human skin. Venom contains a family of proteins of about 1000 amino acid residues, latrotoxins. α-Latrotoxin is a presynaptic toxin that exerts its toxic effects on the vertebrate central nervous system, depolarizing neurons by increasing [Ca²⁺] and by stimulating exocytosis of neurotransmitters from nerve terminals.

Bites by the black widow are described as sharp and pinprick-like, followed by a dull, occasionally numbing pain in the affected extremity and by pain and cramps in one or several of the large muscle masses. Rarely is there any local skin reaction except during the first 60 min following the bite. Muscle fasciculations frequently can be seen within 30 min of the bite. Sweating is common, and the patient may complain of weakness and pain in the regional lymph nodes, which are often tender on palpation and occasionally enlarged; lymphadenitis is frequently observed. Pain in the low back, thighs, or abdomen is a common complaint, and rigidity of the abdominal muscles is seen in most cases in which envenomation has been severe. Severe paroxysmal muscle cramps may occur, and arthralgia has been reported. Hypertension is common, particularly in the elderly, after moderate to severe envenomations.

***Loxosceles* Species (Brown or Violin Spiders)—**Variously known in North America as the fiddle-back spider or the brown recluse, the abdomen of these spiders varies in color from grayish through orange and reddish-brown to blackish and is distinct from the pale yellow to reddish-brown background of the cephalothorax. Both males and females are venomous.

Loxosceles venom may contain phospholipase, protease, esterase, collagenase, hyaluronidase, deoxyribonuclease, ribonuclease, dipeptides, dermonecrosis factors, and sphingomyelinase D.

TABLE 26–3 Comparison of clinical effects of bites by some spiders of Australia.

Clinical Effects	*Lactrodectus* Redback Spiders	*Steatoda* Cupboard Spiders	Lamponidae White-tail Spiders	Mygalomorphae FWS, Mouse Spiders, Trapdoor Spiders
Severe pain (percent)	62	26	27	49
Duration of pain	36 h	6 h	5 min	60 min
Fang marks (percent)	6	17	17	58
Initial erythema	74	96	83	36
Swelling (percent)	7	9	8	13
Itchiness (percent)	38	48	44	0
Nausea, vomiting, headache, malaise (percent)	35	30	9	36
Distal limb bite (percent)	46	52	82	91

The bite of this spider produces about the same degree of pain as does the sting of an ant. A local burning sensation may last for 30 to 60 min around the injury along with slight redness and minimal swelling. In more severe bites, pruritus over the area occurs, and the area becomes red, with a small blanched area surrounding the reddened bite site. Skin temperature usually is elevated over the lesion area. The reddened area enlarges and becomes purplish during the subsequent 1 to 8 h. Hemorrhages may develop throughout the area. A small bleb or vesicle, which forms at the bite site, increases in size until it ruptures and a pustule forms. The red hemorrhagic area continues to enlarge, as does the pustule. The whole area may become swollen and painful, and lymphadenopathy is common.

In serious bites, systemic effects include fever, malaise, stomach cramps, nausea, vomiting, jaundice, spleen enlargement, hemolysis, hematuria, and thrombocytopenia. Fatalities, while rare, are preceded by intravascular hemolysis, hemolytic anemia, thrombocytopenia, hemoglobinuria, and renal failure.

***Steatoda* Species**—These spiders are variously known as the false black widow, comb-footed, cobweb, or cupboard spiders. Bites by *S. grossa* or *S. fulva* have been followed by local pain, often severe; induration; pruritus; and occasional breakdown of tissue at the bite site.

***Cheiracanthium* Species (Running Spiders)**—*C. punctorium, C. inclusum, C. mildei, C. diversum,* and *C. japonicum* are common biting spiders. The abdomen is convex and egg-shaped and varies in color from yellow, green, or greenish-white to reddish-brown; the cephalothorax is usually slightly darker than the abdomen. The chelicerae are strong, and legs are long, hairy, and delicate. *Cheiracanthium* tends to be tenacious and sometimes must be removed from the bite area. The venom has a highly toxic 60 kDa protein and high concentrations of norepinephrine and serotonin.

The bite is sharp and painful, with the pain increasing during the first 30 to 45 min. A reddened wheal with a hyperemic border develops. Small petechiae may appear near the center of the wheal. Lymphadenitis and lymphadenopathy may develop. *C. japonicum* produces more severe effects that include severe local pain, nausea, vomiting, severe pruritus, headache, chest discomfort, and shock.

***Theraphosidae* Species (Tarantulas)**—Tarantulas feed on various vertebrate and invertebrate preys, which are captured after envenomation with venoms that act rapidly and irreversibly on the central and peripheral nervous systems. In humans, reported bites elicit mild-to-severe local pain, strong itching, and tenderness that may last for several hours. Edema, erythema, joint stiffness, swollen limbs, burning feelings, and cramps are common. In more severe cases, strong cramps and muscular spasms lasting up to several hours may be observed.

Ticks

Tick paralysis is caused by the saliva of at least 60 species of ticks of the families Ixodidae, Argasidae, and Nuttalliellidae. The tick bite involves insertion of cutting, tube-like mouthparts through the host's skin with anchoring so that the tick can feed for hours, days, or weeks. Saliva from the salivarium flows outward initially and the blood meal flows inward afterward. Saliva contains several active constituents including apyrase, kininase, glutathione peroxidase, an anticomplement protein, amine-binding proteins (that bind serotonin and histamine) and prostanoids. Ticks are known to transmit organisms causing Lyme disease, Rocky Mountain spotted fever, babesiosis, leptospirosis, Q fever, ehrlichiosis, typhus, tick-borne encephalitis, and others.

Tick bites are often not felt; the first evidence of envenomation may not appear until several days later, when small macules develop. The patient often complains of difficulty with gait, followed by paresis and eventually locomotor paresis and paralysis. Problems in speech and respiration may ensue and lead to respiratory paralysis if the tick is not removed. Removal of the tick usually results in a rapid and complete recovery, although regression of paralysis may resolve slowly.

The ticks that cause the paralysis in humans and domestic animals may be the same, and it is the length of the exposure to the feeding tick that determines the degree of poisoning. These comments are specific only for tick venom poisoning and not for allergic reactions, transmission of disease states, or other complications of tick bites.

CHILOPODA (CENTIPEDES)

These elongated, many-segmented brownish-yellow arthropods are found worldwide. The first pair of legs behind the head is modified into poison jaws. The venom is concentrated within the intracellular granules, discharged into vacuoles of the cytoplasm of the secretory cells, and moved by exocytosis into the lumen of the gland; from thence ducts carry the venom to the jaws.

The venoms of centipedes contain high-molecular-weight proteins, proteinases, esterases, 5-hydroxytryptamine, histamine, lipids, and polysaccharides. Such venom contains a heat-labile cardiotoxic protein of 60 kDa that produces changes associated with acetylcholine release. The bite produces immediate bleeding, redness, and swelling often lasting 24 h. Localized tissue changes and necrosis have been reported, and severe envenomations may cause nausea and vomiting, changes in heart rate, vertigo, and headache. In the most severe cases, there can be mental disturbances.

DIPLOPODA (MILLIPEDES)

Ranging in length from 20 to 300 mm, these arthropods are cylindrical, wormlike creatures, mahogany to dark brown or black in color, bearing two pairs of jointed legs per segment. The lesions produced by millipedes consist of a burning or prickling sensation and development of a yellowish or brown-purple lesion; subsequently a blister containing serosanguineous fluid forms, which may rupture. Eye contact can cause acute conjunctivitis, periorbital edema, keratosis, and much pain.

INSECTA

Heteroptera (True Bugs)

The clinically most important of the true bugs are the Reduviidae (the reduviids): the kissing bug, assassin bug, wheel bug, or cone-nose bug. The most commonly involved species appear to be *Triatoma protracta, T. rubida, T. magista, Reduvius personatus,* and *Arilus cristatus.* The venom of these bugs has apyrase activity and is fairly rich in protease properties. It inhibits collagen-induced platelet aggregation.

The bites of *Triatoma* species are definitely painful and give rise to erythema, pruritus, increased temperature in the bitten part, localized swelling, and—in those allergic to the saliva—systemic reactions such as nausea, vomiting, and angioedema. With some bites, the wound area will slough, leaving a depression.

The water bugs are water-dwelling true bugs of which at least three families, Belostomatidae, Naucordiae, and Notonectidae, are capable of biting and envenomating humans. Water bug saliva contains digestive enzymes, neurotoxic components, and hemolytic fractions. Water bug bites give rise to immediate pain, some localized swelling, and possibly induration and formation of a small papule.

There are some arthropods that are poisonous and the poison must come through their being crushed or eaten. These would include, among others, darkling beetles (stink bugs, *Eleodes*) and the blister beetles (*Epicauta*), from whom cantharidin is obtained.

Hymenoptera (Ants, Bees, Wasps, and Hornets)

Formicidae (Ants)—Most ants have stings, but those that lack them can spray a defensive secretion from the tip of the gaster, which is often placed in the wound of the bite. The clinically important stinging ants are the harvesting ants (*Pagonomyrmex*), fire ants (*Solenopsis*), and little fire ants (*Ochetomyrmex*). Harvester ants are large red, dark brown, or black ranging in size from 6 to 10 mm and have fringes of long hairs on the back of their heads.

Ant venoms vary considerably. The venoms of the Ponerinae, *Pseudomyrmex*, and Ecitoninae are proteinaceous in character. The Myrmecinae venoms are a mixture of amines, enzymes and proteinaceous materials, histamine, hyaluronidase, phospholipase A, and hemolysins, which hemolyze erythrocytes and mast cells. Formicinae ant venom contains about 60 percent formic acid. Fire ant venoms are poor in polypeptides and proteins, but are rich in alkaloids such as solenopsine. The sting of the fire ant gives rise to a painful burning sensation, after which a wheal and localized erythema develop, leading in a few hours to a clear vesicle. Within 12 to 24 h, the fluid becomes purulent and the lesion turns into a pustule. It may break down or become a crust or fibrotic nodule. In multiple stingings there may be nausea, vomiting, vertigo, increased perspiration, respiratory difficulties, cyanosis, coma, and even death.

Apidae (Bees)—The commonest stinging bees are *Apis mellifera* and the Africanized bee, *Apis mellifer adansonii.* The venom contains biologically active peptides, such as melittin, apamine, phospholipase A_2 (PLA_2) and B, hyaluronidase, histamine, dopamine, mast cell-degranulating peptide, monosaccharides, and lipids. Bee stings typically produce immediate, sharp or burning pain, slight local erythema, and edema followed by itching. It is said that 50 stings can lead to respiratory dysfunction, intravascular hemolysis, hypertension, myocardial damage, hepatic changes, shock, and renal failure. With 100 or more stings, death can occur.

Vespidae (Wasps)—This family includes wasps and hornets. These venoms contain a high content of peptide, which include mastoparan in wasps and hornets and crabolin from hornet venom. Other peptides named waspkinins cause immediate pain, vasodilation, and increased vascular permeability leading to edema. These venoms also contain phospholipases and hyaluronidases, which contribute to the breakdown of membranes and connective tissue to facilitate diffusion of the venom.

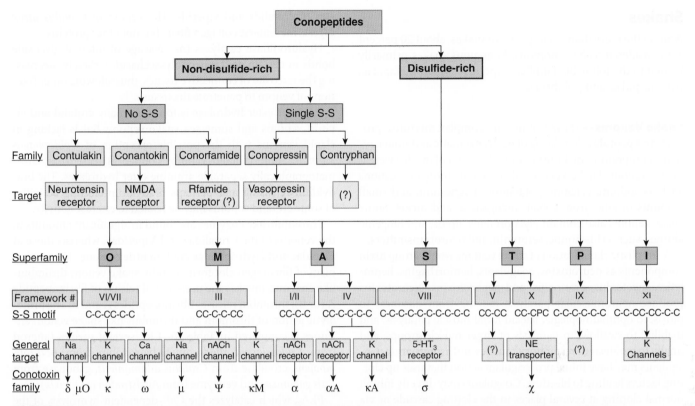

FIGURE 26–2 Organizational diagram for *Conus* peptides, indicating gene superfamilies, disulfide patterns, and known pharmacologic targets. Only the superfamilies of the disulfide-rich peptides are shown. (Used with permission from Terlau H, Olivera BM: Conus venoms: a rich source of novel ion channel-targeted peptides. *Physiol Rev* 84:41–68, 2004.)

Lepidoptera (Caterpillars, Moths, and Butterflies)

The urticating hairs, or setae, of caterpillars are attached to unicellular poison glands at the base of each hair. The toxic material contains aristolochic acids, cardenolides, histamine, and a fibrinolytic protein. After envenomation, coagulation defects such as prolonged prothrombin and partial thromboplastin times have been detected, and decreases in fibrinogen and plasminogen have been noted.

Stings of *Megalopygidae*, *Dioptidae*, *Automeris*, and *Hermileucinae* species of Lepidoptera give rise to a bleeding diathesis. In more severe cases, there is localized pain as well as papules (sometimes hemorrhagic) and hematomas; on occasion there may also be headache, nausea, vomiting, hematuria, lymphadenitis, and lymphadenopathy.

MULLOSCA (CONE SNAILS)

The genus *Conus* is a group of some 500 species of carnivorous predators found in marine habitats that use venom as a weapon for prey capture. There are probably over 100 different venom components per species (Figure 26–2). Components have become known as conotoxins, which may be rich in disulfide bonds, and conopeptides. After injection, conopeptides act synergistically to affect the targeted prey, often resulting in total inhibition of neuromuscular transmission. Various conotoxins inhibit presynaptic calcium channels that control neurotransmitter release, the postsynaptic neuromuscular nicotinic receptors, and the sodium channels involved in muscle action potential. Conotoxins also target ligand-gated ion channels that mediate fast synaptic transmission.

REPTILES

Lizards

The Gila monster (*Heloderma suspectum*) and the beaded lizards (*Heloderma horridum*) are far less dangerous than is generally believed. Their venom is transferred from venom glands in the lower jaw through ducts that discharge their contents near the base of the larger teeth of the lower jaw. The venom is then drawn up along grooves in the teeth by capillary action. The venom of this lizard has serotonin, amine oxidase, phospholipase A, a bradykinin-releasing substance, helodermin, gilatoxin, and low proteolytic as well as high-hyaluronidase activities. Helotherime, a 25-kDa protein, appears to inhibit calcium ion influx from the sarcoplasmic reticulum. The 35 amino acid peptide helodermin produces hypotension by activating potassium channels in vascular smooth muscle. The clinical presentation of a helodermatid bite can include pain, edema, hypotension, nausea, vomiting, weakness, and diaphoresis.

Snakes

Among the more than 2700 species of snakes, about 20 percent are considered to be venomous. Venomous snakes primarily belong to the following families: Viperidae (vipers), Elapidae, Atractaspidae, and Colubridae.

Snake Venoms—These venoms are complex mixtures: proteins and peptides, consisting of both enzymatic and nonenzymatic compounds, making up over 90 percent of the dry weight of the venom. Snake venoms also contain inorganic cations such as sodium, calcium, potassium, magnesium, and small amounts of zinc, iron, cobalt, manganese, and nickel. Some snake venoms also contain glycoproteins, lipids, and biogenic amines, such as histamine, serotonin, and neurotransmitters.

A simplistic classification of snake venoms would group toxin components as neurotoxins, coagulants, hemorrhagins, hemolytics, myotoxins, cytotoxins, and nephrotoxins. Neurotoxins produce neuromuscular paralysis ranging from dizziness to ptosis; to ophthalmoplegia, flaccid facial muscle paralysis, and inability to swallow; to paralysis of larger muscle groups; and finally to paralysis of respiratory muscles and asphyxiation. Coagulants may have initial procoagulant action that uses up clotting factors leading to bleeding. Coagulants may directly inhibit normal clotting at several places in the clotting cascade or via inhibition of platelet aggregation. In addition, some venom components may damage the endothelial lining of blood vessels leading to hemorrhage. Bite victims may show bleeding from nose or gums, the bite site, and in saliva, urine, and stools. Myotoxins can directly impact muscle contraction leading to paralysis or cause rhabdomyolysis or the breakdown of skeletal muscle. Myoglobinuria, or a dark brown urine, and hyperkalemia may be noted. Cytotoxic agents have proteolytic or necrotic properties leading to the breakdown of tissue. Typical signs include massive swelling, pain, discoloration, blistering, bruising, and wound weeping. Sarafotoxins, which are found only in burrowing asps of Afro-Arabia, cause coronary artery constriction, reduced coronary blood flow, angina, and myocardial infarction. Finally, nephrotoxins can cause direct damage to kidney structures, leading to bleeding, damage to several parts of the nephron, tissue oxygen deprivation, and renal failure.

Enzymes—Snake venoms contain at least 26 enzymes, although no single snake venom contains all of them (Figure 26–1). Proteolytic enzymes, also known as peptide hydrolases, proteases, endopeptidases, peptidases, and proteinases, catalyze the breakdown of tissue proteins. Multiple proteolytic enzymes may be in a single venom. Metals are involved in the activity of certain proteases and phospholipases.

The crotalid venoms examined so far appear to be rich in proteolytic enzyme activity. Viperid venoms have lesser amounts, whereas elapid and sea snake venoms have little or no proteolytic activity. Venoms that are rich in proteinase activity are associated with marked tissue destruction.

Collagenase activity, a specific proteinase that digests collagen, has been demonstrated in the venoms of a number of species of crotalids and viperids. The venom of *Crotalus atrox* digests mesenteric collagen fibers but not other proteins.

Hyaluronidase catalyzes the cleavage of internal glycoside bonds in certain acid mucopolysaccharides, thereby decreasing the viscosity of connective tissues, thus allowing other fractions of venom to penetrate the tissues.

Arginine ester hydrolase is found in many crotalid and viperid venoms and some sea snake venoms but is lacking in elapid venoms with the possible exception of *Ophiophagus hannah*. Some crotalid venoms contain at least three chromatographically separable arginine ester hydrolases. The bradykinin-releasing and perhaps bradykinin-clotting activities of some crotalid venoms may be related to esterase activity.

Thrombin-like enzymes are found in significant amounts in the venoms of the Crotalidae and Viperidae, whereas those of Elapidae and Hydrophiidae contain little or none. The mechanism of fibrinogen clot formation by snake venom thrombin-like enzymes invokes the preferential release of fibrinopeptide A (or B); thrombin releases fibrinopeptides A and B. The proteolytic action of thrombin and thrombin-like snake venom enzymes is compared in Table 26–4 for several species (ancrod from *Calloselasma rhodostoma*, batroxobin from *Bothrops moojeni*, crotalase from *Crotalus adamanteus*, gabonase from *Bitis gabonica*, and venzyme from *Agkistrodon contortrix*).

PLA_2, which catalyzes the Ca^{2+}-dependent hydrolysis of the 2-acyl ester bond producing free fatty acids and lysophospholipid, is widely distributed in the venoms of elapids, vipers, crotalids, sea snakes, atractaspids, and several colubrids. PLA_2 interact with other toxins in venom, often resulting in synergistic reactions. Although mammalian PLA_2s are nontoxic, the snake venom enzymes differ widely in their pharmacologic properties.

Phosphomonoesterase (phosphatase) is found in the venoms of all families of snakes except colubrids. It has the properties of an orthophosphoric monoester phosphohydrolase. There are two nonspecific phosphomonoesterases; many venoms contain both acid and alkaline phosphatases, whereas other venoms contain one or the other.

Phosphodiesterase, found in the venoms of all families of poisonous snakes, is an orthophosphoric diester phosphohydrolase that attacks DNA, RNA, and derivatives of arabinose.

There are other enzymes for which their toxicologic contribution to snake venoms is not understood. These include acetylcholinesterase, RNase, DNase, 5′-nucleotidase, nicotinamide adenine dinucleotide (NAD) nucleotidase, L-amino acid, and lactate dehydrogenase.

Polypeptides—More than 80 snake venom polypeptides are low-molecular-weight proteins and have toxic actions. Erabutoxin a, erabutoxin b, alpha-cobratoxin, crotactin, and crotamine are examples of neurotoxins. Disintegrins are short cysteine-rich polypeptides that exhibit affinities for many ligand receptors. The mycotoxins can induce skeletal muscle spasms and paralysis by altering sodium channel function.

Toxicology—In general, the venoms of rattlesnakes and other New World crotalids produce alterations in the resistances (and

TABLE 26-4 Comparison of thrombin and thrombin-like snake venom enzyme actions.

Enzymes	Action on Human Fibrinogen		Activation of Factor XIII	Prothrombin Fragment Cleavage	Platelet Aggregation and Release
	Fibrinopeptides Released	Chain Degradation			
Thrombin	A – B	α(A)	Yes	Yes	Yes
Thrombin-like enzymes	A[1]	α(A)[2] or β(B)[3]	No	Yes or no[4]	No
Agkistrodon c. contortrix Venom	B	ND	Incomplete	ND	No
Bitis gabonica Venom	A + B	ND	Yes	ND	ND

[1]Includes ancrod, batroxobin, crotalase, and the enzyme from *T. okinavensis*.
[2]Ancrod [batroxobin degrades α(A) chain of bovine but not human fibrinogen].
[3]Crotalase.
[4]Fragment I released by crotalase and *Agkistrodon contortrix* venom, but not by ancrod or batroxobin.
ND = not determined.

often the integrity) of blood vessels, changes in blood cells and blood coagulation mechanisms, direct or indirect changes in cardiac and pulmonary dynamics, and—with crotalids like *C. durrissus terrificus* and *C. scutulatus*—serious alterations in the nervous system and changes in respiration. In humans, the course of the poisoning is determined by the kind and amount of venom injected; the site where it is deposited; the general health, size, and age of the patient; and the kind of treatment. Death in humans may occur within less than 1 h or after several days, with most deaths occurring between 18 and 32 h. Hypotension or shock is the major clinical problem in North American crotalid bites.

Snakebite Treatment—The treatment of bites by venomous snakes is so highly specialized that almost every envenomation requires specific recommendations. However, three general principles for every bite should be kept in mind: (1) snake venom poisoning is a medical emergency requiring immediate attention and the exercise of considerable judgment; (2) the venom is a complex mixture of substances of which the proteins contribute the major deleterious properties, and the only adequate antidote is the use of specific or polyspecific antivenom; (3) not every bite by a venomous snake ends in an envenomation. In almost 1000 cases of crotalid bites, 24 percent did not end in a poisoning. The incidence with the bites of cobras and perhaps other elapids is probably higher.

Snake Venom Evolution—Considerable efforts are being expended to examine the complex process by which snake venom components are thought to have changed over the years. In general, the toxins from ancestral proteins that were constructed of dense networks of cysteine cross-linkages are considered among the most diverse today in terms of toxicologic insult.

ANTIVENOM

Antivenoms have been produced against most medically important snake, spider, scorpion, and marine toxins. Animals immunized with venom develop various antibodies to the many antigens in venom. Antivenom consists of venom-specific antisera or antibodies concentrated from immune serum to the venom. Antisera contain neutralizing antibodies: one antigen (monospecific) or several antigens (polyspecific). The serum is harvested, partially or fully purified, and further processed before being administered to the patient. The antibodies bind to the venom molecules, rendering them ineffective.

Antivenoms are available in several forms: intact IgG antibodies or fragments of IgG such as F(ab)$_2$ and Fab. The molecular weight of the intact IgG is about 150,000, whereas that of Fab is approximately 50,000. IgG has a volume of distribution much smaller than that of Fab and is too large for renal excretion. The elimination half-life of IgG is approximately 50 h. Its ultimate fate is not known, but most IgG is probably taken up by the reticuloendothelial system and degraded with the antigen attached. Fab fragments have an elimination half-life of about 17 h, and undergo renal excretion.

All antivenom products are produced through the immunization of animals, which increases the possibility of hypersensitivity. The risks of anaphylaxis should always be considered when deciding whether to administer antivenom.

BIBLIOGRAPHY

Dart RC (ed): *Medical Toxicology*, 3rd ed. Philadelphia: Lippincott, 2004.

Dias JH: *Color Atlas of Human Poisoning and Envenoming*. Boca Raton, FL: CRC Press, 2006.

Meier J, White J: *Handbook of Clinical Toxicology of Animal Venoms and Poisons*. Boca Raton, FL: CRC Press, 1995.

Menez A (ed): *Perspectives in Molecular Toxicology*. New York: Wiley, 2002.

Russell FE, Nagabhushanam R: *The Venomous and Poisonous Marine Invertebrates of the Indian Ocean*. Enfield, NH: Science Publications, 1996.

QUESTIONS

1. Which of the following statements regarding animal toxins is FALSE?
   a. Animal venoms are strictly metabolized by the liver.
   b. The kidneys are responsible for the excretion of metabolized venom.
   c. Venoms can be absorbed by facilitated diffusion.
   d. Most venom fractions distribute unequally throughout the body.
   e. Venom receptor sites exhibit highly variable degrees of sensitivity.

2. Scorpion venoms do NOT:
   a. affect potassium channels.
   b. affect sodium channels.
   c. affect chloride channels.
   d. affect calcium channels.
   e. affect initial depolarization of the action potential.

3. Which of the following statements regarding widow spiders is TRUE?
   a. Widow spiders are exclusively found in tropical regions.
   b. Both male and female widow spiders bite and envenomate humans.
   c. The widow spider toxin decreases calcium concentration in the synaptic terminal.
   d. Alpha-latrotoxin stimulates increased exocytosis from nerve terminals.
   e. A severe alpha-latrotoxin envenomation can result in life-threatening hypotension.

4. Which of the following diseases is not commonly caused by tick envenomation?
   a. Rocky Mountain spotted fever.
   b. Lyme disease.
   c. Q fever.
   d. ehrlichiosis.
   e. cat scratch fever.

5. Which of the following is NOT characteristic Lepidoptera envenomation?
   a. increased prothrombin time.
   b. decreased fibrinogen levels.
   c. decreased partial thromboplastin time.
   d. increased risk of hemorrhaging.
   e. decreased plasminogen levels.

6. A species of which of the following animals produces a venom that contains 60 percent formic acid?
   a. snakes.
   b. lizards.
   c. ants.
   d. spiders
   e. scorpions.

7. Which of the following animals has a venom containing histamine and mast cell-degranulating peptide that is known for causing hypersensitivity reactions?
   a. bees.
   b. ants.
   c. snakes.
   d. spiders.
   e. reduviids.

8. Which of the following enzymes is not typically found in snake venoms?
   a. hyaluronidase.
   b. lactate dehydrogenase.
   c. collagenase.
   d. phosphodiesterase.
   e. histaminase.

9. Which of the following statements regarding snakes is FALSE?
   a. Inorganic anions are often found in snake venoms.
   b. About 20 percent of snake species are venomous.
   c. Snake venoms often interfere with blood coagulation mechanisms.
   d. Proteolytic enzymes are common constituents of snake venoms.
   e. Snakebite treatment is often specific for each type of envenomation.

10. The production of antivenoms requires neutralizing antibodies of which type?
    a. IgA.
    b. IgG.
    c. IgM.
    d. IgE.
    e. IgD.

Toxic Effects of Plants, Fungi, and Algae

Stata Norton

KEY POINTS

- Different portions of the plant (root, stem, leaves, and seeds) often contain different concentrations of a chemical.
- The age of the plant contributes to variability. Young plants may contain more or less of some constituents than mature plants.
- Climate and soil influence the synthesis of some chemicals.
- Plants contain chemicals that may exert toxic effects on skin, lung, cardiovascular system, liver, kidney, bladder, blood, central and peripheral nervous systems, bone, and the reproductive system.

- Contact dermatitis and photosensitivity are common skin reactions with many plants.
- Gastrointestinal effects range from local irritation to emesis and/or diarrhea.
- Cardiac glycosides in the leaves or seeds of many plants cause nausea, vomiting, and cardiac arrhythmias in animals and humans.

INTRODUCTION

Of the many species of plants that contain toxic chemicals, only a few are described here. Selection has been based on three considerations: frequency with which contact occurs, importance and seriousness of toxic effect, and scientific understanding of the nature of the action of the chemical.

Toxic effects of the same species of plant may vary with differences in production of the toxic chemical by plants. The reasons for variability in concentration of toxic chemicals are several:

1. Different portions of the plant (root, stem, leaves, and seeds) often contain different concentrations of a chemical.
2. The age of the plant contributes to variability. Young plants may contain more or less of some constituents than mature plants.
3. Climate and soil influence the synthesis of some chemicals.
4. Genetic differences within a species may alter the ability of individual plants to synthesize a chemical. Synthesis of related toxic chemicals often is found in taxonomically related species as a characteristic of a genus and sometimes as a familial characteristic.

TOXIC EFFECT BY ORGAN

Skin

Contact Dermatitis—Many plants common to temperate regions worldwide contain compounds that produce irritation on contact with the intact plant. Several species of *Ranunculus* (buttercup) cause contact dermatitis. These plants contain ranunculin, which releases toxic protoanemonin, also present in *Anemone*, another genus of the buttercup family. Protoanemonin is readily converted to anemonin, which has marked irritant properties. Ingestion of plants containing protoanemonin may result in severe irritation of the gastrointestinal tract.

Contact of the eye or tongue to the juice of the *Dieffenbachia* plant results in pain and rapid development of edema and inflammation, which may take days or weeks to subside. The toxicity is due to: (1) release of a histamine- or serotonin-like chemical that may be involved in the immediate pain and (2) release of raphides, the needle-like crystals of irritating calcium oxalate that are coated with a trypsin-like inflammatory protein, from ampule-shaped ejector cells throughout the surface of the leaf.

Contact with the trichomes of species of *Urtica* (nettles) causes pain and erythema after penetration of the skin. In the stinging nettles, *Urtica urens* and *Urtica dioica* (family Urticaceae), the trichomes covering the leaves and stems consist of fine tubes with bulbs at the end that break off in the skin and release fluid containing histamine, acetylcholine, and serotonin, causing the acute response.

Allergic Dermatitis—Most people are familiar with allergic dermatitis caused by plants such as poison ivy. Species of both *Philodendron* (family Araceae, arum family) and *Rhus* (Anacardiaceae, cashew family) cause allergic contact dermatitis. *Philodendron scandens* is a common houseplant, while *Rhus radicans* (poison ivy) is native to North America. In addition to poison ivy, the toxicodendron group of plants contains *Rhus diversiloba* (poison oak) and *Rhus vernix* (poison sumac). The active ingredients in *P. scandens* are resorcinols. In *R. radicans,* the allergenic component is a mixture of catechols called urushiol. Allergic dermatitis also develops with repeated exposures to the sap of mango fruit, because the skin of the fruit contains oleoresins that cross-react with allergens of poison ivy.

Flower growers and other individuals who handle bulbs and cut flowers of daffodils, hyacinths, and tulips sometimes develop dermatitis from contact with the sap. The rashes are due to irritation from alkaloids (masonin, lycorin, and other alkaloids)

biologicals (dust mites, fungi, molds, etc.) may also lead to un-expected interactions that are virtually unstudied and thus are not appreciated in the assessment of indoor pollution.

POLLUTANTS OF OUTDOOR AMBIENT AIR

Classic Reducing-type Air Pollution

Reducing-type air pollution, characterized by SO_2 and smoke, is capable of producing disastrous human health effects. Empirical studies in human subjects and animals have long stressed the irritancy of SO_2 and its role in these incidents, whereas the full potential for interactions among the copollutants in the smoky, sulfurous mix has a mixed record of replication in the human exposure laboratory. Nevertheless, the irritancy of most S-oxidation products in the atmosphere is well documented, and there are both empirical and theoretical reasons to suspect that such products act to amplify the irritancy of fossil fuel emission atmospheres via chemical transformations.

Sulfur Dioxide

General toxicology—Sulfur dioxide is a water-soluble irritant gas that is absorbed predominantly in the upper airways and stimulates bronchoconstriction and mucus secretion in a number of species, including humans. The concentrations of SO_2 likely to be encountered in the United States average less than 0.1 ppm. Mandated use of cleaner (low-S) fossil fuels, emission control devices, and tall emission stacks has largely been responsible for the reductions. However, rare down-drafting of smokestack plumes due to meteorological inversions near point sources may result in levels of SO_2 that may pose a health hazard. A 2-min exposure to 0.4 to 1.0 ppm can elicit bronchoconstriction in exercising asthmatics within 5 to 10 min. However, it is the low-level, long-term effects that erode pulmonary defenses that continue to worry some regulators. Studies have shown that SO_2 is capable of impairing macrophage-dependent bacterial killing in murine models. Exposed mice have a greater frequency and severity of infection, which has been suggested to be linked to diminished ability to generate endogenous oxidants for bacterial killing.

The penetration of SO_2 into the lungs is greater during mouth breathing as opposed to nose breathing. An increase in the air-flow rate further augments penetration of the gas into the deeper lung. As a result, persons exercising would inhale more SO_2 and, as noted with asthmatics, are likely to experience greater irritation. Once deposited along the airway, SO_2 dissolves into surface-lining fluid as sulfite or bisulfite and is readily distributed throughout the body. Sulfite interacts with sensory receptors in the airways to initiate bronchoconstriction.

Pulmonary Function Effects—The basic pulmonary response to inhaled SO_2 is mild bronchoconstriction, which is reflected as a measurable increase in airflow resistance due to narrowing of the airways. Concentration-related increases in resistance have been observed in guinea pigs, dogs, cats, and humans.

Sulfuric Acid and Related Sulfates

The conversion of SO_2 to sulfate is favored in the environment. During oil and coal combustion or the smelting of metal ores, sulfuric acid condenses downstream of the combustion processes with available metal ions and water vapor to form submicrometer sulfated fly ash. Photochemical reactions in the troposphere also promote acid sulfate formation via both metal-dependent and independent mechanisms. These sulfates may contribute to health hazards and acid rain (Figure 28–3).

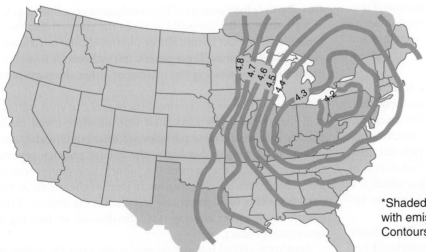

*Shaded areas indicate individual states with emissions of 1000 kilotonnes of SO_2 and greater. Contours connect points of equal precipitation pH.

FIGURE 28–3 **Areas in 1988 where precipitation in the east fell below pH 5: acid rain.** The acidity of the air in the east is thought to result from air mass transport of fine sulfated particulate matter from the industrial centers of the Midwest. (*National Air Pollutant Emission Trends Report,* 1998.)

General Toxicology—Sulfuric acid irritates respiratory tissues by virtue of its ability to protonate (H⁺) receptor ligands and other biomolecules. This action can either directly damage membranes or activate sensory reflexes that initiate inflammation.

Pulmonary Function Effects—Sulfuric acid produces an increase in flow resistance in guinea pigs due to reflex airway narrowing, which impedes the flow of air into and out of the lungs. This response can be thought of as a defensive measure to limit the inhalation of air containing noxious gases. The magnitude of the response is related to both acid concentration and particle size. Small particles are able to penetrate deep into the lung, reaching receptors that stimulate bronchoconstriction and mucus secretion. The thicker mucus blanket of the nose may blunt (by dilution or neutralization by mucus buffers) much of the irritancy of the deposited acid, thus limiting its effects to mucous cell stimulation and a minor increase in nasal flow resistance. In contrast, the less shielded distal airway tissues, with their higher receptor density, would be expected to be more sensitive to the acid particles reaching that area.

Asthmatics appear to be more sensitive to the bronchoconstrictive effects of sulfuric acid than are healthy individuals, owing to hyperresponsive airways. Asthmatic airways are also sensitive to nonspecific airway smooth muscle agonists (e.g., carbachol, histamine, and exercise). The general correlation between airway responsiveness and inflammation that appears to be important in grading asthma severity and risk of negative clinical outcomes may also be predictive of responses to environmental stimuli.

Effects on Mucociliary Clearance and Macrophage Function—Sulfuric acid alters the clearance of particles from the lung and thus can interfere with a major defense mechanism. The impact on mucus clearance appears to vary directly with the acidity ([H⁺]) of the acid sulfate, with sulfuric acid having the greatest effect and ammonium sulfate the smallest. Acidification of mucus is the primary metric to associate with population health effects affecting mucus rheology, viscosity, and secretion and ciliary function.

Chronic Effects—As might be expected, sulfuric acid induces qualitatively similar effects along the airways as are found with high concentrations of SO_2. As a fine aerosol, sulfuric acid deposits deeper along the respiratory tract, and high specific acidity imparts greater injury on phagocytes and epithelial cells. Thus, a primary concern with regard to chronic inhalation of acidic aerosols is its potential to cause bronchitis, which is a problem in occupational settings in which employees are exposed to sulfuric acid mists (e.g., battery plants).

Inhaled sulfuric acid does not appear to stimulate a classic neutrophilic inflammation. Rather, disturbed eicosanoid homeostasis results in macrophage dysfunction and altered host defense. In fact, chronic daily exposure of humans to sulfuric acid at levels of about 100 μg/m³ may lead to impaired clearance and mild chronic bronchitis. As this is less than an order of magnitude above haze levels of sulfuric acid, the possibility that chronic irritancy may elicit bronchitic-like disease in susceptible individuals appears to be reasonable.

Particulate Matter

Particulate matter (PM) in the atmosphere is a mélange of organic, inorganic, and biological materials whose compositional matrix can vary significantly depending on local point sources. A large epidemiologic database contends that PM elicits both short- and long-term health effects at current ambient levels.

Metals—There have been many standard acute and subchronic rodent inhalation studies with specific metal compounds, often oxides, chlorides, or sulfates. Virtually any metal can be found at some concentration in ambient PM and many have toxic or prooxidant potential. The most common are metals released during oil and coal combustion (e.g., transition and heavy metals), metals derived from the earth's crust as dust (e.g., iron, sodium, and magnesium), and metals released from engine wear. Metals derived from anthropogenic combustion sources tend to enrich the fine fraction (<2.5 μm) of PM, whereas coarse (2.5 to 10 μm) PM is made up of metal compounds of crustal origin (e.g., Fe_2O_3 and SiO_2).

Solubility appears to play a role in the toxicity of many inhaled metals by enhancing metal bioavailability (e.g., nickel from nickel chloride versus nickel oxide), but insolubility can also be a critical factor in determining toxicity by increasing pulmonary residence time within the lung (e.g., insoluble cadmium oxide versus soluble cadmium chloride). Moreover, some metals, either in their soluble forms or when coordinated on the surface of silicate or bioorganic materials, can promote electron transfer to induce the formation of reactive oxidants. These and other mechanisms may be involved in the action of inhaled PM-associated metals.

Gas–Particle Interactions—The coexistence of pollutant gases and particles in the atmosphere raises the concern that these phases may interact chemically or physiologically to yield unpredictable outcomes. These generic interactions are feasible as mechanisms for altering the toxicity of either the particle or the gas.

Metal smelting or the combustion of coal can emit sulfuric acid that is physically associated with ultrafine metal oxide particles. These ultrafine particles are distributed widely and deeply in the lung and enhance the irritant potency beyond that predicted on the basis of the sulfuric acid concentration alone. Moreover, the combination of inert or chemically active particles with a toxic gas is able to enhance the impact of the gas alone, by either altering dose distribution or forming a more toxic product.

Another potential interaction may result from the ability of gaseous pollutants to influence the clearance of particles from the lung or alter the metabolism or cellular interactions with lung-deposited particles. Gaseous and particulate pollutants can interact through either chemical or physiologic mechanisms to enhance either immediate or associated long-term risks of complex polluted atmospheres.

Ultrafine Carbonaceous Matter—Carbonaceous material often forms the core of fine PM. The organic materials, which can be of a semivolatile or nonvolatile nature, are more often dispersed within the structure of PM, forming layers or sheaths. Estimates of the carbonaceous content vary considerably but are nominally considered to be about 30 to 60 percent of the total mass of fine PM.

Ultrafine carbon (<0.1 μm) has been suggested to be more toxic than the same substance in the larger range (2.5 μm). Diesel PM is made up of aggregated ultrafine carbon with small amounts of various combustion-derived complex polycyclic and nitroaromatic compounds and only a trace of metals. However, whole diesel exhaust also contains significant amounts of NO_x, CO, SO_x, formaldehyde, acrolein, and other aldehyde compounds, which are known irritants. Diesel exhaust mix is inflammogenic and cytotoxic to airway cells.

Photochemical Air Pollution

Photochemical air pollution arises from a series of complex reactions in the troposphere activated by the ultraviolet (UV) spectrum of sunlight. It consists of a mixture of ozone, nitric oxides, aldehydes, peroxyacetyl nitrates (PANs), and myriad reactive hydrocarbon radicals. If SO_2 is present, sulfuric acid PM may also be formed; likewise, the complex chemistry can generate organic PM, nitric acid vapor, and condensate. Of the photochemical air pollutant gases, O_3 is the toxicant of greatest concern, being highly reactive and more toxic than NO_x. Ozone generation is fueled through cyclic hydrocarbon radicals, and it reaches greater concentrations than the hydrocarbon radical intermediates. In general, concentrations of the hydrocarbon precursors in ambient air do not reach levels high enough to produce acute toxicity. Their importance stems largely from their roles in the chain of photochemical reactions that leads to the formation of oxidant smog or haze.

Although O_3 is of toxicologic importance in the troposphere, in the stratosphere it plays a critical protective role. About 10 km above the earth's surface, there is sufficient short-wave UV light to directly split molecular O_2 to atomic $O\bullet$, which can then recombine with O_2 to form O_3. This O_3 accumulates to several hundred ppm within a thin strip of the stratosphere and absorbs incoming short-wavelength UV radiation. The O_3 forms and decomposes and reforms to establish a "permanent" barrier to UV radiation, which lately has become an issue of concern. This barrier had, in recent years, been threatened by various anthropogenic emissions (Cl_2 gas and certain fluorocarbons) that enhance O_3 degradation. Recent restrictions in the use of these degrading chemicals seem to have been effective in reversing this process. The benefits are believed to be reduction of excess UV light infiltration to the earth's surface and a reduced skin cancer risk and less risk of immune system dysfunction.

The issue is different in the troposphere, where accumulation of O_3 serves no known purpose and poses a threat to the respiratory tract. Near the earth's surface, NO_2 from combustion processes efficiently absorbs longer-wavelength UV light, cleaving a free O atom and initiating the following simplified series of reactions:

$$NO_2 + h\nu \text{ (UV light)} \rightarrow O\bullet + NO\bullet \qquad (1)$$
$$O\bullet + O_2 \rightarrow O_3 \qquad (2)$$
$$O_3 + NO\bullet \rightarrow NO_2 \qquad (3)$$

This process is inherently cyclic, with NO_2 regenerated by the reaction of the $NO\bullet$ and O_3. In the absence of unsaturated hydrocarbons, this series of reactions would approach a steady state with no excess or buildup of O_3. The hydrocarbons, especially olefins and substituted aromatics, are attacked by the free atomic $O\bullet$, resulting in oxidized compounds and free radicals that react with $NO\bullet$ to produce more NO_2. Thus, the balance of the reactions shown in equations (1) to (3) is tipped to the right, leading to buildup of O_3. This reaction is particularly favored when the sun's intensity is greatest at midday, utilizing the NO_2 provided by morning traffic. Aldehydes are also major byproducts of these reactions. Formaldehyde and acrolein account for about 50 and 5 percent, respectively, of the total aldehyde in urban atmospheres. PAN (CH_3COONO_2) and its homologs also arise in urban air, most likely from the reaction of the peroxyacyl radicals with NO_2.

Chronic Exposures to Smog

Studies in animals and human populations have attempted to link degenerative lung disease with chronic exposure to photochemical air pollution. Cross-sectional and prospective field studies have suggested an accelerated loss of lung function in people living in areas of high pollution. However, as with many studies of this type, there are problems with confounding factors (meteorology, imprecise exposure assessment, and population variables). Studies conducted in children living in Mexico City, with very high oxidant and PM levels, found severe epithelial damage and metaplasia as well as permanent remodeling of the nasal epithelium. When children who migrated into Mexico City from cleaner, nonurban regions were evaluated, even more severe damage was observed, suggesting that the remodeling in the permanent residents imparted some degree of incomplete adaptation. Because the children were of middle-class origin, these observations were not likely confounded by socioeconomic variables. These dramatic nasal effects have raised concerns for the more fragile, deep lung tissues, where substantial deposition of oxidant air pollutants may occur.

Ozone

General toxicology—Current mitigation strategies for O_3 have been largely unsuccessful as a result of population growth. With the spread of suburbia and the downwind transport of air masses from populated areas to more rural environments, the geographic distribution of those exposed has spread, as has the temporal profile of potential exposure. In other words, O_3 exposures are no longer stereotyped as brief 1- to 2-h peaks.

Instead, there are prolonged periods of exposure of 6 h or more at or near the NAAQS level that may occur either downtown or in the formerly cleaner suburban or rural areas downwind.

Ozone induces a variety of effects in humans and experimental animals at concentrations found in many urban areas. These effects include morphologic, functional, immunologic, and biochemical alterations. Because of its low water solubility, a substantial portion of inhaled ozone penetrates deep into the lung, but its reactivity is such that about 17 and 40 percent is scrubbed by the nasopharynx of resting rats and humans, respectively. However, regardless of species, the region of the lung that is predicted to have the greatest O_3 deposition (dose per surface area) is the centriacinar region, from the terminal bronchioles to the alveolar ducts. Because O_3 penetration increases with increased tidal volume and flow rate, exercise increases the dose to the target area. Thus, it is important to consider the role of exercise in a study of O_3 or any inhalant before making cross-study comparisons, especially if that comparison is across species.

The acute morphologic response to O_3 involves epithelial cell injury along the entire respiratory tract, resulting in cell loss and replacement. Ciliated cells appear to be most sensitive to O_3, whereas Clara cells and mucus-secreting cells are the least sensitive.

As a powerful oxidant, O_3 seeks to extract electrons from other molecules. The surface fluid lining the respiratory tract and cell membranes that underlie the lining fluid contain a significant quantity of polyunsaturated fatty acids (PUFA), either free or as part of the lipoprotein structures of the cell. The double bonds within these fatty acids have a labile, unpaired electron that is easily attacked by O_3 to form ozonides that ultimately recombine or decompose to lipohydroperoxides, aldehydes, and hydrogen peroxide. These pathways are thought to initiate propagation of lipid radicals and autoxidation of cell membranes and macromolecules (Figure 28–4).

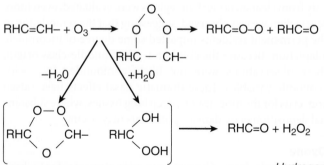

FIGURE 28–4 **Major reaction pathways of O_3 with lipids in lung-lining fluid and cell membranes.** (Adapted with permission from the *Air Quality Criteria Document for Ozone and Photochemical Oxidants*, 600/P-93/004cF, NCEA. Research Triangle Park, NC: U.S. EPA, 1996.)

Pulmonary Function Effects—Exercising human subjects exposed to 0.12 to 0.4 ppm O_3 experience reversible concentration-related decrements in forced vital capacity (FVC) and forced expiratory volume in 1 s (FEV_1) after 2 to 3 h of exposure. Interestingly, the human lung dysfunction resulting from O_3 does not appear to be vagally mediated, but the response can be abrogated by analgesics such as ibuprofen and opiates, which also reduce pain and inflammation. Thus, pain reflexes involving C-fiber networks are thought to be important in the reductions in forced expiratory volumes. On the other hand, animal studies show a prominent role for vagal reflexes in altered airway reactivity and bronchoconstriction. It is widely thought that hyperreactive airways may predispose responses to other pollutants such as sulfuric acid or aeroallergens.

Ozone Interactions with Copollutants—An approach simplifying the complexity of synthetic smog studies yet addressing the issue of pollutant interactions involves the exposure of animals or humans to binary or tertiary mixtures of pollutants known to occur together in ambient air. Such studies have had a number of permutations, but most have attempted to address the interactions of O_3 and nitrogen dioxide or O_3 and sulfuric acid. Depending on study design, there has been evidence supporting either augmentation or antagonism of lung function impairments, lung pathology, or other indices of injury. This apparent conflict only emphasizes the need to carefully consider the myriad factors that might affect studies involving multiple determinants and the nature of the exposure that is most relevant to reality.

As the number of interacting variables increases, so does the difficulty in interpretation. Studies of complex atmospheres involving acid-coated carbon combined with O_3 at near-ambient levels show variable strength of evidence of interaction on lung function and macrophage receptor activities. The statistical separation of the interacting variables and responses from the individual or combined components is difficult. However, it is the complex mixture to which people are exposed that we wish to evaluate. Creative approaches to understanding mixture responses must be addressed in the next decade.

Nitrogen Dioxide

General Toxicology—Nitrogen dioxide, like O_3, is a deep lung irritant that can produce pulmonary edema if it is inhaled at high concentrations. Potential life-threatening exposure is a real-world problem for farmers, as sufficient amounts of NO_2 can be liberated from fermenting fresh silage. Typically, shortness of breath ensues rapidly with exposures nearing 75 to 100 ppm NO_2, with delayed edema and symptoms of pulmonary damage, collectively characterized as silo-filler's disease. Nitrogen dioxide is also an important indoor pollutant, especially in homes with unventilated gas stoves or kerosene heaters. Under such circumstances, very young children and their caregivers who spend considerable time indoors may be especially at risk. Sidestream tobacco smoke can also be a source of low levels of indoor NO_2.

Damage to the respiratory tract is most apparent in the terminal bronchioles. At high concentrations, the alveolar ducts and alveoli are also affected, with type I cells again showing their sensitivity to oxidant challenge. There is also damage to epithelial cells in the bronchioles, notably with loss of ciliated cells, as well as a loss of secretory granules in Clara cells.

Inflammation of the Lung and Host Defense—NO$_2$ does not induce significant neutrophilic inflammation in humans at exposure concentrations approximating those in the ambient outdoor environment. There is some evidence for bronchial inflammation after 4 to 6 h at 2.0 ppm, which approximates the likely highest transient peak indoor level of this oxidant. Exposures at 2.0 to 5.0 ppm have been shown to affect T lymphocytes, particularly CD8$^+$ cells and natural killer cells that function in host defenses against viruses. Although these concentrations may be high, epidemiologic studies variably show enhanced viral infection associated with NO$_2$ exposure, especially during seasonal use of unvented gas-heating indoors. Susceptibility to infection appears to be governed more by the peak exposure concentration than by exposure duration. The effects are ascribed to suppression of macrophage function and clearance from the lung.

Other Oxidants—Whereas a number of reactive oxidants have been identified in photochemical smog, most are short-lived because of their reaction with copollutants. One reactive, irritating constituent of the oxidant atmosphere is PAN, which is thought to be responsible for much of the eye-stinging activity of smog. More soluble and reactive than ozone, PAN rapidly decomposes in mucous membranes before it can get to tissues deep into the lungs. The cornea has many irritant receptors and responds readily, whereas the PAN absorbed into the thicker mucous fluids of the proximal nose and mouth presumably never reaches its target.

Aldehydes—Various aldehydes in polluted air are formed as reaction products of the photooxidation of hydrocarbons. Formaldehyde (HCHO) and acrolein (H$_2$C=CHCHO) contribute to the odor as well as eye and sensory irritations of photochemical smog. Formaldehyde accounts for about 50 percent of the estimated total aldehydes in polluted air, whereas acrolein, the more irritating of the two, may account for about 5 percent of the total. Acetaldehyde (C$_3$HCHO) and many other longer chain aldehydes make up the remainder, but they are not as irritating because of their low concentration and lesser solubility in airway fluids. Formaldehyde and acrolein are found in mainstream tobacco smoke (about 90 and 8 ppm, respectively, per puff) and in sidestream smoke as well. Formaldehyde is also an important indoor air pollutant and can often achieve higher concentrations indoors than outdoors due to outgassing by new upholstery or other furnishings.

Empirical studies have shown that formaldehyde and acrolein are competitive agonists for similar irritant receptors in the airways. Thus, irritation may be related not to "total aldehyde" concentration but to specific ratios of acrolein and formaldehyde. Their relative difference in solubility, with formaldehyde being somewhat more water-soluble and thus having more nasopharyngeal uptake, may distort this relationship under certain exposure conditions (e.g., exercise). Acrolein is very reactive and may interact easily with many tissue macromolecules.

Formaldehyde—Formaldehyde is a primary sensory irritant. It is absorbed in mucous membranes in the nose, upper respiratory tract, and eyes. The dose–response curve for formaldehyde is steep: 0.5 to 1 ppm yields a detectable odor; 2 to 3 ppm produces mild irritation; and 4 to 5 ppm is intolerable to most people. Formaldehyde is thought to act via sensory nerve fibers that signal through the trigeminal nerve (CN-V) to reflexively induce bronchoconstriction through the vagus nerve (CN-X). The introduction of formaldehyde through a tracheal cannula to bypass nasal scrubbing greatly augments the irritant response, indicating that deep lung irritant receptors can also be activated. Formaldehyde can interact with water-soluble salts, such as submicrometer sodium chloride, and with carbon-based particles during inhalation and produce irritancy beyond that expected for the gas alone.

Two aspects of formaldehyde toxicology have brought it to the forefront of attention in recent years. One is its presence in indoor atmospheres as an off-gassed product of construction materials such as plywood, furniture, or improperly polymerized urea-formaldehyde foam insulation. This irritant vapor has the potential to cause respiratory effects at commonly experienced exposure levels. Formaldehyde is also a weak allergen. Recent findings suggest that formaldehyde causes nasopharyngeal cancer in humans and could be linked to leukemia and sinonasal cancer.

Acrolein—Acrolein is an unsaturated aldehyde that is more irritating than formaldehyde. Concentrations below 1 ppm cause irritation of the eyes and the mucous membranes of the respiratory tract. The mechanism of increased pulmonary flow resistance after acrolein appears to be mediated through both a C-fiber and centrally mediated cholinergic reflex. Ablation of the C-fiber network and atropine (muscarinic blocker) block this response. On the other hand, aminophylline, isoproterenol, and epinephrine (sympathetic agonists) partially or completely reversed the changes, whereas the antihistamines pyrilamine and tripelennamine had no effect.

Carbon Monoxide—Carbon monoxide is classed toxicologically as a chemical asphyxiant because its toxic action stems from its formation of carboxyhemoglobin, preventing oxygenation of the blood for systemic transport (see Chapter 11).

Analysis of data from air-monitoring programs in California indicates that 8-h average values can range from 10 to 40 ppm CO. Depending on the location in a community, CO concentrations can vary widely. Concentrations predicted inside the passenger compartments of motor vehicles in downtown traffic were almost three times those for central urban areas and five times those expected in residential areas. Occupants of vehicles traveling on expressways had CO exposures somewhere between those in central urban areas and those in downtown traffic. Concentrations above 87 ppm have been measured in underground garages, tunnels, and buildings over highways.

No overt human health effects have been demonstrated for COHb levels below 2 percent, and levels above 40 percent can be fatal due to asphyxia. At COHb levels of 2.5 percent resulting from about 90-min exposure to about 50 ppm CO, there is an impairment of time-interval discrimination; at approximately 5 percent COHb, there is an impairment of other psychomotor faculties. Cardiovascular changes also may be produced by exposures sufficient to yield COHb in excess of 5 percent.

WHAT IS AN ADVERSE HEALTH EFFECT?

The goal of air-quality management is clearly to avoid or, at worse, limit negative impacts of air pollution on public health. However, one must appreciate the distinction between risk to the individual and to a population. Clearly, risk to an individual can be beyond an acceptable limit and can put that person's health in jeopardy, but this response may be lost in a population index. On the other hand, risk to a population is the summation of individual risks such that there is a shift in the normal distribution putting unspecified individuals at risk. These two forms of risk are clearly related, but most often, the population risk is considered most appropriate and most reasonably quantifiable.

The American Thoracic Society issued a position paper that attempted to define an adverse effect related to air pollution. This statement considers seven broad areas: biomarkers, quality of life, physiologic impacts, symptoms, clinical outcomes, mortality, and population health versus individual risk. The summary states that caution should be exercised in evaluating the many new biomarkers of effect (especially cell and molecular markers), as there is need for validation that *small* changes in these markers represent a progression along a course to disease or permanent impairment. Admittedly, in the clinical environment, many of these markers may appear as salient features of a disease or injury, but the health implications of minor changes in these biomarkers remain uncertain. A common thread through all of these subject areas is the influential role of susceptibility, which can take the form of hyperresponsiveness or loss of reserve. What was a minor reversible effect may now be a dysfunction that cannot be reversed or compensated

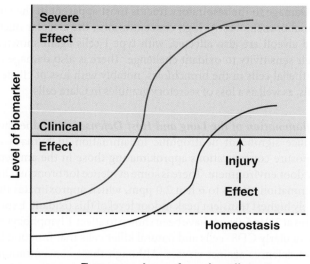

FIGURE 28–5 Schematic illustration of the elements of a dose–response to an air pollutant(s) by a susceptible versus a healthy individual. The hypothetical susceptible individual has both a *loss of reserve* and an *inability to maintain homeostasis*. The *leftward shift in the slope* of the dose–response curve also suggests an increase in responsiveness. These response elements of the susceptible individual may contribute to apparent sensitivity to challenge and the likelihood of progressing from subtle to severe effects.

(Figure 28–5). Obvious examples would be cardiopulmonary-compromised individuals who function with little or no reserve.

CONCLUSION

This chapter relates the breadth and complexity of the problem of air pollution, from the development of credible databases to supporting regulatory action and decision making. The classic and still most important air pollutants provide a foundation for understanding and appreciating the nuances of the issues and strategies for air pollution control and protection of public health.

BIBLIOGRAPHY

Foster WM, Costa DL (eds): *Air Pollutants and the Respiratory Tract*, 2nd ed. Boca Raton: Taylor & Francis, 2005.

Vallero DA (ed): *Fundamental of Air Pollution*, 4th ed. Boston: Elsevier, 2008.

QUESTIONS

1. Which of the following compounds is NOT an oxidant-type air pollutant?
   a. NO_2.
   b. SO_2.
   c. O_3.
   d. radical hydrocarbons.
   e. aldehydes.

2. Which of the following pollutants contributes most to nontobacco-smoking lung cancer?
   a. asbestos.
   b. vinyl chloride.
   c. benzene.
   d. products of incomplete combustion.
   e. formaldehyde.

3. Inhalants, such as NO_2 and trichloroethylene, can increase proliferation of opportunistic pathogens in the lungs by:
   a. destroying goblet cells in the respiratory tract.
   b. damaging the alveolar septa.
   c. inactivating cilia in the respiratory tract.
   d. killing alveolar macrophages.
   e. dampening the immune system.

4. Which of the following is NOT a characteristic of SO_2 toxicology?
   a. SO_2 is a major reducing-type air pollutant.
   b. Increased airflow rate increases the amount of SO_2 inhaled.
   c. SO_2 inhalation causes vasoconstriction and increased blood pressure.
   d. SO_2 is predominately absorbed in the conducting airways.
   e. SO_2 inhalation increases mucus secretion in humans.

5. Which of the following would be MOST likely to occur on sulfuric acid exposure?
   a. vasoconstriction.
   b. decreased mucus secretion.
   c. an anti-inflammatory response.
   d. vasodilation.
   e. bronchoconstriction.

6. All of the following statements regarding particulate matter are true EXCEPT:
   a. Metals are most commonly released into the environment during coal and oil combustion.
   b. The interaction of gases and particles in the atmosphere can create a more toxic product than the gas or particle alone.
   c. Solubility does not play a role in the bioavailability of a metal.
   d. The earth's crust is an important source of atmospheric magnesium.
   e. Diesel exhaust contains reducing- and oxidant-type air pollutants.

7. Which of the following statements is NOT true?
   a. Ozone (O_3) combines with a nitric oxide radical to form NO_2.
   b. O_2 combines with an oxygen radical to form ozone.
   c. O_3 can cause damage to the respiratory tract.
   d. Accumulation of O_3 in the stratosphere is important for protection against UV radiation.
   e. Cl_2 gas is known to cause O_2 degradation.

8. Which of the following is NOT a likely symptom of NO_2 exposure?
   a. increased secretion by Clara cells.
   b. pulmonary edema.
   c. shortness of breath.
   d. loss of ciliated cells in bronchioles.
   e. decreased immune response.

9. Which of the following statements regarding aldehyde exposure is FALSE?
   a. The major aldehyde pollutants are formaldehyde and acrolein.
   b. Formaldehyde is found in tobacco smoke, but acrolein is not.
   c. Acrolein causes increased pulmonary flow resistance.
   d. Formaldehyde exposure induces bronchoconstriction.
   e. The water solubility of formaldehyde increases its nasopharyngeal absorption.

10. Carbon monoxide (CO) exerts its toxic effects via its interaction with which of the following?
    a. DNA polymerase.
    b. actin.
    c. kinesin.
    d. hemoglobin.
    e. microtubules.

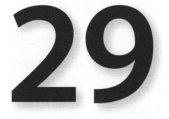
Ecotoxicology

Richard T. Di Giulio and Michael C. Newman

KEY POINTS

- Ecotoxicology is the study of the fate and effects of toxic substances on an ecosystem.
- Chemodynamics is, in essence, the study of chemical release, distribution, degradation, and fate in the environment.
- A chemical can enter any of the four matrices: the atmosphere by evaporation, the lithosphere by adsorption, the hydrosphere by dissolution, or the biosphere by absorption, inhalation, or ingestion (depending on the species). Once in a matrix, the toxicant can enter another matrix by these methods.

- The *biological availability* (or bioavailability) of a chemical is the portion of the total quantity of chemical present that is potentially available for uptake by organisms.
- Pollution may result in a cascade of events, beginning with effects on homeostasis in individuals and extending through populations, communities, ecosystems, and landscapes.
- Terrestrial toxicology is the science of the exposure to and effects of toxic compounds in terrestrial ecosystems.
- Aquatic toxicology is the study of effects of anthropogenic chemicals on organisms in the aquatic environment.

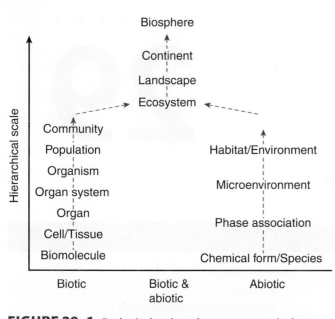

FIGURE 29-1 Ecological scales relevant to ecotoxicology.
Solely biological scales relevant to ecotoxicology range from the molecular to the community levels: solely abiotic scales range from the chemical to the entire habitat. Biotic and abiotic components are usually combined at levels above the ecological community and habitat. The ecological community and physicochemical habitat combine to form the ecosystem. Ecological systems can be considered at the landscape scale, that is, the combination of marine, freshwater, and terrestrial systems at a river's mouth. Recently, the continental and biospheric scales have become relevant as in the cases of ozone depletion, acid precipitation, and global warming.

INTRODUCTION

Ecotoxicology is the study of contaminants in the biosphere and their effects on constituents of the biosphere. It has an overarching goal of explaining and predicting effect or exposure phenomena at several levels of biological organization (Figure 29–1). Relevant effects to nonhuman targets range from biomolecular to global. As the need to predict major effects to populations, communities, ecosystems, and other higher level entities has become increasingly apparent, more cause–effect models relevant to these higher levels of biological organization are added to the conventional set of toxicology models applied by pioneering ecotoxicologists. Contaminant chemical form, phase association, and movement among components of the biosphere are also central issues in ecotoxicology because they determine exposure, bioavailability, and realized dose.

SOME DISTINCT ASPECTS OF EXPOSURE

Relevant exposure routes are the conventional ingestion, inhalation, and dermal absorption. But, unique features of exposure pathways must be accommodated for species that ingest a wide range of materials using distinct feeding mechanisms, breathe gaseous or liquid media using different structures, and come into dermal contact with a variety of gaseous, liquid, and solid media.

Prediction of oral exposure can be limited because species feed on different materials; however, conventional principles about oral bioavailability remain relevant. Many techniques applied to determining human oral bioavailability are available to the ecotoxicologist. As an example, some birds are uniquely at high risk of lead poisoning because they ingest and then use lead shot as grit. The birds grind shot in their gizzards under acidic conditions, releasing significant amounts of dissolved lead.

Estimation of chemical speciation is central to predicting bioavailability of water-associated contaminants. Speciation can determine the bioavailability of dissolved metals. Movements of nonionic and ionizable organic compounds across the gut or gills are strongly influenced by lipid solubility and pH partitioning, respectively. Consequently, determination of a compound's lipophilicity or calculation of pH- and pK_a-dependent ionization facilitates some predictive capability for bioavailability. The free ion activity model (FIAM) states that uptake and toxicity of cationic trace metals are best predicted from their free ion activity or concentration, although exceptions exist.

Bioavailability, bioaccumulation, or exposure concentrations for sediment-associated toxicants are also approached by considering chemical speciation and phase partitioning. Metals in sediments are either incorporated into one of the many solid phases or dissolved in the interstitial waters surrounding the sediment particles. Bioavailable metals have been estimated by normalizing sediment metal concentrations to easily extracted iron and manganese concentrations because solid iron and manganese oxides sequester metals in poorly bioavailable solid forms.

Another issue of importance to the ecotoxicologist is the possibility of biomagnification, the increase in contaminant concentration as it moves through a food web. Biomagnification can result in harmful exposures to species situated high in the food web such as birds of prey.

TOXICANT EFFECTS

One approach to this complex topic of ecotoxicologic effects is to organize effects according to biological levels of organization. One may consider effects, in ascending order, at the subcellular (molecular and biochemical), cellular, organismal, population, community, and ecosystem levels of organization. Ecotoxicology deals with, theoretically at least, all species, and in line with other aspects of natural resource management, the primary concern is one of sustainability. The policies and regulations surrounding chemical effects in natural ecosystems are designed to protect ecological features such as population dynamics, community structures, and ecosystem functions.

Molecular and Biochemical Effects

This lowest level of organization includes fundamental processes associated with the regulation of gene transcription and translation, biotransformation of xenobiotics, and the deleterious biochemical effects of xenobiotics on cellular constituents including proteins, lipids, and DNA.

Gene Expression and Ecotoxicogenomics

Xenobiotics can affect gene transcription through interactions with transcription factors and/or the promoter regions of genes. In the context of environmental toxicology, perhaps the most studied xenobiotic effects involve ligand-activated transcription factors. These intracellular receptor proteins recognize and bind specific compounds, thus forming a complex that binds to specific promoter regions of genes, thereby activating transcription of mRNAs, and ultimately translation of the associated protein.

Estrogen Receptor—The dominant natural ligand for this nuclear receptor is estradiol (E2). Binding of E2 with estrogen receptor (ER) produces a complex that can then bind to estrogen response elements (ERE) of specific genes that contain one or more EREs, thereby causing gene transcription. Genes regulated in this manner by E2–ER play various important roles in sexual organ development, behavior, fertility, and bone integrity.

A number of chemicals can serve as ligands for ER; in most cases these "xenoestrogens" activate gene transcription acting as receptor agonists. Some of these xenoestrogens include diethylstilbestrol (DES), DDT, methoxychlor, endosulfan, surfactants (nonyl-phenol), some PCBs, bisphenol A, and ethinyl E2, a synthetic estrogen observed in municipal effluents and surface waters. Environmental exposures to these chemicals are sufficient to perturb reproduction or development.

Aryl Hydrocarbon Receptor—The aryl hydrocarbon receptor (AHR) is a member of the basic helix–loop–helix Per ARNT Sim (bHLH-PAS) family of receptors/transcription factors that is involved in development, as sensors of the internal and external environment in order to maintain homeostasis, and in establishment and maintenance of circadian clocks. Characterized genes that are upregulated by the AHR system code for enzymes involved in the metabolism of lipophilic chemicals, including organic xenobiotics and some endogenous substrates such as steroid hormones. These enzymes include mammalian CYP1A1, 1A2, and 1B1 and their counterparts in other vertebrates, glutathione transferase, glucuronosyltransferase, alcohol dehydrogenase, and quinone oxidoreductase.

Some ubiquitous pollutants that act as AHR ligands and markedly upregulate gene transcription via the AHR–ARNT signaling pathway include the polycyclic aromatic hydrocarbons (PAHs) and the polyhalogenated aromatic hydrocarbons (pHAHs). In general, pHAH-type AHR ligands are more potent AHR ligands and enzyme inducers than PAHs.

Genomics and Ecotoxicogenomics—Ecotoxicogenomics has great potential for elucidating impacts of chemicals of ecological concern and ultimately for playing an important role in ecological risk assessments (ERA) and regulatory ecotoxicology. Specific areas to which this emerging field can contribute include prioritization of chemicals investigated in ERA, identification of modes of action of pollutants, identification of particularly sensitive species, and effect prediction at higher levels of organization.

Protein Damage—Acetylcholinesterase (AChE) degrades the neurotransmitter acetylcholine, and controls nerve transmission in cholinergic nerve tracts. The widely used organophosphate and carbamate classes of insecticides kill by inhibiting AChE, and this mechanism is operative for "nontarget" organisms including invertebrates, wildlife, and humans. Of particular ecological concern have been the ingestion of AChE-inhibiting insecticides with food items or granular formulations (mistaken as seed or grit) by birds and aquatic animal exposures from agricultural run-off. In addition to enzyme inhibition, chemicals can damage proteins in other ways, including oxidative damage and the formation of stable adducts similar to those formed with DNA.

Oxidative Stress—Oxidative stress has been defined as the point at which production of ROS exceeds the capacity of antioxidants to prevent damage. Numerous environmental contaminants act as prooxidants and enhance production of ROS. The resulting oxidative damage can account wholly or partially for toxicity. Mechanisms by which chemicals enhance ROS production include redox cycling, interactions with electron transport chains (notably in mitochondria, microsomes, or chloroplasts), and photosensitization. Redox cycling chemicals include diphenols and quinones, nitroaromatics and azo compounds, aromatic hydroxylamines, paraquat, and certain metal chelates, particularly of copper and iron.

Photosensitization is an important mechanism in aquatic systems. Ultraviolet (UV) radiation (specifically UVB and UVA) can penetrate surface waters to varying depths, depending on the wavelength of the radiation and the clarity of the water. The UV radiation generates ROS and other free radicals via excitation of photosensitizing chemicals, including common pollutants of aquatic systems.

ROS can drive redox status to a more oxidized state, potentially reducing cell viability. These ROS-mediated impacts and others have been associated with several human diseases including atherosclerosis, arthritis, cancer, and neurodegenerative diseases such as Alzheimer's disease, Parkinson's disease, and amyotrophic lateral sclerosis. With the exception of cancer, the role of ROS in specific diseases in wildlife has received little attention. It is reasonable to assume that oxidative stress accounts in part for the toxicity of diverse pollutants to free-living organisms.

DNA Damage—Cancer is an important health outcome associated with chemical exposures in wildlife. In the context of ecotoxicology, the most widely studied form of damage has been the formation of stable DNA adducts, particularly by PAHs. PAHs must be activated to reactive metabolites to form these adducts.

Cellular, Tissue, and Organ Effects

Cells—Most free-living organisms routinely experience energy deficits. For example, food resources are often scarce during the winter for many animals, which adapt by conserving energy (by hibernating or lowering metabolism) or by storing energy beforehand (as is the case for many migratory birds). Thus, the effects of pollutants on mitochondrial energy metabolism can be of particular importance to wildlife.

Lysosomes, which are involved in the degradation of damaged organelles and proteins, sequester many environmental contaminants, including metals, PAHs, and nanoparticles. The accumulation of xenobiotics by lysosomes can elicit membrane damage, which warns of pathological effects in both invertebrates and vertebrates.

Chemical effects on nuclei have been examined in ecological contexts. Micronuclei are chromosomal fragments that are not incorporated into the nucleus at cell division, and chemical exposures can markedly increase their frequency. Elevated micronuclei numbers have been observed in erythrocytes in fish and in hemocytes in clams from a PCB-polluted harbor.

Target Organs—An important target organ in ecotoxicology of nonmammalian aquatic vertebrates and many invertebrates is the gill, which is the major site of gas exchange, ionic regulation, acid–base balance, and nitrogenous waste excretion. Gills are immersed in a major exposure medium for these animals (surface water), so metabolically active epithelial cells are in direct contact with this medium. They also receive blood supply directly from the heart. Common structural lesions in gills include cell death (via necrosis and apoptosis), rupture of the epithelium, hyperplasia, and hypotrophy of various cell populations that can lead to lamellar fusion, epithelial swelling, and lifting of the respiratory epithelium from the underlying tissue.

Organismal Effects

Mortality—Chemical pollution of the environment does not generally attain levels sufficient to outright kill wildlife. The ecotoxicologic concerns are the long-term, chronic impacts of chemicals on organismal variables such as reproduction and development, behavior, and disease susceptibility, and how such impacts parlay into effects at the population and higher levels of organization. However, mortality is an endpoint in exposure studies.

Reproduction and Development—Contaminant effects on development are often difficult to discern in field studies, due to the small size of embryos and the fact that developmental impacts are generally either lethal or greatly reduce survival. Because early life stages of most organisms are generally more sensitive to xenobiotics than other life stages, developmental impacts merit careful attention by ecotoxicologists.

Chlorinated hydrocarbons continue to generate concerns although many (DDT and other insecticides, and PCBs) have had their production and use sharply curtailed. The dioxins (TCDD) and coplanar PCBs compromise cardiac development, among other effects in vertebrates, and these developmental perturbations are largely receptor-mediated and dependent on binding of the chemical (such as TCDD) with the AHR.

Hydrocarbons, in large part PAHs, associated with oil spills, contaminated sediments, paper mill effluents, and creosote used for wood treatment have profound developmental effects in fish embryos. In many cases, the effects observed visually appear similar to those observed in fish embryos exposed to dioxins and coplanar PCBs, and include malformed hearts ("tube hearts"), craniofacial deformities, hemorrhaging, and edema of the pericardium and yolk sac, the latter resulting in a distended, faintly blue yolk sac that gives this syndrome the name "blue sac disease."

Disease Susceptibility—The potential impacts of environmental contaminants on immune systems that render organisms more susceptible to disease are of great concern. Numerous laboratory studies have demonstrated chemical impacts on immune systems in animals of ecological relevance. These include pesticides in amphibians, PCBs in channel catfish, heavy metals in rainbow trout, PAHs in bivalves, and flame retardants (polybrominated diphenyl ethers) in American kestrels.

Behavior—Relatively subtle effects on behaviors associated with mating and reproduction, foraging, predator–prey interactions, preference/avoidance of contaminated areas, and migration have potentially important ramifications for population dynamics. In some cases, the biochemical mechanisms underlying behavioral effects have been elucidated, which may assist our understanding of these issues and provide useful biomarkers for behavioral toxicants in field studies.

Chemicals causing behavioral effects in wildlife are known to be neurotoxicants. Behavioral effects of insecticides have been observed in fish. For example, impacts of the organophosphate diazinon on olfactory-mediated behaviors such as the alarm response and homing in the Chinook salmon have been observed, as well as similar thresholds for the effects of another organophosphate (chlorpyrifos) on swimming and feeding behaviors and on AChE inhibition in coho salmon (*O. kistich*). Mercury, particularly as methylmercury, comprises another potent neurotoxin that has been shown to perturb behavior in wildlife.

Environmental contaminants not generally thought of as neurotoxicants have also been shown to perturb behavior. For example, cadmium and copper have been shown to impact olfactory neurons and associated behaviors (preference/avoidance to chemicals, including pheromones) in several fish species. Copper exposure in zebrafish also led to loss of neurons in the peripheral mechanosensory system ("lateral line"), which could lead to altered behaviors associated with schooling, predator avoidance, and rheotaxis (physical alignment of fish in a current). Clearly, numerous mechanisms of chemical toxicity can result in behavioral impacts, including direct toxicity to neurons, alterations in hormones that modulate behav-

TABLE 29-1 A summary of one popular set of rules of thumb for assessing plausibility of a causal association in an ecological epidemiology.

Rule	Description
1. Strength of association	How strong the association is between the possible cause and the effect, for example, a very large relative risk
2. Consistency of association	How consistently is there an association between the possible cause and the effect, for example, consistent among several studies with different circumstances
3. Predictive performance	How good is the prediction of effect made from the presence/level of the possible cause
4. Monotonic trend	How consistent is the association between possible cause and effect to a monotonic trend (i.e., either a consistent increase or decrease in effect level/prevalence with an increase in exposure)
5. Inconsistent temporal sequence	The effect, or elevated level of effect, occurs before exposure to the hypothesized cause
6. Factual implausibility	The hypothesized association is implausible given existing knowledge
7. Inconsistency with replication	Very poor reproducibility of association during repeated field assessments encompassing different circumstances or repeated formal laboratory testing

iors, and impaired energy metabolism. Also, impaired behavior may comprise a sublethal impact with substantive ecological consequence.

Cancer—Beginning in the 1960s, numerous cases of cancer epizootics in wildlife that are associated with chemical pollution, particularly in specific fish populations, have been reported in North America and northern Europe. As in humans, cancer in these animals occurs largely in relatively older age classes and therefore is oftentimes considered a disease unlikely to directly impact population dynamics or other ecological parameters. However, this may not always be the case, particularly in species that require many years to attain sexual maturity and/or have low reproductive rates.

Lifestyle is a major contributor to differential cancer susceptibility; benthic (bottom-dwelling) species such as brown bullhead (*Ameiurus nebulosus*) and white sucker (*Catostomus commersoni*) in freshwater systems and English sole (*Parophrys vetulus*) and winter flounder (*Pseudopleuronectes americanus*) in marine systems generally exhibit the highest cancer rates in polluted systems. The bulk of chemicals in these systems associated with cancer epizootics, such as PAHs, PCBs, and other halogenated compounds, reside in sediments; benthic fish live in contact with these sediments and prey in large measure on other benthic organisms.

It is noteworthy that many reports of elevated cancer rates in free-living animals occur in fish, with few reports of potentially chemically related cancers to our knowledge in other vertebrates. It is likely that elevated exposures play an important role in the relatively high frequency of reports of cancers in benthic fish; relative inherent sensitivities among mammals, birds, reptiles, and amphibians, and fish are unclear.

Population

A population is a collection of individuals of the same species that occupy the same space and within which genetic informa-

tion can be exchanged. Population ecotoxicology covers a wide range of topics with core research themes being (1) epidemiology of chemical-related diseases, (2) effects on general population qualities including demographics and persistence, and (3) population genetics.

The level of belief warranted for possible contaminant-related effects in nonhuman populations is assessed by applying routine epidemiological methods. Rules of thumb for gauging the level of belief warranted by evidence that emerged from human epidemiology are also applied in population ecotoxicology (Table 29–1).

Some species populations fluctuate within a range of densities. These fluctuations are characteristic of the species' strategy for maintaining itself in various types of habitats and toxicant exposure could potentially change this range. Combined with decreases in population densities driven by external forces such as weather events, these toxicant-induced modifications of the average population densities and dynamics can increase the risk of a population's density falling so low that local extinction occurs. Toxicants can change a species population's vital rates, such as age- and sex-dependent death, birth, maturation, and migration rates. Combined, these changes determine the population density and distribution of individuals among ages and sexes during exposure.

Individuals of the same species often are grouped into subpopulations within a habitat and all of these subpopulations together comprise a metapopulation (Figure 29–2). Subpopulations in the metapopulation have different levels of exchange and different vital rates that depend on the nature of their habitat. Spatial distances and obstacles or corridors for migration influence migration among patches; habitat quality determines vital rates.

The genetics of exposed populations are studied to understand changes in tolerance to toxicants and to document toxicant influence on field populations. Some populations have the capacity to become more tolerant of toxicants via selection. Genetic qualities are also used to infer past toxicant influence

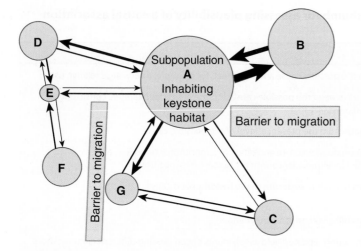

FIGURE 29-2 **Metapopulations are composed of subpopulations that differ in their vital rates and tendency to exchange individuals.** In this illustration, subpopulation A occupies a keystone habitat. The loss of subpopulation A would devastate the metapopulation. Also, loss of the migration corridor between subpopulations A, B, and D would devastate the metapopulation. In contrast, the loss of subpopulation F would not influence the metapopulation to the same degree.

in an exposed population. Another piece of evidence demonstrating past toxicant influence on populations can be a change in genetic diversity. A drop in genetic diversity in populations is thought to be an adverse effect because genetic diversity is required in populations to evolutionarily adapt to environmental changes. Toxicants can influence genetic diversity by purely stochastic means.

Community

An ecological community is an interacting assemblage of populations occupying a defined habitat at a particular time. Populations in a community interact in many ways and, because these many interactions are complex, a community has properties that are not predictable from those of its component populations.

Communities take on characteristic structures as predicted by the Law of Frequencies: the number of individual organisms in a community is related by some function to the number of species in the community. Ecotoxicants can alter the resulting community structure in predictable ways by either directly impacting the fitness of individuals in populations that make up the community or by altering population interactions.

Recently, structural and functional qualities in communities have been combined to generate multimetric indices such as the Index of Biotic Integrity (IBI). Ecological insight is used to select and then numerically combine community qualities such as species richness, health of individual animals in a sample, and the number of individuals in a sample belonging to a particular functional group, such as number of piscivorous fish. The IBI score for a study site is calculated and compared

with that expected for an unimpacted site in order to estimate its biological integrity.

Another central theme in community ecotoxicology is toxicant transfer during trophic interactions. Toxicant concentrations can decrease (biodiminution), remain constant, or increase (biomagnification) with each trophic transfer within a food web. Metals that biomagnify are mercury and the alkali metals, cesium and rubidium. Zinc, an essential metal that is actively regulated in individuals, can exhibit biomagnification or biominification depending on whether ambient levels are below or above those required by the organism to function properly.

Most individuals in a community can feed on different species depending on their life stage, seasons, and relative abundances of prey species. These trophic interactions are best described as occurring in a trophic web, not a trophic chain.

Ecosystem to Biosphere

Ecosystems, the functional unit of ecology, are composed of the ecological community and its abiotic habitat. The ecotoxicologist is interested in understanding how toxicants diminish an ecosystem's capacity to perform essential functions and to understand toxicant movement within different ecosystem components enough to assess exposure.

Conventional ecosystem studies involve descriptions of contaminant concentrations and movements in easily defined ecosystems such as lakes, forests, or fields. Some toxicants, especially those subject to wide dispersal by air or water, cannot be completely understood in this framework, so a landscape scale might be chosen instead. As an example, acid precipitation might be examined in the context of an entire watershed, mountain range, or even a continental region. Still other ecotoxicants require a global context in order to fully understand their movements and accumulation. As an example, hexachlorobenzene concentration in tree bark collected worldwide showed a clear latitudinal gradient.

APPROACHES

Toxicity Tests

Toxicity testing encompassing representative animals and plants at different levels of organization offers a practical approach to characterize chemical effects on biological systems. Toxicity tests address the potential direct effects of toxic substances on individual ecosystem components in a controlled and reproducible manner. Ecotoxicology tests feature a wide variety of aquatic (including algae, invertebrates, tadpoles, bivalves, shrimp, and fish), avian (quail and duck), and terrestrial (soil microorganisms, crops, honey bees, earthworms, and wild mammals) species. Species are selected based on their traditional use as laboratory animals, but also on ecological relevance, which further complicates global harmonization of ecological testing. In addition, testing of aquatic species requires monitoring of water quality, investigation of the solubility and stability of the test substance under the conditions of testing, and determination of nominal versus measured concentrations.

In acute toxicity testing, single species are exposed to various concentrations of the test agent. The most common endpoint in acute tests is death. Abnormal behavior and other gross observations are commonly noted, and nonlethal endpoints occasionally apply. Data from different test concentrations are used to derive concentration–response curves. The LC_{50} represents the concentration of test substance killing 50 percent of the tested animals and EC_{50} the concentration of test substance affecting 50 percent of the test population during a specified period of time, such as growth; the IC_{50} is the concentration causing a 50 percent reduction in a nonquantal measurement (such as movement) for the test population. Other quantitative values are the lowest observed effect concentration (LOEC), that is, the lowest concentration where an effect is observed, and the no observed effect concentration (NOEC), the highest concentration resulting in no adverse effects.

Short-term laboratory studies conducted with single species are useful for rapid screening, provide information on thresholds for effects, selective and comparative toxicity, and can be used as range finders to guide subsequent, often more involved, studies. Long-term and reproductive studies evaluate the effects of substances on organisms over extended periods of time and/or sequential generations (chronic toxicity, life cycle, and reproduction).

Unique to ecotoxicology are the more elaborate microcosm, mesocosm, and field studies. Microcosms are representative aquatic or terrestrial ecosystems created under laboratory conditions that include a number of relevant species (such as protozoa, plankton, algae, plants, and invertebrates). Simulated field studies or mesocosms can be created in the laboratory or in the field (e.g., artificial streams and ponds) or consist of enclosures of existing habitats, containing representative soil, water, and biota. Lastly, full-scale field studies (aquatic organisms, terrestrial wildlife, and pollinators) evaluate the effects of a substance on wildlife under real-life scenarios of actual use conditions of a product (e.g., pesticide field usage rate), and thus are more complicated, subject to considerable variability, and require extensive knowledge of the local population and community dynamics.

As a final point, plant studies are a significant component of ecological toxicity testing, particularly for pesticide registration, and involve tiered testing of both target area and nontarget terrestrial and aquatic plants.

Biomarkers

The term "biomarker" is most often employed to refer to molecular, physiologic, and organismal responses to contaminant exposure that can be quantified in organisms inhabiting or captured from natural systems. Biomarkers do not directly provide information concerning impacts on the higher levels of organization that ecotoxicology ultimately endeavors to discern. Nevertheless, biomarkers often provide important ancillary tools

for discerning contaminant exposures and potential impacts of ecological importance. Biomarkers can provide sensitive early warning signals of incipient ecological damage.

Chemical specificity among biomarkers is also highly variable and is imbued with trade-offs. Many biomarkers are invasive and require sacrifice of the organism in order to obtain needed tissues. This can be problematic, particularly in cases involving rare species or charismatic species such as marine mammals. In such cases, and in others where feasible, the use of noninvasive biomarkers is either preferred or required. Biomarkers can provide powerful tools as early warning signals of ecological damage, to assist in assessments of environmental contamination, and in determining the effectiveness of various environmental management decisions such as clean-ups. However, careful case-specific thought is required for the selection of biomarkers.

Population

Demographic surveys or experiments can be conducted for exposed populations. Some studies explore age-specific vital rates but others are designed to explore vital rates for different ages such as nestling, fledgling, juvenile, and adult. Most result in data sets that can be analyzed profitably using either a simple life table or more involved matrix analysis. The matrix method allows one to describe the population state and also to understand the sensitivity of the population to effects on vital rates for various ages or stages. The value of such studies lies in the ability to integrate effects on several factors into a projection of population consequences. Demographic studies are becoming more common in ecotoxicology, especially with species amenable to laboratory manipulation.

Conventional studies of increased tolerance after generations of exposure and molecular genetic surveys of exposed populations are the primary approaches by which genetic consequences are assessed. Increased tolerance is usually detected by subjecting individuals from the chronically exposed population and a naïve population to toxicant challenge and formally testing for tolerance differences. Alternatively, a change associated with a tolerance mechanism might be examined in chronically exposed and naïve populations. Close examinations of population genetics associated with contaminated habitats are also used to infer consequences of multigenerational exposure.

Community and Ecosystem

Most studies of community and ecosystem effects use modified methods developed in community and systems ecology. The approach affording the most control and ability to replicate treatments involves laboratory microcosms. A microcosm is a simplified system that is thought to possess the community or ecosystem qualities of interest. The experimental control and reproducibility associated with microcosms come at the cost of losing ecological realism. Gaining back some realism by giving up some degree of tractability, outdoor mesocosms are also applied to community and ecosystem ecotoxicology. Mesocosms are larger experimental systems, usually constructed outdoors that also attempt to simulate some aspect of an ecosystem such as community species composition. Field studies are the third means of exploring effects at the community or ecosystem level. The high realism of associated findings from field studies is balanced against the difficulty of achieving true replication and sufficient control of other factors influencing the system's response. Field studies can involve manipulations such as introducing toxicant into replicate water bodies; however, the majority of field studies involve biomonitoring of an existing, notionally impacted, community or ecosystem.

Landscape to Biosphere

Technologies for acquiring, processing, and analyzing large amounts of information have been essential. Archived and new imagery from satellites and high-altitude platforms are now integrated with off-the-shelf geographic information systems (GIS) software with affordable computers. Remote sensing data from satellites or aircraft provide information for wide spatial areas and the rapidly emerging, ground- or water-based observing system networks have begun to produce extremely rich data streams.

ECOLOGICAL RISK ASSESSMENT

ERA applies ecotoxicologic knowledge to support environmental decision making. A widely dispersed ecotoxicant such as acid precipitation or widely used product such as an herbicide might require assessment of risk at a landscape or subcontinental scale. Ecotoxicants requiring a global ERA might include greenhouse gases contributing to global warming, hydrofluorocarbons depleting the ozone layer, and persistant organic pollutants that accumulate to harmful concentrations in polar regions far from their release point at industrialized latitudes.

Adaptations are based on the context of an ERA. Some ERAs address existing situations. Considerable field information might be available for such a retroactive ERA and epidemiological methods might be applied advantageously. In contrast, predictive ERAs assess possible risk associated with a future or proposed toxicant exposure.

Exposure characterization describes or predicts contact between the toxicant and the assessment endpoint. Depending on the ERA context, this could involve a simple calculation of average exposure, or a temporally and spatially explicit description of amounts present in relevant media. Toxicant sources, transport pathways, kinds of contact, and potential costressors are also defined.

Ecological effects characterization describes the qualities of any potential effects of concern, the connection between the potential effects and the assessment endpoint, and how changes in the level of exposure might influence the effects manifesting in the assessment endpoint. Normally, a statement about the strength of evidence associated with the descriptions and uncertainties is presented in the ecological effects characterization.

INTERCONNECTIONS BETWEEN ECOSYSTEM INTEGRITY AND HUMAN HEALTH

It is important to consider interconnections between human health and ecological integrity, or health. By determining how chemicals and other anthropogenic stressors degrade ecosystems and impact human health and well-being, and vice versa, a holistical understanding of the results of environmental contamination is obtained. For example, a conceptual model attempts to elucidate the interconnections linking natural and social systems in a circular manner with continuous feedbacks. The natural system produces both positive outputs (such as natural resources and raw materials) and negative outputs (such as hurricanes and disease vectors) to the social system. The culture and institution of the social system in turn transform the natural system outputs in various ways and subsequently deliver various positive outputs (consumer goods and conservation efforts) and negative outputs (pollution and deforestation) to the natural system. These outputs influence the quantity and quality of life (human and nonhuman) of the natural system, and the circular flow of resources continually creates conditions that influence the well-being of individuals, societies, and ecosystems.

This rather abstract model formalizes the interconnections between human and ecological health that most of us intuitively sense. Some of these connections are obvious. Chemical contamination of seafoods valued by humans is one example. Others are less clear but potentially very significant, such as human impacts on aquatic systems that foster the propagation of human disease vectors, or human impacts on global climate that may concomitantly impact humans and ecosystems in varied and complex ways. Collaboration among biomedical, environmental, and social scientists and policy-makers will catalyze the integrated protection of human and ecosystem health.

BIBLIOGRAPHY

Benson WH, Di Giulio RT (eds): *Emerging Molecular and Computational Approaches for Cross-species Extrapolations.* New York: Taylor & Francis, 2006.

Newman MC (ed): *Fundamentals of Ecotoxicology,* 3rd ed. Boca Raton: CRC Press, 2009.

Walker, CH, Hopkin SP, Sibly RM, Peakall DB: *Principles of Ecotoxicology.* Boca Raton: CRC Press/Taylor & Francis, 2006.

QUESTIONS

1. What is the mode by which a chemical enters the lithosphere?
   a. evaporation.
   b. adsorption.
   c. dissolution.
   d. absorption.
   e. diffusion.

2. The bioavailability of contaminants in the hydrosphere is directly related to:
   a. chemical concentration.
   b. amount of chemical.
   c. water solubility of chemical.
   d. toxicity of chemical.
   e. molecular size of chemical.

3. All of the following regarding biomarkers are true EXCEPT:
   a. Dermal absorption is considered an external dose.
   b. Biomarkers of susceptibility are useful in extrapolating wildlife disease to human diseases.
   c. Induction of certain enzymes is an important biomarker.
   d. The biologically effective dose is the amount of internal dose needed to elicit a certain response.
   e. The effects of chemical exposure can be different across species.

4. Which of the following processes is LEAST likely to be affected by endocrine-disrupting agents?
   a. enzyme activity.
   b. transcription.
   c. hormone secretion.
   d. signal transduction.
   e. DNA replication.

5. Estrogen exposure has been shown to cause all of the following in wildlife species EXCEPT:
   a. sexual imprinting.
   b. altered sex hormone levels.
   c. immune suppression.
   d. gonadal malformations.
   e. sex reversal.

6. Which of the following is FALSE regarding terrestrial ecotoxicology?
   a. Terrestrial organisms are generally exposed to contaminants via ingestion.
   b. Predation is an important confounder of measurements in terrestrial toxicology field studies.
   c. Reproductive tests are not important in measuring endpoints in toxicity tests.
   d. Enclosure studies are better able to control for environmental factors in field studies.
   e. Toxicity tests usually test the effects of an oral chemical dose.

7. An important type(s) of compound that is far more toxic in water than in air is/are:
   a. organic compounds.
   b. photochemicals.
   c. vapors.
   d. lipid-soluble xenobiotics.
   e. metals.

8. Which of the following are used to record endpoint toxicity of aquatic toxicity tests?
   a. LD_{50} and ED_{50}.
   b. LC_{50} and EC_{50}.
   c. reproductive tests.
   d. LD_{50} and LC_{50}.
   e. LD_{50} and EC_{50}.

9. Biological availability is:
   a. the total amount of chemical within an organism.
   b. the concentration of chemical in an environmental reservoir.
   c. the threshold concentration of a chemical needed for toxic effect.
   d. the concentration of chemical within an organism.
   e. the proportion of chemical potentially available for uptake.

10. Chemodynamics does NOT study:
    a. the fate of chemicals in the environment.
    b. the rate at which chemicals are metabolized.
    c. the distribution of chemicals in the environment.
    d. the effects of toxic substances on the environment.
    e. the release of chemicals into the environment.

CHAPTER

30

Food Toxicology

Frank N. Kotsonis and George A. Burdock

- Food is an exceedingly complex mixture of nutrient and nonnutrient substances.
- A substance listed as Generally Recognized as Safe (GRAS) achieves this determination on the adequacy of safety, as shown through scientific procedures or through experience based on common use.
- An estimated daily intake (EDI) is based on two factors: the daily intake of the food in which the substance will be used and the concentration of the substance in that food.
- Food hypersensitivity (allergy) refers to a reaction involving an immune-mediated response, including cutaneous reactions, systemic effects, and even anaphylaxis.
- The vast majority of food-borne illnesses in developed countries are attributable to microbiologic contamination of food.

UNIQUENESS OF FOOD TOXICOLOGY

The nature of food is responsible for the uniqueness of food toxicology. Food cannot be commercially produced in a definable environment under strict quality controls and thus cannot meet the rigorous standards of chemical identity, purity, and good manufacturing practice met by most consumer products. The fact that food is harvested from the soil, the sea, or inland waters or is derived from land animals subject to the unpredictable forces of nature makes the constancy of raw food unreliable. Food is more complex and variable in composition than all other substances to which humans are exposed, and humans are exposed more to food than to any other chemicals!

Nature and Complexity of Food

Food is an exceedingly complex mixture whether it is consumed in the "natural" (unprocessed) form or as a highly processed "Meal Ready to Eat" (MRE). Nonnutrient substances (substances other than carbohydrates, proteins, fats, or vitamins/minerals) may be contributed by food processing, but nature provides the vast majority of nonnutrient constituents. Table 30–1 indicates that natural, or minimally processed, foods contain far more nonnutrient than nutrient constituents.

Importance of the Gastrointestinal Tract

The constituents of food and other ingesta (e.g., drugs, contaminants, and inhaled pollutants dissolved in saliva and swallowed) are physicochemically heterogeneous, and the primary mechanisms for intestinal absorption are passive or simple diffusion, active transport, facilitated diffusion, and pinocytosis. Each mechanism characteristically transfers a defined group of constituents from the lumen into the body (Table 30–2).

TABLE 30–1 Nonnutrient substances in food.

Food	Number of Identified Nonnutrient Chemicals
Cheddar cheese	160
Orange juice	250
Banana	325
Tomato	350
Wine	475
Coffee	625
Beef (cooked)	625

Source: Smith RL: Does one man's meat become another man's poison? *Trans Med Soc Lond* (November 11):6, 1991. With permission from Medical Society of London.

TABLE 30–2 Systems transporting enteric constituents.

System	Enteric Constituent
Passive diffusion	Sugars (e.g., fructose, mannose, and xylose, which may also be transported by facilitated diffusion), lipid-soluble compounds, water
Facilitated diffusion	D-Xylose, 6-deoxy-1,5-anhydro-D-glucitol, glutamic acid, aspartic acid, short-chain fatty acids, xenobiotics with carboxy groups, sulfates, glucuronide esters, lead, cadmium, zinc
Active transport	Cations, anions, sugars, vitamins, nucleosides (pyrimidines, uracil, and thymine, which may be in competition with 5-fluorouracil and 5-bromouracil), cobalt, manganese (which competes for the iron transportation system)
Pinocytosis	Long-chain lipids, vitamin B_{12} complex, azo dyes, maternal antibodies, botulinum toxin, hemagglutinins, phalloidins, *E. coli* endotoxins, virus particles

SAFETY STANDARDS FOR FOODS, FOOD INGREDIENTS, AND CONTAMINANTS

The Food, Drug, and Cosmetics Act

The FD&C Act presumes that traditionally consumed foods are safe if they are free of contaminants. To ban such foods, the FDA must have clear evidence that death or illness can be traced to the consumption of a particular food. The FD&C Act permits the addition of substances to food to accomplish a specific technical effect if the substance is determined to be Generally Recognized as Safe (GRAS). The act requires that scientific experts base a GRAS determination on the adequacy of safety, as shown through scientific procedures or through experience based on common use. If a food contains an unavoidable contaminant even with the use of Current Good Manufacturing Practices (CGMP), it may be declared unfit as food if the contaminant may render the food injurious to health. Foods containing *unavoidable* contaminants are not automatically banned, but the FDA has set some informal limits (called action levels) on the tolerable quantity of unavoidable contaminants.

In addition to allowing GRAS substances to be added to food, the act provides for a class of substances that are regulated food additives, which must be approved and regulated for their intended use by the FDA. Two distinct types of color additives have been approved for food use: those requiring certification by FDA chemists and those exempt from certification. Most certified colors approved for food use bear the prefix FD&C (such as FD&C Blue No. 1). Such color additives consist of structures that cannot be synthesized without a variety of impurities, and so must be carefully monitored and certified as safe before use in food products. Food colors that are exempt from certification are derived primarily from natural sources.

Methods Used to Evaluate the Safety of Foods, Ingredients, and Contaminants

Safety Evaluation of Direct Food and Color Additives—
The safety of any substance added to food must be established on the basis of specific intended conditions of use or uses in food. Factors that need to be considered include (1) the purpose for use of the substance, (2) the food to which the substance is added, (3) the concentration level used in the proposed foods, and (4) the population expected to consume the substance.

Exposure: The Estimated Daily Intake—
Exposure is most often referred to as an estimated daily intake (EDI) and is based on two factors: the daily intake (I) of the food in which the substance will be used and the concentration (C) of the substance in that food. In estimates of consumption and/or exposure, one must also consider other sources of consumption for the proposed intended use of the additive if it already is used in food for another purpose, occurs naturally in foods, or is used in nonfood sources (e.g., drugs, toothpaste, and lipstick).

Before approval, regulatory agencies require evidence that a food additive is safe for its intended use(s) and that the EDI is less than its acceptable daily intake (ADI). The ADI is generally based on results from animal toxicology studies.

Assignment of Concern Level (CL) and Required Testing—
Structures of functional groups in food additives are assigned to categories (A, B, and C) based on their relative harmful nature (category A is least harmful and category C is most harmful). Based on structure assignment and calculated exposure, a CL for a certain additive can be assigned (Table 30–3). An additive with a higher CL (CLIII) is more likely to be dangerous than one with a lower CL (CLI). Once the CL is established, a specific test battery is prescribed, as shown in Table 30–4.

Safety Determination of Indirect Food Additives—
Indirect food additives are substances that are not added directly to food but enter food by migrating from surfaces that contact food. These surfaces may be from packaging material (cans, paper, and plastic) or surfaces used in processing, holding, or transporting food. The level of overall consumption of these materials determines the testing required by the FDA to allow certain foods to be packaged in certain ways.

Safety Requirements for GRAS Substances—
The FD&C Act regards foods as GRAS when they are added to other food,

TABLE 30–3 Assignment of concern level.

Structure Category A	Structure Category B	Structure Category C	Concern Level
<0.05 ppm in the total diet (<0.0012 mg/kg per day)	<0.025 ppm in the total diet (<0.00063 mg/kg per day)	<0.0125 ppm in the total diet (<0.00031 mg/kg per day)	I
≥0.05 ppm in the total diet (≥0.0012 mg/kg per day)	≥0.025 ppm in the total diet (≥0.00063 mg/kg per day)	≥0.0125 ppm in the total diet (≥0.00031 mg/kg per day)	II
≥1 ppm in the total diet (≥0.025 mg/kg per day)	≥0.5 ppm in the total diet (≥0.0125 mg/kg per day)	≥0.25 ppm in the total diet (≥0.0063 mg/kg per day)	III

TABLE 30–4 **Summary of the toxicity tests recommended for different levels of concern.**[1]

Toxicity Studies[2]	Concern Levels		
	I	II	III
Short-term tests for genetic toxicity	X	X	X
Metabolism and pharmacokinetic studies		X	X
Short-term (28-day) toxicity studies with rodents	X[3]		
Subchronic (90-day) toxicity studies with rodents		X[3]	X[3]
Subchronic (90-day) toxicity studies with nonrodents		X[3]	
Reproduction studies with teratology phase		X[3]	X[3]
One-year toxicity studies with nonrodents			X
Carcinogenicity studies with rodents			X[4]
Chronic toxicity/carcinogenicity studies with rodents			X[4,5]

[1] http://www.cfsan.fda.gov/~redbook/redtoc93.html.
[2] Not including dose range-finding studies, if appropriate.
[3] Including neurotoxicity and immunotoxicity screens.
[4] An in utero phase is recommended for one of the two recommended carcinogenicity studies with rodents, preferably the study with rats.
[5] Combined study may be performed as separate studies.

such as green beans in vegetable soup. It also regards a number of food ingredients as GRAS. A list of examples of substances regarded as GRAS is given in Table 30–5. It is important to re-emphasize that GRAS substances, though *used* like food additives, are *not* food additives; this allows GRAS substances to be exempt from the premarket clearance restrictions applied to food additives.

Importance of the GRAS Concept

Transgenic Plant (and New Plant Varieties) Policy—Over the past decade, scientists have employed biotechnology to add one or more specific genes into crops like soybeans, corn, cotton, and canola, to improve pest and disease management, resulting in agronomic, economic, environmental, health, and social benefits for farmers. Irrespective of the breeding method used to produce a new plant variety, tests must be done to ensure

that the levels of nutrients or toxins in the plants have not changed and that the food is still safe to consume. In particular, tests on new plant varieties must demonstrate that any new proteins produced in the plant by genetic engineering are nontoxic and nonallergenic.

Nanotechnology—Nanotechnology offers some distinct advantages in delivery systems using micelles and liposomes and other technological advantages such as nanoemulsions (emulsion stability), biopolymeric nanoparticles (encapsulation technology), and cubosomes (solubilized hydrophobic, hydrophilic, and amphiphilic molecules, among other uses). Nanotechnology allows new and more efficient uses of old products by enhancing solubility, facilitating controlled release, improving bioavailability, and protecting labile substances (including micronutrients and bioactive substances) during processing, storage, and distribution.

TABLE 30–5 **Examples of GRAS substances and their functionality.**

CFR Number	Substance	Functionality
Substances Generally Recognized as Safe 21 CFR 182		
182.2122	Aluminum calcium silicate	Anticaking agent
182.8985	Zinc chloride	Nutrient supplement
Direct food substances affirmed as Generally Recognized as Safe 21 CFR 184		
184.1005	Acetic acid	Several
184.1355	Helium processing aid	
Indirect food substances affirmed as Generally Recognized as Safe 21 CFR 186		
186.1025	Caprylic acid	Antimicrobial
186.1374	Iron oxides	Ingredient of paper and paperboard

Bovine Spongiform Encephalopathy

Bovine spongiform encephalopathy (BSE, or mad cow disease) is transmitted by an infectious protein called a prion. Present in diseased cows, prions are transmitted to humans in meat that is improperly handled. BSE manifests clinically as neurologic deterioration leading to death.

CONCLUSION

Food consists of myriad chemical substances in addition to the macro- and micronutrients that are essential to life. The vast majority of food-borne illnesses are attributable to microbiologic contamination of food. Thus, the overwhelming concern for food safety must be directed toward preserving the microbiologic integrity of food.

BIBLIOGRAPHY

Barceloux DG: *Medical Toxicology of Natural Substances: Foods, Fungi, Medicinal Herbs, Plants, and Venomous Animals.* Hoboken, NJ: John Wiley & Sons, 2008.

Kotsonis F, Mackey M (eds): *Nutritional Toxicology.* New York: Taylor & Francis, 2002.

Omaye ST: *Food and Nutritional Toxicology.* Boca Raton, FL: CRC Press, 2004.

Pussa T: *Principles of Food Toxicology.* Boca Raton, FL: CRC Press, 2008.

QUESTIONS

1. Which of the following statements regarding food complexity is FALSE?
   a. Many flavor additives are nonnutrient substances.
   b. Foods are subjected to environmental forces that alter their chemical composition.
   c. There are more nonnutrient chemicals in food than nutrient chemicals.
   d. A majority of nonnutrient chemicals are added to food by humans.
   e. Food is more variable and complex than most other substances to which humans are exposed.

2. Which of the following foods contains the most nonnutrient chemicals?
   a. beef.
   b. banana.
   c. tomato.
   d. orange juice.
   e. Cheddar cheese.

3. Which of the following is considered an indirect food additive?
   a. nitrites.
   b. plastic.
   c. food coloring.
   d. EDTA.
   e. citric acid.

4. Estimated daily intake (EDI) is based on which of the following?
   a. metabolic rate.
   b. daily intake.
   c. substance concentration in a food item.
   d. body mass index.
   e. concentration of substance in a food item and daily intake.

5. Which of the following is NOT characteristic of IgE-mediated food allergies?
   a. urticaria.
   b. wheezing.
   c. hypertension.
   d. nausea.
   e. shock.

6. Which of the following wheat proteins is famous for being allergenic?
   a. casein.
   b. ovalbumin.
   c. livetin.
   d. gluten.
   e. glycinin.

7. Which of the following foods contains a chemical that causes hypertension by acting as a noradrenergic stimulant?
   a. cheese.
   b. peanuts.
   c. shrimp.
   d. chocolate.
   e. beets.

8. What is the mechanism of saxitoxin, found in shellfish?
   a. interference with ion channels.
   b. direct neurotoxicity.
   c. interference with DNA replication.
   d. binding to hemoglobin.
   e. interference with a stimulatory G protein.

9. Which of the following foods can cause a reaction that mimics iodine deficiency?
   a. chocolate.
   b. shellfish.
   c. peanuts.
   d. fava beans.
   e. cabbage.

10. Improperly canned foods can be contaminated with which of the following bacteria, causing respiratory paralysis?
    a. *C. perfringens.*
    b. *R. rickettsii.*
    c. *S. aureus.*
    d. *C. botulinum.*
    e. *E. coli.*

Analytic/Forensic Toxicology

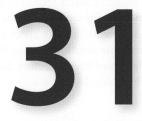

Alphonse Poklis

ANALYTIC TOXICOLOGY

ANALYTIC ROLE IN FORENSIC TOXICOLOGY

TOXICOLOGIC INVESTIGATION OF A POISON DEATH

CRIMINAL POISONING OF THE LIVING

FORENSIC URINE DRUG TESTING

HUMAN PERFORMANCE TESTING

COURTROOM TESTIMONY

ANALYTIC ROLE IN CLINICAL TOXICOLOGY

ANALYTIC ROLE IN THERAPEUTIC MONITORING

ANALYTIC ROLE IN BIOLOGICAL MONITORING

CONCLUSION

K E Y   P O I N T S

- Analytic toxicology involves the application of the tools of analytic chemistry to the qualitative and/or quantitative estimation of chemicals that may exert adverse effects on living organisms.
- Forensic toxicology involves the use of toxicology for the purposes of the law; by far the most common application is to identify any chemical that may serve as a causative agent in inflicting death or injury on humans or in causing damage to property.

- The toxicologic investigation of a poison death involves (1) obtaining the case history in as much detail as possible and gathering suitable specimens, (2) conducting suitable toxicologic analyses based on the available specimens, and (3) the interpretation of the analytic findings.
- The toxicologist as an expert witness may provide two objectives: testimony and opinion. Objective testimony usually involves a description of analytic methods and findings. When a toxicologist testifies as to the interpretation of analytic results, that toxicologist is offering an "opinion."

ANALYTIC TOXICOLOGY

Analytic toxicology applies the tools of analytic chemistry to the qualitative and/or quantitative estimation of chemicals that may exert adverse effects on living organisms. Forensic toxicology involves the use of toxicology for the purposes of the law; by far the most common application is to identify any chemical that may serve as a causative agent in inflicting death or injury on humans or in causing damage to property. A systematic approach, a reliance on the practical experience of generations of forensic toxicologists, and use of the sophisticated tools of analytic chemistry provide the data needed to understand better the hazards of toxic substances.

In 1873 in his *Elements de Toxicologie*, Chapuis described a system of classifying toxic agents by their origin or nature into several categories: gases, volatile substances, corrosive agents, metals, anions and nonmetals, nonvolatile organic substances, and miscellaneous. Closely related to this descriptive classification is the method for separating a toxic agent from the matrix in which it is embedded. The agent of interest may exist in a matrix of a simple solution or may be bound to protein and other cellular constituents; before analysis can be done, the agent must be isolated.

ANALYTIC ROLE IN FORENSIC TOXICOLOGY

The duties of a forensic toxicologist in postmortem investigations include the qualitative and quantitative analyses of drugs or poisons in biological specimens collected at autopsy and the interpretation of the analytic findings in regard to the physiologic and behavioral effects of the detected chemicals on the deceased at the time of death.

Establishing the cause of death rests with the medical examiner, coroner, or pathologist, but success in arriving at the correct conclusion often depends on the combined efforts of the pathologist and the toxicologist. The cause of death in cases of poisoning cannot be proved beyond contention without a toxicologic analysis that establishes the presence of the toxicant in the tissues and body fluids of the deceased. Additionally, a toxicologist can furnish valuable evidence concerning the circumstances surrounding a death. Such cases commonly involve demonstrating the presence of intoxicating concentrations of ethanol in victims of automotive or industrial accidents, or determining concentrations of carbon monoxide in fire victims in order to determine whether the deceased died as a result of the fire or was dead before the fire started.

TOXICOLOGIC INVESTIGATION OF A POISON DEATH

The toxicologic investigation of a poison death may be divided into three steps: (1) obtaining the case history in as much detail as possible and gathering suitable specimens, (2) conducting suitable toxicologic analyses based on the available specimens, and (3) the interpretation of the analytic findings. Knowledge of drug biotransformation often is essential before analysis is performed because the metabolites may provide the only evidence that a drug or poison has been administered. Specific questions may be answered, such as the route of administration, the dose administered, and whether the concentration of the toxicant present was sufficient to cause death or alter the decedent's actions enough to cause his or her death.

CRIMINAL POISONING OF THE LIVING

Forensic toxicologists have become more and more involved in the analysis of specimens obtained from living victims of criminal poisonings. This increase in testing has arisen from two types of cases: (1) administration of drugs to incapacitate

TABLE 31–1 Distribution of drugs of abuse encountered in urine specimens in 578 cases of alleged sexual assault.

Rank	Drug/Drug Group	Incidence	Percent of Cases[*]
1	No drugs found	167	29
2	Ethanol	148	26
3	Benzodiazepines	70	12
4	Marijuana	67	12
5	Amphetamines	41	7
6	Gamma-hydroxybutyrate	24	4
7	Opiate (morphine/codeine)	20	4
8	Other drugs	13	3

Source: Data from ElSohly MA, et al: *Analysis of flunitrazepam metabolites and other substances in alleged cases of sexual assault. Presentation at the 50th Anniversary Meeting of the American Academy of Forensic Sciences*, San Francisco, CA, February 13, 1997.
[*]Percentages do not add to 100% due to rounding.

victims of kidnapping, robbery, or sexual assault and (2) poisoning as a form of child abuse.

Common drugs of abuse or other psychoactive drugs that are often involved in cases of alleged sexual assault are listed in Table 31–1. The many potent inductive agents administered prior to general anesthesia are of particular concern. Many of these drugs, such as benzodiazepines and phenothiazines, are available today through illegal and legal sources. When administered surreptitiously, they cause sedation and incapacitate the victim in addition to producing amnesia, without causing severe central nervous system depression. These cases often present a difficult analytic challenge to the toxicologist because the drug has usually been eliminated from the body by the time the victim can bring forth an allegation.

Poisoning as a form of child abuse involves the deliberate administration of toxic or injurious substances to a child. Common agents used to intentionally poison children have included syrup of ipecac, table salt, laxatives, diuretics, antidepressants, sedative-hypnotics, and narcotics. The poison may be given to an infant to stop its crying or be force-fed to older children as a form of punishment. Sophisticated gas chromatograph/mass spectroscopy testing methods may be required to detect such agents.

FORENSIC URINE DRUG TESTING

Concerns about the potentially adverse consequences of substance abuse both for the individual and for society have led to widespread urine analysis for the detection of controlled or illicit drugs. Forensic urine drug testing (FUDT) differs from other areas of forensic toxicology in that urine is the only specimen analyzed and testing is performed for a limited number of drugs. Initial testing is performed by immunoassays on high-speed, large-throughput analyzers. A confirmation analysis in FUDT-certified laboratories is then performed.

Many individuals who are subject to regulated urine testing have devised techniques to mask their drug use either by physiologic means such as the ingestion of diuretics or by attempting to adulterate the specimen directly with bleach, vinegar, or other products that interfere with the initial immunoassay tests. Thus, specimens are routinely tested for adulteration by checking urinary pH, creatinine, and specific gravity and noting any unusual color or smell. Recently a mini-industry has developed to sell various products that are alleged to "fool drug testers" by interfering with the initial or confirmatory drug test. Thus, FUDT laboratories now routinely test not only for drugs of abuse, but also for a wide variety of chemical adulterants. In most instances, a positive test result for adulteration has as serious a consequence as a positive drug test.

HUMAN PERFORMANCE TESTING

Forensic toxicology activities also include the determination of the presence of ethanol and other drugs and chemicals in blood, breath, or other specimens and the evaluation of their role in modifying human performance and behavior. The most common application of human performance testing is to determine driving under the influence of ethanol (DUI) or drugs (DUID). The threshold blood alcohol concentration (BAC) for diminished driving performance of these complex functions in many individuals is as low as 0.04 g/dL, the equivalent of ingestion of two beers within an hour's time. The statutory definition of DUI in the United States is a BAC of either 0.08 or 0.10 g/dL, depending on the particular state law. These concentrations are consistent with diminished performance of complex driving skills in the vast majority of individuals.

During the past decade, there has been growing concern about the deleterious effects of drugs other than ethanol on driving performance. The highest drug-use accident rates are associated with the use of such illicit or controlled drugs as cocaine, benzodiazepines, marijuana, and phencyclidine. Proving that drug use was important in a driving accident is difficult, and there are legal and scientific problems concerning drug concentrations and driving impairment that need to be resolved.

COURTROOM TESTIMONY

The forensic toxicologist often is called upon to testify in legal proceedings. The toxicologist is referred to as an "expert witness." An expert witness may provide two types of testimony: objective testimony and "opinion." Objective testimony by a toxicologist usually involves a description of his or her analytic methods and findings. When a toxicologist testifies as to the interpretation of his or her analytic results or those of others, that toxicologist is offering an "opinion." An expert witness is called to provide informed assistance to the jury. The jury, not the expert witness, determines the guilt or innocence of the defendant.

ANALYTIC ROLE IN CLINICAL TOXICOLOGY

In a clinical setting, analytic toxicology can aid in the diagnosis and treatment of toxic incidents as well as in monitoring the effectiveness of treatment regimens by clearly identifying the nature of the toxic exposure and measuring the amount of the toxic substance that has been absorbed. This information, together with the clinical state of the patient, permits a clinician to relate the signs and symptoms observed to the anticipated effects of the toxic agent.

A cardinal rule in the treatment of poisoning cases is to remove any unabsorbed material, limit the absorption of additional poison, and hasten its elimination. The clinical toxicology laboratory assists by monitoring the amount of the toxic agent remaining in circulation or measuring what is excreted. Commonly encountered intoxicants in emergency toxicology testing and the rapid methodologies to detect their presence in serum and/or urine specimens are presented in Table 31–2.

Primary examples of the usefulness of emergency toxicology testing are the rapid quantitative determination of acetaminophen, salicylate, alcohols, and glycol serum concentrations in instances of suspected overdose. Ethanol is the most common agent encountered in emergency toxicology; serum values are important in the assessment of behavioral and neurologic function. Intoxications from accidental or deliberate ingestion of other alcohols or glycols—such as methanol from windshield deicer or paint thinner, isopropanol from rubbing alcohol, and ethylene glycol from antifreeze—are also encountered in emergency departments.

The utilization of the analytic clinical toxicology laboratory has increased enormously in recent years. Typically, the laboratory performs testing for the emergency department and other medical departments, because drugs and toxic agents may be a consideration in diagnosis in many medical problems.

ANALYTIC ROLE IN THERAPEUTIC MONITORING

Historically, the administration of drugs for long-term therapy was based largely on experience. If the drug seemed ineffective, the dose was increased; if toxicity developed, the dose was decreased or the frequency of dosing was altered. The factors responsible for individual variability in responses to drug therapy include the rate and extent of drug absorption, distribution and binding in body tissues and fluids, rate of metabolism and excretion, pathological conditions, and interaction with other drugs. Monitoring of the plasma or serum concentration at regular intervals will detect deviations from the average serum concentration, which indicates that dosage correction is needed.

In a given patient, the administration of the same dose of a drug at regular intervals eventually produces a steady-state

TABLE 31–2 Commonly encountered drugs and methods for analysis in emergency toxicology.

Drug/Drug Group	Specimen	Analytic Method
Drugs of <u>abuse</u> (amphetamines, cocaine, opiates, phencyclidine)	Urine	Immunoassays
Ethanol	Serum	GC
Benzodiazepines	Urine/serum	Immunoassay/GC/MS
Acetaminophen, salicylates	Serum	Immunoassay/HPLC
Tricyclic antidepressants	Serum	Immunoassay/HPLC
Ibuprofen	Urine/serum	TLC/HPLC
Dextropropoxyphene	Urine	Immunoassay
Fluoxetine	Urine/serum	TLC/HPLC
Barbiturates (50 percent phenobarbital)	Urine/serum	Immunoassay/GC
Diphenhydramine	Urine	TLC

Note: GC = gas chromatography; GC/MS = gas chromatography/mass spectrometry; HPLC = high-pressure liquid chromatography; TLC = thin-layer chromatography.
Source: Data from Year-End 1998 Emergency Department Data from the Drug Abuse Warning Network, Department of Health and Human Services, December 1999.

condition (Figure 31–1). Monitoring of steady-state drug concentrations assures that an effective concentration is present. Appropriate situations for therapeutic drug monitoring are presented in Table 31–3.

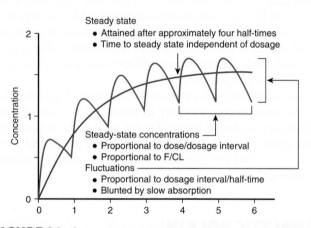

FIGURE 31–1 Fundamental pharmacokinetic relationships for the repeated administration of drugs. The red line is the pattern of drug accumulation during the repeated administration of a drug at intervals equal to its elimination half-time, when drug absorption is 10 times as rapid as elimination. As the relative rate of absorption increases, the concentration maxima approach 2 and minima approach 1 during steady state. The blue line depicts the pattern during administration of equivalent dosage by continuous intravenous infusion. Curves are based on the one-compartment model. Average concentration (Css) when steady state is attained during intermittent drug administration is Css = $F \times$ dose/Cl $\times T$, where F is the fractional bioavailability of the dose and T the dosage interval (time). By substitution of infusion rate for $F \times$ dose/T, the formula provides the concentration maintained at steady state during continuous intravenous infusion. (Reproduced with permission from Brunton LL, Lazzo JS, Parker KL: *Goodman & Gilman's the pharmacological basis of therapeutics*, 11th edition. New York: McGraw-Hill, 2006.)

Because the nature of drugs is varied, many different analytic techniques may be applied. Drugs that are commonly monitored during therapy, usual effective therapeutic serum concentrations, panic values, and typical analytic methodologies applied to serum measurements are presented in Table 31–4. The term *panic value* denotes a serum drug concentration associated with potentially serious toxicity. In clinical laboratories, the panic value alerts the toxicologist to *immediately* notify the treating physician of the test result.

TABLE 31–3 Appropriate use of therapeutic drug monitoring.

Use	Examples
Optimize efficacy while minimizing toxicity	
Optimal SDC for clinical effect	
Routine, prophylactic peak serum	Aminoglycosides
Poor patient response Suspected toxicity	Antiarrhythmics, antidepressants
Resolve complicating factors	
Patient characteristics	Age, smoking, noncompliance
Disease	Renal failure, hepatic disorders
Drug interactions	Induction or inhibition of drug metabolism
Sudden change in physiologic state	Improved cardiac function on lidocaine therapy increases clearance
Dosage regimen design	
Individualize future dosing (single SDC)	
Pharmacokinetic profiling (multiple SDC)	Ideal dosage for aminoglycosides
Follow-up SDC	Single steady-state lidocaine
Verify therapy	Medicolegal lithium

Note: SDC = serum drug concentration.

TABLE 31–4 Drugs commonly indicated for therapeutic monitoring.

Therapeutic Use Drug	Effective Serum Range, mg/L	Panic Value, mg/L	Analytic Methodology
Antiarrythmic			
Digoxin	0.0005–0.002	0.0024	Immunoassay
Procainamide	4–10	12	Immunoassay
NAPA	5–30	40	Immunoassay
Anticonvulsant			
Carbamazepine	4–12	15	Immunoassay
Gabapentin	2–15	20	GC
Lamotrigine	0.5–8	10	HPLC
Phenobarbital	15–30	50	Immunoassay
Phenytoin	10–20	40	Immunoassay
Tropiramate	2–10	Undetermined	GC
Valproic acid	50–100	200	GC
Antidepressants			
Amitriptyline	0.08–0.250	0.5	HPLC
Desipramine	0.125–0.30	0.4	HPLC
Nortriptyline	0.08–0.250	0.5	HPLC
Antimicrobials			
Tobramycin	0.5–1.5 (trough)	2	Immunoassay
	5–10 (peak)	12	Immunoassay
Vancomycin	5–10 (trough)		Immunoassay
	30–40 (peak)	90	Immunoassay
Immunosuppressant			
Cyclosporine	0.1 (trough, whole blood)		HPLC
Neonatal apnea			
Caffeine	8–20	50	HPLC

Note: GC = gas chromatography; HPLC = high-pressure liquid chromatography.

ANALYTIC ROLE IN BIOLOGICAL MONITORING

Biological monitoring of a worker directly can be a better indicator of exposure than simply monitoring the environment, because the monitoring can show what has actually been absorbed. Often, environmental exposures are to a mixture of chemicals and/or those compounds that are converted to physiologically important metabolites. Thus, analytic methods must be capable of separating a family of chemical agents and their major metabolites. Additionally, methods must be sufficiently specific and sensitive to measure minute concentrations of the compounds in complex biological matrices.

Besides measuring the chemical or its metabolites in the body fluids, hair, or breath of the worker, other, more indirect methods may be employed. Agents that interact with macromolecules may form adducts that persist for long periods. These adducts can be sampled periodically and potentially can serve as a means of integrating exposure to certain substances over long periods. For example, adducts of ethylene oxide with DNA or hemoglobin have been noted in workers. Another approach that is useful in biological monitoring is to measure changes of normal metabolites induced by xenobiotics. Although monitoring the alteration of the urinary excretion of these metabolites may not indicate exposure to specific substances, this technique can be used in a generic fashion to flag a potentially harmful exposure. The early recognition of a toxicologic problem may permit the protection of a worker before irreversible effects occur.

CONCLUSION

Though analytic techniques expand in complexity and improve in reliability, forensic toxicologists continue focusing on conducting unequivocal identification of toxic substances in such a manner that the results can withstand a legal challenge. Substance abuse, designer drugs, increased potency of therapeutic agents, and concern about pollution and the safety and health of workers will continue to present challenges to the analyst's skills.

BIBLIOGRAPHY

Flanagan RJ, Taylor AA, Watson ID, Whelpton R: *Fundamentals of Analytical Toxicology.* Hoboken, NJ: John Wiley & Sons, 2007.

Jickells S, Negrusz (eds): *Clarke's Analytical Forensic Toxicology.* Chicago: Pharmaceutical Press, 2008.

Kulpmann WR (ed): *Clinical Toxicological Analysis: Procedures, Results, Interpretation.* Hoboken, NJ: John Wiley & Sons, 2009.

QUESTIONS

1. Which of the following is most commonly used as a drug of sexual assault?
   a. narcotics.
   b. amphetamines.
   c. benzodiazepines.
   d. ethanol.
   e. antidepressants.

2. All of the following statements regarding analytic/forensic toxicology are true EXCEPT:
   a. Analytic toxicology uses analytic chemistry to characterize a chemical's adverse effect on an organism.
   b. Medical examiners and coroners are most important in determining cause of death.
   c. Tissues and body fluids are vital in forensic toxicology.
   d. Forensic toxicology is used for purposes of the law.
   e. Chapuis first characterized a system for classifying toxic agents.

3. Which of the following criteria is NOT routinely used to check for adulteration of drug urine analysis?
   a. urea.
   b. pH.
   c. color.
   d. specific gravity.
   e. creatinine.

4. Which blood alcohol concentration (BAC) is most commonly used as the statutory definition of DUI?
   a. 0.04.
   b. 0.06.
   c. 0.08.
   d. 0.12.
   e. 0.16.

5. Which of the following drugs is NOT properly matched with its most common analytic method?
   a. benzodiazepines—GC/MS.
   b. ibuprofen—TLC/HPLC.
   c. amphetamines—immunoassays.
   d. barbiturates—GC/immunoassays.
   e. ethanol—immunoassays.

6. For which of the following drugs is serum NOT used during toxicology testing?
   a. ethanol.
   b. cocaine.
   c. aspirin.
   d. barbiturates.
   e. ibuprofen.

7. Which of the following is LEAST important in determining variability in response to drug therapy?
   a. drug interactions.
   b. distribution in body tissue.
   c. body mass index.
   d. pathological conditions.
   e. rate of metabolism.

8. Which of the following statements is FALSE regarding steady state?
   a. Steady-state concentrations are proportional to the dose/dosage interval.
   b. Steady state is attained after approximately four half-lives.
   c. The steady-state concentrations are proportional to F/Cl.
   d. Monitoring of steady-state drug concentration assumes that an effective concentration is present.
   e. Fluctuations in concentration are increased by slow drug absorption.

9. Which of the following is an indirect method of measuring a chemical or its metabolite?
   a. blood test.
   b. hair sample.
   c. urinalysis.
   d. hemoglobin adduct detection.
   e. breath analysis.

10. Which of the following statements regarding analytic/forensic toxicology is TRUE?
    a. Antidepressants are commonly used to incapacitate victims.
    b. It is easy to test for and prove that marijuana is a factor in an automobile accident.
    c. Heroin is the drug most commonly encountered in emergency toxicology.
    d. Toxicologists can play an important role in courtroom testimonies.
    e. Ethanol intoxication often results in death.

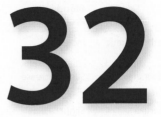

Clinical Toxicology

Louis R. Cantilena Jr.

KEY POINTS

- Clinical toxicology encompasses the expertise in the specialties of medical toxicology, applied toxicology, and clinical poison information.

- Important components of the initial clinical encounter with a poisoned patient include stabilization of the patient, clinical evaluation (history, physical, laboratory, and radiology), prevention of further toxin absorption, enhancement of toxin elimination, administration of antidote, and supportive care with clinical follow-up.

CLINICAL STRATEGY FOR TREATMENT OF THE POISONED PATIENT

The following general steps represent important components of the initial clinical encounter with a poisoned patient:

1. stabilization of the patient;
2. clinical evaluation (history, physical, laboratory, and radiology);
3. prevention of further toxin absorption;
4. enhancement of toxin elimination;
5. administration of antidote;
6. supportive care and clinical follow-up.

Clinical Stabilization

The first priority in the treatment of the poisoned patient is stabilization. Assessment of the vital signs and the effectiveness of respiration and circulation are the initial concerns. Some toxins or drugs can cause seizures early in the course of presentation. The steps and clinical procedures incorporated to stabilize a

TABLE 32–1   Clinical features of toxic syndromes.

	Blood Pressure	Pulse	Temperature	Pupils	Lungs	Abdomen	Neurologic
Sympathomimetic	Increase	Increase	Slight increase	Mydriasis	NC	NC	Hyperalert, increased reflexes
Anticholinergic	Slight increase or NC	Increase	Increase	Mydriasis	NC	Decreased bowel sounds	Altered mental status
Cholinergic	Slight decrease or NC	Decrease	NC	Miosis	Increased bronchial sounds	Increased bowel sounds	Altered mental status
Opioid	Decrease	Decrease	Decrease	Miosis	NC or rales (late)	Decreased bowel sounds	Decreased level of consciousness

critically ill, poisoned patient are numerous and include, if appropriate, support of ventilation, circulation, and oxygenation. In critically ill patients, sometimes treatment interventions must be initiated before a patient is truly stable.

Clinical History in the Poisoned Patient

The primary goal of taking a medical history in poisoned patients is to determine, if possible, the substance ingested or the substance to which the patient has been exposed as well as the extent and time of exposure. In the setting of a suicide attempt, patients may not provide any history or may give incorrect information so as to increase the possibility that they will successfully bring harm to themselves. Information sources commonly employed in this setting include family members, emergency medical technicians who were at the scene, a pharmacist who can sometimes provide a listing of prescriptions recently filled, or an employer who can disclose what chemicals are available in the work environment.

In estimating the level of exposure to the poison, one generally should maximize the possible dose received. That is, one should assume that the entire prescription bottle contents were ingested, that the entire bottle of liquid was consumed, or that the highest possible concentration of airborne contaminant was present in the case of a patient poisoned by inhalation.

With an estimate of dose, the toxicologist can refer to various information sources to determine what the range of expected clinical effects might be from the exposure. The estimation of expected toxicity greatly assists with the triage of poisoned patients. Estimating the timing of the exposure to the poison is frequently the most difficult aspect of the clinical history in the setting of treatment of the poisoned patient.

Taking an accurate history in the poisoned patient can be challenging and in some cases unsuccessful. When the history is unobtainable, the clinical toxicologist is left without a clear picture of the exposure history. In this setting, the treatment proceeds empirically as an "unknown ingestion" poisoning.

Physical Examination

A thorough physical examination is required to assess the patient's condition, categorize the patient's mental status, and, if altered, determine possible additional causes such as trauma or central nervous system infection. Whenever possible, the patient's physical examination parameters are categorized into broad classes referred to as *toxic syndromes,* constellations of clinical signs that, taken together, are likely associated with exposure from certain classes of toxicologic agents. Categorization of the patient's presentation into toxic syndromes allows for the initiation of rational treatment based on the most likely category of toxin responsible, even if the exact nature of the toxin is unknown. Table 32–1 lists clinical features of the major toxic syndromes. Occasionally a characteristic odor detected on the poisoned patient's breath or clothing may point toward exposure or poisoning by a specific agent (Table 32–2).

Laboratory Evaluation

Table 32–3 lists drugs or other chemicals that are typically available for immediate measurement in a hospital facility. As one can see, the number of agents for which detection is possible in the rapid-turnaround clinical setting is extremely limited compared with the number of possible agents that can poison patients. This further emphasizes the importance of recognizing clinical syndromes for poisoning and for the clinical toxicologist to initiate general treatment and supportive care for the patient with poisoning from an unknown substance.

TABLE 32–2   Characteristic odors associated with poisonings.

Odor	Potential Poison
Bitter almonds	Cyanide
Eggs	Hydrogen sulfide, mercaptans
Garlic	Arsenic, organophosphates, DMSO, thallium
Mothballs	Naphthalene, camphor
Vinyl	Ethchlorvynol
Wintergreen	Methylsalicylate

TABLE 32–3 Drugs commonly measured in a hospital setting on a stat basis.

Acetaminophen	Osmolality
Acetone	Phenobarbital
Carbamazepine	Phenytoin
Carboxyhemoglobin	Procainamide/NAPA
Digoxin	Quinidine
Ethanol	Salicylates
Gentamycin	Theophylline
Iron	Tobramycin
Lithium	Valproic acid
Methemoglobin	

TABLE 32–4 Differential diagnosis of metabolic acidosis with elevated anion gap: "AT MUD PILES."

A	Alcohol (ethanol ketoacidosis)
T	Toluene
M	Methanol
U	Uremia
D	Diabetic ketoacidosis
P	Paraldehyde
I	Iron, isoniazid
L	Lactic acid
E	Ethylene glycol
S	Salicylate

For the substances that can be measured on a rapid-turnaround basis in an emergency department setting, the quantitative measurement can often provide both prognostic and therapeutic guidance.

Predictive relationships of drug plasma concentration and clinical outcome and/or suggested concentrations that require therapeutic interventions are available for several agents including salicylates, lithium, digoxin, iron, phenobarbital, and theophylline. Some authors have identified "action levels" or toxic threshold values for the measured plasma concentrations of various drugs or chemicals. Generally, these values represent mean concentrations of the respective substance that have been retrospectively shown to produce a significant harmful effect.

Because of the limited clinical availability of "diagnostic" laboratory tests for poisons, toxicologists utilize specific, routinely obtained clinical laboratory data—especially the anion gap and the osmol gap—to determine what poisons may have been ingested. An abnormal anion or osmol gap suggests a differential diagnosis for significant exposure. Both calculations are used as diagnostic tools when the clinical history suggests poisoning and the patient's condition is consistent with exposure to agents known to cause elevations of these parameters (i.e., metabolic acidosis, altered mental status, etc.).

The anion gap is calculated as the difference between the serum Na ion concentration and the sum of the serum Cl and HCO$_3$ ion concentrations. A normal anion gap is <12. When there is laboratory evidence of metabolic acidosis, the finding of an elevated anion gap would suggest systemic toxicity from a relatively limited number of agents (Table 32–4).

The second calculated parameter from clinical chemistry values is the osmol gap. The osmol gap is calculated as the numerical difference between the measured serum osmolality and the serum osmolarity calculated from the clinical chemistry measurements of the serum sodium ion, glucose, and blood urea nitrogen (BUN) concentrations. The normal osmol gap is <10 mOsm. An elevated osmol gap suggests the presence of an osmotically active substance (methanol, ethanol, ethylene glycol, and isopropanol) in the plasma that is not accounted for by the sodium ion, glucose, or BUN concentrations.

Radiographic Examination

The use of clinical radiographs to visualize drug overdose or poison ingestions is relatively limited. Generally, plain radiographs can detect a significant amount of ingested oral medication containing ferrous or potassium salts. In addition, certain formulations that have an enteric coating or certain types of sustained release products are radiopaque as well.

The most useful radiographs ordered in a case of overdose or poisoning include the chest and abdominal radiographs and the computed tomography (CT) study of the head. The abdominal radiograph has been used to detect recent lead paint ingestion in children, and ingestion of halogenated hydrocarbons, such as carbon tetrachloride or chloroform, that may be visualized as a radiopaque liquid in the gut lumen. Finally, abdominal plain radiographs have been helpful in the setting where foreign bodies are detected in the gastrointestinal tract, such as would be seen in a "body packer," or one who smuggles illegal substances by swallowing latex or plastic storage vesicles filled with cocaine or some other substance. Occasionally these storage devices rupture and the drug is released into the gastrointestinal tract, with serious and sometimes fatal results.

Plain radiography and other types of diagnostic imaging in clinical toxicology can also be extremely valuable for the diagnosis of toxin-induced pathology. For example, the detection of drug-induced noncardiac pulmonary edema is associated with serious intoxication with salicylates and opioid agonists. Another example of the use of radiologic imaging in clinical toxicology is with CT of the brain. Significant exposure to carbon monoxide (CO) has been associated with CT lesions of the brain consisting of low-density areas in the cerebral white matter and in the basal ganglia, especially the globus pallidus.

Prevention of Further Poison Absorption

During the early phases of poison treatment or intervention for a toxic exposure via the oral, inhalational, or topical route, a significant opportunity exists to prevent further absorption of the poison by minimizing the total amount that reaches the systemic circulation. For toxins presented by the inhalational route, the main intervention used to prevent further absorption involves removing the patient from the environment where the toxin is found and providing adequate ventilation and oxygenation for the patient. For topical exposures, clothing containing the toxin must be removed and the skin washed with water and mild soap.

The four primary methods to prevent continued absorption of an oral poison are induction of emesis with syrup of ipecac, gastric lavage, oral administration of activated charcoal, and whole bowel irrigation. Although potentially indicated for individuals who are hours away from a medical facility, syrup of ipecac use for induction of emesis in the treatment of a potentially toxic ingestion has declined. Risk of cardio- and neurotoxicity and lower effectiveness at removing the toxicant than desired limit its use. Likewise, gastric lavage, which involves placing an orogastric tube into the stomach and aspirating fluid, and then cyclically instilling fluid and aspirating until the effluent is clear, is limited by the risk of aspiration during the lavage procedure and evidence of limited effectiveness.

For many years, orally administered activated charcoal has been routinely incorporated into the initial treatment of a patient poisoned by the oral route. The term *activated* means that the charcoal has been specially processed to be more efficient at adsorbing toxins.

The usefulness of whole bowel irrigation for a poisoned patient is very limited. Considerable absorption of the toxicant can occur before the procedure "washes" the lumen of the GI tract clear of unabsorbed material.

Enhancement of Poison Elimination

There are several methods available to enhance the elimination of specific poisons or drugs once they have been absorbed into the systemic circulation. The primary methods employed for this use today include alkalinization of the urine, hemodialysis, hemoperfusion, hemofiltration, plasma exchange or exchange transfusion, and serial oral activated charcoal.

The use of urinary alkalinization results in enhancement of the renal clearance of weak acids. The basic principle is to increase the pH of urinary filtrate to a level sufficient to ionize the weak acid and prevent renal tubule reabsorption of the molecule. Although there are potentially similar advantages to be gained from acidification of the urine in order to enhance the clearance of weak bases, this method is not used because acute renal failure and acid–base and electrolyte disturbances are associated with acidification.

The dialysis technique, either peritoneal dialysis or hemodialysis, relies on passage of the toxic agent through a semipermeable dialysis membrane so that it can subsequently be

TABLE 32–5 Agents for which hemodialysis has been shown effective as a treatment modality for poisoning.

Alcohols	Meprobamate
Antibiotics	Metformin
Boric acid	Paraldehyde
Bromide	Phenobarbital
Calcium	Potassium
Chloral hydrate	Salicylates
Fluorides	Strychnine
Iodides	Theophylline
Isoniazid	Thiocyanates
Lithium	Valproic acid

removed. Hemodialysis incorporates a blood pump to pass blood next to a dialysis membrane, which allows agents permeable to the membrane to pass through and reach equilibrium. Some drugs are bound to plasma proteins and so cannot pass through the dialysis membrane; others are distributed mainly to the tissues and so are not concentrated in the blood, making dialysis impractical. Hemodialysis has been shown to be clinically effective in the treatment of poisoning by the drugs and toxins shown in Table 32–5.

The technique of hemoperfusion is similar to hemodialysis except there is no dialysis membrane or dialysate involved in the procedure. The patient's blood is pumped through a perfusion cartridge, where it is in direct contact with adsorptive material (usually activated charcoal). Protein binding does not significantly interfere with removal by hemoperfusion.

The technique of hemofiltration is relatively new in clinical toxicology applications. As in the case of hemodialysis, the patient's blood is delivered through hollow fiber tubes and an ultrafiltrate of plasma is removed by hydrostatic pressure from the blood side of the membrane. The perfusion pressure for the technique is generated either by the patient's blood pressure (for arteriovenous hemofiltration) or by a blood pump (for venovenous hemofiltration). Needed fluid and electrolytes removed in the ultrafiltrate are replaced intravenously with sterile solutions.

The use of either plasma exchange or exchange transfusions has been relatively limited in the field of clinical toxicology. Although the techniques afford the potential advantage of being able to remove high-molecular-weight and/or plasma protein-bound toxins, their clinical utility in poison treatment has been limited. Plasma exchange, or pheresis, involves removal of plasma and replacement with frozen donor plasma, albumin, or both with intravenous fluid. The risks and complications of this technique include allergic-type reactions, infectious complications, and hypotension. Exchange transfusion involves replacement of a patient's blood volume with donor blood. The use of this technique in poison treatment is uncommon and

TABLE 32–6 Agents for which activated charcoal has been shown as an effective means of enhanced body clearance.

Carbamazepine
Dapsone
Digoxin
Digitoxin
Nadolol
Phenobarbital
Salicylates
Theophylline

mostly confined to inadvertent drug overdose in a neonate or premature infant.

Serial oral administration of activated charcoal, also referred to as Multiple-dose Activated Charcoal (MDAC), has been shown to increase the systemic clearance of various drug substances. The mechanism for the observed augmentation of nonrenal clearance caused by repeated doses of oral charcoal is thought to be transluminal efflux of the drug from the blood to the charcoal passing through the gastrointestinal tract. The activated charcoal in the gut lumen serves as a "sink" for the toxin. A concentration gradient is maintained and the toxin passes continuously into the gut lumen, where it is adsorbed to charcoal. In addition, MDAC is thought to produce its beneficial effect by interrupting the enteroenteric–enterohepatic circulation of drugs. The technique involves continuing oral administration of activated charcoal beyond the initial dosage every 2 to 4 h. An alternative technique is to give a loading dose of activated charcoal via an orogastric tube or nasogastric tube, followed by a continuous infusion intragastrically. A list of agents for which MDAC has been shown to be an effective means of enhanced body clearance is given in Table 32–6.

Use of Antidotes in Poisoning

A relatively small number of specific antidotes are available for clinical use in the treatment of poisoning. The U.S. Food and Drug Administration (FDA) has placed incentives for sponsors to develop drugs for rare diseases or conditions through the Orphan Drug Act.

The mechanism of action of various antidotes is quite different. For example, a chelating agent or Fab fragments specific to digoxin will work by physically binding the toxin, preventing the toxin from exerting a deleterious effect in vivo, and, in some cases, facilitating body clearance of the toxin. Other antidotes pharmacologically antagonize the effects of the toxin. Atropine, an antimuscarinic, anticholinergic agent, is used to pharmacologically antagonize at the receptor level the effects of organophosphate insecticides that produce lethal cholin-

ergic, muscarinic effects. Certain agents exert their antidote effects by chemically reacting with biological systems to increase detoxifying capacity for the toxin. For example, sodium nitrite is given to patients poisoned with cyanide to cause formation of methemoglobin, which serves as an alternative binding site for the cyanide ion, thereby making it less toxic to the body.

Supportive Care of the Poisoned Patient

The supportive care phase of poison treatment is very important. Not only are there certain poisonings that have delayed toxicity, but there are also toxins that exhibit multiple phases of toxicity. Close clinical monitoring can detect these later-phase poisoning complications and allow for prompt medical intervention.

Another important component of the supportive care phase of poison treatment is the psychiatric assessment. For intentional self-poisonings, a formal psychiatric evaluation of the patient should be performed prior to discharge. In many cases, it is not possible to perform a psychiatric interview of the patient during the early phases of treatment and evaluation. Once the patient has been stabilized and is able to communicate, a psychiatric evaluation should be obtained.

CONCLUSION

Clinical toxicology encompasses the expertise in the specialties of medical toxicology, applied toxicology, and clinical poison information specialists. The clinical science has significantly evolved to the present state of the discipline over the past 50 years or more. The incorporation of evidence-based, outcome-driven practice recommendations has significantly improved the critical evaluation of treatment modalities and methods for poison treatment. A careful diagnostic approach to a poisoned patient is essential, as important medical history is often absent or unreliable. Skillful use of antidotes is an important component of the practice of medical toxicology. Continued research will increase the repertoire of effective treatments for poisoning and ultimately improve clinical practice.

EXAMPLES OF POISONING CASES

There are many cases in the literature that describe clinical problems associated with toxic substances. A few are excerpted below. It is imperative that readers understand that medicine is constantly changing and the therapeutic approaches mentioned in the cases may not reflect current standard practice. The reader wanting a full discussion of clinical cases is referred to the following references:

1. Bates N, Edwards N, Roper J, Volans G (eds): *Paediatric Toxicology. Handbook of Poisoning in Children.* New York: Stockton Press, 1997.

2. Erickson TB (ed): *Pediatric Toxicology: Diagnosis and Management of the Poisoned Child*. New York: McGraw-Hill, 2005.
3. Gossel TA, Bricker JD: *Principles of Clinical Toxicology*, 3rd ed. New York: Raven Press, 1994.
4. Osterhoudt KC, Perrone J, DeRoos F, Henretiz FM: *Toxicology Pearls*. Philadelphia: Elsevier Mosby, 2004.

Aspirin

A 25-year-old woman with a history of depression is currently taking sertraline daily. Approximately 3 h prior to admission to the emergency room, she swallowed an entire bottle (potentially 100 tablets) of aspirin (325 mg acetylsalicylate per tablet). She vomited twice, bringing up remnants of the ingested tablets each time. The patient's vital signs were blood pressure 180/90 mmHg, heart rate 100 beats/min, and respirations around 30/min. Her temperature was 104°F, and she complained of tinnitus. Her laboratory values were consistent with metabolic acidosis and respiratory alkalosis. Supportive care and intravenous electrolytes were initiated. Ice packs were used to lower body temperature.

Iron Poisoning

A 23-year-old female ingested 50 to 60 ferrous sulfate tablets. Within 1 h, she developed abdominal cramping, and vomited a dark brown liquid. Several hours later, she vomited bright red blood. Approximately 8 h postingestion, she was admitted. Her vitals included blood pressure 90/60 mmHg, heart rate 95 beats/min, respirations 16/min, and oral temperature 97°F. Physical examination revealed slight epigastric tenderness, but normal bowel sounds. Abnormal laboratory values included low hemoglobin and hematocrit, slight acidosis, and an elevated serum iron. After gastric lavage with 5 percent sodium bicarbonate and normal saline for approximately an hour, deferoxamine infusion at 15 mg/kg/h intravenously was initiated and continued for 24 h until urine was no longer tinged red. She was discharged on the third day.

Lead Poisoning

A 39-year-old female was admitted to the hospital with diffuse pains and anemia. She had injured her back in an automobile accident 6 months previously, and was taking a natural product she obtained from an Internet source for analgesia. With continued dosing, she became irritable and now had pain in her knees and hips. It was difficult for her to hold objects in her hands and she often felt constipated. Abnormal laboratory values included low hematocrit and elevated reticulocyte count, and peripheral blood smears showed hypochromic, microcytic anemia with basophilic stippling. Symptoms and laboratory values suggested lead poisoning. Her serum lead concentration was 9 times higher than the reference value. The patient was started on $CaNa_2$-EDTA intravenously, along with intravenous fluids, and then switched to succimer 24 h later. Her serum lead levels had normalized by day 7.

Naphtha

A 40-year-old homeless man injected himself intravenously with 3 mL of charcoal lighter fluid. Shortly thereafter, he had burning chest pains and dyspnea. The following morning he had severe pleuritic chest pain, epigastric discomfort, and shortness of breath. On admission, his temperature was 100°F, blood pressure 115/65 mmHg, respirations 41/min with bibasilar rales, and pulse 90 beats/min, and chest x-ray showed diffuse fluffy infiltrates. On the second day after admission, respirations varied from 35 to 55/min, and his sputum was bloody and contained numerous PMNs. He was treated with a glucocorticoid. The final x-ray at 6 months revealed no residual abnormalities.

Methanol

A 55-year-old female complained of a whiteness in her vision. The previous evening she had consumed three glassfuls of home-made wine. On admission, she had irregular, rapid respirations 31/min, blood pressure 170/110 mmHg, and pulse 114 beats/min. Laboratory values indicated acidosis and a high blood methanol concentration. After treatment with fomepizole, sodium bicarbonate, and hemodialysis, blood methanol levels returned to baseline. Ophthalmologic examination revealed only slight pallor of the optic disc; otherwise, recovery was complete.

Organophosphate

During his afternoon nap, a 4-year-old male vomited. A few hours later, he complained of abdominal pain and headache, and became tremulous and limp. At the hospital, the boy became flaccid and then comatose. His pupils were constricted to 1 mm. No seizures were noted, but he did have fasciculations on one thigh. There was no evidence suggesting the ingestion of any toxic substance or prior trauma. The remaining family members remained well. The young boy had a blood pressure of 125/58 mmHg, pulse of 128 beats/min, and respirations of 28/min. Laboratory findings were unremarkable and a toxicology screen was negative for sedative-hypnotic drugs, alcohol, heavy metals, salicylates, phenothiazines, and opiates. Two hours after admission, he was given 0.15 mg atropine i.v. and 500 mg pralidoxime (2-PAM). An increase in EEG activity was noted within 2 min, and eventually consciousness was restored. Further discussion with the mother revealed that she had had the child with her as she applied parathion to control aphids on the plants in her garden.

Jimson Weed Poisoning

A 19-year-old male college student was found with a flushed face, incoherent behavior, and symptoms of hallucinations. On arrival to the emergency department, he was comatose, his blood pressure was 165/95 mmHg, pulse 46 beats/min, and body temperature 99°F. His pupils were dilated and equal, but contracted minimally to light. His skin was hot and dry. Doll's eye movements were intact. Hyperactive deep tendon reflexes were noted. He occasionally displayed episodes of myoclonic jerks. Within 1 h after admission, the patient's vital signs began to diminish. Poisoning by an anticholinergic-type substance was suspected, so physostigmine salicylate was administered i.v. Within 15 min, he began to respond to this treatment. He became more alert and responsive to verbal commands. He then admitted to ingesting "loco seeds." His neurologic status improved and he was released without apparent neurologic damage.

Multiple Drug Interaction

A 76-year-old white male was brought by ambulance to the ER after his wife watched him collapse on the stairs at home. The unconscious patient is hypotensive (BP 90/55 mmHg), tachycardic (pulse 100 beats/min), and tachypneic (22 respirations/min). There is a very slow capillary refill and his extremities are cool. A 20-cm vertical scar centered over the sternum is exposed and the patient's wife related that the patient had undergone his second CABG procedure about 8 weeks ago. An EKG is essentially normal, except for significant Q waves in leads II, III, and aVf indicating a prior inferior MI. The rest of the physical exam is normal except for 1+ pretibial edema to the midcalf and a heme-positive rectal exam. The patient is stabilized with i.v. fluids.

The patient's wife has a bag containing all of her husband's medications: alprazolam 0.5 mg po bid prn, digoxin 0.250 mg po q daily, enalapril 20 mg po q daily, naproxen sodium 500 mg po bid, furosemide 20 mg po bid, simvastatin 20 mg po q daily, and warfarin 5 mg po qhs. The patient's wife relates that her husband's "stomach had gotten so upset" that he had been having "really black, tarry stools for the past 2 days" and had started taking cimetidine OTC regularly. The following questions then arise:

1. What drug is most responsible for the patient's upset stomach prior to taking cimetidine?
2. Why is the patient in shock? Is he bleeding?
3. What test could confirm your suspicions?

A 21-year-old male was brought to the emergency room following ingestion of an estimated 2.2 g amphetamine sulfate that he took in a suicide gesture. On examination 1 h after ingestion, he was fully oriented and agitated. He quickly became hyperkinetic and incoherent. Physical findings included: pulse, 168 beats/min; blood pressure, 160/80 mmHg; temperature, 108.4°F; and respirations, rapid and shallow at 48/min. His skin was blanched and slightly moist. Pupils were dilated to about 6 mm, and reacted minimally to light. The conjunctivae were edematous. It was not possible to move his head in any direction, but all extremities were easily moved and reflexes were normally reactive. Treatment consisted of vigorous gastric lavage, followed by diazepam. His temperature de-

creased to 101.6°F following immersion in an ice bath and massage. By 12 h after admission, his temperature had returned to normal.

Thyroid Hormone

A 3-year-old boy was taken to the hospital after his father found him playing with his Synthroid prescription bottle. Based on the number of missing tablets, it was estimated that the boy had consumed 12 mg of thyroxine. His stomach was emptied of fragments by nasogastric lavage until returns were clear, and he was given 30 g activated charcoal with 8.3 g magnesium sulfate. Blood T4 concentration was 180 μg/dL and T3 was 67 μg/dL. On the next day, the child had a supraventricular tachycardia of 160 beats/min. Propranolol was given to control the tachycardia. On the third day, the child experienced persistent sweating and diarrhea. Propranolol was discontinued on day 7 and he was discharged later with a resting pulse of 120 beats/min.

Clitocybe dealbata Mushrooms

A 25-year-old woman picked wild mushrooms. After cooking and eating, she became nauseated and diaphoretic. Her family noticed that she was confused and transported her to a hospital. On arrival 30 min later, she was vomiting, had profuse diarrhea, was agitated and disoriented, and had visual hallucinations. Her vital signs were blood pressure 100/60 mmHg, pulse rate 60 beats/min, and temperature 98°F. Physical examination showed generalized muscular fasciculation and pallor. Pupils were constricted. After gastric lavage and activated charcoal, all gastrointestinal symptoms and confusion had resolved. She reported paresthesia in her hands. These symptoms resolved over the next 24 h and she had no further problems. The mushrooms were identified as *C. dealbata*.

Anticholinergic Poisoning

A 33-year old woman was brought to the emergency room after being found in her apartment bound and gagged. On admission she was alert, but could remember only her name. Vital signs included blood pressure 155/105 mmHg, pulse 120 beats/min, respirations 16/min, and rectal temperature 100°F. Pupils were dilated (8 mm) and not reactive to light. Examination of the abdomen indicated there were no bowel sounds. Abdominal muscles were relaxed and the abdomen distended. The remainder of the physical examination was unremarkable. Therapy consisted of oral 50 percent dextrose in water and 50 g activated charcoal. About 12 h later, her mental status began to improve. It was then revealed that she had been drinking wine from a glass that was contaminated very likely with an anticholinergic drug by a guest, who drugged, and then robbed her. Several days later, she reported no adverse sequella.

Phenylpropanolamine

An 18-year-old girl ingested eight diet tablets, each containing 50 mg phenylpropanolamine and 200 mg caffeine. She was seen approximately 2 h later in an emergency facility. Blood pressure was 145/95 mmHg, and pulse 55 beats/min. Neurologic examination failed to disclose abnormalities. She was given atropine sulfate, and gastrointestinal decontamination with lavage. Shortly thereafter, she experienced several generalized convulsions. She was lethargic, but awake and oriented. Within a couple of hours, there was an abrupt decline in the patient's mental state. She lost all brainstem reflexes. Examination of spinal fluid revealed blood. She quickly deteriorated and died. Autopsy revealed right intracerebral hematoma with rupture into the lateral ventricle and subarachnoid space. The brain was diffusely swollen.

BIBLIOGRAPHY

Dart RC: *Medical Toxicology*, 3rd ed. Philadelphia: Williams & Wilkins, 2004.

Goldfrank NR, Flomenbaum NE, Lewin NA, et al (eds): *Goldfrank's Toxicologic Emergencies*, 8th ed. New York: McGraw-Hill, 2008.

Tintinalli JE, Kelen GD, Stapczynski JS (eds): *Emergency Medicine: A Comprehensive Study Guide*, 6th ed. New York: McGraw-Hill, 2004.

QUESTIONS

1. What is the primary goal in taking a history in a poisoned patient?
   a. determining drug allergies.
   b. determining susceptibility to drug overdose.
   c. determining likelihood of an attempted suicide.
   d. determining the ingested substance.
   e. determining the motive behind the poisoning.

2. Who is most likely to give incorrect information while taking a history of a poisoned patient?
   a. patient.
   b. EMT.
   c. employer.
   d. pharmacist.
   e. family members.

3. Which of the following sets of clinical features characterizes an anticholinergic toxic syndrome?
   a. increased blood pressure, decreased heart rate, decreased temperature.
   b. decreased blood pressure, increased heart rate, decreased temperature.
   c. increased blood pressure, increased heart rate, increased temperature.
   d. decreased blood pressure, decreased heart rate, decreased temperature.
   e. increased blood pressure, decreased heart rate, increased temperature.

4. Which of the following sets of clinical features characterizes a sympathomimetic toxic syndrome?
   a. miosis, decreased bowel sounds, decreased alertness.
   b. decreased heart rate, increased temperature, mydriasis.
   c. hyperalertness, decreased blood pressure, miosis.
   d. increased temperature, increased heart rate, miosis.
   e. mydriasis, increased blood pressure, hyperalertness.

5. Which of the following drugs CANNOT be tested for in a hospital on a stat basis?
   a. ethanol.
   b. cocaine.
   c. aspirin.
   d. phenytoin.
   e. digoxin.

6. Which is NOT included in the differential diagnosis of an elevated anion gap?
   a. ethanol.
   b. methanol.
   c. diabetes.
   d. ethylene glycol.
   e. diarrhea.

7. An elevated osmol gap might suggest which of the following?
   a. methanol poisoning.
   b. chronic vomiting.
   c. lactic acidosis.
   d. diabetic ketoacidosis.
   e. chronic diarrhea.

8. Which of the following is LEAST likely to prevent further poison absorption?
   a. induction of emesis.
   b. activated charcoal.
   c. gastric lavage.
   d. syrup of ipecac.
   e. parasympathetic agonist.

9. Which of the following would NOT be used to enhance poison elimination?
   a. oral activated charcoal.
   b. hemoperfusion.
   c. acidification of urine.
   d. hemodialysis.
   e. plasma exchange.

10. Which of the following might be used as an antidote for patients with cyanide poisoning?
    a. syrup of ipecac.
    b. atropine.
    c. chelating agents.
    d. sodium nitrite.
    e. quinine.

Occupational Toxicology

Peter S. Thorne

KEY POINTS

- Occupational toxicology is the application of the principles and methodology of toxicology toward chemical and biological hazards encountered at work.

- In occupational environments, exposure is often used as a surrogate for dose.

- Occupational exposure limits do not correspond to the level of exposure below which the probability of impairing the health of the exposed workers is acceptable.

- Diseases arising in occupational environments involve exposure primarily through inhalation, ingestion, or dermal absorption.

INTRODUCTION

Occupational toxicology is the application of the principles and methodology of toxicology toward chemical and biological hazards encountered at work. The objective of the occupational toxicologist is to prevent adverse health effects in workers that result from their work environment. Because the work environment often presents exposures to complex mixtures, the occu-

pational toxicologist must also recognize exposure combinations that are particularly hazardous.

It is often difficult to establish a causal link between a worker's illness and job. First, the clinical expressions of occupationally induced diseases are often indistinguishable from those arising from nonoccupational causes. Second, there may be a long interval between exposure and the expression of disease. Third, diseases of occupational origin may be multifactorial

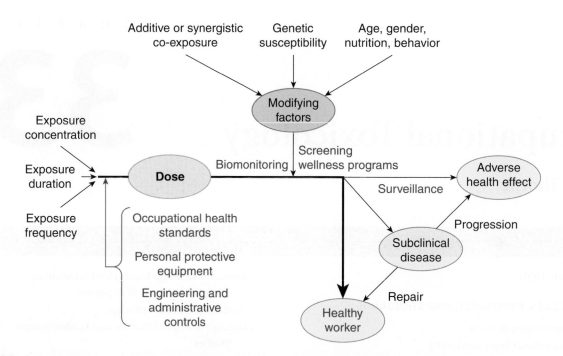

FIGURE 33-1 Pathway from exposure to disease, showing modifying factors and opportunities for intervention.

with personal or other environmental factors contributing to the disease process.

WORKPLACES, EXPOSURES, AND STANDARDS

Determinants of Dose

Dose is defined as the amount of toxicant that reaches the target tissue over a defined time span. In occupational environments, *exposure* is often used as a surrogate for *dose*. The response to a toxic agent is dependent on both host factors and dose. Figure 33–1 illustrates the pathway from exposure to subclinical disease or adverse health effect and suggests that there are important modifying factors: contemporaneous exposures, genetic susceptibility, age, gender, nutritional status, and behavioral factors. These modifying factors can influence whether a worker remains healthy, develops subclinical disease that is repaired, or progresses to illness. As illustrated in Figure 33–1, the dose is a function of exposure concentration, exposure duration, and exposure frequency. Individual and environmental characteristics also can affect dose. Table 33–1 indicates determinants of dose for exposure via the inhalation and dermal routes.

Occupational Exposure Limits

Workplace exposure limits exist for chemical, biological, and physical agents in order to promote worker health and safety. For chemical and biological agents, exposure limits are expressed as acceptable ambient concentration levels (occupational exposure limits [OELs]) or as concentrations of a toxicant,

its metabolites, or a specific marker of its effects (biological exposure indices [BEIs]).

OELs are established as standards by regulatory agencies or as guidelines by research groups or trade organizations. In the United States, the Occupational Safety and Health Administration under the Department of Labor promulgates legally enforceable standards known as permissible exposure limits (PELs). The National Institute for Occupational Safety and Health (NIOSH), under the Centers for Disease Control and Prevention, publishes recommended exposure limits that are frequently updated and are generally more stringent than PELs.

TABLE 33-1 Determinants of toxicant dose.

Inhalation exposure
- Airborne concentration
- Particle size distribution
- Respiratory rate
- Tidal volume
- Other host factors
- Duration of exposure
- Chemical, physical, or biological properties of the hazardous agent
- Effectiveness of personal protective devices

Dermal exposure
- Concentration in air, droplets, or solutions
- Degree and duration of wetness
- Integrity of skin
- Percutaneous absorption rate
- Region of skin exposed
- Surface area exposed
- Preexisting skin disease
- Temperature in the workplace
- Vehicle for the toxicant
- Presence of other chemicals on skin

The American Conference of Governmental Industrial Hygienists is a trade organization that annually publishes OELs for chemicals and for physical agents. These take the form of threshold limit values (TLVs) and BEIs. They are developed as guidelines and are not enforceable standards.

OELs correspond to the level of exposure below which the probability of impairing the health of the exposed workers is acceptable. To determine that the risks from an occupational hazard are acceptable, it is necessary to characterize the hazard, identify the potential diseases or adverse outcomes, and establish the relationship between exposure intensity or dose and the adverse health effects.

OCCUPATIONAL DISEASES

Routes of Exposure

Diseases arising in occupational environments involve exposure primarily through inhalation, ingestion, or dermal absorption. Exposures leading to occupational infections may arise through inhalation or ingestion of microorganisms, from needle sticks in health care workers, or from insect bites among those who work outdoors. Additionally, poisonings from toxic plants or venomous animals can occur through skin inoculation (e.g., zookeepers, horticulturists, or commercial skin divers).

Agents Associated with Diseases

Table 33–2 outlines some major occupational diseases and examples of toxicants that cause them. Table 33–3 lists known human carcinogens (group 1), for which there are extensive occupational exposure.

Occupational Respiratory Diseases

Occupational lung diseases (such as coal workers' pneumoconiosis, asbestosis, and occupational asthma) are largely responsible for the creation of the occupational regulatory framework. The crude U.S. death rate and annual deaths noted in Table 33–4 illustrate that death rates are fairly low, but in truth fatalities are just the tip of the iceberg. Hypersensitivity pneumonitis is rarely fatal but is often debilitating. Moreover, there are 20,000 yearly hospital discharges related to cases of asbestosis and 188,000 coal workers receive federal black lung benefits.

Toxic gas injuries are often characterized by leakage of both fluid and osmotically active proteins from the vascular tissue into the interstitium and airways. The vapors of anhydrous ammonia combine with water in the tissues of the eyes, sinuses, and upper airways and form ammonium hydroxide, quickly producing liquefaction necrosis. Chemicals with lower solubility, such as nitrogen dioxide, act more on the distal airways and alveoli and take longer to induce tissue damage.

Occupational asthma occurs when airways restrict in response to some stimulus present in the workplace. Stimuli include plastic and rubber polymers, reactive dyes, and acid anhydrides, biocides and fungicides, metals, latex, and some enzymes. Exposure to plants, animals, or fungi may also induce asthma.

Other Occupational Diseases

Occupational toxicants may induce diseases in a variety of sites distant from the lung or skin. These include tumors arising in the liver, bladder, gastrointestinal tract, or hematopoietic system and are attributable to a variety of chemical classes. Nervous system damage can be central, peripheral, or both. It may be acute, as with some organophosphate exposures, or chronic, as with organomercury poisoning or acrylamide-induced neuropathy. Immune system injury may arise from the immunosuppressive effects of chemicals or from hypersensitivity leading to respiratory or dermal allergy or systemic hypersensitivity reactions. Autoimmune syndromes have been associated with occupational exposures to crystalline silica and vinyl chloride.

Occupational diseases of the cardiovascular system include atherosclerosis, various arrhythmias, impaired coronary blood supply, systemic hypotension, and right ventricular hypertrophy usually due to pulmonary hypertension. Liver diseases include carbon tetrachloride-induced fatty liver. Occupational diseases of the reproductive system can be gender- and organ-specific, or may affect both sexes. Disease due to exposures to infectious agents occurs in such occupations as veterinarians, health care workers, biomedical researchers, and farmers.

Both industrial and nonindustrial indoor environments may pose occupational hazards due to the presence of chemical or biological agents. Problems with ventilation and use of synthetic building materials have led to a rise in complaints associated with occupancy in buildings. Volatile and semivolatile chemicals are released from process materials in manufacturing, building materials, floor coverings, furniture, cleaning products, biocides, and microorganisms. In some cases, the occupied space of a building may be clean and dry, but local amplification sites for molds, such as damp closets or subfloors, may develop. Airborne viruses, bacteria, and fungi are responsible for a variety of building-related illnesses.

TOXICOLOGIC EVALUATION OF OCCUPATIONAL AGENTS

Evaluation of Occupational Risks

To recommend an acceptable exposure level to an industrial chemical, one must attempt to define the risks associated with adverse effects in the most sensitive exposed populations. It then remains to decide what proportion of exposed subjects may still develop an adverse effect at the proposed acceptable exposure level.

TABLE 33–2 Examples of occupational diseases and the toxicants that cause them.

Organ System or Disease Group	Disease	Causative Agent
Lung and airways	Acute pulmonary edema, bronchiolitis obliterans	Nitrogen oxides, phosgene
	Allergic rhinitis	Pollens, fungal spores
	Asphyxiation	Carbon monoxide, hydrogen cyanide, inert gas dilution
	Asthma	Toluene diisocyanate, α-amylase, animal urine proteins
	Asthma-like syndrome	Swine barn environments, cotton dust, bioaerosols
	Bronchitis, pneumonitis	Arsenic, chlorine
	Chronic bronchitis	Cotton dust, grain dust, welding fumes
	Emphysema	Coal dust, cigarette smoke
	Fibrotic lung disease	Silica, asbestos
	Hypersensitivity pneumonitis	Thermophilic bacteria, avian proteins, pyrethrum, *Penicillium, Aspergillus*
	Metal fume fever	Zinc, copper, magnesium
	Mucous membrane irritation	Hydrogen chloride, swine barn environments
	Organic dust toxic syndrome	"Moldy" silage, endotoxin
	Upper respiratory tract inflammation	Endotoxin, peptidoglycan, glucans, viruses
Cancer	Acute myelogenous leukemia	Benzene, ethylene oxide
	Bladder cancer	Benzidine, 2-naphthylamine, 4-biphenylamine
	Gastrointestinal cancers	Asbestos
	Hepatic hemangiosarcoma	Vinyl chloride
	Hepatocellular carcinoma	Aflatoxin, hepatitis B virus
	Mesothelioma, lung carcinoma	Asbestos, arsenic, radon, bis(chloromethyl) ether
	Skin cancer	Polycyclic aromatic hydrocarbons, ultraviolet irradiation
Skin	Allergic contact dermatitis	Natural rubber latex, isothiazolins, poison ivy, nickel
	Chemical burns	Sodium hydroxide, hydrogen fluoride
	Chloracne	TCDD,[1] polychlorinated biphenyls
	Irritant dermatitis	Sodium dodecyl sulfate
Nervous system	Cholinesterase inhibition	Organophosphate insecticides
	Neuronopathy	Methyl mercury
	Parkinsonism	Carbon monoxide, carbon disulfide
	Peripheral neuropathy	*N*-Hexane, trichloroethylene, acrylamide
Immune system	Autoimmune disease	Vinyl chloride, silica
	Hypersensitivity	See entries for allergic rhinitis, asthma, hypersensitivity pneumonitis, allergic contact dermatitis
	Immunosuppression	TCDD,[1] lead, mercury, pesticides
Renal disease	Indirect renal failure	Arsine, phosphine, trinitrophenol
	Nephropathy	Paraquat, 1,4-dichlorobenzene, mercuric chloride
Cardiovascular disease	Arrhythmias	Acetone, toluene, methylene chloride, trichloroethylene
	Atherosclerosis	Dinitrotoluene, carbon monoxide
	Coronary artery disease	Carbon disulfide
	Cor pulmonale	Beryllium
	Systemic hypotension	Nitroglycerine, ethylene glycol dinitrate
Liver disease	Fatty liver (steatosis)	Carbon tetrachloride, toluene
	Cirrhosis	Arsenic, trichloroethylene
	Hepatocellular death	Dimethylformamide, TCDD[1]
Reproductive system	Male	Chlordecone (kepone), dibromochloropropane, hexane
	Female	Aniline, styrene
	Both sexes	Carbon disulfide, lead, vinyl chloride
Infectious diseases	Arboviral encephalitides	Alphavirus, bunyavirus, flavivirus
	Aspergillosis	*Aspergillus niger, A. fumigatus, A. flavus*
	Cryptosporidiosis	*Cryptosporidium parvum*
	Hepatitis B	Hepatitis B virus
	Histoplasmosis	*Histoplasma capsulatum*
	Legionellosis	*Legionella pneumophila*
	Lyme disease	*Borrelia burgdorferi*
	Psittacosis	*Chlamydia psittaci*
	Tuberculosis	*Mycobacterium tuberculosis hominis*

[1]TCDD = 2,3,7,8-tetrachlorodibenzo-*para*-dioxin.

TABLE 33–3 Occupational exposure agents classified by IARC as definite human carcinogens.

Agent	Industries and Occupations Where Some Workers May Be Exposed
Particulate matter	
Asbestos	Miners, abatement workers, construction workers, sheet metal workers, steam fitters, shipyard workers
Crystalline silica	Stone and ceramics industry, foundries, construction, abrasives manufacturing
Talc containing asbestiform fibers	Ceramics industry
Erionite	Waste treatment workers, building materials manufacturing
Wood dust	Wood and wood products industries, pulp and paper industry, wood working trades
Metals	
Arsenic and arsenic compounds	Miners, nonferrous metal smelting, arsenical pesticide manufacturers and applicators
Beryllium	Specialty metallurgy workers, avionics, electronics, nuclear industry
Cadmium and cadmium compounds	Cadmium smelting, battery production, dyes and pigment making, electroplating
Hexavalent chromium compounds, nickel compounds[1]	Chromate production plants, dye and pigment making, welders, tanners, nickel smelting, welding
Organic chemicals	
Benzene	Refineries, shoe industry; chemical, pharmaceutical, and rubber industry; printing industry
Coal tars and pitches	Coke production, coal gasification, refineries, foundries, road paving, hot tar roofing
Mineral oils, untreated and mildly treated	Metal machining and honing, roll steel production, printing
Shale oils or shale-derived lubricants	Mining and processing, cotton textile industry
Soot	Chimney sweeps, heating and ventilation contractors, firefighters, metallurgical workers
Vinyl chloride	Plastics industry, production of polyvinyl chloride products and copolymers
Bis(chloromethyl) ether and chloromethyl ether (technical grade)	Chemical industry, laboratory reagent, plastic manufacturing
4-Aminobiphenyl	Chemical industry, dyestuffs and pigment manufacturing
Benzidine	Chemical industry, dyestuffs and pigment manufacturing
2-Naphthylamine	Chemical industry, dyestuffs and pigment manufacturing
Ethylene oxide	Chemical industry, dry vegetable fumigation, hospital sterilizing
2,3,7,8-Tetrachlorodibenzo-*para*-dioxin (TCDD)	Hazardous waste processing, chlorophenoxy herbicide production and use, pulp and paper industry
Aflatoxin	Animal feed industry, grain handling and processing
Other agents with occupational exposure	
Environmental tobacco smoke	Restaurant, bar, and entertainment industry; other smoke-exposed workers
Mustard gas	Production, soldiers, some research laboratories
Strong inorganic acid mists containing sulfuric acid	Steel industry, petrochemical industry, fertilizer industry, pickling industry
Physical agents	
Ionizing radiation[2]	Radiology and nuclear medicine staff, nuclear workers, miners, hazardous waste workers
Solar radiation	Farmers, gardeners and landscapers, lifeguards, construction workers

[1]Certain combinations of nickel oxides and sulfides.
[2]Includes x-rays, γ-rays, neutrons, and radon gas.
IARC = International Agency for Research on Cancer.

TABLE 33–4 U.S. deaths and crude death rates attributed to selected occupational lung diseases.

Disease	Number of Deaths	Death Rate Per Million Working-age People
Asbestosis	1265	6.0
Coal workers' pneumoconiosis	1003	4.7
Silicosis	187	0.9
Byssinosis	7	0.03
Other pneumoconiosis[1]	318	1.5
Malignant mesothelioma	2485	11.7
Hypersensitivity pneumonitis	57	0.3

[1]This includes aluminosis, berylliosis, stannosis, siderosis, and fibrosis from bauxite, graphite fibers, wollastonite, cadmium, Portland cement, emery, kaolin, antimony, and mica.
Source: NIOSH Worker Health Chartbook 2004, U.S. Bureau of Labor Statistics.

	Assessment of exposure to specific agents	Consideration or control of confounders	Evidence of a dose–response relationship	Consistent results from different studies	Objective clinical data	Endpoints related to human pathology	Appropriate subjects or models
In vitro studies							
Animal studies							
Human challenge studies							
Case studies							
Epidemiology studies							

For each type of study listed in the first column weight the quality of data from existing studies based on the criteria listed in the column headings as follows:

    0   No evidence or condition is not met
    1   Equivocal evidence or condition is partially met
    2   Some evidence or condition is mostly met
    3   Clear evidence or condition is convincingly met

FIGURE 33–2 Matrix for assessing the strength of an association between a toxicant and an occupational disease.

Establishing Causality—In complex occupational environments, it may be difficult to establish a causal relationship between a toxic substance and a disease. A matrix was developed to evaluate the weight of evidence for a causal association between a toxicant and an occupational disease (Figure 33–2). Evidence from well-conducted in vitro studies, animal studies, human challenge studies (intentional clinical exposure to humans), case reports, and epidemiologic investigations are evaluated. This evaluation is guided by seven criteria. If a chemical were thoroughly studied in animals, humans, and in vitro studies and produced clear and convincing evidence of an exposure–response relationship in controlled studies that used appropriate models and relevant endpoints, then that would constitute compelling evidence of a causal relationship between that chemical and that disease.

Animal Toxicology Testing for Establishing Acceptable Levels of Exposure

Animal studies provide valuable data from which to estimate the level of exposure at which the risk of health impairment is acceptable. The duration of tests necessary to establish an acceptable level for occupational exposure is primarily a function of the type of toxic action suspected. It is generally recognized that for systemically acting chemicals, subacute and short-term toxicity studies are usually insufficient for proposing OELs. Subacute and short-term toxicity tests are usually performed to find out whether the compound exhibits immunotoxic properties and cumulative characteristics. They also aid in selection of the doses for long-term exposures. Studies designed to evaluate reproductive effects and teratogenicity should also be considered.

Information derived from exposure routes similar to those sustained by workers is clearly most relevant. The choice of what studies to perform using which routes of administration must be evaluated scientifically for each toxicant. Important considerations include its target sites and mechanism of action, metabolism, the nature of its adverse effects, and how workers are exposed to the toxicant.

Worker Health Surveillance

The primary objective of occupational toxicology is to provide both periodic screening of general health and wellness and health exposure monitoring tailored to recognized hazards of the workplace. Monitoring of exposures to toxicants in the workplace may be important in detecting excessive exposures before the occurrence of significant biological disturbances and health impairment. When a new chemical is being used on a large scale, careful clinical surveillance of workers and monitoring of workplaces should be instituted. Evaluation of the validity of the proposed OEL derived from animal experiments through workplace surveillance is the major goal.

Epidemiologic studies designed to assess exposure–response relationships will have more validity if both the target dose and the critical biological changes are monitored in exposure–response studies. Knowledge of the fate of the chemical in the organism and its mechanism of action are required. Because early biomarkers of effect are subtle and individual variations exist in the response to a chemical insult, results generally require a statistical comparison between a group of exposed workers and a similar group of workers without the exposure of interest. If exposure induces an adverse effect, it is expected that these studies may permit establishment of the relationship between integrated exposure (intensity × time) and frequency of abnormal results and, consequently, a redefinition of the OEL.

In cases where a surveillance program was not instituted before the introduction of a new chemical, it is more difficult to establish the efficacy of the exposure limit. In this situation, evaluation depends on retrospective cohort studies or case–control studies or on cross-sectional studies on workers who have already sustained exposure.

Case reports of isolated overexposures resulting from specific incidents such as containment breaches, chemical spills, or vessel or pipe ruptures can provide useful information. Such observations may indicate whether human symptomatology is similar to that found in animals and may suggest functional or biological tests that might prove useful for routine monitoring of exposed workers.

Linkage of Animal Studies and Epidemiologic Studies

In the field of occupational toxicology, close cooperation between those conducting animal studies and those conducting studies of workers is essential for examining risks associated with overexposure to chemicals and other toxicants. Several occupational carcinogens have been identified clearly through combined epidemiologic and experimental approaches. For example, the carcinogenicity of vinyl chloride was first demonstrated in rats, and a few years later, epidemiologic studies confirmed the same carcinogenic risk for humans. This observation stimulated several investigations on the metabolism of vinyl chloride in animals and on its mutagenic activity in in vitro systems, leading to a better understanding of its mechanism of carcinogenicity.

Studies of the metabolic handling of occupational toxicants in animals are instrumental in the characterization of reactive intermediates and may suggest unsuspected risks or indicate new methods of biological monitoring. Conversely, clinical observations on workers may stimulate studies of the metabolism or the mechanism of toxicity of a toxicant in animals, thereby revealing the health significance of a biological disturbance.

Arsenic is one of the very few compounds for which there are limited data of predictive value from animal studies to human health effects. Inorganic arsenic has been shown conclusively to cause human cancers of many organs, but not to cause cancer in animals. This demonstrates that the occupational toxicologist cannot rely solely on animal or epidemiologic studies. A combined approach is necessary in order to identify, elucidate, and prioritize risks and to develop interventions and techniques for worker health surveillance.

EXPOSURE MONITORING

Environmental Monitoring for Exposure Assessment

A critical element of establishing OELs is the accurate and uniform assessment of exposure. Methodology for exposure assessment must be specifically tailored to the agent under study and the environment in which it appears. To assess airborne exposures, personal samples taken in the breathing zone are generally used. Repeated random sampling is usually the best approach to developing unbiased measures of exposure. Recent studies have demonstrated that group-based approaches, assessing exposures to groups rather than to individuals, are more efficient in terms of measurement effort for obtaining a desired level of accuracy.

Although one cannot assess dose directly through exposure monitoring, it has distinct advantages over biomonitoring, which cannot provide route-specific exposure data. Environmental monitoring techniques are generally less expensive and less invasive than techniques involving the collection and analysis of biological samples such as blood or urine. Spatial, temporal, and work practice associations can be established by air monitoring and can suggest better interventions and engineering controls.

Biological Monitoring for Exposure Assessment

Biomonitoring consists of the measurement of toxicants, their metabolites, or molecular signatures of effect in specimens from humans or animals, including urine, blood, feces, exhaled breath, hair, fingernails or toenails, bronchial lavage, breast milk, and adipose tissue. These may serve as biomarkers of exposure, biological effect, or susceptibility. Emerging technologies will allow measurement and monitoring of chemicals in the body and transmission of the data from indwelling biosensors. Biomonitoring data provide a measurement of exposure based on internalized dose, or the amount of chemical stored in one or in several body compartments or in the whole body, and, thus, account for all exposures by all routes for the assessed analyte.

The greatest advantage of using biological measurements is that the biological parameter of exposure is more directly related to the adverse health effects than environmental measurements. It may offer a better estimate of the risk than can be determined from ambient monitoring. Biological monitoring accounts for uptake by all exposure routes.

Several factors can influence uptake. Personal hygiene habits vary from one person to another, and there is some degree of individual variation in the absorption rate of a chemical through the lungs, skin, or gastrointestinal tract. Because of its ability to encompass and evaluate the overall exposure (whatever the route of entry), biological monitoring also can be used to test the overall efficacy of personal protective equipment such as respirators, gloves, or barrier creams. Another consideration with biological monitoring is the fact that the nonoccupational exposures (hobbies, residential exposures, dietary habits, smoking, and second jobs) also may be expressed in the biological sample.

Relationships between air monitoring and biological monitoring may be modified by factors that influence the fate of an occupational toxicant in vivo. Metabolic interactions can occur when workers are exposed simultaneously to chemicals that are biotransformed through identical pathways or that modify the activity of the biotransformation enzymes. Furthermore, metabolic interferences may occur between occupational toxicants and alcohol, tobacco, food additives, prescription drugs, natural product remedies, or recreational drugs.

In summary, environmental and biological monitoring should be regarded as complementary elements in an occupational health and safety program.

CONCLUSION

The working environment will always present the risk of overexposure of workers to various toxicants. Recognition of these risks should not wait until epidemiologic studies have defined hazardous levels. A combined experimental, clinical, and epidemiologic approach is the most effective for evaluating the potential risks, promulgating scientifically based occupational health standards, and implementing workplace controls to ensure adherence to the standards.

BIBLIOGRAPHY

ACGIH: *2008 TLVs and BEIs: Threshold Limit Values for Chemical Substances and Physical Agents and Biological Exposure Indices.* Cincinnati, OH: American Conference of Governmental Industrial Hygienists, 2008.

Aw TC, Gardiner K, Harrington JM, et al (eds): *Occupational Health.* Malden, MA: Blackwell, 2006.

Gantt P, Schnepp R: *Hazardous Materials: Regulations, Response and Site Operations,* 2nd ed. Clifton Park, NY: Delmar Cengage Learning, 2009.

QUESTIONS

1. Which of the following is NOT a modifying factor that can influence the likelihood of disease?
   a. age.
   b. dose.
   c. nutritional status.
   d. gender.
   e. genetic susceptibility.

2. Which of the following is LEAST likely to increase occupational inhalation of a chemical?
   a. increased airborne concentration.
   b. increased respiratory rate.
   c. increased tidal volume.
   d. increased particle size.
   e. increased length of exposure.

3. Which would increase the likelihood of toxic dosage through dermal exposure?
   a. no preexisting skin disease.
   b. toxic exposure to thick skin.
   c. increased percutaneous absorption rate.
   d. low surface area of exposure.
   e. high epidermal intercellular junction integrity.

4. Prolonged arsenic exposure could cause:
   a. infertility.
   b. cirrhosis.
   c. cor pulmonale.
   d. skin cancer.
   e. nephropathy.

5. Which of the following lung diseases has the highest occupational death rate?
   a. asbestosis.
   b. coal workers' pneumoconiosis.
   c. byssinosis.
   d. hypersensitivity pneumonitis.
   e. silicosis.

6. Lyme disease is caused by which of the following?
   a. *B. burgdorferi.*
   b. *H. capsulatum.*
   c. *M. tuberculosis.*
   d. *L. pneumophila.*
   e. *C. psittaci.*

7. Asbestos exposure is unlikely to cause:
   a. lung cancer.
   b. GI cancer.
   c. emphysema.
   d. pulmonary fibrosis.
   e. mesothelioma.

8. Exposure to which of the following can cause autoimmune disease?
   a. mercury.
   b. nitrogen dioxide.
   c. vinyl chloride.
   d. lead.
   e. flavivirus.

9. Which of the following might be linked to parkinsonism?
   a. nitrogen dioxide.
   b. zinc.
   c. copper.
   d. magnesium.
   e. carbon monoxide.

10. Which of the following infectious agents can cause hepatocellular carcinoma?
    a. flavivirus.
    b. bunyavirus.
    c. alphavirus.
    d. hepatitis C virus.
    e. hepatitis B virus.

Answers to Chapter Questions

Chapter 1
1. b.
2. a.
3. a.
4. d.
5. b.

Chapter 2
1. b.
2. c.
3. b.
4. d.
5. e.
6. e.
7. b.
8. c.
9. d.
10. a.

Chapter 3
1. b.
2. e.
3. a.
4. c.
5. d.
6. e.
7. b.
8. a.
9. e.
10. c.
11. b.
12. b.

Chapter 4
1. d.
2. c.
3. c.
4. c.
5. e.
6. c.
7. c.
8. d.
9. c.
10. b.

Chapter 5
1. a.
2. e.
3. d.
4. b.
5. e.
6. c.
7. c.
8. d.
9. b.
10. d.

Chapter 6
1. b.
2. c.
3. c.
4. e.
5. b.
6. d.
7. d.
8. a.
9. e.
10. d.

Chapter 7
1. c.
2. a.
3. d.
4. d.
5. e.
6. c.
7. b.
8. d.
9. b.
10. c.

Chapter 8
1. d.
2. e.
3. e.
4. b.
5. c.
6. a.
7. d.
8. e.
9. c.
10. b.

Chapter 9
1. c.
2. d.
3. b.
4. c.
5. e.
6. b.
7. e.
8. c.
9. c.
10. d.

Chapter 10
1. d.
2. c.
3. a.
4. c.
5. d.
6. b.
7. e.
8. c.
9. e.
10. e.

Chapter 11
1. c.
2. a.
3. d.
4. d.
5. a.
6. c.
7. d.
8. c.
9. e.
10. b.

Chapter 12
1. d.
2. b.
3. c.
4. b.
5. c.
6. d.
7. e.
8. b.
9. d.
10. a.

Chapter 13

1. d.
2. d.
3. b.
4. e.
5. a.
6. c.
7. b.
8. d.
9. e.
10. e.

Chapter 14

1. e.
2. b.
3. c.
4. d.
5. d.
6. a.
7. c.
8. e.
9. d.
10. c.

Chapter 15

1. d.
2. b.
3. d.
4. e.
5. d.
6. b.
7. d.
8. a.
9. c.
10. c.

Chapter 16

1. e.
2. d.
3. c.
4. b.
5. d.
6. b.
7. a.
8. d.
9. c.
10. d.

Chapter 17

1. e.
2. c.
3. b.
4. a.
5. d.
6. a.
7. e.
8. d.
9. e.
10. d.

Chapter 18

1. b.
2. b.
3. d.
4. d.
5. e.
6. c.
7. c.
8. a.
9. d.
10. d.

Chapter 19

1. b.
2. e.
3. a.
4. d.
5. b.
6. c.
7. d.
8. c.
9. c.
10. a.

Chapter 20

1. c.
2. d.
3. b.
4. a.
5. e.
6. b.
7. e.
8. d.
9. b.
10. c.

Chapter 21

1. c.
2. d.
3. b.
4. c.
5. e.
6. b.
7. c.
8. d.
9. a.
10. b.

Chapter 22

1. a.
2. c.
3. b.
4. a.
5. e.
6. d.
7. b.
8. c.
9. d.
10. d.

Chapter 23

1. c.
2. d.
3. d.
4. b.
5. a.
6. e.
7. c.
8. d.
9. a.
10. c.

Chapter 24

1. d.
2. c.
3. c.
4. b.
5. d.
6. b.
7. d.
8. b.
9. a.
10. d.

Chapter 25

1. b.
2. c.
3. a.
4. e.
5. d.
6. c.
7. c.
8. d.
9. a.
10. e.

Chapter 26

1. a.
2. d.
3. d.
4. e.
5. c.
6. c.
7. a.
8. e.
9. a.
10. b.

Chapter 27

1. b.
2. d.
3. a.
4. c.
5. c.
6. e.
7. b.
8. c.
9. a.
10. e.

Chapter 28

1. b.
2. d.
3. e.
4. c.
5. e.
6. c.
7. d.
8. a.
9. b.
10. d.

Chapter 29

1. b.
2. c.
3. a.
4. e.
5. c.
6. c.
7. e.
8. b.
9. e.
10. d.

Chapter 30

1. d.
2. a.
3. b.
4. e.
5. c.
6. d.
7. d.
8. a.
9. e.
10. d.

Chapter 31

1. d.
2. b.
3. a.
4. c.
5. e.
6. b.
7. c.
8. e.
9. d.
10. d.

Chapter 32

1. d.
2. a.
3. c.
4. e.
5. b.
6. e.
7. a.
8. e.
9. c.
10. d.

Chapter 33

1. b.
2. d.
3. c.
4. b.
5. b.
6. a.
7. c.
8. c.
9. e.
10. e.

Index

NOTE: Pages in **boldface** refer to major discussions; page numbers followed by *f* indicate figures; those followed by *t* indicate tables.